Johannes W. Rohen
Chihiro Yokochi
Elke Lütjen-Drecoll

Color Atlas
of Anatomy

A Photographic Study
of the Human Body

Seventh Edition

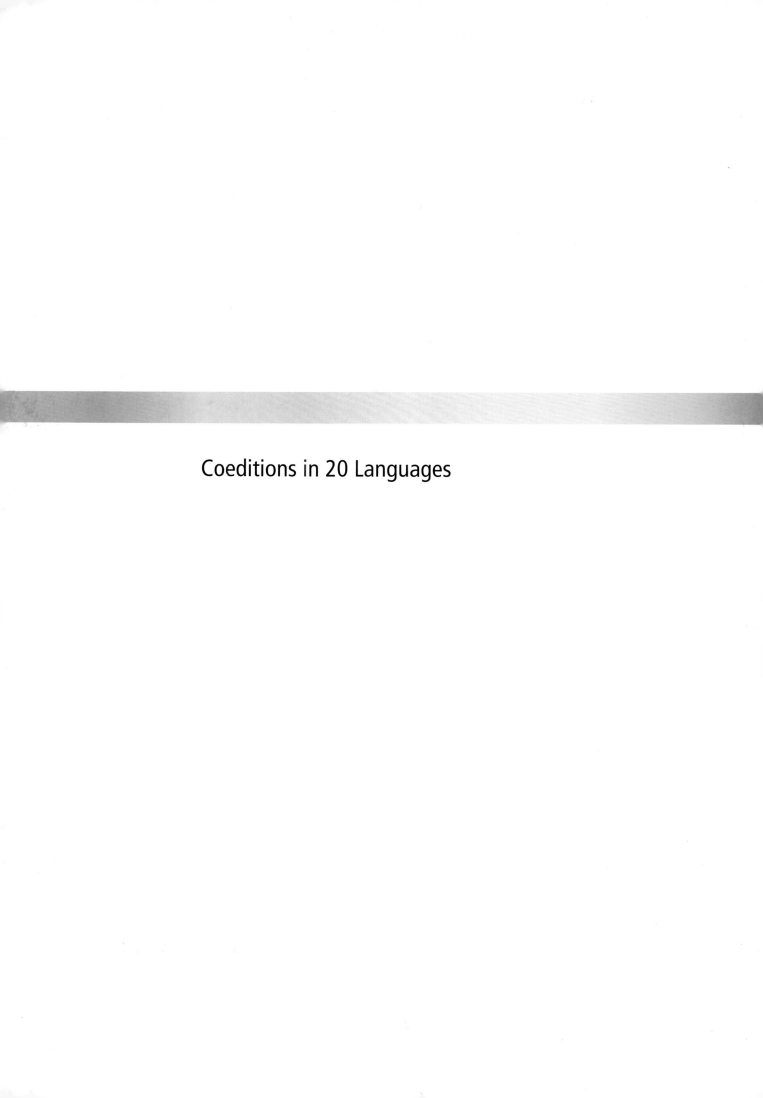

Coeditions in 20 Languages

Johannes W. Rohen
Chihiro Yokochi
Elke Lütjen-Drecoll

Color Atlas
of Anatomy

A Photographic Study
of the Human Body

Seventh Edition

With 1211 Figures,
1117 in Color,
and 94 Radiographs, CT and MRI Scans

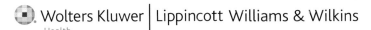

Wolters Kluwer | Lippincott Williams & Wilkins
Health
Philadelphia · Baltimore · New York · London
Buenos Aires · Hong Kong · Sydney · Tokyo

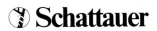
Schattauer

Prof. Dr. med. Dr. med. h.c. Johannes W. Rohen
Anatomisches Institut II der Universität Erlangen-Nürnberg
Universitätsstraße 19, 91054 Erlangen, Germany

Chihiro Yokochi, M.D.
Professor emeritus, Department of Anatomy
Kanagawa Dental College, Yokosuka, Kanagawa, Japan
Correspondence to:
Prof. Chihiro Yokochi, c/o Igaku-Shoin Ltd., 1-28-23 Hongo,
Bunkyo-ku Tokyo 113-8719, Japan

Prof. Dr. med. Elke Lütjen-Drecoll
Anatomisches Institut II der Universität Erlangen-Nürnberg
Universitätsstraße 19, 91054 Erlangen, Germany

With Collaboration of
Kyung W. Chung, Ph.D.
David Ross Boyd Professor & Vice Chairman
Samuel Roberts Noble Foundation Presidential Professor
Director, Advanced Human Anatomy
University of Oklahoma, College of Medicine
Department of Cell Biology

Copyright ©
Fourth Edition, 1998
Fifth Edition, 2002
Sixth Edition, 2006
Seventh Edition, 2011 by
Schattauer GmbH,
Hölderlinstraße 3, 70174 Stuttgart, Germany; http://www.schattauer.de, and
Lippincott Williams & Wilkins, a Wolters Kluwer business

351 West Camden Street   530 Walnut Street
Baltimore, MD 21201   Philadelphia, PA 19106

9 8 7 6 5 4 3

Library of Congress Cataloging-in-Publication data has been applied for and is available upon request.

DISCLAIMER
Care has been taken to confirm the accuracy of the information present and to describe generally accepted practices. However, the authors, editors, and publisher are not responsible for errors or omissions or for any consequences from application of the information in this book and make no warranty, expressed or implied, with respect to the currency, completeness, or accuracy of the contents of the publication. Application of this information in a particular situation remains the professional responsibility of the practitioner; the clinical treatments described and recommended may not be considered absolute and universal recommendations.

The authors, editors, and publisher have exerted every effort to ensure that drug selection and dosage set forth in this text are in accordance with the current recommendations and practice at the time of publication. However, in view of ongoing research, changes in government regulations, and the constant flow of information relating to drug therapy and drug reactions, the reader is urged to check the package insert for each drug for any change in indications and dosage and for added warnings and precautions. This is particularly important when the recommended agent is a new or infrequently employed drug.

Some drugs and medical devices presented in this publication have Food and Drug Administration (FDA) clearance for limited use in restricted research settings. It is the responsibility of the health care provider to ascertain the FDA status of each drug or device planned for use in their clinical practice.

To purchase additional copies of this book, call our customer service department at **(800) 638-3030** or fax orders to **(301) 223-2320**. International customers should call **(301) 223-2300**.

Visit Lippincott Williams & Wilkins on the Internet: http://www.lww.com. Lippincott Williams & Wilkins customer service representatives are available from 8:30 am to 6:00 pm, EST.

ISBN: 9781582558561

Preface to the Seventh Edition

This new edition was revised and structured anew in different ways. Each chapter is provided with an introductory front page to give an overview of the topics of the chapter and short descriptions. The whole introductory chapter "General Anatomy" was newly arranged and supported with introductory texts, thus facilitating students to better understand the complicated "world" of gross anatomy. The large chapter 2 "Head and Neck" was split into 5 sub-chapters with an introductory page each. Furthermore, the drawings were revised and improved in many chapters and depicted more consistently. In most of the chapters new photographs taken from newly dissected specimens were incorporated.

The general structure and arrangement of the Atlas were maintained. The chapters of regional anatomy are consequently placed behind the systematic descriptions of the anatomical structures so that students can study – e.g. before dissecting an extremity – the systematic anatomy of bones, joints, muscles, nerves and vessels. For studying the photographs of the specimens the use of a magnifier might be helpful. The enormous plasticity of the photos is surprising, especially at higher magnifications.

In many places new MRI and CT scans were added to give consideration to the new imaging techniques which become more and more important for the student in preclinics. We would like to express our sincere thanks to Prof. Heuck, Munich, who provided us with the MRI scans.

In the underlying seventh edition photographs of the surface anatomy of the human body were included again. We omitted marks and indications in order not to affect the quality of the pictures.

Despite numerous additions and amendments the size of the volume did not increase so that students both in preclinics and in clinics are offered an atlas easy to handle and cope with.

While preparing this new edition, the authors were reminded of how precisely, beautifully, and admirably the human body is constructed. If this book helps the student or medial doctor to appreciate the overwhelming beauty of the anatomical architecture of tissues and organs in the human, then it greatly fulfils its task. Deep interest and admiration of the anatomical structures may create the "love for man", which alone can be considered of primary importance for daily medical work.

We would like to express our great gratitude to all coworkers for their skilled work. Without their help the improvements of the *Color Atlas of Anatomy* would not have been possible. We would also like to express our sincere thanks to those at Schattauer GmbH, Stuttgart, Germany, Lippincott, Williams & Wilkins, Baltimore, Maryland, USA, and Igaku-Shoin, Tokyo, Japan, who always listened to our suggestions and invested again a great deal of their effort into improving this book.

Acknowledgements

We would like to express our great gratitude to all coworkers who helped to make the *Color Atlas of Anatomy* a success. We are particularly indebted to those who dissected new specimens with great skill and knowledge, particularly to Jeff Bryant (member of our staff) and Dr. Martin Rexer (now Klinikum Fürth, Germany), who prepared most of the new specimens of the fifth, sixth and seventh edition. We would also like to thank Dr. K. Okamoto (now Nagasaki, Japan), who dissected many excellent specimens of the fourth edition, also included in the fifth edition. Furthermore, we are greatly indebted to Prof. W. Neuhuber and his coworkers for their great efforts in supporting our work.

The specimens of the previous editions also depicted in this volume were dissected with great skill and enthusiasm by Prof. Dr. S. Nagashima (now Nagasaki, Japan), Dr. Mutsuko Takahashi (now Tokyo, Japan), Dr. Gabriele Lindner-Funk (Erlangen, Germany), Dr. P. Landgraf (Erlangen, Germany), and Miss Rachel M. McDonnell (now Dallas, Texas, USA).

We are greatly indebted to Prof. Kyung Won Chung, Ph.D., Director of Medical Gross Anatomy, University of Oklahoma, USA, Dept. of Cell Biology, for his careful corrections of the proofs of the new edition.

We would also like to express our many thanks to Prof. W. Bautz (Radiologisches Institut, University Erlangen-Nürnberg, Germany) and Prof. A. Heuck (Radiologisches Zentrum, München-Pasing, Germany), who provided the newly included excellent CT and MRI scans.

We are also greatly indebted to Mr. Hans Sommer (SOMSO Co., Coburg, Germany), who kindly provided a number of excellent bone specimens.

Finally, we would like to express our great gratitude to our photographer, Mr. Marco Gößwein, who contributed the very excellent macrophotos. Excellent and untiring work was done by our secretaries, Mrs. Lisa Köhler and Elisabeth Wascher, and as well by our artists, Mr. Jörg Pekarsky and Mrs. Annette Gack, who not only performed excellent new drawings but revised effectively the layout of the new edition.

Last but not least, we would like to express our sincere thanks to all scientists, students, and other coworkers, particularly to the ones at the publishing companies themselves.

Erlangen, Germany; Spring 2010

J. W. Rohen
C. Yokochi
E. Lütjen-Drecoll

Preface to the First Edition

Today there exist any number of good anatomic atlases. Consequently, the advent of a new work requires justification. We found three main reasons to undertake the publication of such a book.

First of all, most of the previous atlases contain mainly schematic or semischematic drawings which often reflect reality only in a limited way; the third dimension, i.e., the spatial effect, is lacking. In contrast, the photo of the actual anatomic specimen has the advantage of conveying the reality of the object with its proportions and spatial dimensions in a more exact and realistic manner than the "idealized", colored "nice" drawings of most previous atlases. Furthermore, the photo of the human specimen corresponds to the student's observations and needs in the dissection courses. Thus he has the advantage of immediate orientation by photographic specimens while working with the cadaver.

Secondly, some of the existing atlases are classified by systemic rather than regional aspects. As a result, the student needs several books each supplying the necessary facts for a certain region of the body. The present atlas, however, tries to portray macroscopic anatomy with regard to the regional and stratigraphic aspects of the object itself as realistically as possible. Hence it is an immediate help during the dissection courses in the study of medical and dental anatomy.

Another intention of the authors was to limit the subject to the essential and to offer it didactically in a way that is self-explanatory. To all regions of the body we added schematic drawings of the main tributaries of nerves and vessels, of the course and mechanism of the muscles, of the nomenclature of the various regions, etc. This will enhance the understanding of the details seen in the photographs. The complicated architecture of the skull bones, for example, was not presented in a descriptive way, but rather through a series of figures revealing the mosaic of bones by adding one bone to another, so that ultimately the composition of skull bones can be more easily understood.

Finally, the authors also considered the present situation in medical education. On one hand there is a universal lack of cadavers in many departments of anatomy, while on the other hand there has been a considerable increase in the number of students almost everywhere. As a consequence, students do not have access to sufficient illustrative material for their anatomic studies. Of course, photos can never replace the immediate observation, but we think the use of a macroscopic photo instead of a painted, mostly idealized picture is more appropriate and is an improvement in anatomic study over drawings alone.

The majority of the specimens depicted in the atlas were prepared by the authors either in the Dept. of Anatomy in Erlangen, Germany, or in the Dept. of Anatomy, Kanagawa Dental College, Yokosuka, Japan. The specimens of the chapter on the neck and those of the spinal cord demonstrating the dorsal branches of the spinal nerves were prepared by Dr. K. Schmidt with great skill and enthusiasm. The specimens of the ligaments of the vertebral column were prepared by Dr. Th. Mokrusch, and a great number of specimens in the chapter of the upper and lower limb was very carefully prepared by Dr. S. Nagashima, Kurume, Japan.

Once again, our warmest thanks go out to all of our coworkers for their unselfish, devoted and highly qualified work.

Erlangen, Germany; Spring 1983

J. W. Rohen
C. Yokochi

Contents

1 General Anatomy 1

Architectural Principles of the Human Body _____ 1
**Position of the Inner Organs, Palpaple Points,
and Regional Lines** _____ 2
Planes and Directions of the Body _____ 4
Osteology _____ 6
   Skeleton of the Human Body _____ 6
   Bone Structure _____ 8
   Ossification of the Bones _____ 9
Arthrology _____ 10
   Types of Joints _____ 10
   Architecture of the Joint _____ 12
Myology _____ 13
   Shapes of Muscles _____ 13
   Structure of the Muscular System _____ 14
**Comparative Imaging of Skeletal
and Muscular Structures in MRI and X-Ray** _____ 15
Organization of the Circulatory System _____ 16
Organization of the Lymphatic System _____ 17
Organization of the Nervous System _____ 18

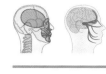

2 Head and Neck 19

2.1 Skull and Muscles of the Head _____ 19

Bones of the Skull _____ 20
Disarticulated Skull I _____ 24
   Sphenoidal and Occipital Bones _____ 24
   Temporal Bone _____ 26
   Frontal Bone _____ 28
Calvaria _____ 29
Base of the Skull _____ 30
Skull of the Newborn _____ 35
Median Sections through the Skull _____ 36
Disarticulated Skull II _____ 38
   Ethmoidal Bone _____ 38
   Ethmoidal and Palatine Bones _____ 39
   Palatine Bone and Maxilla _____ 40
   Sphenoidal, Ethmoidal, and Palatine Bones _____ 43
   Maxilla, Zygomatic Bone, and Bony Palate _____ 45
   Pterygopalatine Fossa and Orbit _____ 46
   Orbit, and Nasal and Lacrimal Bones _____ 47
Bones of the Nasal Cavity _____ 48
Septum and Cartilages of the Nose _____ 49
Maxilla and Mandible with Teeth _____ 50
Deciduous and Permanent Teeth _____ 51
Mandible and Dental Arch _____ 52
Ligaments of the Temporomandibular Joint _____ 53
Temporomandibular Joint _____ 54
Temporomandibular Joint and Masticatory Muscles __ 55
Masticatory Muscles _____ 56
   Temporalis and Masseter Muscles _____ 56
   Pterygoid Muscles _____ 57
Facial Muscles _____ 58
Supra- and Infrahyoid Muscles _____ 60
Section through the Cavities of the Head _____ 62
Maxillary Artery _____ 63

2.2 Cranial Nerves _____ 64

Brain and Cranial Nerves _____ 64
   Trigeminal Nerve _____ 68
   Facial Nerve _____ 70
   Connection with the Brain Stem _____ 71
   Nerves of the Orbit _____ 72
   Base of the Skull with Cranial Nerves _____ 74
Regions of the Head _____ 76
   Lateral Region _____ 76
   Retromandibular Region _____ 80
   Para- and Retropharyngeal Regions _____ 83

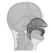

2 Head and Neck

2.3 Brain and Sensory Organs _____ 84

Position of Brain and Great Sensory Organs _____ 84
Scalp and Meninges _____ 85
Meninges _____ 86
    Dura Mater and Dural Venous Sinuses _____ 86
    Dura Mater _____ 88
    Pia Mater and Arachnoid _____ 89
Brain _____ 90
    Median Sections _____ 90
    Arteries and Veins _____ 92
    Arteries _____ 93
    Arteries and the Arterial Circle of Willis _____ 98
    Cerebrum _____ 99
    Cerebellum _____ 102
    Dissections _____ 104
    Limbic System _____ 107
    Hypothalamus _____ 108
    Subcortical Nuclei _____ 109
    Ventricular System _____ 112
    Brain Stem _____ 114
    Coronal and Cross Sections _____ 116
    Horizontal Sections _____ 118
Auditory and Vestibular Apparatus _____ 122
    Temporal Bone _____ 125
    Middle Ear _____ 126
    Auditory Ossicles _____ 128
    Internal Ear _____ 129
    Auditory Pathway and Areas _____ 131
Visual Apparatus and Orbit _____ 132
    Eyeball _____ 133
    Vessels of the Eye _____ 134
    Extra-ocular Muscles _____ 135
    Visual Pathway and Areas _____ 137
    Layers of the Orbit _____ 140
    Lacrimal Apparatus and Lids _____ 142

2.4 Oral and Nasal Cavities _____ 143

Position of Oral and Nasal Cavities _____ 143
Nasal Cavity _____ 144
    Paranasal Sinuses _____ 144
    Nerves and Arteries _____ 146
Sections through the Nasal and Oral Cavities _____ 148
Oral Cavity _____ 150
    Muscles _____ 150
    Submandibular Triangle _____ 152
    Salivary Glands _____ 153

2.5 Neck and Organs of the Neck _____ 154

Organization and Regions of the Neck _____ 154
Muscles of the Neck _____ 156
Larynx _____ 158
    Cartilages and Hyoid Bone _____ 158
    Muscles _____ 160
    Vocal Ligament _____ 161
    Nerves _____ 162
Larynx and Oral Cavity _____ 163
Pharynx _____ 164
    Muscles _____ 166
Vessels of the Head and Neck _____ 168
    Arteries _____ 168
    Arteries and Veins _____ 170
    Veins _____ 171
    Lymph Vessels and Nodes _____ 172
Regions of the Neck _____ 174
    Anterior Region _____ 174
    Lateral Region _____ 178
Cervical and Brachial Plexuses _____ 186

3 Trunk
187

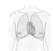

4 Thoracic Organs
243

Segmental Structure of the Trunk _____ 187
Skeleton _____ 188
Vertebrae _____ 190
Vertebral Column and Thorax _____ 192
   Vertebral Joints _____ 195
   Costovertebral Joints and Intercostal Muscles _____ 196
   Costovertebral Joints _____ 197
   Ligaments _____ 198
   Joints Connecting to the Head _____ 200
   Vertebral Column of the Neck _____ 203
Surface Anatomy of the Anterior Body _____ 204
   Female _____ 204
   Male _____ 205
Thoracic Wall _____ 206
Thoracic and Abdominal Walls _____ 209
   Vessels and Nerves _____ 214
Inguinal Region _____ 217
   Male _____ 217
   Female _____ 220
Back _____ 221
   Muscles _____ 221
   Nerves _____ 226
Vertebral Canal and Spinal Cord _____ 230
Nuchal Region _____ 234

Position of the Thoracic Organs _____ 243
Respiratory System _____ 246
   Bronchial Tree _____ 246
   Projections of Lungs and Pleura _____ 248
   Lungs _____ 249
   Bronchopulmonary Segments _____ 250
Heart _____ 252
   Myocardium _____ 257
   Valves _____ 258
   Function _____ 260
   Conducting System _____ 261
   Arteries and Veins _____ 262
Regional Anatomy of the Thoracic Organs _____ 264
   Thymus _____ 266
   Heart _____ 268
   Pericardium _____ 272
   Epicardium _____ 273
Posterior Mediastinum _____ 274
   Mediastinal Organs _____ 274
Posterior and Superior Mediastinum _____ 281
   Mediastinal Organs _____ 281
Diaphragm _____ 282
Coronal Sections through the Thorax _____ 284
Horizontal Sections through the Thorax _____ 286
Fetal Circulatory System _____ 288
Mammary Gland _____ 290

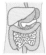

5 Abdominal Organs   291

Position of the Abdominal Organs _____ 291
Anterior Abdominal Wall _____ 293
Stomach _____ 294
Pancreas and Bile Ducts _____ 296
Liver _____ 298
Spleen _____ 300
Upper Abdominal Organs _____ 301
Vessels of the Abdominal Organs _____ 302
   Superior Mesenteric Vessels _____ 302
   Portal Circulation _____ 303
   Superior Mesenteric Artery _____ 304
   Inferior Mesenteric Artery _____ 305
Dissection of the Abdominal Organs _____ 306
   Mesenteric Arteries _____ 308
   Mesentery _____ 310
   Upper Abdominal Organs _____ 311
Posterior Abdominal Wall _____ 316
   Pancreas and Bile Ducts _____ 316
   Duodenum, Pancreas, and Spleen _____ 317
   Root of the Mesentery and Peritoneal Recesses ____ 318
Horizontal Sections through the Abdominal Cavity __ 320
Midsagittal Sections through the Abdominal Cavity __ 322

6 Retroperitoneal Organs   323

Position of the Urinary Organs _____ 323
Sections through the Retroperitoneal Region _____ 325
Kidney _____ 326
   Arteries _____ 328
   Arteries and Veins _____ 329
Retroperitoneal Region _____ 330
   Urinary System _____ 330
   Lymph Vessels and Nodes _____ 332
   Vessels and Nerves _____ 333
   Autonomic Nervous System_____ 334
Male Urogenital System_____ 336
Male Genital Organs (isolated) _____ 337
Male External Genital Organs _____ 340
   Penis _____ 342
Male Internal Genital Organs _____ 343
   Testis and Epididymis _____ 343
   Accessory Glands _____ 344
Pelvic Cavity in the Male _____ 345
   Coronal Sections _____ 345
   Vessels of the Pelvic Organs _____ 346
   Abdominal Aorta _____ 348
   Vessels and Nerves of the Pelvic Organs _____ 349
Urogenital and Pelvic Diaphragms in the Male _____ 350
Female Urogenital System _____ 354
Female Genital Organs (isolated) _____ 356
Female Internal Genital Organs_____ 358
   Uterus and Related Organs _____ 359
   Arteries and Lymph Vessels _____ 360
Female External Genital Organs _____ 361
**Urogenital Diaphragm
and External Genital Organs in the Female** _____ 363
Pelvic Cavity in the Female _____ 366
   Coronal and Horizontal Sections _____ 367

7 Upper Limb   368

Skeleton of the Shoulder Girdle and Thorax _____ 368
Scapula _____ 371
Skeleton of the Shoulder Girdle and Humerus _____ 372
Humerus _____ 373
Skeleton of the Forearm _____ 374
Skeleton of the Forearm and Hand _____ 375
Skeleton of the Hand _____ 376
Joints and Ligaments of the Shoulder _____ 378
Ligaments of the Elbow Joint _____ 379
Ligaments of the Hand and Wrist _____ 380
Muscles of the Shoulder and Arm _____ 382
    Dorsal Muscles _____ 382
    Pectoral Muscles _____ 384
Muscles of the Arm _____ 386
Muscles of the Forearm and Hand _____ 388
    Flexor Muscles _____ 388
    Extensor Muscles _____ 392
Muscles of the Hand _____ 394
Arteries _____ 396
Veins _____ 398
Nerves _____ 399
Surface Anatomy of the Upper Limb _____ 401
    Posterior and Lateral Aspects _____ 401
    Anterior Aspect _____ 402
Neck and Shoulder _____ 403
Shoulder _____ 404
    Posterior Region _____ 404
    Anterior Region _____ 406
Shoulder and Arm _____ 408
Axillary Region _____ 410
Brachial Plexus _____ 413
Arm _____ 414
Cubital Region _____ 416
Forearm and Hand _____ 420
    Posterior Region _____ 420
    Anterior Region _____ 422
Hand _____ 424
    Posterior Region _____ 424
    Anterior Region _____ 426
Sections through the Upper Limb _____ 430

8 Lower Limb   432

Skeleton of the Pelvic Girdle and Lower Limb _____ 432
Bones of the Pelvis _____ 433
Skeleton of the Pelvis _____ 435
Bones of the Hip Joint _____ 438
Femur _____ 439
Skeleton of the Leg _____ 440
Bones of the Knee Joint _____ 441
Skeleton of the Foot _____ 442
Ligaments of the Pelvis and Hip Joint _____ 444
Knee Joint _____ 446
Ligaments of the Knee Joint _____ 447
Joints of the Ankle _____ 449
Ligaments of the Foot _____ 450
Muscles of the Thigh _____ 452
    Adductor Muscles _____ 452
    Gluteal Muscles _____ 454
    Flexor Muscles _____ 455
Muscles of the Leg _____ 457
    Flexor Muscles _____ 457
Muscles of the Leg and Foot _____ 458
    Deep Flexor Muscles _____ 460
    Extensor Muscles _____ 462
Muscles of the Foot _____ 463
Arteries _____ 466
Veins _____ 468
Nerves _____ 470
    Lumbosacral Plexus _____ 471
Lumbar Part of the Vertebral Canal and Spinal Cord __ 472
Spinal Cord with Intercostal Nerves _____ 474
Spinal Cord and Lumbar Plexus _____ 475
Surface Anatomy of the Lower Limb _____ 476
    Posterior Aspect _____ 476
    Anterior Aspect _____ 477
Thigh _____ 478
    Anterior Region _____ 478
Gluteal Region _____ 482
Thigh _____ 484
    Posterior Region _____ 484
Knee and Popliteal Fossa _____ 486
Crural Region _____ 489
Crural Region and Foot _____ 492
Coronal Sections through the Foot _____ 495
Sections through the Lower Limb _____ 496
Foot _____ 498
    Posterior Region _____ 498
    Anterior Region _____ 500

Index   503

1 General Anatomy

Three general principles are recognizable in the architecture of the human organism:

1. **The principle of polarity:** Polarity is reflected mainly in the formal and functional contrast between the head (predominantly spherical form) and the extremities (radially arranged skeletal elements). In the phylogenetic development of the upright position of the human body, polarity developed also among the extremities: The lower extremities provide the basis for locomotion whereas the upper extremities are not needed anymore for locomotion, so they can be used for gesture, manual and artistic activities.

2. **The principle of segmentation:** This principle dominates in the trunk. The anatomical structures (vertebrae, pairs of ribs, muscles, and nerves) are arranged segmentally and replicate rhythmically in a similar way.

3. **The principle of bilateral symmetry:** Both sides of the body are separated by a midsagittal plane and resemble each other like image and mirror-image.

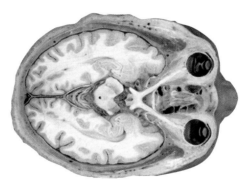

Horizontal section through the head at the level of the eyes.

There are also different principles in the architecture and function of the inner organs:

The **skull** contains the brain and the sensory organs. They are arranged like mirror and mirror-image and are the basis of our consciousness.

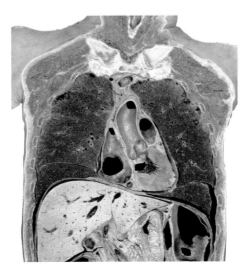

Coronal section through the thoracic and abdominal cavity.

The **thorax** contains the organs of the rhythmic system (heart, lung), which are only to some extent bilaterally organized. The consciousness (feeling, etc.) is located in-between.

In the **abdominal cavity,** the most important abdominal organs (intestinal tract, liver, pancreas) are arranged unpaired. Their functions remain subconscious.

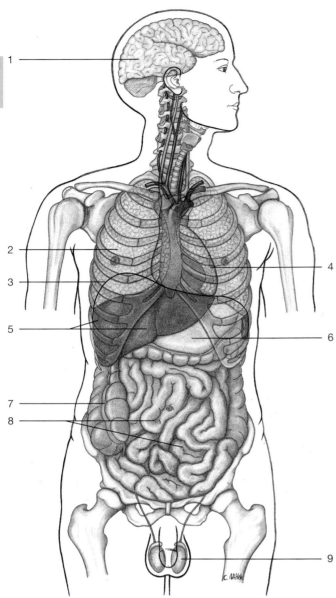

Position of the inner organs of the human body (anterior aspect). The main cavities of the body and their contents.

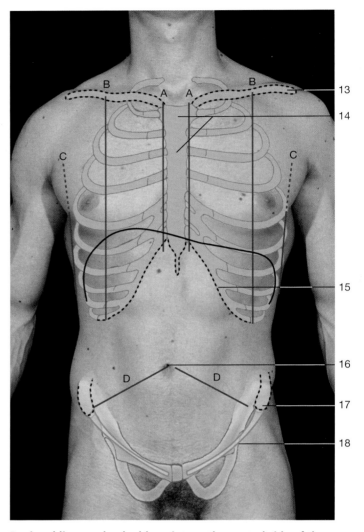

Regional lines and palpable points at the ventral side of the human body.

Regional lines
A = parasternal line
B = midclavicular line
C = anterior axillary line
D = umbilical-pelvic line

The bones of the skeletal system are palpable through the skin at different points. This enables physicians to localize the inner organs. On the **ventral side,** the clavicle, sternum, ribs, and intercostal spaces are palpable. Furthermore, the anterior iliac spine and the symphysis can be localized. For better orientation, several **lines of orientation** are used, e.g., the parasternal line, the midclavicular line, the anterior axillary line, the umbilical-pelvic line.

By means of these lines, the heart and the position of the vermiform process can be localized.

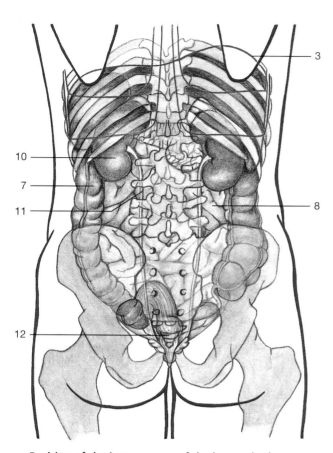

Position of the inner organs of the human body (posterior aspect).

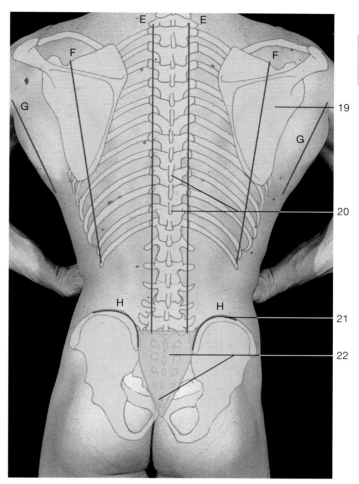

Regional lines and palpable points at the dorsal side of the human body.

Regional lines
E = paravertebral line
F = scapular line
G = posterior axillary line
H = iliac crest

1 Brain
2 Lung
3 Diaphragm
4 Heart
5 Liver
6 Stomach
7 Colon
8 Small intestine
9 Testis
10 Kidney
11 Ureter
12 Anal canal
13 Clavicle
14 Manubrium sterni
15 Costal arch
16 Umbilicus
17 Anterior superior iliac spine
18 Inguinal ligament
19 Scapular spine
20 Spinous processes
21 Iliac crest
22 Coccyx and sacrum

At the **dorsal side** of the body, the posterior spines of the vertebral column, the ribs, the scapula, the sacrum, and the iliac crest are palpable. **Lines of orientation** are the paravertebral line, the scapular line, the posterior axillary line, and the iliac crest.

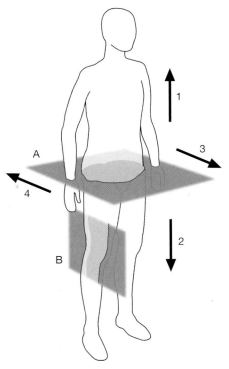

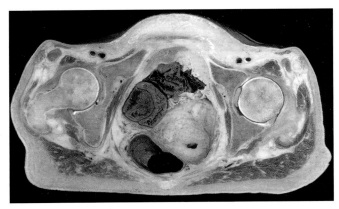

Horizontal section through the pelvic cavity and the hip joints.

Planes of the body:
A = horizontal or axial or transverse plane
B = sagittal plane (at the level of the knee joint)

Directions:
1 = cranial   3 = anterior (ventral)
2 = caudal   4 = posterior (dorsal)

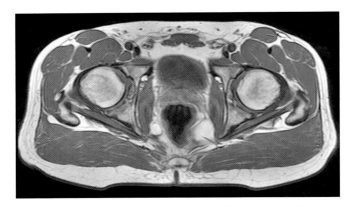

MRI scan through the pelvic cavity and the hip joints (horizontal or axial or transverse plane).

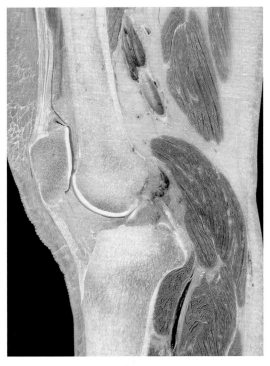

Sagittal section through the knee joint.

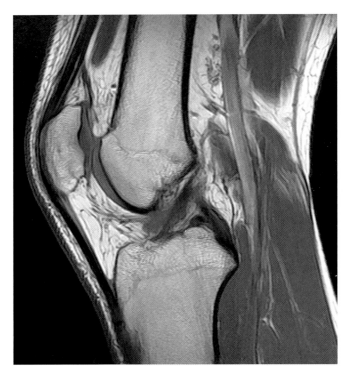

MRI scan through the knee joint (sagittal plane).

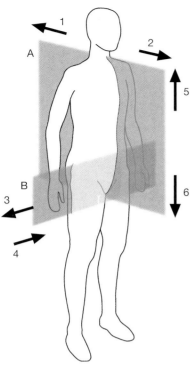

Planes of the body:
A = midsagittal or median plane
B = frontal or coronal plane (through the pelvic cavity)

Directions:
1 = posterior (dorsal)   4 = medial
2 = anterior (ventral)   5 = cranial
3 = lateral   6 = caudal

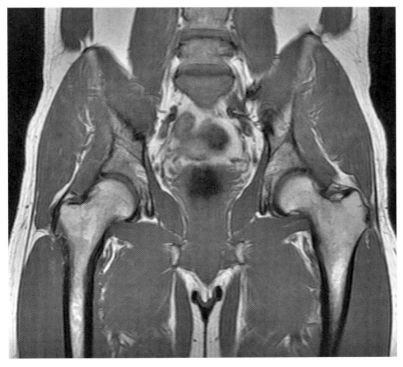

MRI scan through the pelvic cavity and the hip joints (frontal or coronal plane).

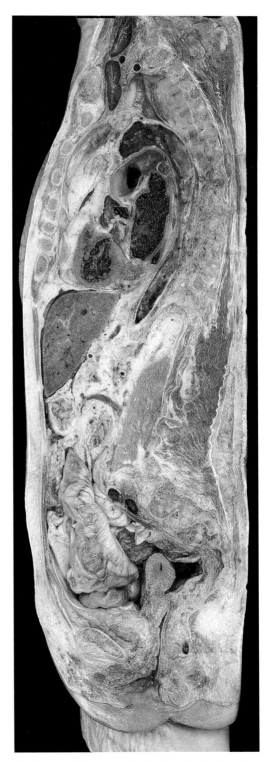

Median section through the trunk of a female.

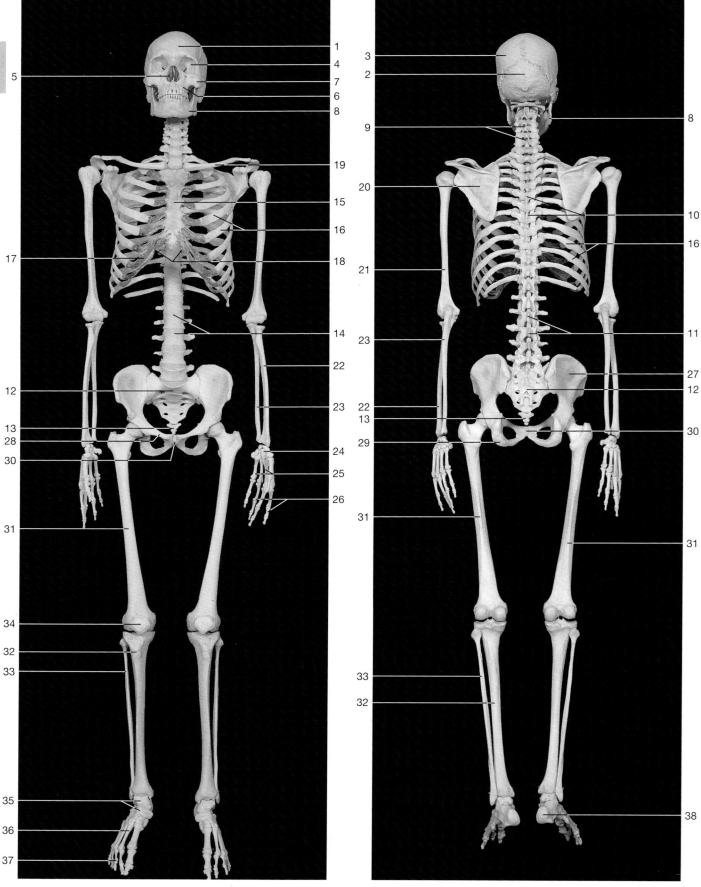

Skeleton of a female adult (anterior aspect).

Skeleton of a female adult (posterior aspect).

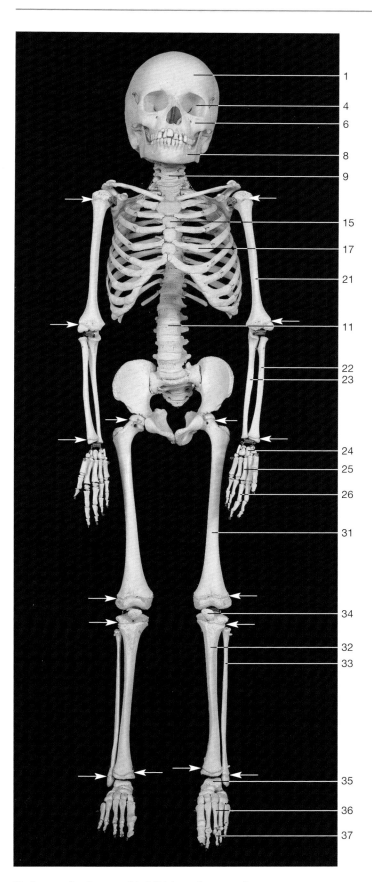

Axial skeleton
Head
1   Frontal bone
2   Occipital bone
3   Parietal bone
4   Orbit
5   Nasal cavity
6   Maxilla
7   Zygomatic bone
8   Mandible

Trunk and thorax
Vertebral column
9   Cervical vertebrae
10   Thoracic vertebrae
11   Lumbar vertebrae
12   Sacrum
13   Coccyx
14   Intervertebral discs
Thorax
15   Sternum
16   Ribs
17   Costal cartilage
18   Infrasternal angle

Appendicular skeleton
Upper limb and shoulder girdle
19   Clavicle
20   Scapula
21   Humerus
22   Radius
23   Ulna
24   Carpal bones
25   Metacarpal bones
26   Phalanges of the hand

Lower limb and pelvis
27   Ilium
28   Pubis
29   Ischium
30   Symphysis pubis
31   Femur
32   Tibia
33   Fibula
34   Patella
35   Tarsal bones
36   Metatarsal bones
37   Phalanges of the foot
38   Calcaneus

Skeleton of a 5-year-old child (anterior aspect).
The zones of the cartilaginous growth plates are seen (arrows).
In contrast to the adult, the ribs show a predominantly
horizontal position.

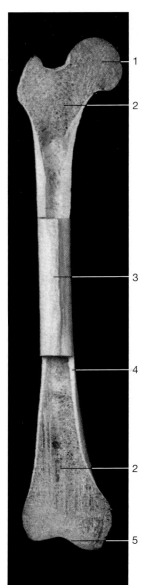

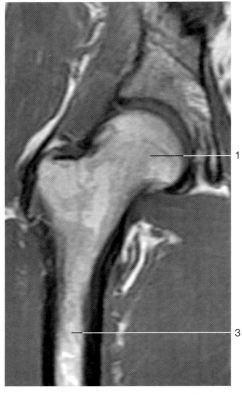

MRI scan of the right femur and the hip joint (coronal section) (from Heuck et al., MRT-Atlas, 2009).

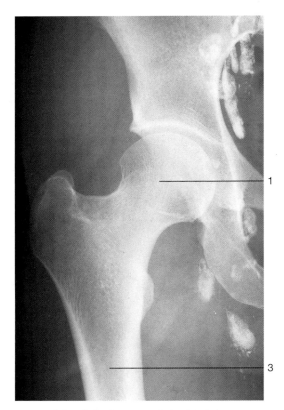

X-ray of the right femur and the hip joint (a.-p. direction).

◁ **Femur of the adult.** Coronal section of the proximal and distal epiphyses displaying the spongy bone and the medullary cavity.

1   Head of the femur
2   Spongy bone
3   Diaphysis of the femur
4   Compact bone
5   Articular cartilage

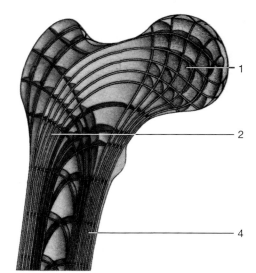

Three-dimensional representation on the trajectorial lines of the femoral head (according to B. Kummer).

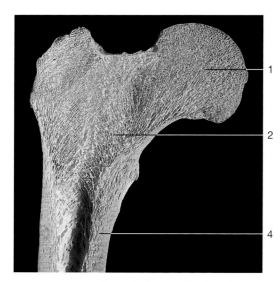

Coronal section through the proximal end of the adult femur showing the characteristic structure of the spongy bone.

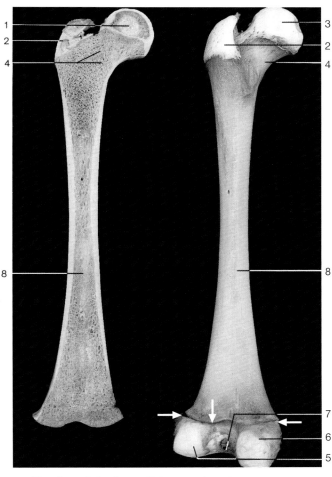

The **ossification of the bones** of the limbs starts within the ossification centers of the primary cartilagenous bones. Here, the medullary cavity develops. The ossification process of limb bones is not finished at birth.

◁ 1 Ossification center in the   5 Lateral condyle
       head of the femur   6 Medial condyle
   2 Greater trochanter   7 Intercondylar notch
   3 Head of the femur   8 Diaphysis
   4 Neck of the femur

Ossification of the femur (left: coronal section, right: posterior view of the femur). Arrows: distal epiphysis.

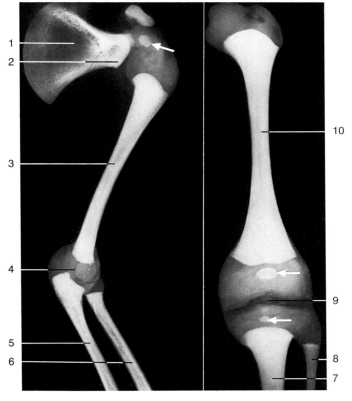

X-ray of the upper and lower limb of a newborn child (left: upper limb, right: lower limb). Arrows: ossification centers.

   1 Scapula   6 Radius
   2 Shoulder joint   7 Tibia
   3 Humerus   8 Fibula
   4 Elbow joint   9 Knee joint
   5 Ulna   10 Femur

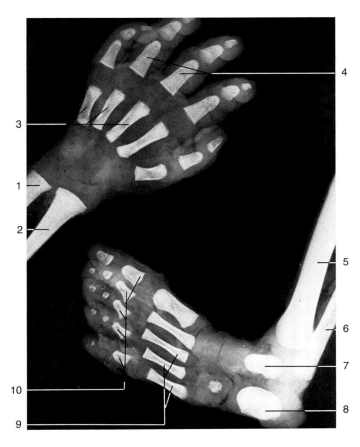

◁ 1 Ulna   6 Fibula
   2 Radius   7 Talus
   3 Metacarpals   8 Calcaneus
   4 Phalanges   9 Metatarsals
   5 Tibia   10 Phalanges

X-ray of hand and foot of a newborn.

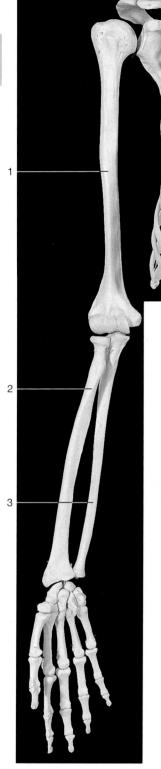

Skeleton of the right arm and shoulder girdle (anterior aspect).

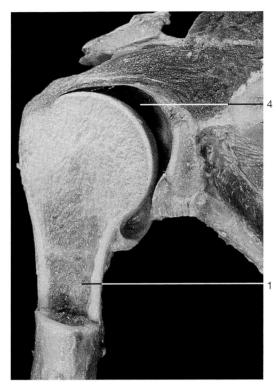

Shoulder joint as an example of a multiaxial ball-and-socket joint (coronal section).

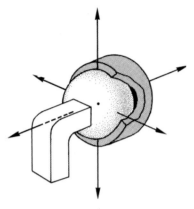

Ball-and-socket joint with its different axes (schematic drawing). Arrows: axes of movement.

1 Humerus
2 Radius
3 Ulna
4 Articular cavity (shoulder joint)
5 Metacarpophalangeal joint
6 Joints of fingers

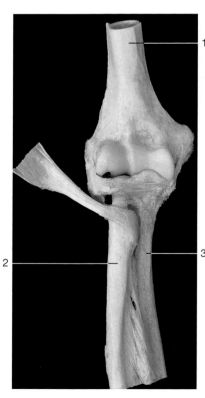

Elbow joint with ligaments as an example of a hinge joint (monaxial humero-ulnar joint) in combination with a pivot joint (monaxial radio-ulnar joint), which allows rotation.

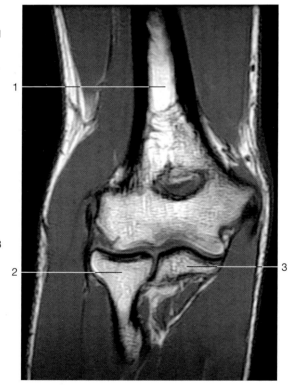

Coronal section of the elbow joint (MRI scan, courtesy of Prof. Heuck, Munich). The possibilities of movement are shown in the schematic drawings on p. 11.

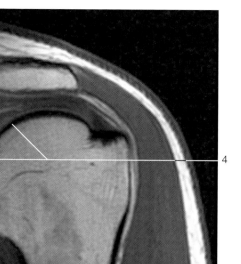

Coronal section of the shoulder joint
(MRI scan, from Heuck et al., MRT-Atlas, 2009).

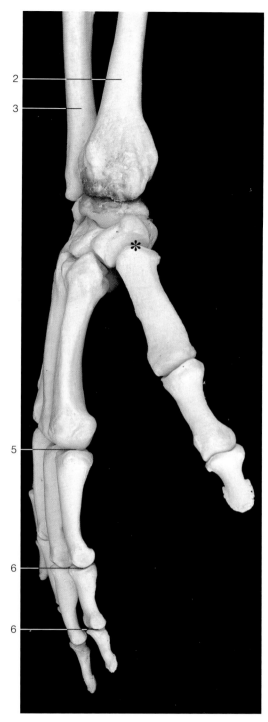

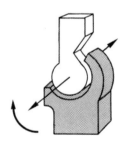

Hinge joint
(e.g. humero-ulnar joint). Left: extension, right: flexion.
Arrows: axes of movement.

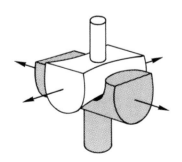

Pivot joint
(e.g. radio-ulnar joint).

Saddle joint
(e.g. carpometacarpal joint of
the thumb).

Skeleton of right wrist and hand (medial aspect).
The metacarpophalangeal joints are biaxial, as is
the carpometacarpal joint of the thumb (✲ in the
figure). The joints of the fingers, however, are
monaxial.

Joints exhibit a variety of functions. In
general, mobility becomes reduced in the
direction from proximal to distal. The hip
joint, e.g., is multiaxial; the knee joint is
biaxial, and the joints of toes and fingers are
monaxial.

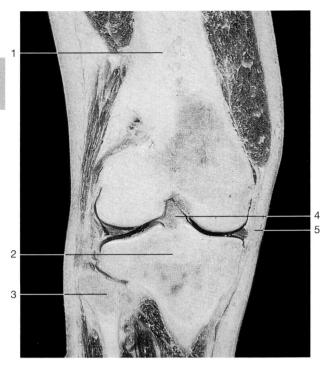

Coronal section through the knee joint (anterior aspect of the right joint in extension).

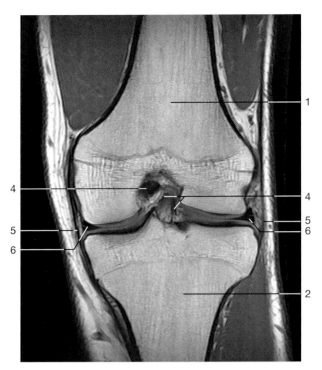

MRI scan of the knee joint (coronal plane) (from Heuck et al., MRT-Atlas, 2009).

1   Femur
2   Tibia
3   Fibula
4   Cruciate ligaments
5   Collateral ligaments
6   Meniscus

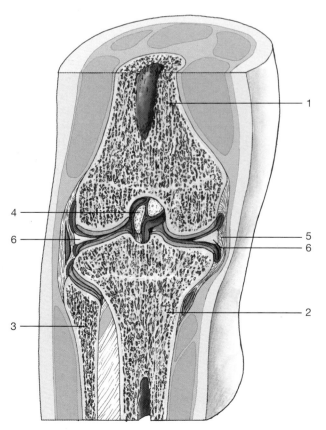

Joints are places of articulation allowing movements between bones. Synovial joints are characterized by a joint cavity enclosed by a joint capsule containing synovial fluid, which is produced by the articular capsule. The kind of movements depends not only on form and structure of the articulating bones but also on ligaments incorporated into the articular capsule. In some synovial joints, fibrocartilagenous articular discs develop, when the articulating surfaces of the bones are incongruous.

Schematic drawing of the knee joint as an example of a synovial joint, characterized by a joint cavity enclosed by a joint capsule (red) containing synovial fluid. Blue = articular cartilage.

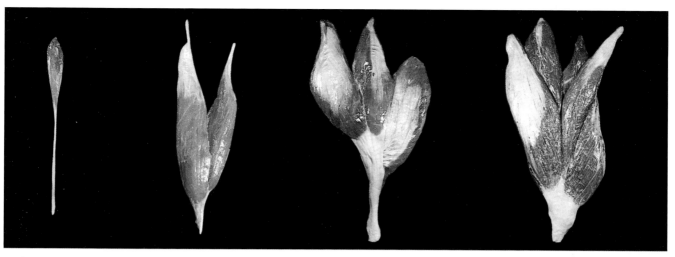

Fusiform
(palmaris longus)

Bicipital
(biceps brachii)

Tricipital (triceps surae,
gastrocnemius, and soleus)

Quadricipital
(quadriceps femoris)

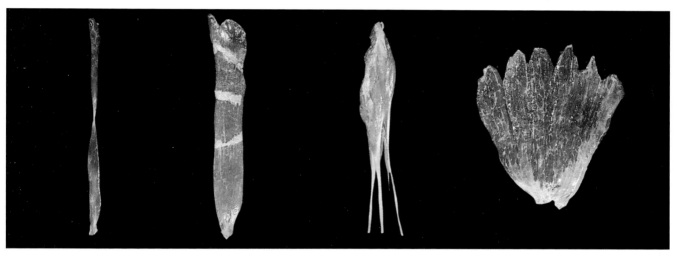

Digastric
(omohyoideus)

Multiventral
(rectus abdominis)

Multicaudal
(flexor digitorum prof.)

Serrated
(serratus anterior)

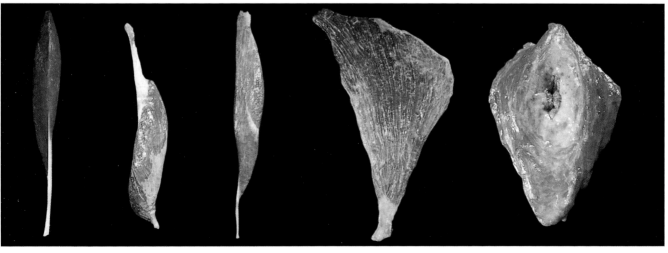

Bipennate
(tibialis anterior)

Unipennate
(semimembranosus)

Semitendinous
(semitendinosus)

Broad, flat muscle
(latissimus dorsi)

Ring-like
(sphincter ani externus)

The human body possesses **a great variety of muscles.** The architecture of the muscles depends on the functional systems in which they are involved, i.e., the kind of movements, the form of the joints with their specific ligaments, etc. The movements themselves vary to a great extent individually.

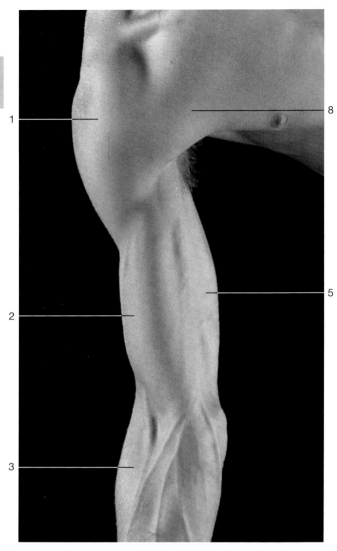

Ventral aspect of the right arm. The biceps muscle appears slightly contracted. In the area of the elbow joint, several subcutaneous veins can be recognized.

1   Deltoid muscle
2   Biceps brachii muscle
3   Brachioradialis muscle
4   Humerus
5   Triceps brachii muscle
6   Elbow joint
7   Brachialis muscle
8   Pectoralis major muscle
9   Radius
10 Ulna

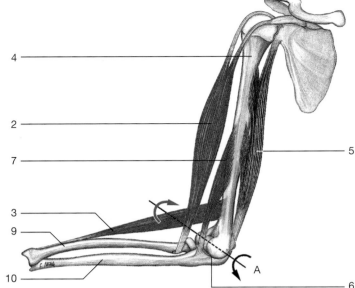

Diagram illustrating the position of the flexor and extensor muscles of the arm and their effect on the elbow joint.
A = axis of humero-ulnar joint; arrows = direction of movements; red = flexion; black = extension.

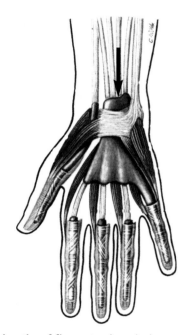

Synovial sheaths of flexor tendons (palmar aspect of right hand, semischematic drawing). **The flexor retinaculum** protects the flexor tendons passing through the carpal tunnel (arrow).

Joints are moved by muscles. The highly differentiated movements are coordinated by special groups of muscles (**synergists**). Their counterparts are called **antagonists**. Movements can only be carried out harmoniously if the contraction of the synergists are supported by a corresponding dilatation of the antagonists. This interaction is controlled by the nervous system. In order to carry out certain directions of movements, often the tendons of muscles have to be directed by ligaments. At those places, the tendons often develop synovial sheaths, e.g., at the wrist joint or at the fingers.

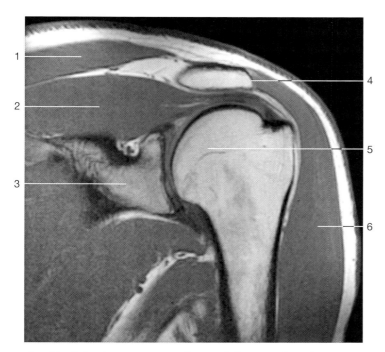

Shoulder joint (MRI scan, coronal section) (from Heuck et al., MRT-Atlas, 2009).

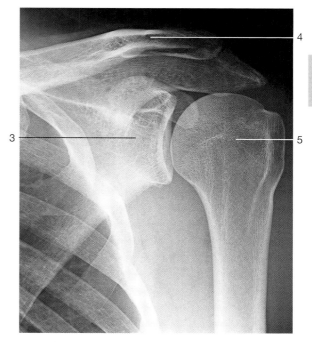

Shoulder joint (X-ray, a.-p. direction) (courtesy of Dr. Holik, Spardorf).

1	Trapezius muscle	6	Deltoid muscle
2	Supraspinatus muscle	7	Cavity of shoulder joint
3	Scapula	8	Articular cartilage
4	Acromion	9	Articular cavity
5	Head of humerus	10	Humerus

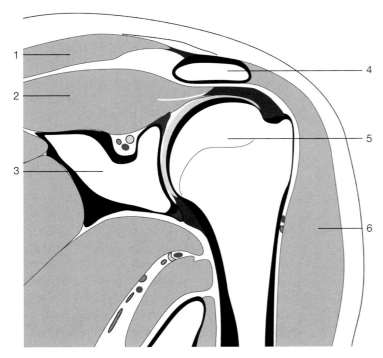

Shoulder joint (schematic drawing of the MRI scan above) (from Heuck et al., MRT-Atlas, 2009).

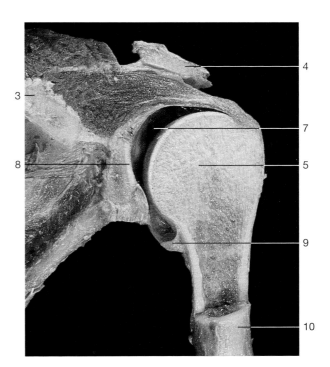

Frontal section of the shoulder joint (compare with the two pictures above).

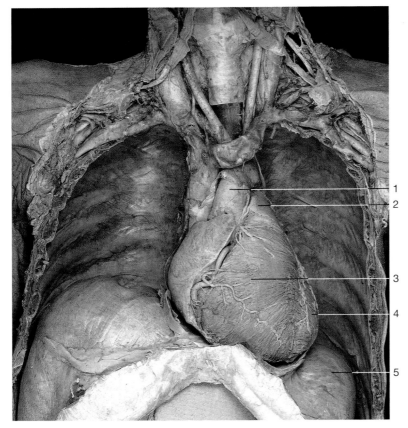

Heart and related vessels in situ (anterior aspect). Anterior thoracic wall, pericardium, and epicardium have been removed. The trachea is divided.

1	Aorta	4	Left heart
2	Pulmonary artery	5	Diaphragm
3	Right heart	6	Abdominal aorta

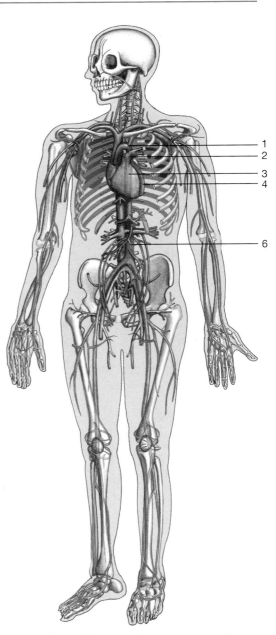

Organization of the circulatory system with the heart in the center. Red = arteries; blue = veins (from Lütjen-Drecoll, Rohen, Innenansichten des menschlichen Körpers, 2010).

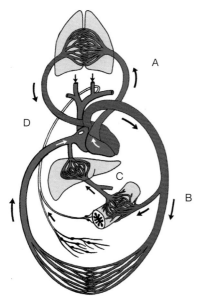

Organization of the circulatory systems in the human body. The center of this system represents the heart. Red = arteries; blue = veins (from Lütjen-Drecoll, Rohen, Innenansichten des menschlichen Körpers, 2010).

A = pulmonary circulation   C = portal circulation
B = systemic circulation   D = lymphatic circulation

The center of the circulatory system is the heart, which is situated in the thoracic cavity and in contact with the diaphragm. In the right ventricle, the venous blood is collected and pumped through the pulmonary artery and into the lung where the blood is oxygenated. The veins of the lung transport the blood to the left ventricle, where it is pumped through the aorta and its branches (arteries) in the human body. Arteries and veins mostly run parallel. The venous blood from the intestine reaches the liver via the portal vein.

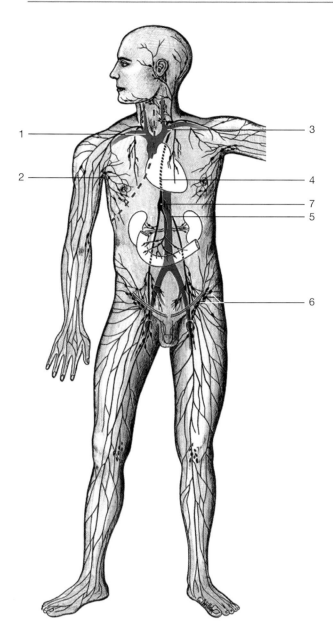

Organization of the lymphatic system.
Course of the main lymphatic vessels and lymph nodes in the body. Dotted red line = border between lymphatic vessels draining toward the right and the left venous angles.

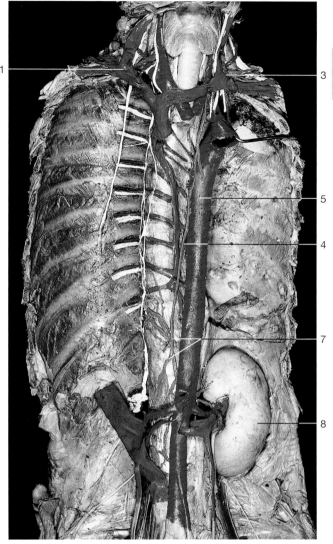

Major lymph vessels of the trunk (green). Blue = veins, red = arteries, white = nerves.

1	Right venous angle	5	Aorta
2	Axillary lymph nodes	6	Inguinal lymph nodes
3	Left venous angle	7	Cisterna chyli
4	Thoracic duct	8	Left kidney

Lymphatic vessels originate in the tissue spaces (lymph capillaries) and unite to form larger vessels (lymphatics). These resemble veins but have a much thinner wall, more valves, and are interrupted by lymph nodes at various intervals. Large groups of lymph nodes are located in the inguinal and axillary regions, deep to the mandible and sternocleidomastoid muscle, and within the root of the mesentery of the intestine. The lymphatic vessels of the right half of the head and neck, the right thorax, and the right upper limb drain toward the right venous angle; those of the rest of the body, toward the left venous angle.

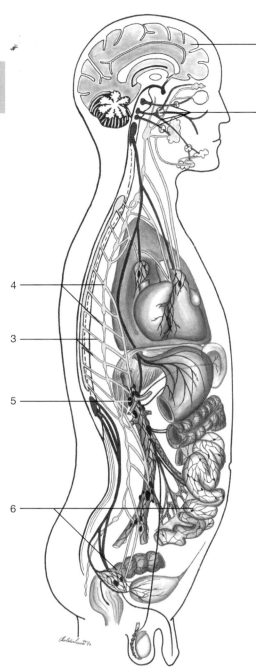

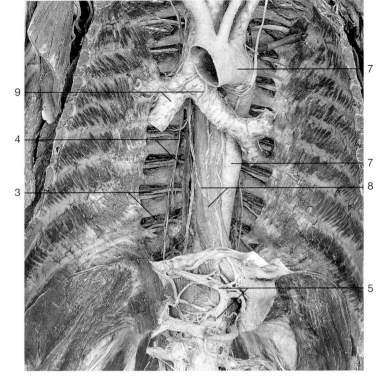

Posterior part of the trunk. The **solar plexus** with its connection to the vagus nerve and the sympathetic trunk has been dissected.

Diagram illustrating the **localization of the three functional portions of the nervous system** (brain, spinal cord and autonomic nervous system). Yellow = sympathetic system; red = parasympathetic system.

1	Cerebrum	6	Nervous plexus of the
2	Cranial nerves		autonomic system
3	Spinal nerves	7	Aorta
4	Sympathetic trunk	8	Vagus nerve and esophagus
5	Solar plexus	9	Bifurcation of trachea

The nervous system can be divided into three functionally distinct parts:
1. The cranial part, which comprises the great sensory organs and the brain.
2. The spinal cord, which shows a segmental structure and serves predominantly as a reflex organ.
3. The autonomic nervous system, which controls the involuntary functions (subconscious control) of organs and tissues. The autonomic part of the nervous system forms many delicate plexuses near or within the organs.

At certain places these plexuses contain aggregations of nerve cells (prevertebral and intramural ganglia).

The spinal nerves leave the spinal cord at regular intervals. The ventral rami of the spinal nerves form the cervical and brachial plexus, which innervates the upper extremity, and the ventral rami of the lumbar and sacral spinal nerves form the lumbosacral plexus, which innervates the pelvis and genital organs and the lower extremity.

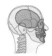

2 Head and Neck

2.1 Skull and Muscles of the Head

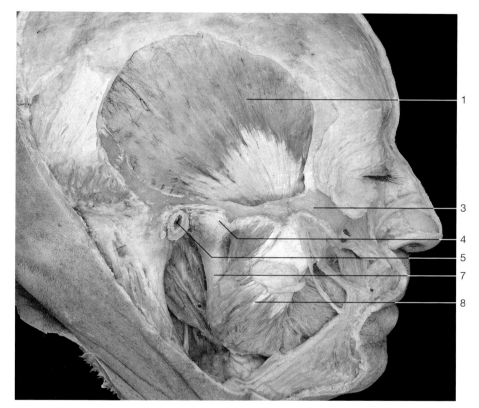

Muscles of mastication and facial muscles (lateral aspect).
The auricle has been removed.

The head contains the brain and the great sensory organs (neurocranium). Anteriorly, the facial bones, the facial muscles, and the muscles of mastication have been developed (viscerocranium). The base of the skull is slightly bent so that the structures of the viscerocranium become located underneath the neurocranium, a specifity of the human head. Therefore mimic movements are possible in the human face.

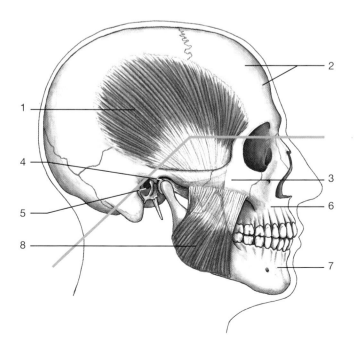

1 Temporalis muscle
2 Frontal bone
3 Zygomatic bone
4 Temporomandibular joint
5 External acoustic meatus
6 Maxilla
7 Mandible
8 Masseter muscle

Lateral aspect of the skull with muscles of mastication
(temporalis and masseter muscles = red).
The base of the skull is bent (grey line).

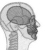

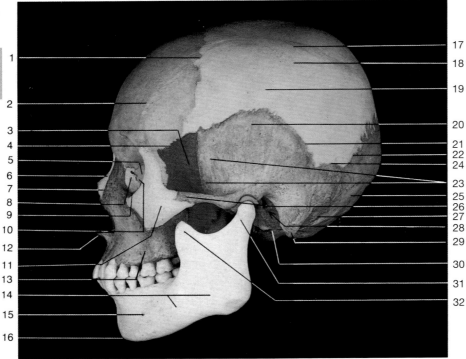

1	Coronal suture
2	Frontal bone
3	Sphenoidal bone
4	Sphenofrontal suture
5	Ethmoidal bone
6	Nasal bone
7	Nasomaxillary suture
8	Lacrimal bone
9	Lacrimomaxillary suture
10	Ethmoidolacrimal suture
11	Zygomatic bone
12	Anterior nasal spine
13	Maxilla
14	Mandible
15	Mental foramen
16	Mental protuberance
17	Superior temporal line
18	Inferior temporal line
19	Parietal bone
20	Temporal bone
21	Squamous suture
22	Lambdoid suture
23	Temporal fossa
24	Parietomastoid suture
25	Occipital bone
26	Zygomatic arch
27	Occipitomastoid suture
28	External acoustic meatus
29	Mastoid process
30	Tympanic portion of temporal bone
31	Condylar process of mandible
32	Coronoid process of mandible

General architecture of the skull (lateral aspect). The different bones are indicated in color (numbers cf. table).

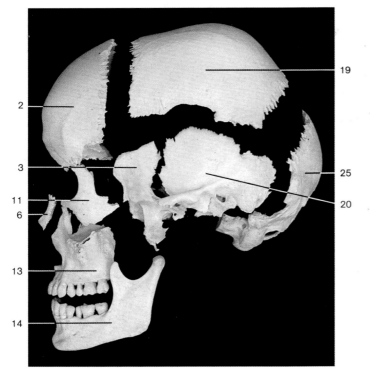

Lateral aspect of the disarticulated skull (palatine bone, lacrimal bone, ethmoidal bone, and vomer are not depicted).

2	Frontal bone (orange)	**Cranial bones**
19	Parietal bone (light yellow)	
3	Greater wing of sphenoidal bone (red)	
25	Squama of occipital bone (blue)	
20	Squama of temporal bone (brown)	
5	Ethmoidal bone (dark green)	**Base of skull**
3	Sphenoidal bone (red)	
	Temporal bone excluding squama (brown)	
30	Tympanic portion of temporal bone (dark brown)	
	Occipital bone excluding squama (blue)	
6	Nasal bone (white)	**Facial bones**
8	Lacrimal bone (light yellow)	
	Inferior nasal concha	
	Vomer	
11	Zygomatic bone (dark yellow)	
	Palatine bone	
13	Maxilla (violet)	
14	Mandible (white)	
	Malleus ⎫	**Auditory ossicles**
	Incus ⎬ within petrous portion of	
	Stapes ⎭ temporal bone	
	Hyoid	

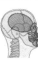

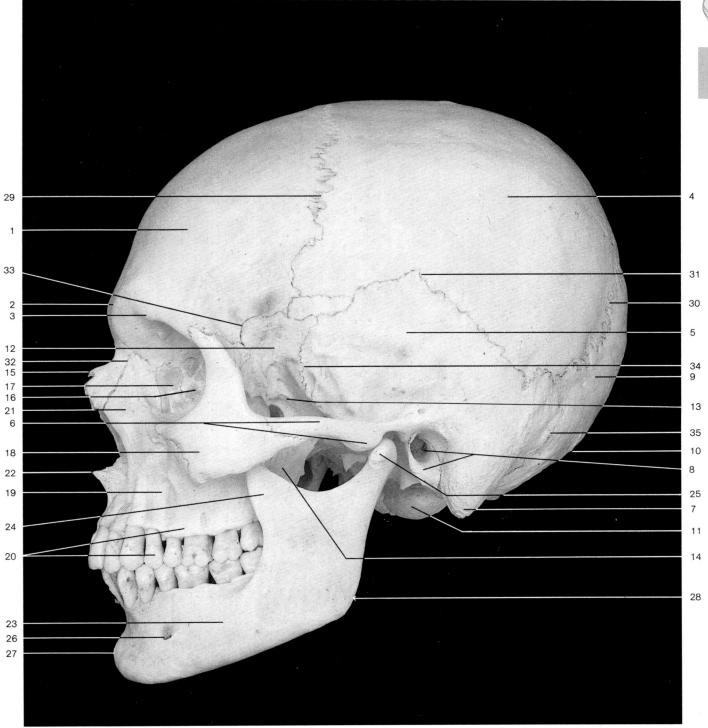

29
1
33
2
3
12
32
15
17
16
21
6
18
22
19
24
20
23
26
27

4
31
30
5
34
9
13
35
10
8
25
7
11
14
28

Lateral aspect of the skull.

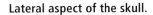

1	Frontal bone	12	Sphenoidal bone (greater wing)
2	Glabella	13	Infratemporal crest of sphenoid
3	Supraorbital margin	14	Pterygoid process (lateral pterygoid plate)
4	Parietal bone	15	Nasal bone
5	Temporal bone (squamous part)	16	Ethmoidal bone (orbital part)
6	Zygomatic process (articular tubercle)	17	Lacrimal bone
		18	Zygomatic bone
7	Mastoid process	19	Maxilla (body)
8	Tympanic part (tympanic plate) and external acoustic meatus	20	Alveolar process and teeth
		21	Frontal process
9	Occipital bone (squamous part)	22	Anterior nasal spine
10	External occipital protuberance	23	Mandible (body)
11	Occipital condyle	24	Coronoid process

25	Condylar process
26	Mental foramen
27	Mental protuberance
28	Angle of the mandible

Sutures
29	Coronal suture
30	Lambdoid suture
31	Squamous suture
32	Nasomaxillary suture
33	Frontosphenoid suture
34	Sphenosquamosal suture
35	Occipitomastoid suture

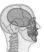

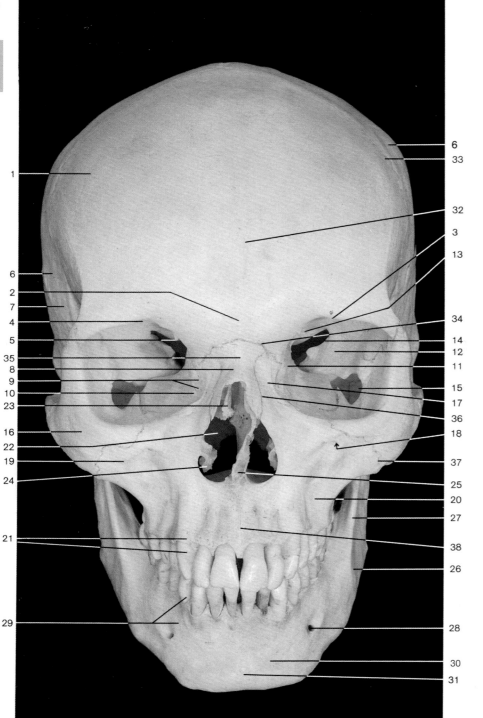

1   Frontal bone
2   Glabella
3   Supra-orbital margin / Foramen
4   Supra-orbital notch
5   Trochlear spine
6   Parietal bone
7   Temporal bone
8   Nasal bone

Orbit
9   Lacrimal bone
10 Posterior lacrimal crest
11 Ethmoidal bone

Sphenoidal bone
12 Greater wing of sphenoidal bone
13 Lesser wing of sphenoidal bone
14 Superior orbital fissure
15 Inferior orbital fissure
16 Zygomatic bone

Maxilla
17 Frontal process
18 Infra-orbital foramen
19 Zygomatic process
20 Body of maxilla
21 Alveolar process with teeth

Nasal cavity
22 Anterior nasal aperture
23 Middle nasal concha
24 Inferior nasal concha
25 Nasal septum, vomer

Mandible
26 Body of mandible
27 Ramus of mandible
28 Mental foramen
29 Alveolar part with teeth
30 Base of mandible
31 Mental protuberance

Sutures
32 Frontal suture
33 Coronal suture
34 Frontonasal suture
35 Internasal suture
36 Nasomaxillary suture
37 Zygomaticomaxillary suture
38 Intermaxillary suture

Anterior aspect of the skull.

The skull comprises a mosaic of numerous complicated bones that form the cranial cavity protecting the brain (**neurocranium**) and several cavities such as the nasal and oral cavities in the facial region. The neurocranium consists of large bony plates that develop directly from the surrounding sheets of connective tissue (**desmocranium**).

The bones of the skull base are formed out of cartilaginous tissue (**chondrocranium**), which ossifies secondarily. The **visceral skeleton,** which in fish gives rise to the gills, has in higher vertebrates been transformed into the bones of the masticatory and auditory apparatus (maxilla, mandible, auditory ossicles, and hyoid bone).

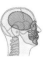

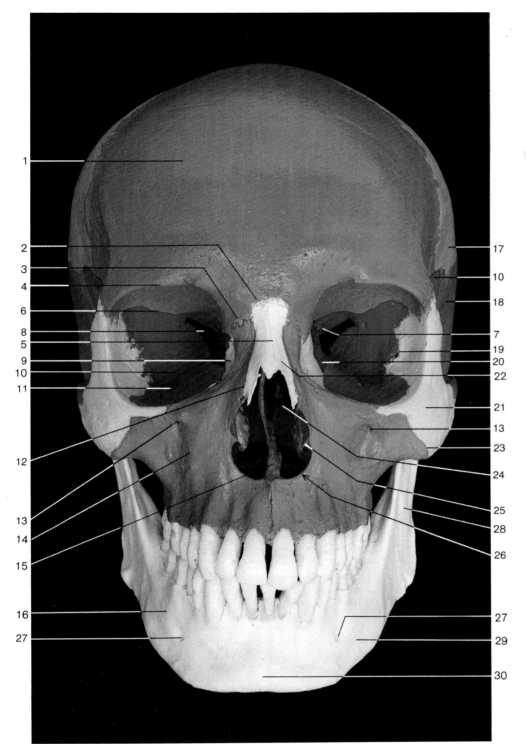

1	Frontal bone
2	Frontonasal suture
3	Frontomaxillary suture
4	Supra-orbital margin
5	Internasal suture
6	Sphenofrontal suture
7	Optic canal in lesser wing of sphenoidal bone
8	Superior orbital fissure
9	Lacrimal bone
10	Sphenoidal bone (greater wing)
11	Inferior orbital fissure
12	Nasomaxillary suture
13	Infra-orbital foramen
14	Maxilla
15	Vomer
16	Body of mandible
17	Parietal bone
18	Temporal bone
19	Sphenozygomatic suture
20	Ethmoidal bone
21	Zygomatic bone
22	Nasal bone
23	Zygomaticomaxillary suture
24	Middle nasal concha
25	Inferior nasal concha
26	Anterior nasal aperture
27	Mental foramen
28	Ramus of mandible
29	Base of mandible
30	Mental protuberance

Bones

Brown	=	frontal bone
Light green	=	parietal bone
Dark brown	=	temporal bone
Red	=	sphenoidal bone
Yellow	=	zygomatic bone
Dark green	=	ethmoidal bone
Yellow	=	lacrimal bone
Orange	=	vomer
Violet	=	maxilla
White	=	nasal bone
White	=	mandible

Anterior aspect of the skull (individual bones indicated by color).

The following series of figures are arranged so that the mosaic-like pattern of the skull becomes understandable. It starts with the bones of the **skull base** (sphenoidal and occipital bones) to which the other bones are added step by step. The facial skeleton is built up by the ethmoidal bone to which the palatine bone and maxilla are attached laterally; the small nasal and lacrimal bones fill the remaining spaces. Cartilages remain only in the external part of the nose.

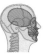

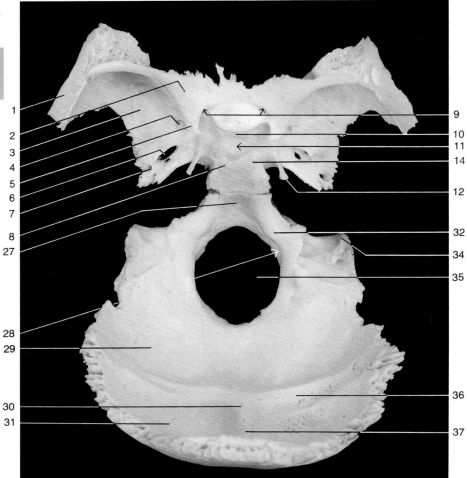

Sphenoidal and occipital bone (from above).

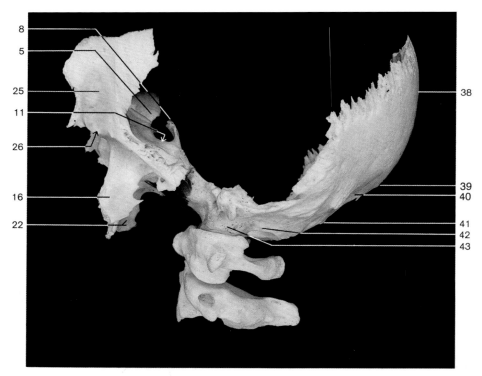

Sphenoidal and occipital bone in connection with the atlas and axis
(1st and 2nd cervical vertebrae) (left lateral view).

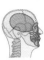

Sphenoidal bone
1 Greater wing
2 Lesser wing
3 Cerebral or superior surface of greater wing
4 Foramen rotundum
5 Anterior clinoid process
6 Foramen ovale
7 Foramen spinosum
8 Dorsum sellae
9 Optic canal
10 Chiasmatic groove (sulcus chiasmatis)
11 Hypophysial fossa (sella turcica)
12 Lingula
13 Opening of sphenoidal sinus
14 Posterior clinoid process
15 Pterygoid canal
16 Lateral pterygoid plate of pterygoid process
17 Pterygoid notch
18 Pterygoid hamulus
19 Orbital surface of greater wing
20 Sphenoidal crest
21 Sphenoidal rostrum
22 Medial pterygoid plate
23 Superior orbital fissure
24 Spine of sphenoid
25 Temporal surface of greater wing
26 Infratemporal crest

Occipital bone
27 Clivus with basilar part of occipital bone
28 Hypoglossal canal
29 Fossa for cerebellar hemisphere
30 Internal occipital protuberance
31 Fossa for cerebral hemisphere
32 Jugular tubercle
33 Condylar canal
34 Jugular process
35 Foramen magnum
36 Groove for transverse sinus
37 Groove for superior sagittal sinus
38 Squamous part of the occipital bone
39 External occipital protuberance
40 Superior nuchal line
41 Inferior nuchal line
42 Condylar fossa
43 Condyle
44 Pharyngeal tubercle
45 External occipital crest

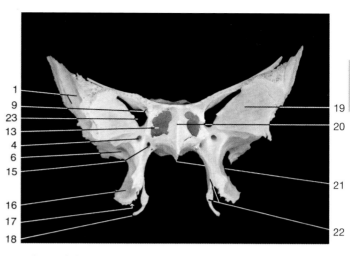

Sphenoidal bone (anterior aspect).

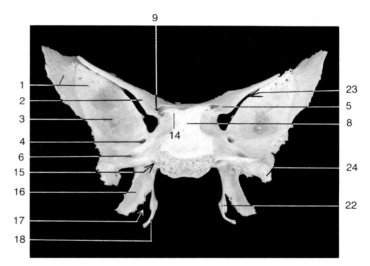

Sphenoidal bone (posterior aspect).

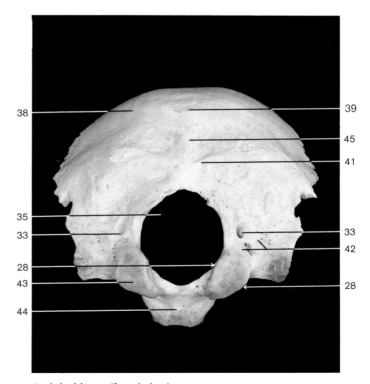

Occipital bone (from below).

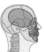

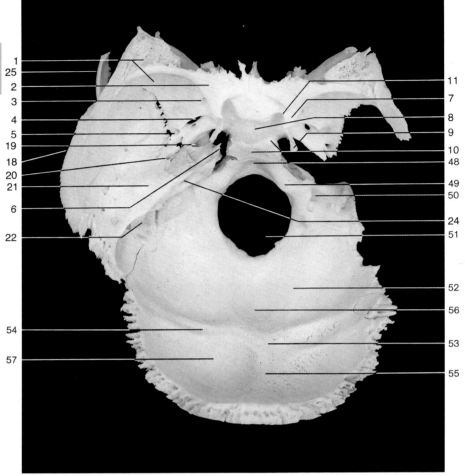

Sphenoidal bone
1   Greater wing
2   Lesser wing
3   Foramen rotundum
4   Foramen ovale
5   Foramen spinosum
6   Foramen lacerum
7   Anterior clinoid process
8   Hypophysial fossa (sella turcica)
9   Lingula
10 Dorsum sellae and posterior clinoid
    process
11 Optic canal
12 Sphenoidal rostrum
13 Medial pterygoid plate
14 Lateral pterygoid plate
15 Pterygoid hamulus
16 Infratemporal crest
17 Body of the sphenoidal bone

Sphenoidal, occipital, and left temporal bone (from above). Internal aspect of the
base of the skull. The left temporal bone has been added to the preceding figure.

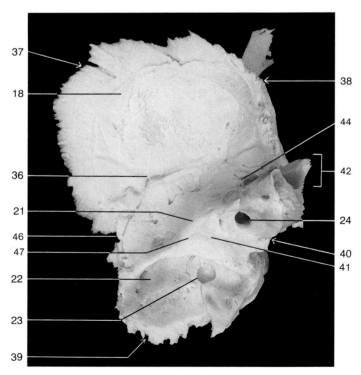

Left temporal bone (medial aspect).

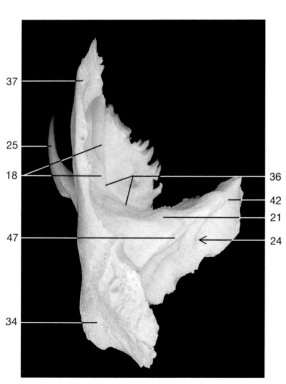

Left temporal bone (from above).

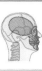

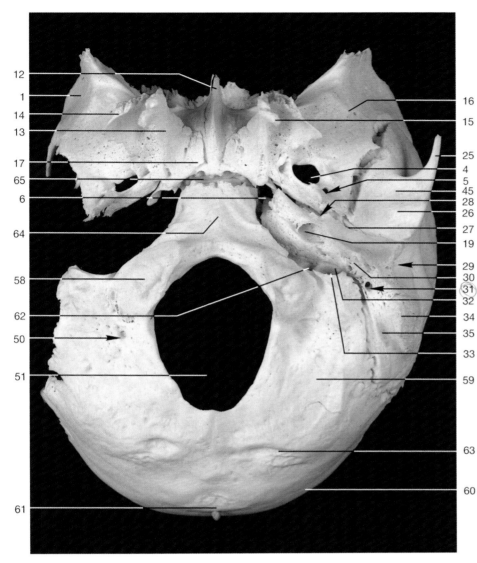

Sphenoidal, occipital, and left temporal bone. Base of the skull (external aspect).

Temporal bone
18 Squamous part
19 Carotid canal
20 Hiatus of facial canal
(for the greater petrosal nerve)
21 Arcuate eminence
22 Groove for the sigmoid sinus
23 Mastoid foramen
24 Internal acoustic meatus
25 Zygomatic process
26 Mandibular fossa
27 Petrotympanic fissure
28 Canalis musculotubarius
(bony part of auditory tube)
29 External acoustic meatus
30 Styloid process (remnant only)
31 Stylomastoid foramen
32 Mastoid canaliculus
33 Jugular fossa
34 Mastoid process
35 Mastoid notch
36 Groove for middle
meningeal vessels
37 Parietal margin
38 Sphenoidal margin
39 Occipital margin
40 Cochlear canaliculus
41 Aqueduct of the vestibule
42 Apex of the petrous part
43 Tympanic part
44 Trigeminal impression
45 Articular tubercle
46 Parietal notch
47 Groove for the superior
petrosal sinus

Occipital bone
48 Clivus
49 Jugular tubercle
50 Condylar canal
51 Foramen magnum
52 Lower part of squamous
occipital bone
(cerebellar fossa)
53 Internal occipital protuberance
54 Groove for the transverse sinus
55 Groove for the superior sagittal sinus
56 Internal occipital crest
57 Upper part of squamous occipital
bone (cerebral fossa)
58 Condyle
59 Nuchal plane
60 Superior nuchal line
61 External occipital protuberance
62 Jugular foramen
63 Inferior nuchal line
64 Pharyngeal tubercle
65 Spheno-occipital synchondrosis

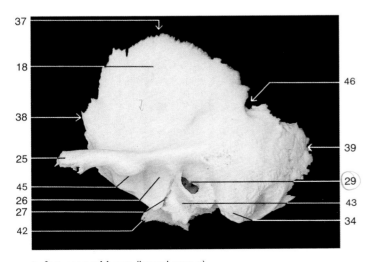

Left temporal bone (lateral aspect).

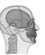

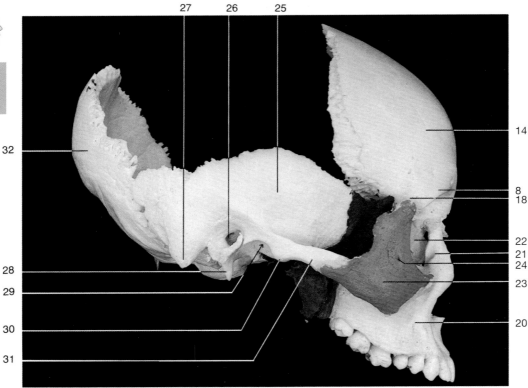

Part of a disarticulated skull (right lateral aspect). The frontal bone and the maxilla are connected with the temporal bone by the zygomatic bone (orange). Sphenoidal bone (black), palatine bone (red), lacrimal bone (yellow).

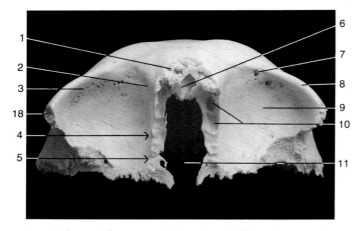

Frontal bone (inferior aspect). The ethmoidal foveolae cover the ethmoidal cavities of the ethmoidal bone.

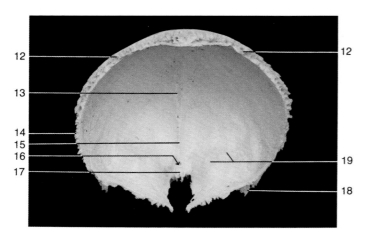

Frontal bone (posterior aspect).

Frontal bone
1 Nasal margin
2 Trochlear fossa
3 Fossa for lacrimal gland
4 Anterior ethmoidal foramen
5 Posterior ethmoidal foramen
6 Nasal spine
7 Supra-orbital notch
8 Supra-orbital margin
9 Orbital plate
10 Roofs of the ethmoidal air cells
11 Ethmoidal notch
12 Parietal margin
13 Groove for superior sagittal sinus
14 Squamous part of frontal bone
15 Frontal crest
16 Foramen cecum
17 Nasal spine
18 Zygomatic process of frontal bone
19 Juga cerebralia

Facial bones
20 Maxilla
21 Frontal process of maxilla
22 Lacrimal bone (yellow)
23 Zygomatic bone (orange)
24 Zygomaticofacial foramen

Temporal bone
25 Squamous part of temporal bone
26 External acoustic meatus
27 Mastoid process
28 Styloid process
29 Mandibular fossa
30 Articular tubercle
31 Zygomatic process

Occipital bone
32 Squamous part of occipital bone

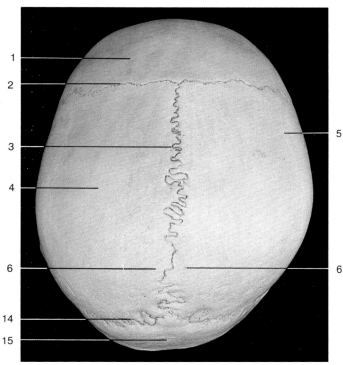

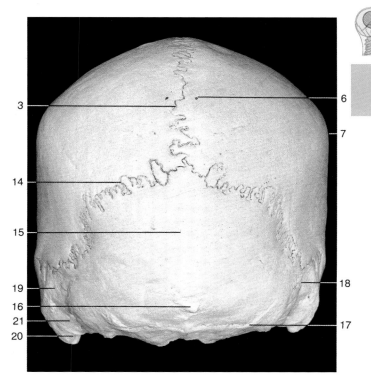

Calvaria (superior aspect).

Calvaria (posterior aspect).

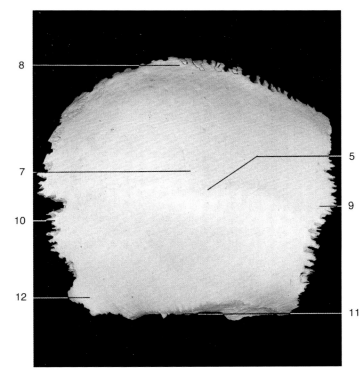

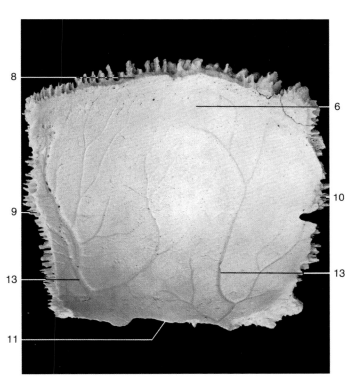

Left parietal bone (external aspect).

Left parietal bone (internal aspect).

1	Frontal bone	8	Sagittal margin	15	Occipital bone
2	Coronal suture	9	Occipital margin	16	External occipital protuberance
3	Sagittal suture	10	Frontal margin	17	Inferior nuchal line
4	Parietal bone	11	Squamous margin	18	Occipitomastoid suture
5	Superior temporal line	12	Sphenoidal angle	19	Temporal bone
6	Parietal foramen	13	Groove for middle meningeal artery	20	Mastoid process
7	Parietal tuber or eminence	14	Lambdoid suture	21	Mastoid notch

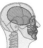

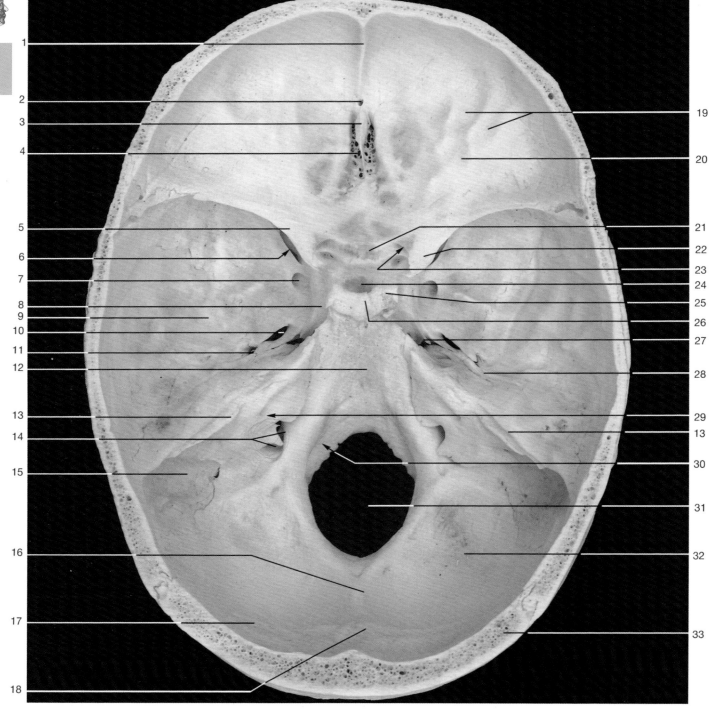

Base of the skull, calvaria removed (internal aspect).

1 Frontal crest	12 Clivus	23 Optic canal
2 Foramen cecum	13 Groove for superior petrosal sinus	24 Sella turcica (hypophysial fossa)
3 Crista galli	14 Jugular foramen	25 Posterior clinoid process
4 Cribriform plate of ethmoidal bone	15 Groove for sigmoid sinus	26 Dorsum sellae
5 Lesser wing of sphenoidal bone	16 Internal occipital crest	27 Foramen lacerum
6 Superior orbital fissure	17 Groove for transverse sinus	28 Groove for greater petrosal nerve
7 Foramen rotundum	18 Internal occipital protuberance	29 Internal acoustic meatus
8 Carotid sulcus	19 Digitate impressions	30 Hypoglossal canal
9 Middle cranial fossa	20 Anterior cranial fossa	31 Foramen magnum
10 Foramen ovale	21 Chiasmatic sulcus	32 Posterior cranial fossa
11 Foramen spinosum	22 Anterior clinoid process	33 Diploe

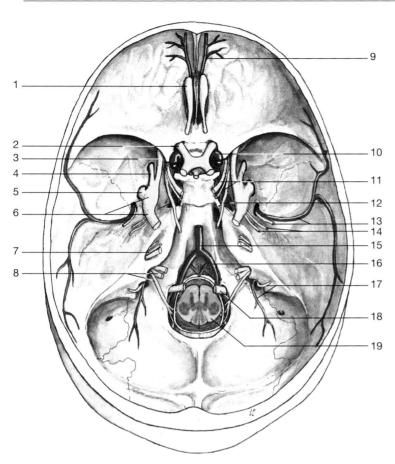

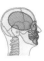

1   Olfactory bulb
2   Optic nerve (n. II)
3   Ophthalmic nerve (n. V₁)
4   Maxillary nerve (n. V₂)
5   Mandibular nerve (n. V₃)
6   Trigeminal nerve (n. V) with trigeminal ganglion
7   Facial nerve (n. VII) and vestibulocochlear nerve (n. VIII)
8   Glossopharyngeal nerve (n. IX), vagus nerve (n. X) and accessory nerve (n. XI)
9   Anterior meningeal artery
10 Internal carotid artery
11 Oculomotor nerve (n. III) and trochlear nerve (n. IV)
12 Abducent nerve (n. VI)
13 Middle meningeal artery and meningeal branch of mandibular nerve
14 Greater and lesser petrosal nerves
15 Basilar artery
16 Vertebral artery
17 Posterior meningeal artery and recurrent meningeal nerve
18 Hypoglossal nerve (n. XII)
19 Medulla oblongata

Base of the skull with cranial nerves and meningeal arteries (internal aspect, schematic drawing).

	Cranial nerves and vessels	**Related foramina**	**Related regions**
Anterior cranial fossa	Olfactory nerves (n. I), Anterior ethmoidal artery, vein, and nerve, Anterior meningeal artery	Lamina cribrosa	Nasal cavity
Middle cranial fossa	Optic nerve (n. II), Ophthalmic artery	Optic canal	Orbit
	Oculomotor nerve (n. III), Trochlear nerve (n. IV), Abducent nerve (n. VI), Ophthalmic nerve (n. V₁), Superior ophthalmic vein	Superior orbital fissure	Orbit
	Maxillary nerve (n. V₂)	Foramen rotundum	Pterygopalatine fossa
	Mandibular nerve (n. V₃)	Foramen ovale	Infratemporal fossa
	Middle meningeal artery, Meningeal branch of mandibular nerve (n. V₃)	Foramen spinosum	Infratemporal fossa
	Internal carotid artery	Carotid canal	Cavernous sinus, Base of skull
Posterior cranial fossa	Facial nerve (n. VII), Vestibulocochlear nerve (n. VIII), Artery and vein of the labyrinth	Internal acoustic meatus, Stylomastoid foramen, Facial canal	Inner ear, Face
	Glossopharyngeal nerve (n. IX), Vagus nerve (n. X), Accessory nerve (n. XI), Internal jugular vein, Posterior meningeal artery	Jugular foramen	Parapharyngeal region
	Hypoglossal nerve (n. XII)	Hypoglossal canal	Tongue
	Accessory nerve (n. XI, spinal root), Vertebral arteries, Anterior and posterior spinal arteries, Medulla oblongata	Foramen magnum	Base of skull

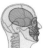

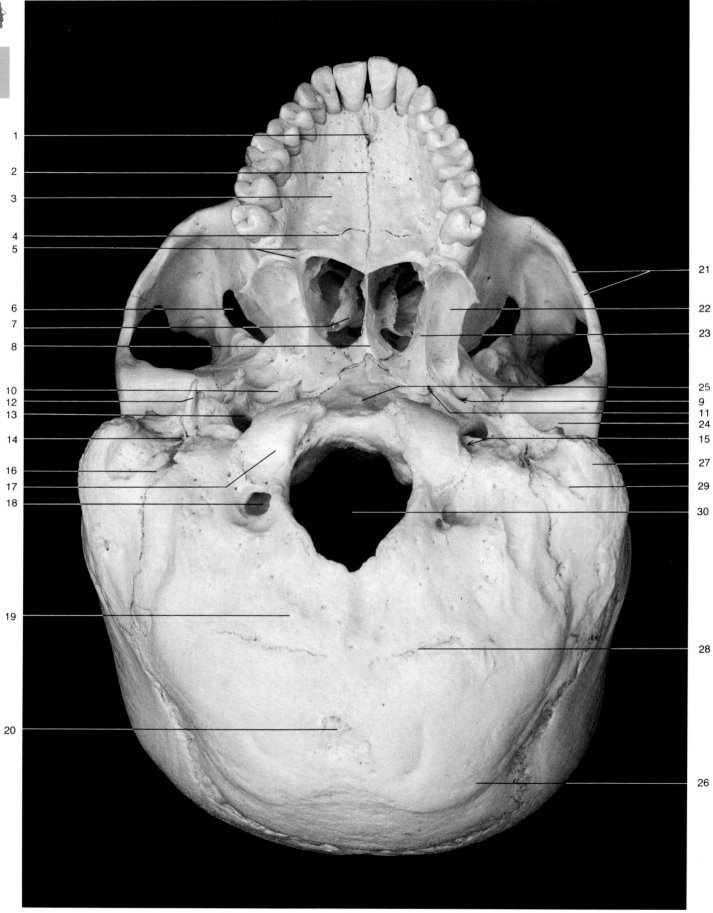

Base of the skull (inferior aspect).

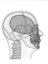

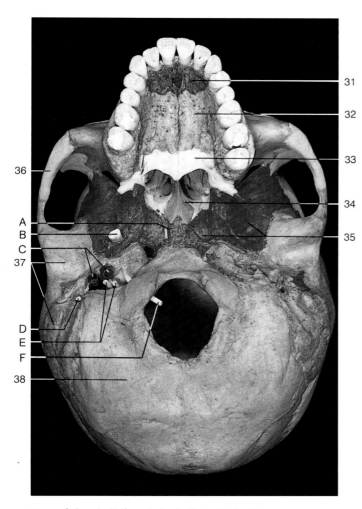

Base of the skull (from below). The individual bones are indicated by different colors.

A = **pterygoid canal**
B = **foramen ovale**
C = internal carotid artery within **carotid canal** and internal jugular vein within the venous part of jugular foramen
D = **stylomastoid foramen** (facial nerve)
E = **jugular foramen** (glossopharyngeal, vagus and accessory nerves)
F = **hypoglossal canal** (hypoglossal nerve)

1 Incisive canal
2 Median palatine suture
3 Palatine process of maxilla
4 Palatomaxillary suture
5 Greater and lesser palatine foramina
6 Inferior orbital fissure
7 Middle concha (process of ethmoidal bone)
8 Vomer
9 Foramen ovale
10 Groove for auditory tube
11 Pterygoid canal
12 Styloid process
13 Carotid canal
14 Stylomastoid foramen
15 Jugular foramen
16 Groove for occipital artery
17 Occipital condyle
18 Condylar canal
19 Nuchal plane
20 External occipital protuberance
21 Zygomatic arch
22 Lateral pterygoid plate
23 Medial pterygoid plate
24 Mandibular fossa
25 Pharyngeal tubercle
26 Superior nuchal line
27 Mastoid process
28 Inferior nuchal line
29 Mastoid notch
30 Foramen magnum
31 Incisive bone or premaxilla (dark violet)
32 Maxilla (violet)
33 Palatine bone (white)
34 Vomer (orange)
35 Sphenoidal bone (red)
36 Zygomatic bone (yellow)
37 Temporal bone (brown)
38 Occipital bone (blue)
39 Palatine process of maxilla
40 Vomer
41 Sphenoidal bone
42 Petrous part of temporal bone
43 Basilar part ⎫
44 Lateral part ⎬ of occipital bone
45 Squamous part ⎭
46 Mandible
47 Zygomatic arch
48 Choana
49 Pterygoid process of sphenoidal bone
50 Carotid canal
51 External acoustic meatus (tympanic anulus)
52 Sphenoidal fontanelle
53 Parietal bone
54 Mastoid fontanelle

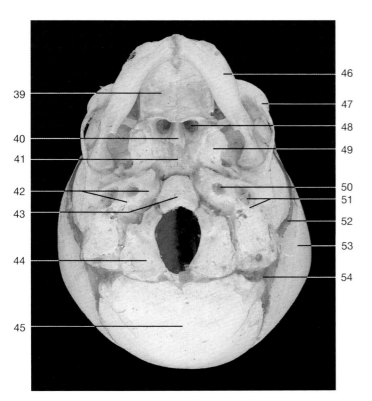

Skull of the newborn (inferior aspect).

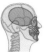

20 3 21 25   26

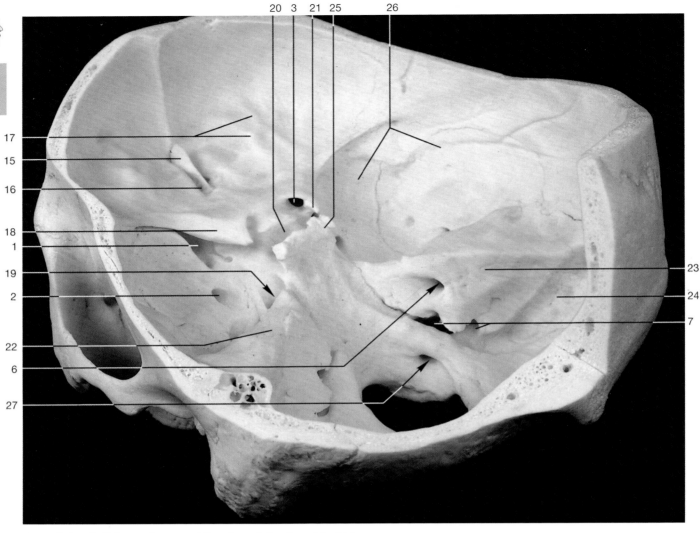

Base of the skull (internal aspect, oblique lateral view from left side).

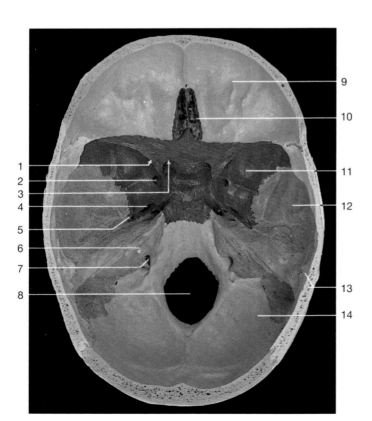

Canals, fissures, and foramina of the base of the skull

1   Superior orbital fissure
2   Foramen rotundum
3   Optic canal
4   Foramen ovale
5   Foramen spinosum
6   Internal acoustic meatus
7   Jugular foramen
8   Foramen magnum

Bones

9   Frontal bone (orange)
10 Ethmoidal bone (dark green)
11 Sphenoidal bone (red)
12 Temporal bone (brown)
13 Parietal bone (yellow)
14 Occipital bone (blue)

Details of bones

15 Crista galli
16 Cribriform plate

17 Digitate impressions (frontal bone)
18 Lesser wing of sphenoidal bone
19 Foramen lacerum
20 Hypophysial fossa (sella turcica)
21 Anterior clinoid process
22 Trigeminal impression
23 Petrous part of temporal bone
24 Groove for sigmoid sinus
25 Dorsum sellae (posterior clinoid process)
26 Greater wing of sphenoidal bone, groove for middle meningeal artery
27 Hypoglossal canal

Base of the skull (internal aspect, superior view). Individual bones indicated by color.

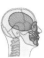

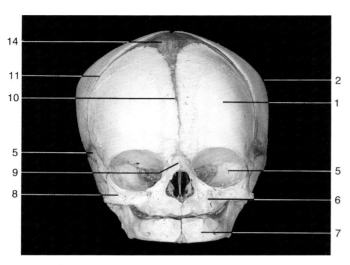

Skull of the newborn (anterior aspect).

Cranial skeleton
1   Frontal tuber or eminence
2   Parietal tuber or eminence
3   Occipital tuber or eminence
4   Squamous part of temporal bone
5   Greater wing of sphenoidal bone

Facial skeleton
6   Maxilla
7   Mandible
8   Zygomatic bone
9   Nasal bone

Sutures and fontanelles
10   Frontal suture
11   Coronal suture
12   Sagittal suture
13   Lambdoid suture
14   Anterior fontanelle
15   Posterior fontanelle
16   Sphenoidal (anterolateral) fontanelle
17   Mastoid (posterolateral) fontanelle

Base of the skull
18   Frontal bone
19   Ethmoidal bone
20   Sphenoidal bone
21   Hypophysial fossa (sella turcica)
22   Dorsum sellae
23   Temporal bone
24   Mastoid (posterolateral) fontanelle
25   Occipital bone

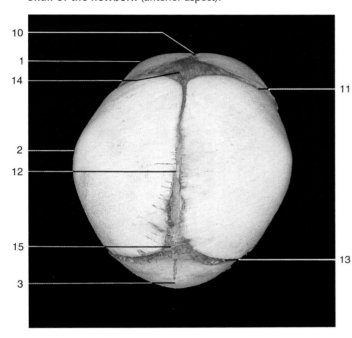

Skull of the newborn (superior aspect). Calvaria.

In the newborn, the facial skeleton, in contrast to the cranial skeleton, appears relatively small. There are no teeth presenting. The bones of the cranium are separated by wide fontanelles.

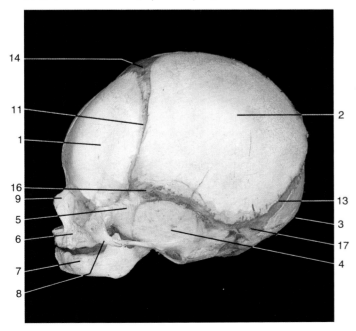

Skull of the newborn (lateral aspect).

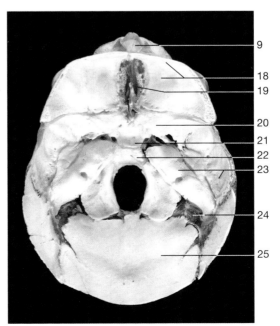

Base of the skull of the newborn (internal aspect).

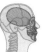

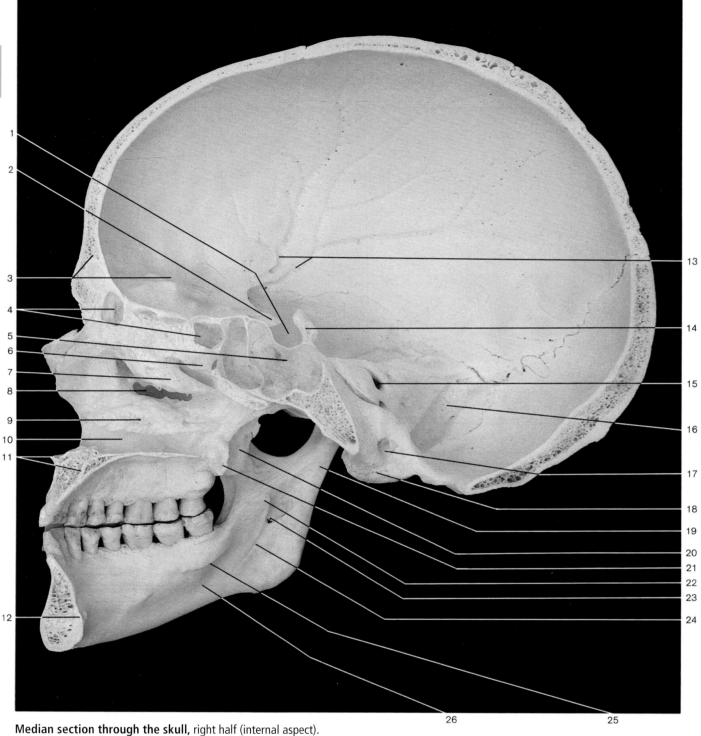

Median section through the skull, right half (internal aspect).

1	Hypophysial fossa (sella turcica)	14	Dorsum sellae
2	Anterior clinoid process	15	Internal acoustic meatus
3	Frontal bone	16	Groove for sigmoid sinus
4	Ethmoidal air cells	17	Hypoglossal canal
5	Sphenoidal sinus	18	Occipital condyle
6	Superior concha	19	Condylar process
7	Middle concha	20	Lateral pterygoid plate ⎫ of pterygoid process
8	Maxillary hiatus	21	Medial pterygoid plate ⎭
9	Inferior concha	22	Lingula of mandible
10	Inferior meatus	23	Mandibular foramen
11	Anterior nasal spine and maxilla	24	Mylohyoid groove
12	Mental spine or genial tubercle	25	Mylohyoid line
13	Groove for middle meningeal artery	26	Submandibular fovea

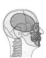

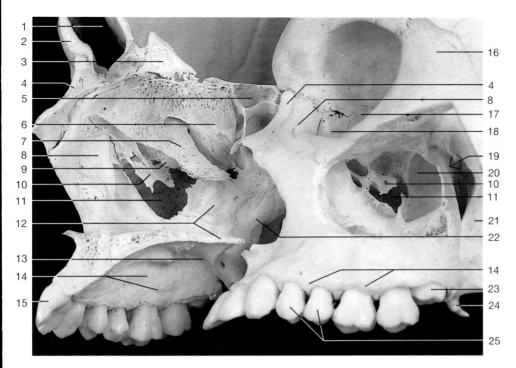

1
2
3
4
5
6
7
8
9
10
11
12
13
14
15

16
4
8
17
18
19
20
10
11
21
22
14
23
24
25

1 Frontal sinus
2 Frontal bone
3 Crista galli
4 Nasal bone
5 Sphenoidal sinus
6 Superior concha } of ethmoidal
7 Middle concha   } bone
8 Frontal process
   of maxilla
9 Ethmoidal bulla
10 Uncinate process
11 Maxillary hiatus
12 Palatine bone
13 Greater palatine foramen
14 Alveolar process of maxilla
15 Central incisor
16 Zygomatic bone
17 Ethmoidal bone
18 Lacrimal bone
19 Pterygopalatine fossa
20 Maxillary sinus
21 Lateral pterygoid plate
22 Medial pterygoid plate
23 Third molar tooth
24 Pterygoid hamulus
25 Two premolar teeth

Facial part of the skull (viscerocranium), divided in two halves (lateral and medial aspect). Right inferior concha has been removed to show the maxillary hiatus.
Left maxillary sinus opened.

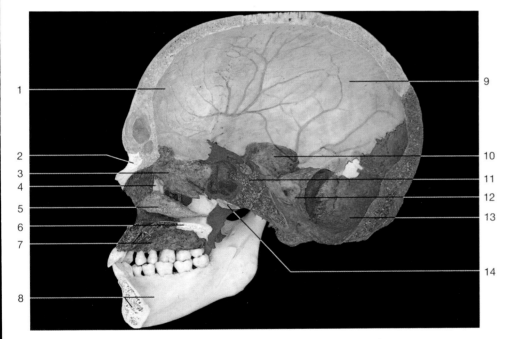

1
2
3
4
5
6
7
8

9
10
11
12
13
14

Bones (indicated by colors)
1 Frontal bone (yellow)
2 Nasal bone (white)
3 Ethmoidal bone (dark green)
4 Lacrimal bone (yellow)
5 Inferior nasal concha (pink)
6 Palatine bone (white)
7 Maxilla (violet)
8 Mandible (white)
9 Parietal bone (light green)
10 Temporal bone (brown)
11 Sphenoidal bone (red)
12 Petrous part of temporal
   bone (brown)
13 Occipital bone (blue)
14 Ala of vomer (light brown)

Median section through the skull. The nasal septum has been removed.
Bones indicated by colors.

Because of the upright posture that the human developed in the course of evolution, the cranial cavity greatly increased in size, whereas the facial skeleton decreased. As a result, the base of the skull developed an angulation of about 120° between the clivus and the cribriform plate (see drawing on page 19). The hypophysial fossa containing the pituitary gland lies at the angle formed between these two planes.

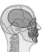

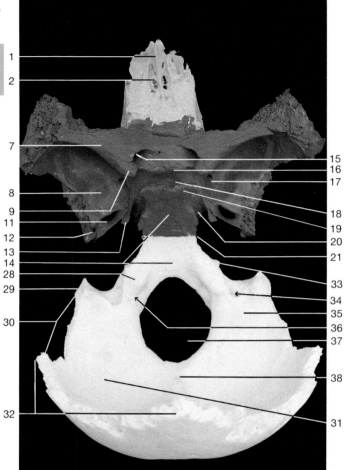

Ethmoidal bone
1 Crista galli
2 Cribriform plate
3 Ethmoidal air cells
4 Middle concha
5 Perpendicular plate (part of nasal septum)
6 Orbital plate

Sphenoidal bone
7 Lesser wing
8 Greater wing
9 Anterior clinoid process
10 Posterior clinoid process
11 Foramen ovale
12 Foramen spinosum
13 Lingula of the sphenoidal bone
14 Clivus
15 Optic canal
16 Tuberculum sellae
17 Foramen rotundum (right side)
18 Hypophysial fossa (sella turcica)
19 Dorsum sellae
20 Carotid sulcus
21 Spheno-occipital synchondrosis
22 Lateral pterygoid plate
23 Greater wing of sphenoidal bone (orbital surface)
24 Greater wing of sphenoidal bone (maxillary surface)
25 Foramen rotundum (left side)
26 Superior orbital fissure
27 Infratemporal crest of the greater wing

Part of the disarticulated base of the skull.
Ethmoidal, sphenoidal, and occipital bones (from above).
Green = sphenoidal bone; yellow = ethmoidal bone.

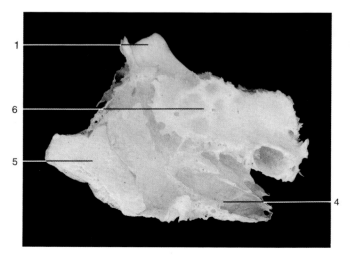

Ethmoidal bone (lateral aspect), posterior portion to the right.

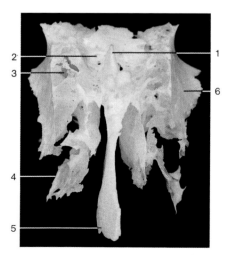

Ethmoidal bone (anterior aspect).

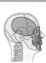

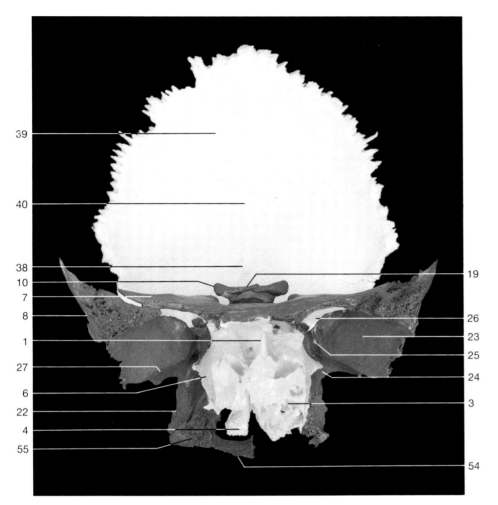

Occipital bone
28 Jugular tubercle
29 Jugular process
30 Mastoid margin
31 Posterior cranial fossa
32 Lambdoid margin
33 Intrajugular process
34 Condylar canal
35 Lateral part of occipital bone
36 Hypoglossal canal
37 Foramen magnum
38 Internal occipital crest
39 Squamous part of occipital bone
40 Internal occipital protuberance

Maxilla
41 Orbital surface
42 Infra-orbital groove
43 Maxillary tuberosity with foramina
44 Frontal process
45 Nasolacrimal groove
46 Infra-orbital margin
47 Anterior nasal spine
48 Zygomatic process
49 Alveolar process

Palatine bone
50 Orbital process
51 Sphenopalatine notch
52 Sphenoidal process
53 Perpendicular plate
54 Horizontal plate
55 Pyramidal process

Disarticulated base of the skull (anterior aspect). Green = sphenoidal bone; yellow = ethmoidal bone; red = palatine bone.

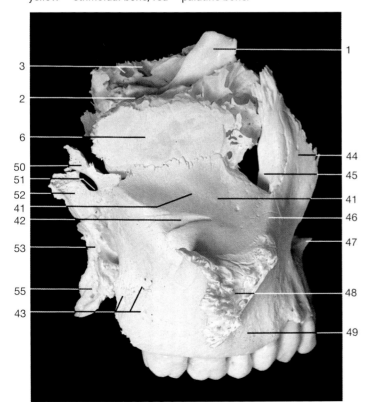

Right maxilla, ethmoidal, and palatine bone (lateral aspect).

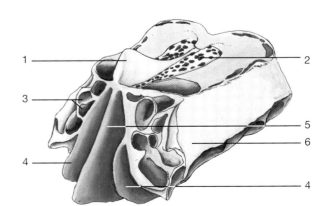

Ethmoidal bone (oblique anterior aspect). (Schematic drawing.)

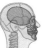

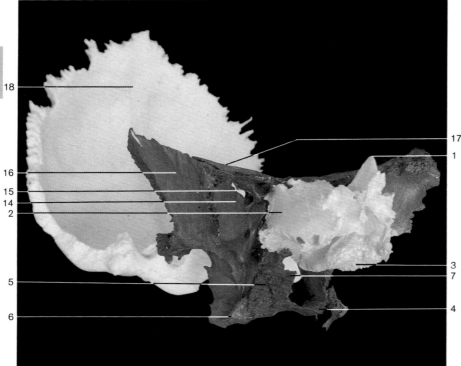

Ethmoidal bone
1 Crista galli
2 Orbital plate
3 Middle concha

Palatine bone
4 Horizontal plate of palatine bone
5 Greater palatine canal
6 Pyramidal process
7 Maxillary process
8 Orbital process
9 Sphenopalatine notch
10 Perpendicular plate of palatine bone
11 Conchal crest
12 Nasal crest
13 Sphenoidal process

Sphenoidal bone
14 Greater wing
15 Superior orbital fissure
16 Greater wing (orbital surface)
17 Lesser wing

Occipital bone
18 Squamous part of occipital bone

Maxilla
19 Maxillary tuberosity
20 Frontal process
21 Orbital surface
22 Infra-orbital margin
23 Infra-orbital groove
24 Zygomatic process
25 Alveolar process

Part of a disarticulated skull base, similar to the preceding figures, but with palatine bone. Green = sphenoidal bone; yellow = ethmoidal bone; red = palatine bone.

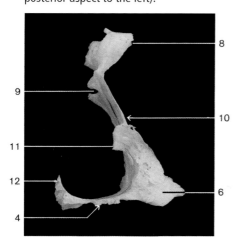

Left palatine bone (medial aspect, posterior aspect to the left).

Left palatine bone (anterior aspect).

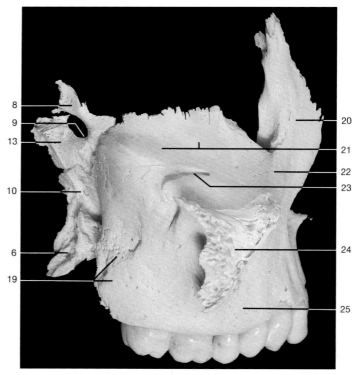

Right maxilla and right palatine bone (lateral aspect).

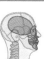

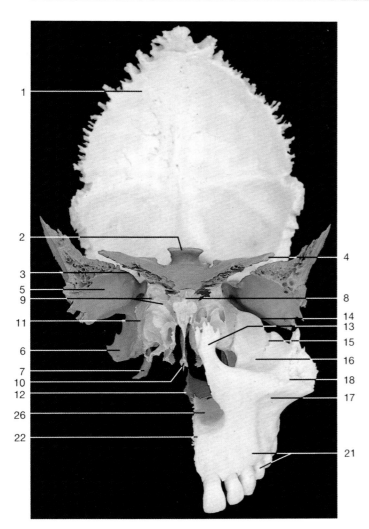

Occipital bone
1   Squamous part

Sphenoidal bone
2   Dorsum sellae
3   Superior orbital fissure
4   Lesser wing
5   Greater wing (orbital surface)
6   Lateral pterygoid plate
7   Medial pterygoid plate

Ethmoidal bone
8   Crista galli
9   Ethmoidal air cells
10 Perpendicular plate
11 Orbital plate

Palatine bone
12 Horizontal plate (nasal crest)

Maxilla
13 Frontal process
14 Inferior orbital fissure
15 Infra-orbital groove
16 Orbital surface
17 Infra-orbital foramen
18 Zygomatic process
19 Anterior lacrimal crest
20 Canine fossa
21 Alveolar process with teeth
22 Anterior nasal spine
23 Juga alveolaria (elevations formed by roots of teeth)
24 Lacrimal groove
25 Maxillary tuberosity with alveolar foramina
26 Palatine process of maxilla

Part of a disarticulated skull.
The left **maxilla** is added to the preceding specimen.

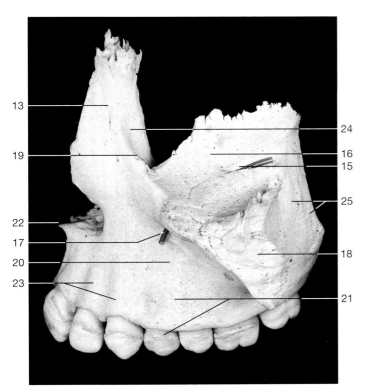

Left maxilla (lateral aspect). Probe = infra-orbital canal.

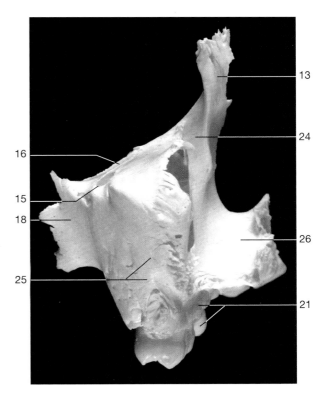

Left maxilla (posterior aspect).

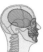

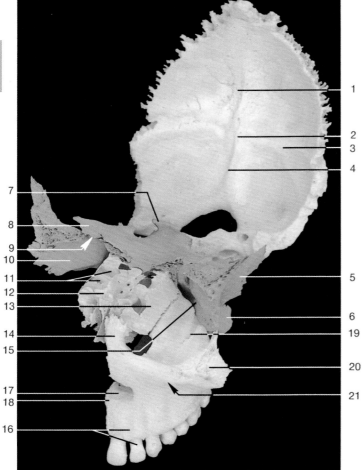

Part of a disarticulated base of skull. The mosaic of the facial bones [sphenoidal bone (green), ethmoidal bone (yellow), and palatine bone (red)] is seen from the antero-lateral aspect.

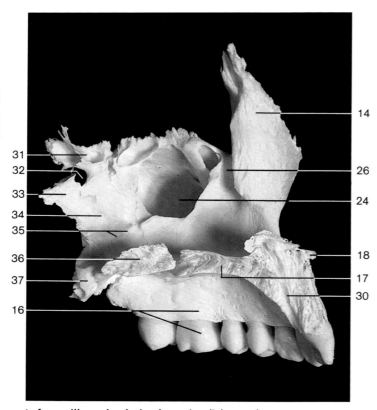

Left maxilla and palatine bone (medial aspect).

Occipital bone
1   Groove for superior sagittal sinus
2   Internal occipital protuberance
3   Groove for transverse sinus
4   Internal occipital crest

Sphenoidal bone
5   Greater wing (temporal surface)
6   Lateral pterygoid plate
7   Dorsum sellae
8   Lesser wing
9   Superior orbital fissure
10 Greater wing (orbital surface)

Ethmoidal bone
11 Ethmoidal air cells
12 Crista galli
13 Orbital plate

Maxilla
14 Frontal process
15 Inferior orbital fissure
16 Alveolar process with teeth
17 Palatine process
18 Anterior nasal spine
19 Infra-orbital groove
20 Zygomatic process
21 Location of infra-orbital foramen
22 Middle nasal meatus
23 Inferior nasal meatus
24 Maxillary hiatus
     (leading to maxillary sinus)
25 Third molar
26 Lacrimal groove
27 Conchal crest
28 Body of maxilla (nasal surface)
29 Nasal crest
30 Incisive canal

Palatine bone
31 Orbital process
32 Sphenopalatine notch
33 Sphenoidal process
34 Perpendicular plate
35 Conchal crest
36 Horizontal plate
37 Pyramidal process

Frontal bone
38 Squamous part
39 Supra-orbital foramen
40 Frontal notch
41 Frontal spine

Inferior nasal concha
42 Inferior nasal concha
     with maxillary process

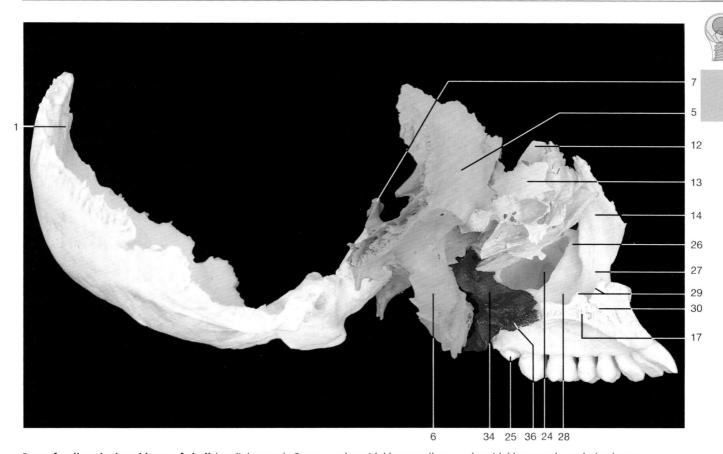

Part of a disarticulated base of skull (medial aspect). Green = sphenoidal bone; yellow = ethmoidal bone; red = palatine bone; natural colored = left maxilla.

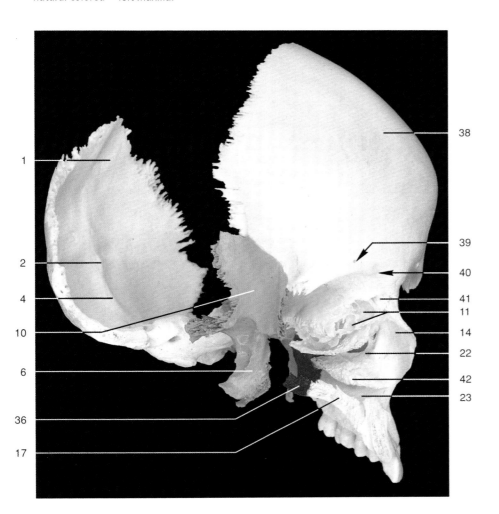

Part of a disarticulated base of skull. The same specimen as shown above but with frontal bone (oblique-lateral aspect).

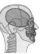

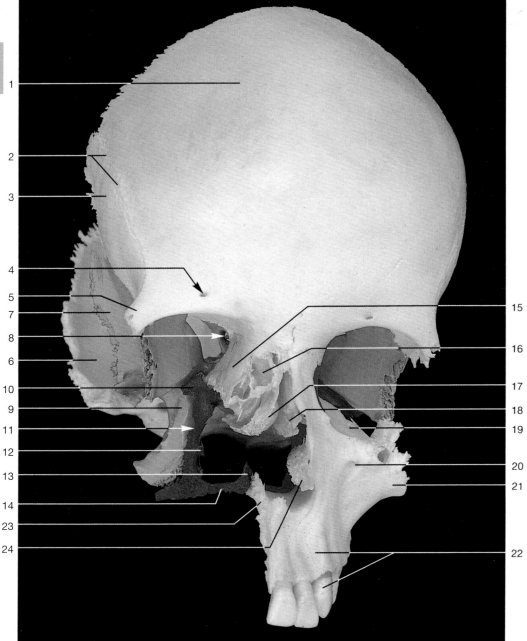

Part of a disarticulated skull showing the connection of the palatine bone (red) and the maxilla with ethmoidal bone (yellow) and sphenoidal bone (green) (anterior aspect).

Frontal bone
1 Squamous part
2 Inferior temporal line
3 Temporal surface
4 Supra-orbital foramen
5 Zygomatic process

Occipital bone
6 Squamous part

Sphenoidal bone
7 Greater wing (temporal surface)
8 Optic canal within the lesser wing
9 Lateral pterygoid plate

Palatine bone
10 Orbital process
11 Perpendicular plate
12 Conchal crest
13 Nasal crest
14 Horizontal plate

Ethmoidal bone
15 Orbital plate
16 Ethmoidal air cell
17 Middle concha
18 Perpendicular plate
    (part of bony nasal septum)

Maxilla
19 Infra-orbital groove
20 Infra-orbital foramen
21 Zygomatic process
22 Alveolar process with teeth
23 Palatine process

Left inferior nasal concha
24 Anterior part of
    inferior concha

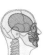

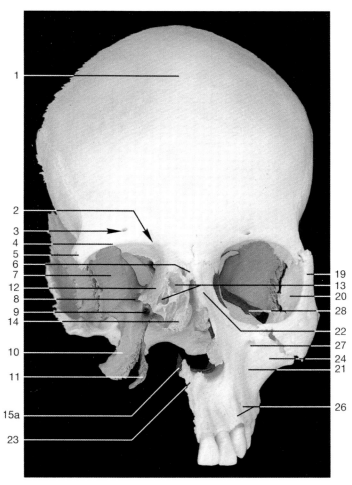

Frontal bone
1 Squamous part
2 Frontal notch
3 Supra-orbital foramen
4 Supra-orbital margin
5 Zygomatic process
6 Frontal spine

Sphenoidal bone
7 Greater wing (orbital surface)
8 Foramen rotundum
9 Pterygoid or Vidian canal
10 Lateral pterygoid plate
11 Medial pterygoid plate

Ethmoidal bone
12 Orbital plate
13 Ethmoidal air cells
14 Middle concha

Palatine bone
15 Horizontal plate
15a Nasal crest
16 Pyramidal process
17 Lesser palatine foramen
18 Greater palatine foramen

Zygomatic bone
19 Frontal process
20 Orbital surface

Maxilla
21 Canine fossa
22 Frontal process
23 Palatine process
24 Zygomatic process
25 Alveolar process and teeth
26 Juga alveolaria
27 Infra-orbital foramen
28 Infra-orbital groove
29 Anterior nasal aperture
30 Anterior nasal spine

Incisive bone
31 Central incisor and incisive bone or premaxilla
32 Incisive fossa

Vomer
33 Ala of the vomer

Sutures and choanae
34 Median palatine suture
35 Transverse palatine suture
36 Choanae

Anterior view of a disarticulated skull showing the connection of the maxilla with the frontal and zygomatic bones. Yellow = ethmoidal bone; red = palatine bone; green = sphenoidal bone.

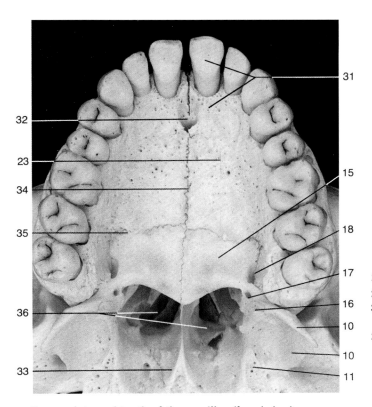

Bony palate and teeth of the maxillae (from below).

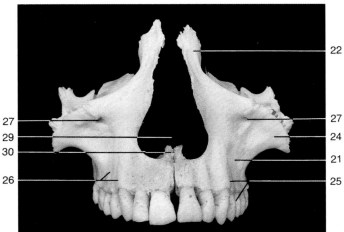

Anterior view of both maxillae forming the anterior bony aperture of the nose.

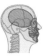

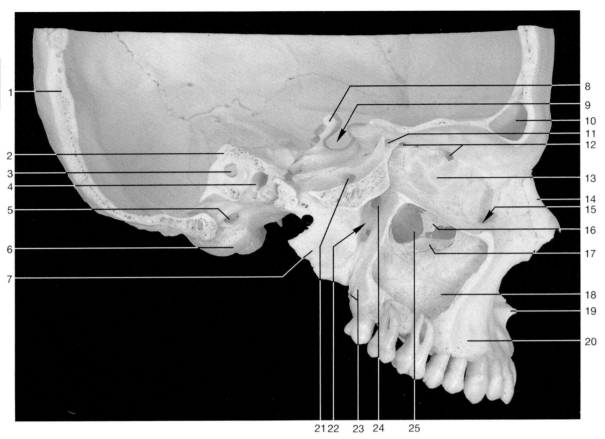

Paramedian section through the skull, right side (lateral aspect). Frontal and maxillary sinuses are opened.

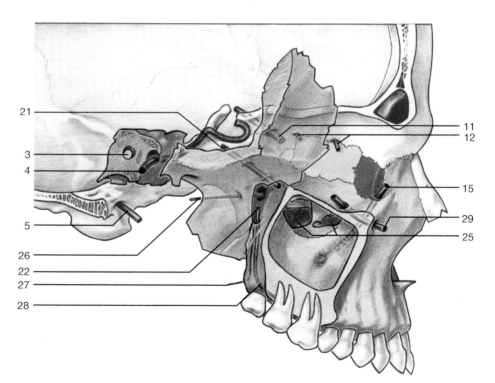

Illustration of canals and foramina connected with the right orbit and pterygopalatine fossa (compare the above figure). The greater wing of sphenoidal bone (green) is shown as being transparent. Brown = temporal bone; yellow = ethmoidal bone; red = lacrimal bone; light red = inferior nasal concha; violet = maxilla; red = palatine bone.

1 Occipital bone
2 Temporal bone (petrous part)
3 Internal acoustic meatus
4 Carotid canal
5 Hypoglossal canal
6 Occipital condyle
7 Lateral plate of pterygoid process
8 Dorsum of sella turcica
9 Sella turcica
10 Frontal sinus
11 Optic canal
12 Posterior and anterior
     ethmoidal foramina
13 Orbital plate of ethmoidal bone
14 Nasal bone
15 Nasolacrimal canal
16 Uncinate process
17 Inferior nasal concha
     (maxillary process)
18 Maxillary sinus
19 Anterior nasal spine
20 Alveolar process of maxilla
21 Foramen rotundum
22 Pterygopalatine fossa
23 Tuberosity of maxilla
     with alveolar foramina
24 Sphenopalatine foramen
25 Maxillary hiatus
26 Pterygoid or Vidian canal
27 Lesser palatine canal
28 Greater palatine canal
29 Infra-orbital canal

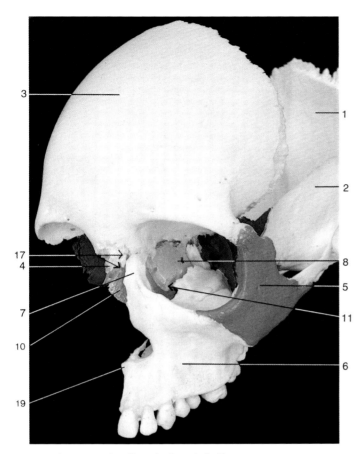

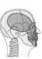

1   Occipital bone
2   Temporal bone
3   Frontal bone
4   Nasal spine of frontal bone
5   Zygomatic bone
6   Maxilla
7   Frontal process of maxilla
8   Ethmoidal bone
9   Orbital plate of ethmoidal bone
10 Perpendicular plate of ethmoidal bone
11 Site of lacrimal bone
12 Lacrimal groove of lacrimal bone
13 Posterior lacrimal crest
14 Fossa for lacrimal sac
15 Lacrimal hamulus
16 Nasolacrimal canal
17 Site of nasal bone
18 Nasal foramina of nasal bone
19 Anterior nasal spine of maxilla
20 Vomer
21 Greater wing of sphenoidal bone
22 Anterior and posterior ethmoidal foramina
23 Optic canal
24 Superior orbital fissure
25 Inferior orbital fissure
26 Infra-orbital groove
27 Infra-orbital foramen

Anterior part of a disarticulated skull.
Orange = zygomatic bone; yellow = ethmoidal bone;
dark green = sphenoidal bone. The arrows indicate the locations
of the lacrimal bone (11) and the nasal bone (17).

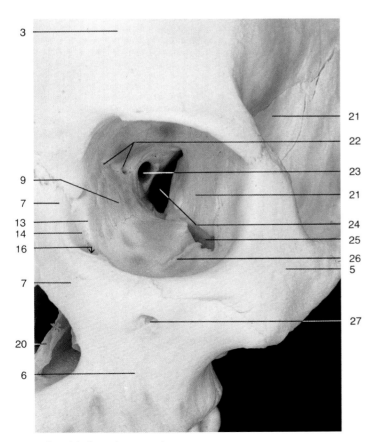

Left orbit (anterior aspect).

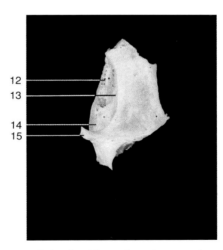

Left lacrimal bone (anterior aspect).

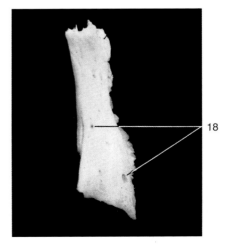

Left nasal bone (anterior aspect).

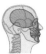

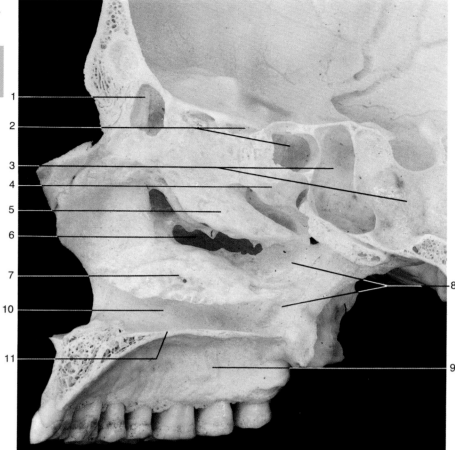

1   Frontal sinus
2   Ethmoidal air cells
3   Sphenoidal sinus
4   Superior nasal concha
5   Middle nasal concha
6   Maxillary hiatus
7   Inferior nasal concha
8   Palatine bone
9   Maxilla
10 Inferior meatus
11 Palatine process of the maxilla

▷

To page 49:

Blue	=	occipital bone
Light green	=	parietal bone
Yellow	=	frontal bone
Dark brown	=	temporal bone
Red	=	sphenoidal bone
Dark green	=	ethmoidal bone
Light blue	=	nasal bone
Pink	=	inferior concha
Orange	=	vomer
Violet	=	maxilla
White	=	palatine bone
White	=	mandible

Lateral wall of the nasal cavity. Median section through the skull.

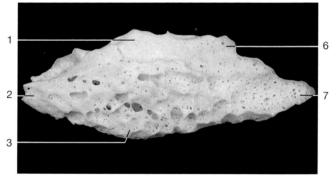

Right inferior nasal concha (medial aspect). Anterior part to the left.

Inferior concha and vomer
1   Ethmoidal process
2   Anterior part of concha
3   Inferior border
4   Ala of vomer
5   Posterior border of nasal septum
6   Lacrimal process
7   Posterior part of concha
8   Maxillary process

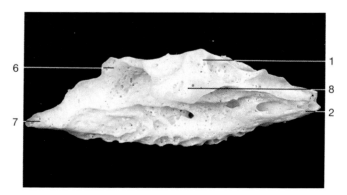

Right inferior nasal concha (lateral aspect). Anterior part to the right.

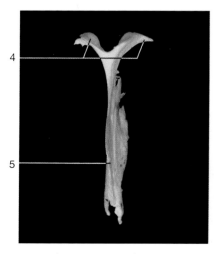

Vomer (posterior aspect).

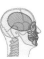

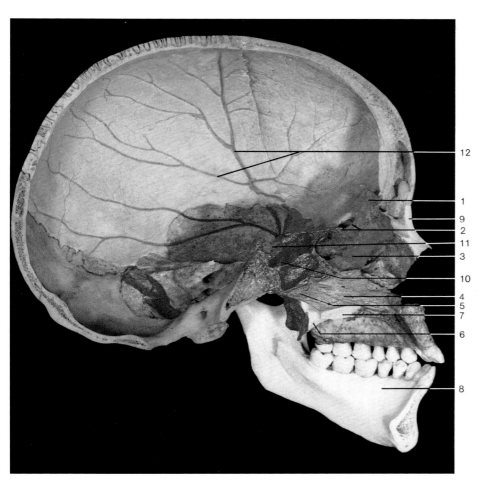

1   Crista galli
2   Cribriform plate
    of ethmoidal bone
3   Perpendicular plate
    of ethmoidal bone
4   Vomer
5   Ala of the vomer
6   Palatine bone
    (perpendicular process)
7   Palatine bone (horizontal plate)
8   Mandible
9   Nasal bone
10 Sphenoidal sinus
11 Hypophysial fossa (sella turcica)
12 Grooves for the middle
    meningeal artery

Cartilages of the nose
13 Lateral nasal cartilage
14 Greater alar cartilage
15 Lesser alar cartilages
16 Septal cartilage
17 Location of nasal bone

Paramedian sagittal section through the skull including the nasal septum.

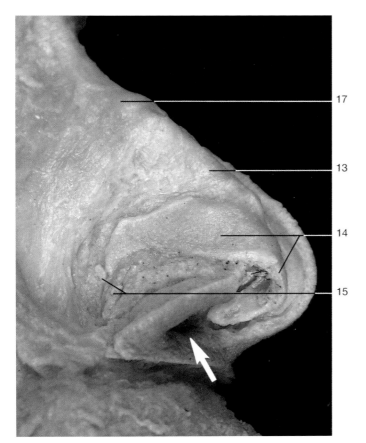

Cartilages of the nose (right anterior aspect). Arrow = nostril, framed by nasal wing.

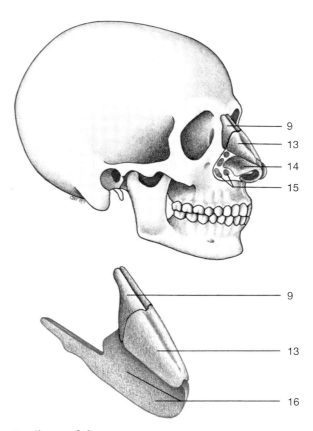

Cartilages of the nose
(schematic diagram of the external nose).

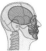

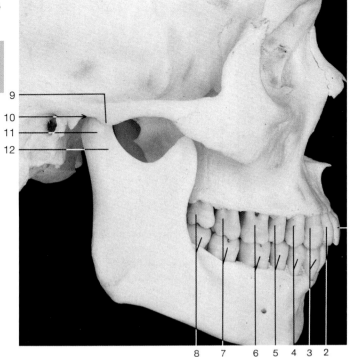

Normal position of teeth. Dentition in centric occlusion (lateral view).

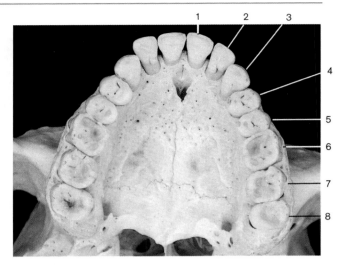

Upper teeth of the adult (inferior aspect).

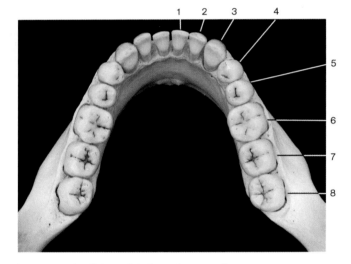

Lower teeth of the adult (superior aspect).

1   Central incisor
2   Lateral incisor
3   Canines
4   First premolars or bicuspids
5   Second premolars or bicuspids
6   First molars
7   Second molars
8   Third molars
9   Articular tubercle
10 Mandibular fossa
11 Head of mandible
12 Condylar process
13 Hard palate and palatine glands
14 Oral cavity
15 Upper molar
16 Oral vestibule
17 Lower molar
18 Platysma muscle
19 Mandible
20 Maxillary sinus
21 Superior longitudinal muscle of tongue
22 Transverse muscle of tongue
23 Buccinator muscle
24 Inferior longitudinal muscle of tongue
25 Sublingual gland
26 Genioglossus muscle

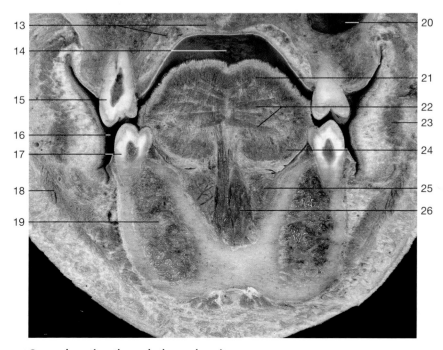

Coronal section through the oral cavity.

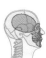

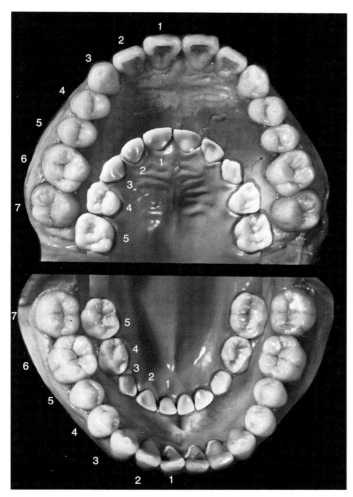

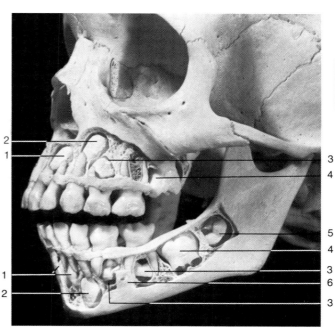

Deciduous teeth in child's skull. The developing crowns of the permanent teeth are displayed in their crypts in the maxilla and mandible.

1   Permanent incisors
2   Permanent cuspid (canine)
3   Premolars
4   First permanent molar
5   Second permanent molar
6   Mental foramen

Comparison of the deciduous and permanent teeth.
Notice that the breadth of the alveolar arch of the child's mandible and maxilla holding the deciduous teeth is nearly the same as the comparable portion in the jaws of the adult. Note the emergence of the third molars. The numbers of the teeth correspond to the numbers in the figure below.

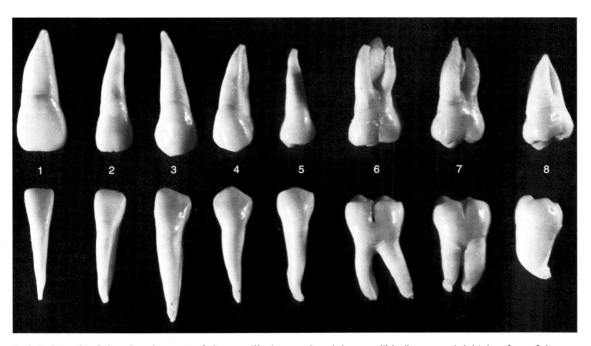

Isolated teeth of the alveolar part of the maxilla (top row) and the mandible (lower row), labial surface of the teeth.

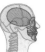

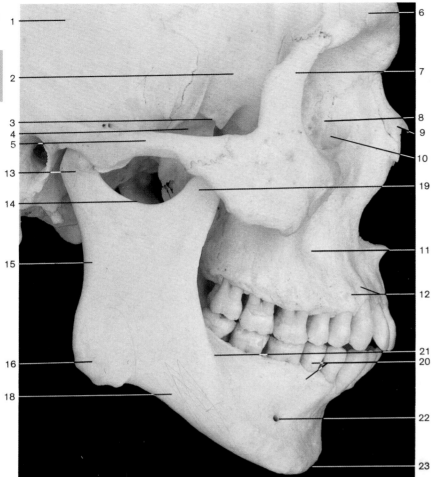

Lateral aspect of the facial bones. Mandible and teeth in the position of occlusion. Upper and lower jaw occluded.

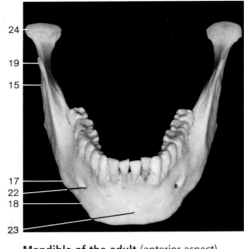

Mandible of the adult (anterior aspect).

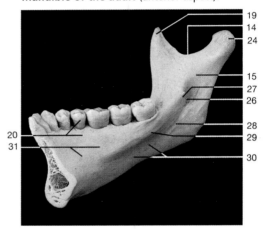

Right half of mandible (medial aspect).

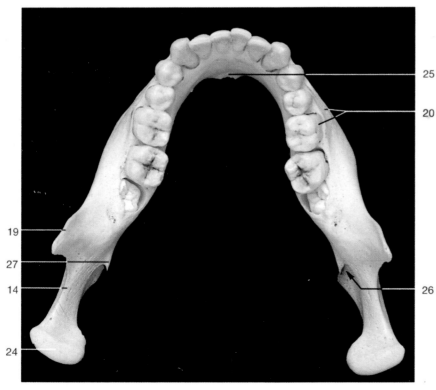

Mandible of the adult (superior aspect).

1 Temporal bone
2 Temporal fossa (greater wing of sphenoidal bone)
3 Infratemporal crest
4 Infratemporal fossa
5 Zygomatic arch
6 Frontal bone
7 Zygomatic bone (frontal process)
8 Lacrimal bone
9 Nasal bone
10 Lacrimal groove
11 Maxilla (canine fossa)
12 Alveolar process of maxilla

Mandible

13 Condylar process
14 Mandibular notch
15 Ramus of the mandible
16 Masseteric tuberosity
17 Angle of the mandible
18 Body of the mandible
19 Coronoid process
20 Alveolar process including teeth
21 Oblique line
22 Mental foramen
23 Mental protuberance
24 Head of the mandible
25 Genial tubercle or mental spine
26 Mandibular foramen (entrance to mandibular canal)
27 Lingula
28 Mylohyoid sulcus
29 Mylohyoid line
30 Submandibular fossa
31 Sublingual fossa

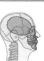

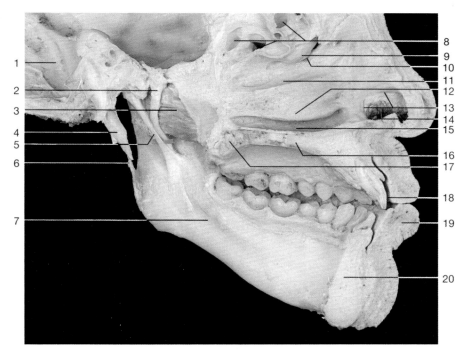

1. Groove for sigmoid sinus
2. Mandibular nerve
3. Lateral pterygoid muscle
4. Styloid process
5. Sphenomandibular ligament
6. Stylomandibular ligament
7. Mylohyoid groove
8. Ethmoidal air cells
9. Ethmoidal bulla
10. Hiatus semilunaris
11. Middle meatus
12. Inferior nasal concha
13. Limen nasi
14. Vestibule with hairs
15. Inferior meatus
16. Hard palate
17. Soft palate
18. Vestibule of oral cavity
19. Lower lip
20. Mandible
21. Calvaria with diploe
22. Sella turcica
23. Internal acoustic meatus
24. Atlanto-occipital articulation
25. Median atlanto-axial articulation
26. Atlas (C$_1$)
27. Dens of axis (C$_2$)
28. Spinous process of axis (C$_2$)
29. Cervical vertebrae (C$_3$, C$_4$)
30. Frontal sinus
31. Crista galli
32. Sphenoidal sinus
33. Nasal septum
34. Mandibular foramen
35. Mylohyoid line
36. Bodies of cervical vertebrae (C$_5$, C$_6$)
37. Articular capsule
38. Lateral ligament
39. Mastoid process
40. Styloid process

Ligaments of temporomandibular joint. Left half of the head (medial aspect).

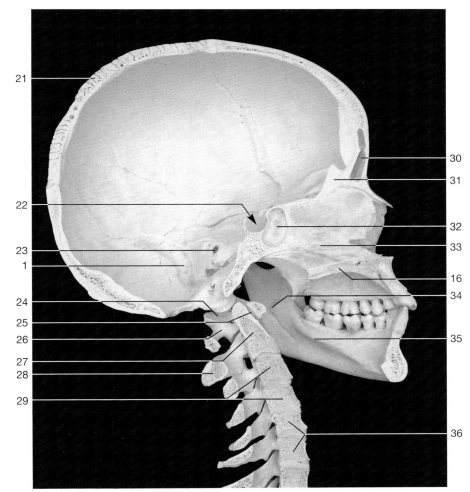

Head and cervical vertebral column (median section through skull and cervical vertebrae, medial aspect).

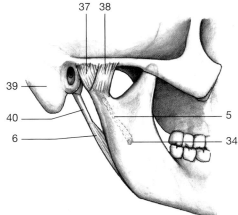

Ligaments related to the temporomandibular joint (schematic drawing).

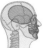

1 Zygomatic arch
2 Articular capsule
3 External acoustic meatus
4 Lateral ligament
5 Mandibular notch
6 Stylomandibular ligament
7 Ramus of the mandible
8 Zygomatic bone
9 Coronoid process
10 Maxilla
11 Articular cartilage of condylar process
12 Styloid process
13 Mandibular fossa
14 Articular disc
15 Articular tubercle
16 Lateral pterygoid muscle
17 Condylar process of mandible
18 Temporalis muscle
19 Digastric muscle, posterior belly
20 Masseter muscle
21 Medial pterygoid muscle
22 Parotid duct
23 Buccinator muscle
24 Mandible

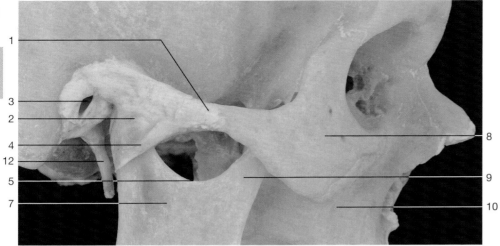

Temporomandibular joint with ligaments.

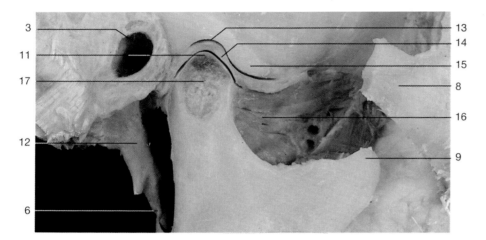

Temporomandibular joint, sagittal section.

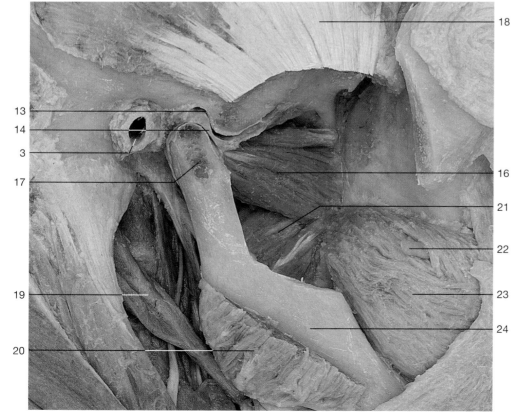

Temporomandibular joint.
Dissection of the articular disc and the related muscles (lateral aspect).

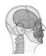

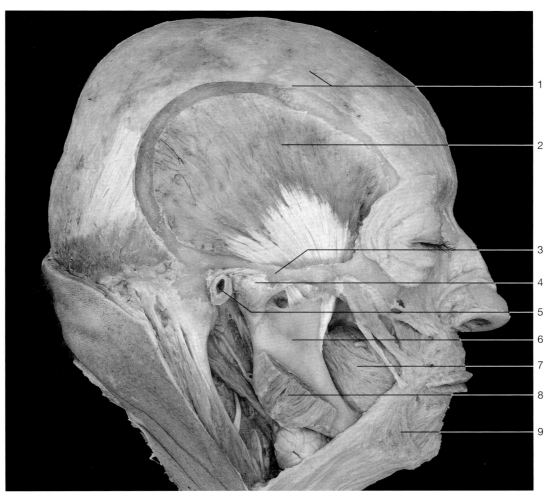

Muscles of mastication and temporomandibular joint. Masseter muscle partly removed.

1   Galea aponeurotica
2   Temporalis muscle
3   Zygomatic arch
4   Temporomandibular joint
5   External acoustic meatus
6   Mandible
7   Buccinator muscle
8   Masseter muscle (cut)
9   Platysma muscle
10 Lateral pterygoid muscle
11 Posterior belly of digastric muscle
12 Stylohyoid muscle
13 Medial pterygoid muscle
14 Anterior belly of digastric muscle
15 Mylohyoid muscle
16 Hyoid bone

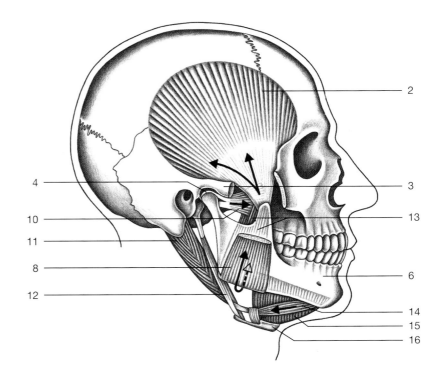

Effect of the masticatory muscles on the temporomandibular joint (arrows).

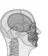

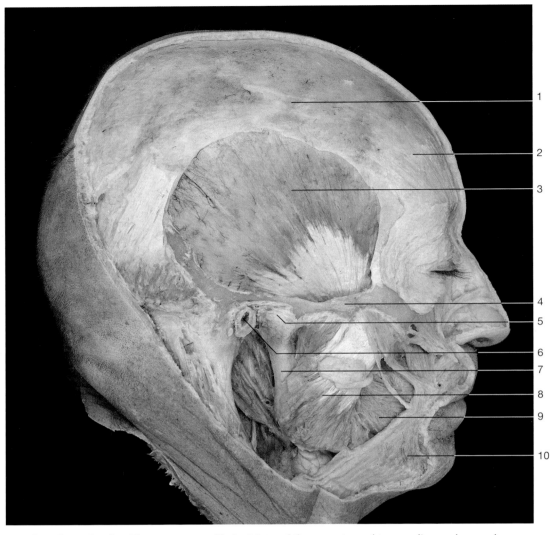

Muscles of mastication. The temporomandibular joint and the masseter and temporalis muscles are shown.

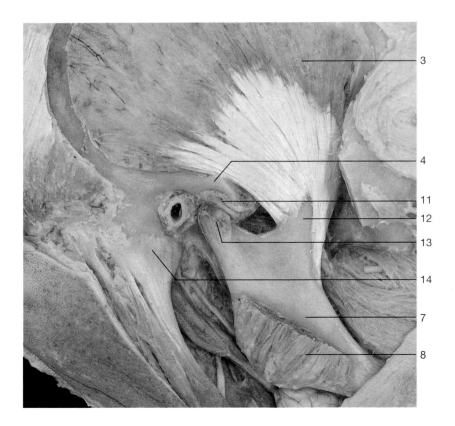

1 Galea aponeurotica
2 Frontal belly of occipitofrontalis muscle
3 Temporalis muscle
4 Zygomatic arch
5 Temporomandibular joint
6 External acoustic meatus
7 Mandible
8 Masseter muscle
9 Buccinator muscle
10 Platysma muscle
11 Articular disc of temporomandibular joint
12 Coronoid process of mandible
13 Condylar process of mandible
14 Mastoid process

Temporalis muscle with insertion at the mandible and the temporomandibular joint. Zygomatic arch and masseter muscle have been partly removed.

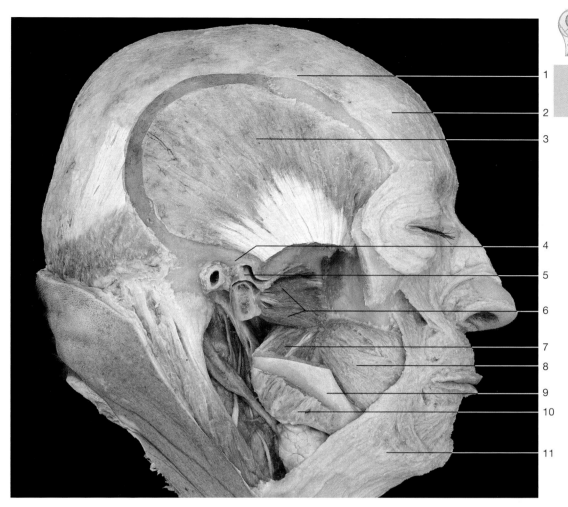

Muscles of mastication. The zygomatic arch and part of the mandible have been removed to reveal the medial and lateral pterygoid muscles.

1 Galea aponeurotica
2 Frontal belly of occipitofrontalis muscle
3 Temporalis muscle
4 Zygomatic arch
5 Articular disc of temporomandibular joint
6 Lateral pterygoid muscle
7 Medial pterygoid muscle
8 Buccinator muscle
9 Mandible
10 Masseter muscle
11 Platysma muscle

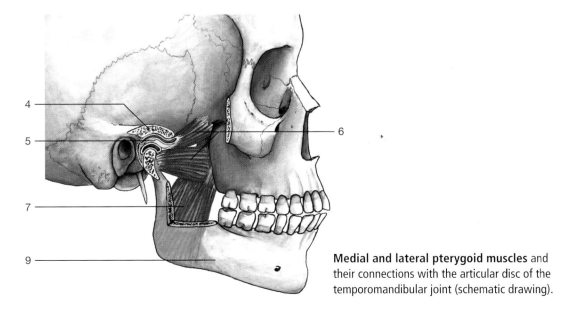

Medial and lateral pterygoid muscles and their connections with the articular disc of the temporomandibular joint (schematic drawing).

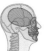

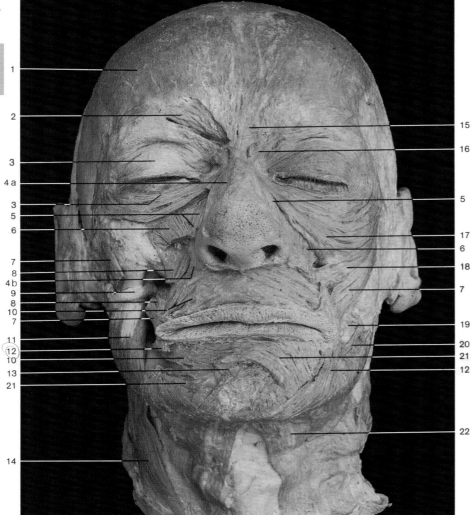

1   Frontal belly of occipitofrontalis muscle
2   Corrugator supercilii muscle
3   Palpebral part of orbicularis oculi muscle
4a Transverse part of nasalis muscle
4b Alar part of nasalis muscle
5   Levator labii superioris alaeque nasi muscle
6   Levator labii superioris muscle
7   Zygomaticus major muscle
8   Levator anguli oris muscle
9   Parotid duct
10 Orbicularis oris muscle
11 Masseter muscle
12 Depressor anguli oris muscle
13 Mentalis muscle
14 Sternocleidomastoid muscle
15 Procerus muscle
16 Depressor supercilii muscle
17 Orbital part of orbicularis oculi muscle
18 Zygomaticus minor muscle
19 Buccinator muscle
20 Risorius muscle
21 Depressor labii inferioris muscle
22 Platysma muscle
23 Galea aponeurotica
24 Temporoparietalis muscle
25 Occipital belly of occipitofrontalis muscle
26 Parotid gland with fascia
27 Temporal fascia
28 Orbicularis oculi muscle
29 Parotid duct and masseter muscle

Facial muscles (anterior aspect). Left side: superficial layer, right side: deeper layer.

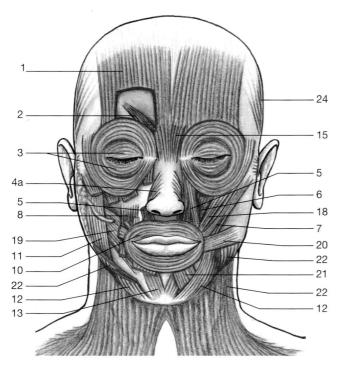

Facial muscles (schematic drawing).
Left side: superficial layer, right side: deeper layer.

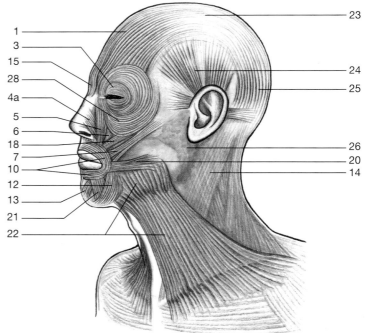

Facial muscles (schematic drawing). Sphincter-like muscles surround the orifices of the head. Radially arranged muscles work as their antagonists.

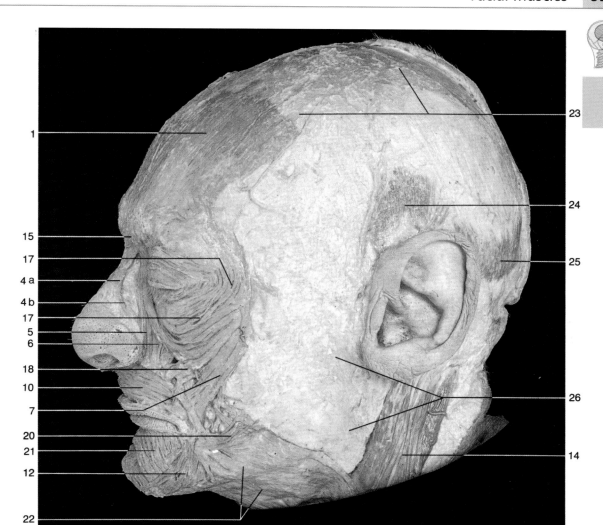

Facial muscles (lateral aspect).

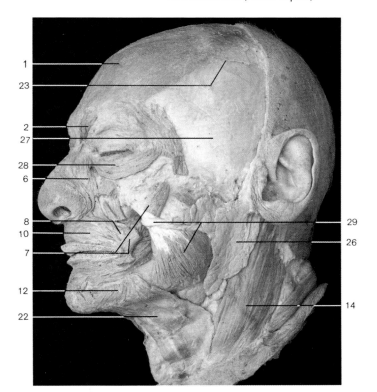

Facial muscles and parotid gland (lateral aspect).

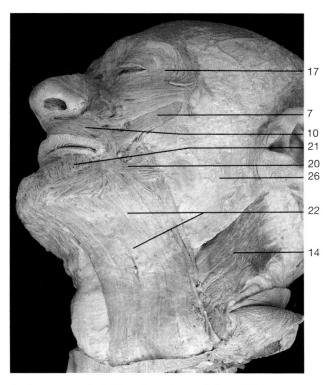

Platysma muscle (oblique lateral aspect). Superficial lamina of cervical fascia partly removed.

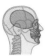

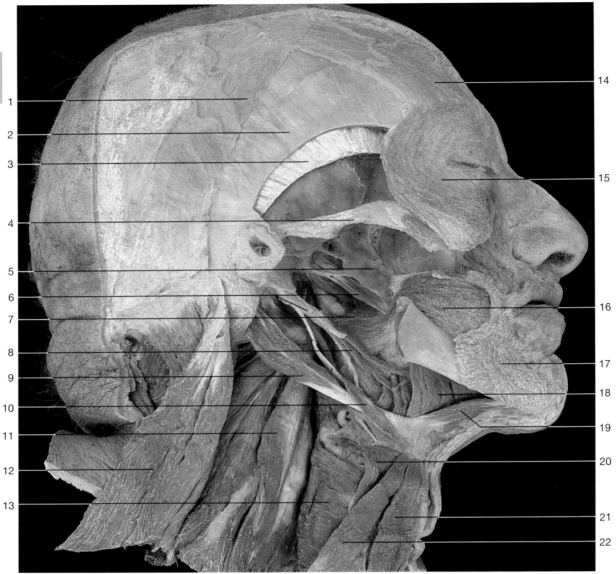

Supra- and infrahyoid muscles and pharynx (lateral aspect). Ramus of mandible, pterygoid muscles, and insertion of temporalis muscle removed.

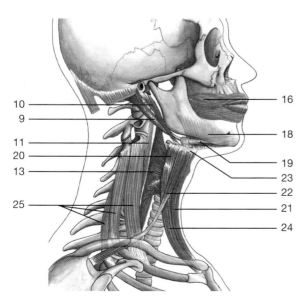

Supra- and infrahyoid muscles (schematic drawing).

1 Galea aponeurotica
2 Temporal fascia
3 Tendon of temporalis muscle
4 Zygomatic arch
5 Lateral pterygoid plate
6 Tensor veli palatini muscle (styloid process)
7 Superior constrictor muscle of pharynx
8 Styloglossus muscle
9 Posterior belly of digastric muscle
10 Stylohyoid muscle
11 Longus capitis muscle
12 Sternocleidomastoid muscle (reflected)
13 Inferior constrictor of pharynx
14 Frontal belly of occipitofrontalis muscle
15 Orbital part of orbicularis oculi muscle
16 Buccinator muscle
17 Depressor anguli oris muscle
18 Mylohyoid muscle
19 Anterior belly of digastric muscle
20 Thyrohyoid muscle
21 Sternohyoid muscle
22 Omohyoid muscle
23 Hyoid bone
24 Sternothyroid muscle
25 Scalenus muscles

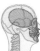

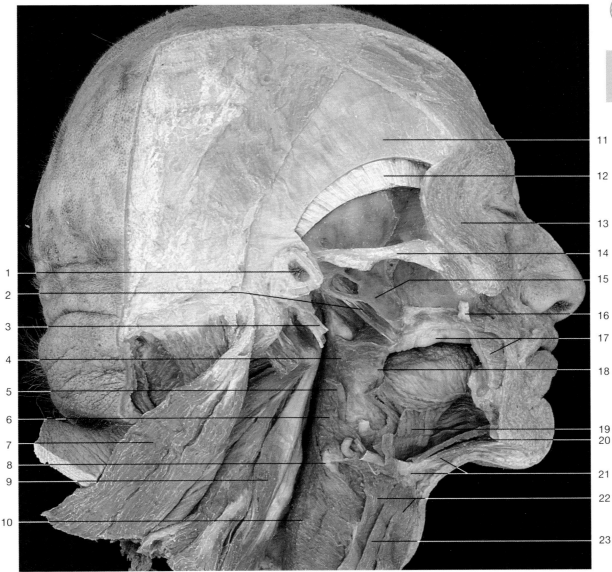

Supra- and infrahyoid muscles and pharynx (lateral aspect). Buccinator muscle removed; oral cavity opened.

1   External acoustic meatus
2   Tensor veli palatini muscle
3   Styloid process
4   Superior constrictor muscle of pharynx
5   Stylopharyngeus muscle (divided)
6   Middle constrictor muscle of pharynx
7   Sternocleidomastoid muscle
8   Greater horn of hyoid bone
9   Longus capitis muscle
10 Inferior constrictor muscle of pharynx
11 Temporal fascia
12 Tendon of temporalis muscle
13 Orbicularis oculi muscle
14 Zygomatic arch
15 Lateral pterygoid plate
16 Parotid duct
17 Gingiva of upper jaw (without teeth),
     buccinator muscle (divided)
18 Pterygomandibular raphe
19 Hyoglossus muscle
20 Mylohyoid muscle
21 Anterior belly of digastric muscle (hyoid bone)
22 Sternohyoid and thyrohyoid muscles
23 Omohyoid muscle

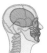

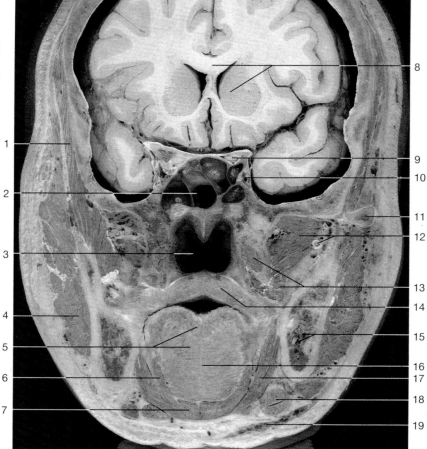

1 Temporalis muscle
2 Sphenoidal sinus
3 Nasopharynx
4 Masseter muscle
5 Superior longitudinal, transverse and vertical muscles of tongue
6 Hyoglossus muscle
7 Geniohyoid muscle
8 Corpus callosum (caudate nucleus)
9 Optic nerve
10 Cavernous sinus
11 Zygomatic arch
12 Cross section of lateral pterygoid muscle and maxillary artery
13 Section of medial pterygoid muscle
14 Soft palate
15 Mandible and inferior alveolar nerve
16 Septum of the tongue
17 Mylohyoid muscle
18 Submandibular gland
19 Platysma muscle
20 Foramen magnum, vertebral artery and spinal cord
21 Internal carotid artery
22 Head of mandible
23 Styloid process
24 Inferior alveolar nerve
25 Lingual nerve and chorda tympani nerve
26 Medial pterygoid muscle
27 Uvula
28 Anterior belly of digastric muscle (cut)
29 Condyle of occipital bone
30 Mastoid process
31 Lateral pterygoid muscle
32 Auditory tube and levator veli palatini muscle
33 Tensor veli palatini muscle

Coronal section through cranial, nasal, and oral cavities at the level of sphenoidal sinus.

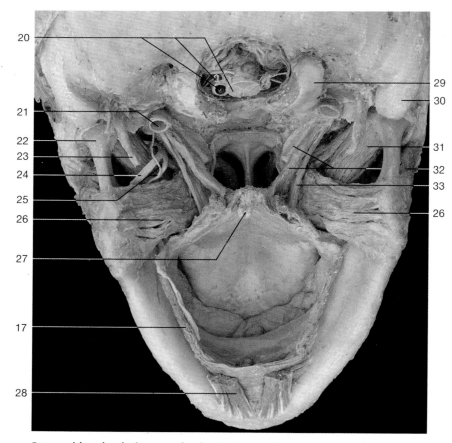

Pterygoid and palatine muscles (posterior aspect).

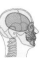

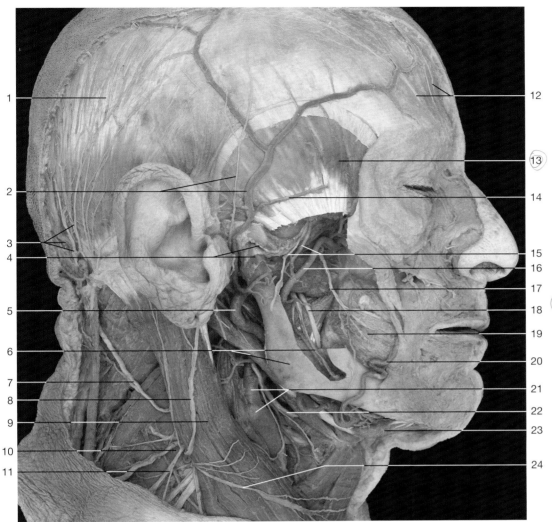

1 Galea aponeurotica
2 Superficial temporal artery and auriculo-temporal nerve
3 Occipital artery and greater occipital nerve (C₂)
4 Temporomandibular joint (opened)
5 External carotid artery
6 Mandible and inferior mandibular artery and nerve
7 Accessory nerve (Var.)
8 Great auricular nerve
9 Sternocleidomastoideus muscle
10 Punctum nervosum
11 Supraclavicular nerves
12 Supra-orbital nerves
13 Temporalis muscle
14 Transverse facial artery
15 Masseteric nerve and deep temporal branch of maxillary artery
16 Maxillary artery
17 Buccal nerve
18 Lingual nerve
19 Buccinator muscle
20 Facial artery
21 External carotid artery and sinus caroticus
22 Hypoglossal nerve
23 Digastric muscle
24 Transverse cervical nerves

Dissection of maxillary artery (lateral aspect). Ramus mandibulae partly removed and canalis mandibulae opened.

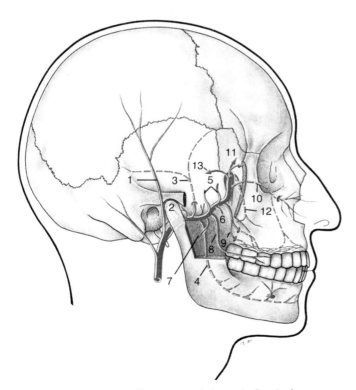

Main branches of maxillary artery (schematic drawing).

1 Superficial temporal artery

Branches of the first part
2 Deep auricular artery and anterior tympanic artery
3 Middle meningeal artery
4 Inferior alveolar artery

Branches of the second part
5 Deep temporal branches
6 Pterygoid branches
7 Masseteric artery
8 Buccal artery

Branches of the third part
9 Posterior superior alveolar artery
10 Infra-orbital artery
11 Sphenopalatine artery and branches to the nasal cavity
12 Descending palatine artery
13 Artery of the pterygoid canal

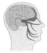

2.2 Cranial Nerves

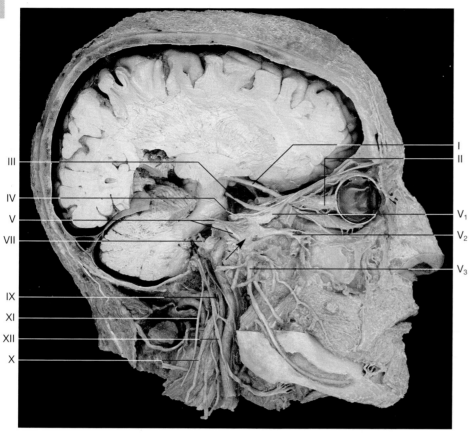

Dissection of the cranial nerves (indicated by I–XII) (lateral aspect). Brain, brain stem, and cerebellum have been partly removed (from Lütjen-Drecoll, Rohen, Innenansichten des menschlichen Körpers, 2010).

The twelve cranial nerves emerge from the brain stem and penetrate the skull at different places. The olfactory nerves (n. I) pass the lamina cribrosa innervating the upper part of the nasal mucous membrane. The optic nerve (n. II) is related to the eye. The external ocular muscles are innervated by the oculomotor, trochlear, and abducent nerves (n. III, n. IV, and n. VI). Facial skin and masticatory muscles are innervated by the trigeminal nerve (n. V) while the facial nerve (n. VII) innervates mainly the mimic musculature. The stato-acoustic organ is related to the vestibulocochlear nerve (n. VIII). The vagus nerve (n. X) is one of the longest cranial nerves, running through the lateral neck region to reach the thoracic and abdominal cavities. It belongs to the parasympathetic part of the autonomic nervous system. The glossopharyngeal (n. IX), accessory (n. XI), and hypoglossal (n. XII) nerves innervate the muscles of the neck, the tongue, and the pharynx. During human evolution, they were incorporated secondarily into the brain cavity.

Schematic drawing of the cranial nerves (indicated by I–XII) (lateral aspect).

Cranial nerves

I	=	Olfactory nerves
II	=	Optic nerve
III	=	Oculomotor nerve
IV	=	Trochlear nerve
V	=	Trigeminal nerve
VI	=	Abducent nerve
VII	=	Facial nerve
VIII	=	Vestibulocochlear nerve
IX	=	Glossopharyngeal nerve
X	=	Vagus nerve
XI	=	Accessory nerve
XII	=	Hypoglossal nerve

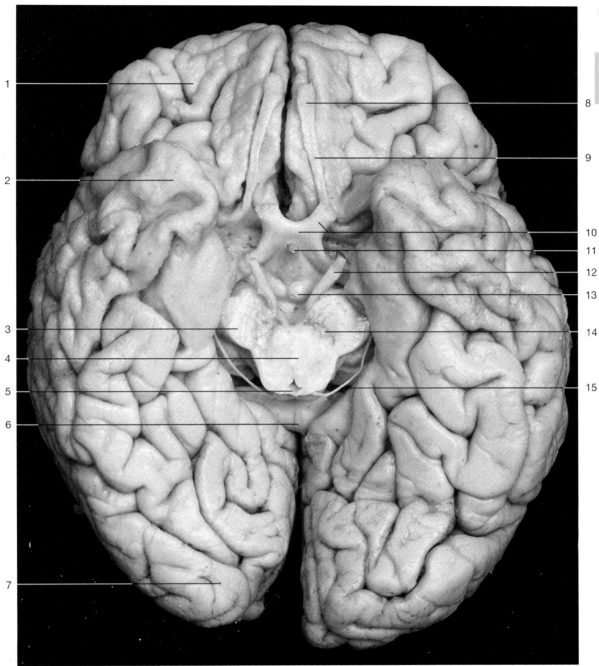

Inferior aspect of the brain with cranial nerves. Midbrain divided.

1	Frontal lobe	9	Olfactory tract
2	Temporal lobe	10	Optic nerve and optic chiasma
3	Pedunculus cerebri	11	Infundibulum
4	Midbrain (divided)	12	Oculomotor nerve (n. III)
5	Cerebral aqueduct	13	Mamillary body
6	Splenium of corpus callosum	14	Substantia nigra
7	Occipital lobe	15	Trochlear nerve (n. IV)
8	Olfactory bulb		

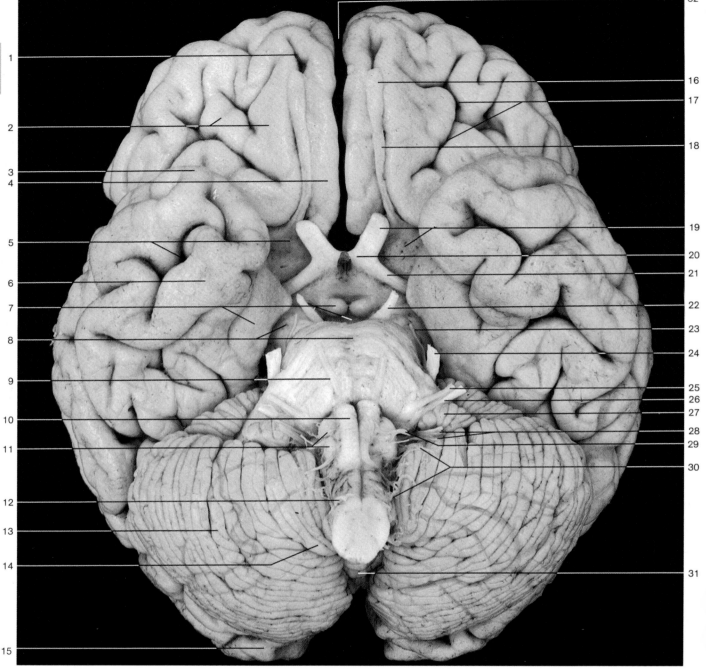

Cranial nerves. Brain (inferior aspect).

1   Olfactory sulcus (termination)
2   Orbital gyri
3   Temporal lobe
4   Straight gyrus
5   Olfactory trigone and inferior temporal sulcus
6   Medial occipitotemporal gyrus
7   Parahippocampal gyrus, mamillary body, and interpeduncular fossa
8   Pons and cerebral peduncle
9   Abducent nerve (n. VI)
10 Pyramid
11 Inferior olive
12 Cervical spinal nerves

13 Cerebellum
14 Tonsil of cerebellum
15 Occipital lobe (posterior pole)
16 Olfactory bulb
17 Orbital sulci of frontal lobe
18 Olfactory tract
19 Optic nerve (n. II) and anterior perforated substance
20 Optic chiasma
21 Optic tract
22 Oculomotor nerve (n. III)
23 Trochlear nerve (n. IV)
24 Trigeminal nerve (n. V)

25 Facial nerve (n. VII)
26 Vestibulocochlear nerve (n. VIII)
27 Flocculus of cerebellum
28 Glossopharyngeal nerve (n. IX) and vagus nerve (n. X)
29 Hypoglossal nerve (n. XII)
30 Accessory nerve (n. XI)
31 Vermis of cerebellum
32 Longitudinal fissure

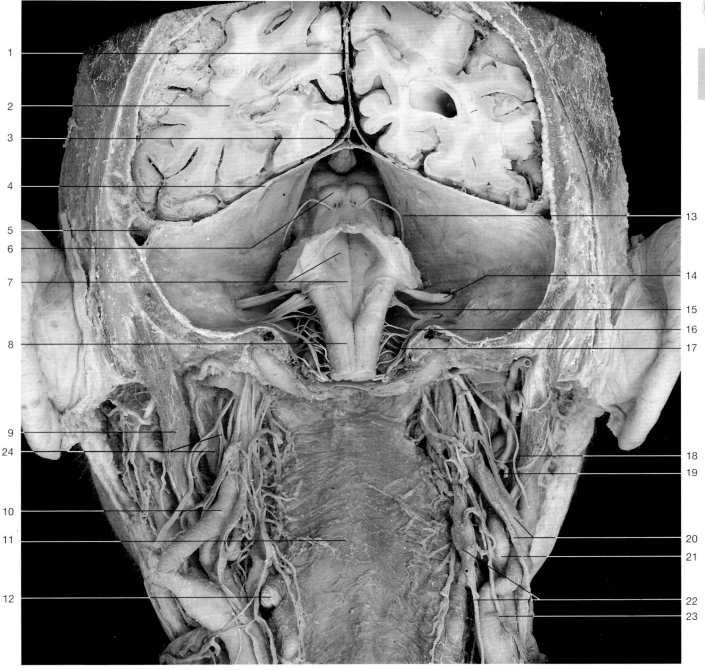

Brain stem and pharynx with cranial nerves (posterior aspect). Cranial cavity opened and cerebellum removed.

1   Falx cerebri
2   Occipital lobe
3   Straight sinus
4   Tentorium cerebelli
5   Transverse sinus
6   Inferior colliculus of midbrain
7   Rhomboid fossa
8   Medulla oblongata
9   Posterior belly of digastric muscle
10 Internal carotid artery

11 Pharynx (middle constrictor muscle)
12 Hyoid bone (greater horn)
13 Trochlear nerve (n. IV)
14 Facial nerve (n. VII) and
    vestibulocochlear nerve (n. VIII)
15 Glossopharyngeal nerve (n. IX)
    and vagus nerve (n. X)
16 Accessory nerve (intracranial portion) (n. XI)
17 Hypoglossal nerve (intracranial portion) (n. XII)
18 Accessory nerve (n. XI)

19 Hypoglossal nerve (n. XII)
20 Vagus nerve (n. X) and internal carotid artery
21 External carotid artery
22 Sympathetic trunk and superior cervical ganglion
23 Ansa cervicalis (superior root of
    hypoglossal nerve)
24 Glossopharyngeal nerve (n. IX) and
    stylopharyngeus muscle

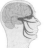

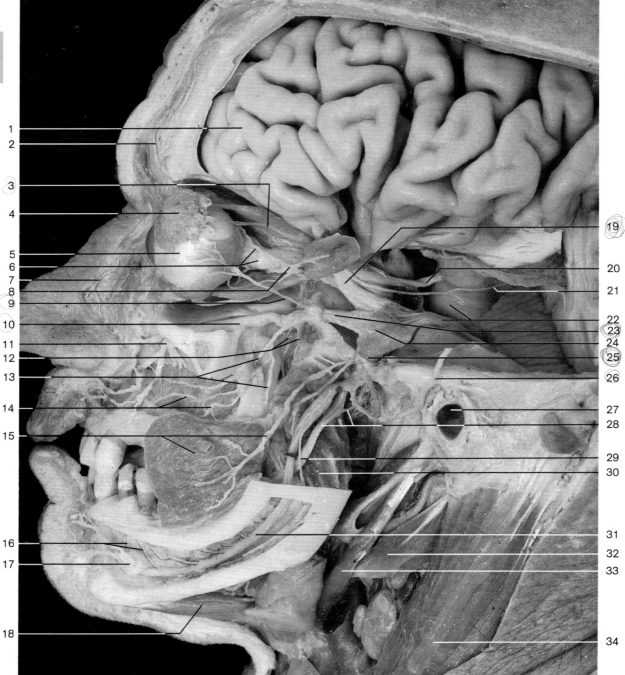

Dissection of the trigeminal nerve in its entirety. Lateral wall of cranial cavity, lateral wall of orbit, zygomatic arch, and ramus of the mandible have been removed and the mandibular canal opened.

1	Frontal lobe of cerebrum	
2	Supra-orbital nerve	
3	Lacrimal nerve	
4	Lacrimal gland	
5	Eyeball	
6	Optic nerve and short ciliary nerves	
7	External nasal branch of anterior ethmoidal nerve	
8	Ciliary ganglion	
9	Zygomatic nerve	
10	Infra-orbital nerve	
11	Infra-orbital foramen and terminal branches of infra-orbital nerve	

12 Pterygopalatine ganglion and pterygopalatine nerves
13 Posterior superior alveolar nerves
14 Superior dental plexus
15 Buccinator muscle and buccal nerve
16 Inferior dental plexus
17 Mental foramen and mental nerve
18 Anterior belly of digastric muscle
19 Ophthalmic nerve (n. V₁)
20 Oculomotor nerve (n. III)
21 Trochlear nerve (n. IV)
22 Trigeminal nerve and pons

23 Maxillary nerve (n. V₂)
24 Trigeminal ganglion
25 Mandibular nerve (n. V₃)
26 Auriculotemporal nerve
27 External acoustic meatus (divided)
28 Lingual nerve and chorda tympani
29 Mylohyoid nerve
30 Medial pterygoid muscle
31 Inferior alveolar nerve
32 Posterior belly of digastric muscle
33 Stylohyoid muscle
34 Sternocleidomastoid muscle

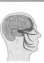

1   Frontal nerve
2   Lacrimal gland and eyeball
3   Lacrimal nerve
4   Lateral rectus muscle
5   Ciliary ganglion lateral to optic nerve
6   Zygomatic nerve
7   Inferior branch of oculomotor nerve
8   Ophthalmic nerve (n. V₁)
9   Maxillary nerve (n. V₂)
10 Trigeminal ganglion
11 Mandibular nerve (n. V₃)
12 Posterior superior alveolar nerves
13 Tympanic cavity, external acoustic meatus, and tympanic membrane
14 Inferior alveolar nerve
15 Lingual nerve
16 Facial nerve (n. VII)
17 Vagus nerve (n. X)
18 Hypoglossal nerve (n. XII) and superior root of ansa cervicalis
19 External carotid artery
20 Olfactory tract (n. I)
21 Optic nerve (n. II) (intracranial part)
22 Oculomotor nerve (n. III)
23 Abducent nerve (n. VI)
24 Trochlear nerve (n. IV)
25 Trigeminal nerve (n. V)
26 Vestibulocochlear nerve (n. VIII) and facial nerve (n. VII)
27 Glossopharyngeal nerve (n. IX) (leaving brain stem)
28 Rhomboid fossa
29 Vagus nerve (n. X) (leaving brain stem)
30 Hypoglossal nerve (n. XII) (leaving medulla oblongata)
31 Accessory nerve (n. XI) (ascending from foramen magnum)
32 Vertebral artery
33 Spinal ganglion and dura mater of spinal cord
34 Accessory nerve (n. XI)
35 Internal carotid artery
36 Lateral and medial branch of supra-orbital nerve
37 Infratrochlear nerve
38 Infra-orbital nerve
39 Pterygopalatine ganglion and middle superior alveolar nerve
40 Middle superior alveolar nerves (entering superior dental plexus)
41 Buccal nerve
42 Mental nerve and mental foramen
43 Auriculotemporal nerve
44 Otic ganglion (dotted line)
45 Chorda tympani
46 Mylohyoid nerve
47 Submandibular gland
48 Hyoid bone

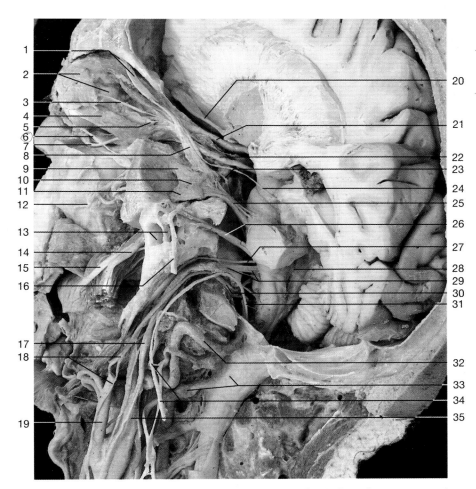

Cranial nerves in connection with the brain stem. Left side (lateral superior aspect). Left half of brain and head partly removed. Notice the location of trigeminal ganglion.

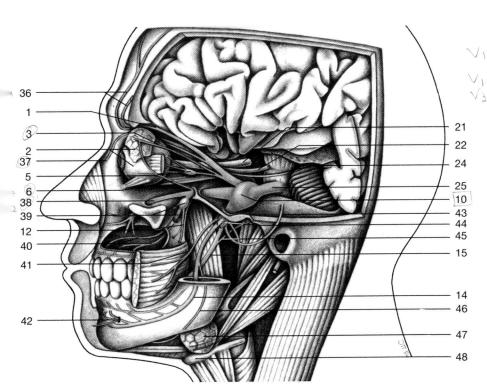

Main branches of trigeminal nerve (schematic drawing of figure on opposite page).

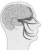

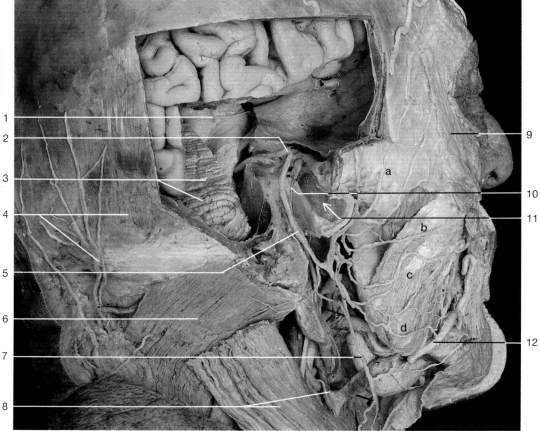

Dissection of facial nerve in its entirety. Cranial cavity fenestrated; temporal lobe partly removed. Facial canal and tympanic cavity opened, posterior wall of external acoustic meatus removed.
Branches of facial nerve: a = temporal branch; b = zygomatic branches; c = buccal branches; d = marginal mandibular branch.

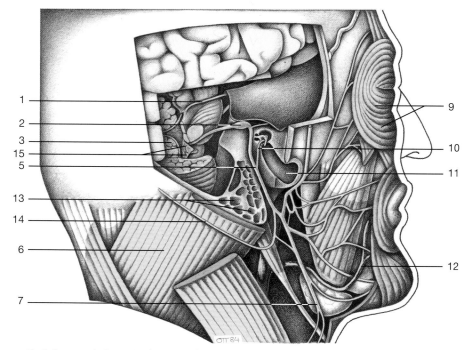

Facial nerve (schematic drawing of the dissection above).

1 Trochlear nerve
2 Facial nerve with geniculate ganglion
3 Cerebellum (right hemisphere)
4 Occipital belly of occipitofrontalis muscle and greater occipital nerve
5 Facial nerve at stylomastoid foramen
6 Splenius capitis muscle
7 Cervical branch of facial nerve
8 Sternocleidomastoid muscle and retromandibular vein
9 Orbicularis oculi muscle
10 Chorda tympani
11 External acoustic meatus
12 Facial artery
13 Mastoid air cells
14 Posterior auricular nerve
15 Nucleus and genu of facial nerve

Cranial nerves in connection with the brain stem (oblique-lateral aspect). Lateral portion of the skull, brain, neck and facial structures, lateral wall of orbit and oral cavity have been removed. The tympanic cavity has been opened. The mandible has been divided and the muscles of mastication have been removed.

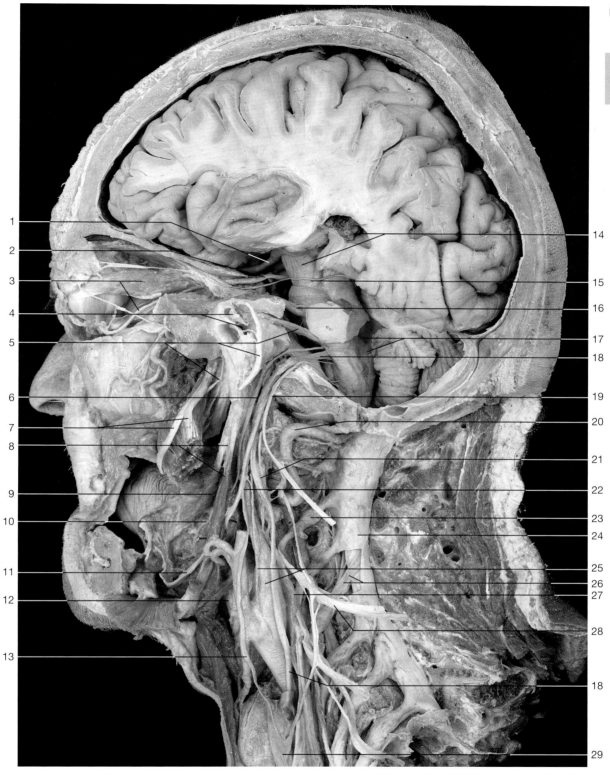
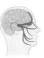

1   Optic tract
2   Oculomotor nerve (n. III)
3   Lateral rectus muscle and inferior branch
    of oculomotor nerve
4   Malleus and chorda tympani
5   Chorda tympani, facial nerve (n. VII), and
    vestibulocochlear nerve (n. VIII)
6   Glossopharyngeal nerve (n. XI)
7   Lingual nerve and inferior alveolar nerve
8   Styloid process and stylohyoid muscle
9   Styloglossus muscle
10 Lingual branches of glossopharyngeal
    nerve

11 Lingual branch of hypoglossal nerve
12 External carotid artery
13 Superior root of ansa cervicalis (branch of
    hypoglossal nerve, derived from C_1)
14 Lateral ventricle with choroid plexus and
    cerebral peduncle
15 Trochlear nerve (n. IV)
16 Trigeminal nerve (n. V)
17 Fourth ventricle and rhomboid fossa
18 Vagus nerve (n. X)
19 Accessory nerve (n. XI)
20 Vertebral artery
21 Superior cervical ganglion

22 Hypoglossal nerve (n. XII)
23 Spinal ganglion with dural sheath
24 Dura mater of spinal cord
25 Internal carotid artery and carotid
    sinus branch of glossopharyngeal
    nerve
26 Dorsal roots of spinal nerve
27 Sympathetic trunk
28 Branch of cervical plexus (ventral
    primary ramus of third cervical
    spinal nerve)
29 Ansa cervicalis

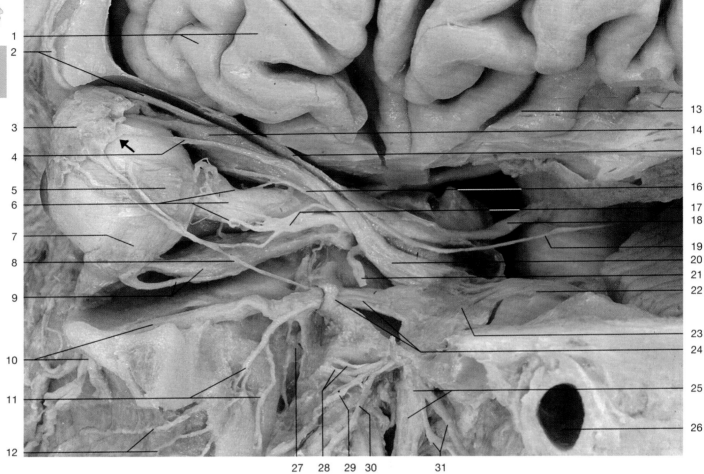

Cranial nerves of the orbit and pterygopalatine fossa. Left orbit (lateral aspect). Note the zygomaticolacrimal anastomosis (arrow).

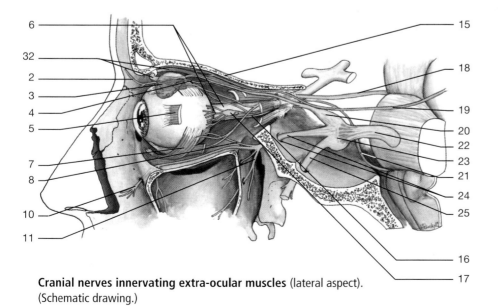

Cranial nerves innervating extra-ocular muscles (lateral aspect).
(Schematic drawing.)

1 Frontal lobe	6 Optic nerve and short ciliary nerves	10 Infra-orbital nerve
2 Supra-orbital nerve	7 Inferior oblique muscle	11 Posterior superior alveolar nerves
3 Lacrimal gland	8 Zygomatic nerve	12 Branches of superior alveolar plexus
4 Lacrimal nerve	9 Inferior branch of oculomotor nerve and	adjacent to mucous membrane of
5 Lateral rectus muscle (divided)	inferior rectus muscle	maxillary sinus

13 Central sulcus of insula
14 Superior rectus muscle
15 Periorbita (roof of orbit)
16 Nasociliary nerve
17 Ciliary ganglion
18 Oculomotor nerve (n. III)
19 Trochlear nerve (n. IV)
20 Ophthalmic nerve (n. V_1)
21 Abducent nerve (n. VI) (divided)
22 Trigeminal nerve (n. V)
23 Trigeminal ganglion
24 Maxillary nerve (n. V_2) and foramen
     rotundum
25 Mandibular nerve (n. V_3)
26 External acoustic meatus
27 Pterygopalatine nerves
28 Deep temporal nerves
29 Buccal nerve
30 Masseteric nerve
31 Auriculotemporal nerve
32 Trochlea and superior oblique muscle

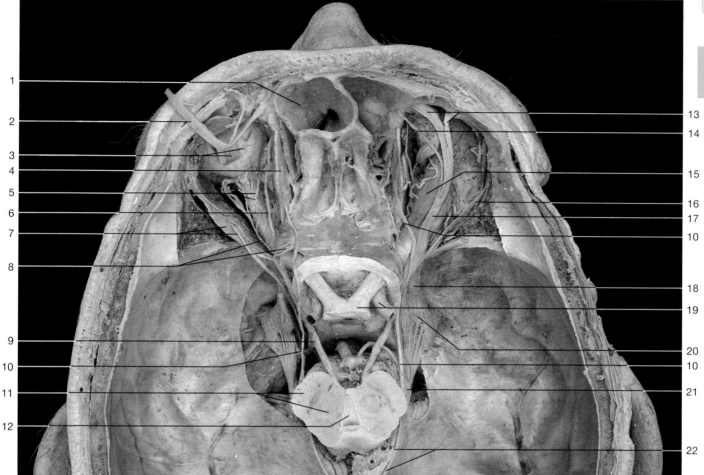

Cranial nerves of the orbit (superior aspect). Right side: superficial layer, left side: middle layer of the orbit (superior rectus muscle and frontal nerve divided and reflected). Tentorium and dura mater partly removed.

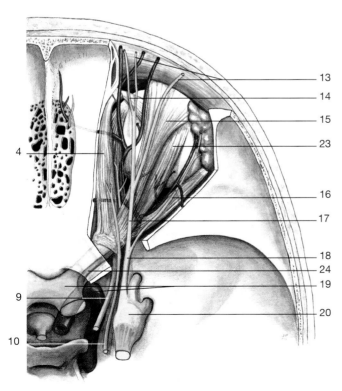

Cranial nerves within the orbit (superior aspect).

1 Frontal sinus (enlarged)
2 Frontal nerve (divided and reflected)
3 Superior rectus muscle (divided) and eyeball
4 Superior oblique muscle
5 Short ciliary nerves and optic nerve (n. II)
6 Nasociliary nerve
7 Abducent nerve (n. VI) and lateral rectus muscle
8 Ciliary ganglion and superior rectus muscle (reflected)
9 Oculomotor nerve (n. III)
10 Trochlear nerve (n. IV)
11 Crus cerebri and midbrain
12 Inferior wall of the third ventricle connected with cerebral aqueduct
13 Lateral and medial branches of supra-orbital nerve
14 Supratrochlear nerve
15 Superior levator palpebrae muscle
16 Lacrimal nerve
17 Frontal nerve
18 Ophthalmic nerve (n. V_1)
19 Optic chiasma and internal carotid artery
20 Trigeminal ganglion
21 Trigeminal nerve (n. V)
22 Tentorial notch
23 Superior rectus muscle
24 Ophthalmic artery

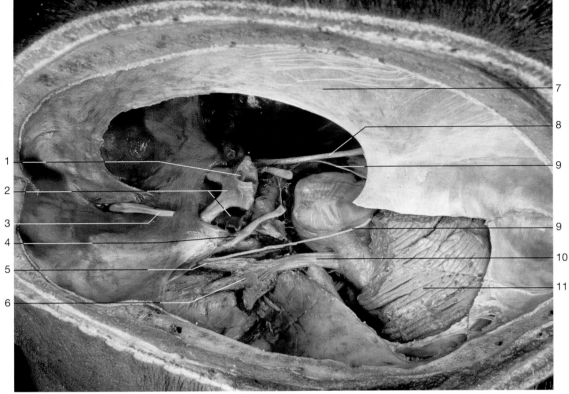

Cranial nerves at the base of the skull. The brain stem was divided and the tentorium fenestrated. Both hemispheres were removed.

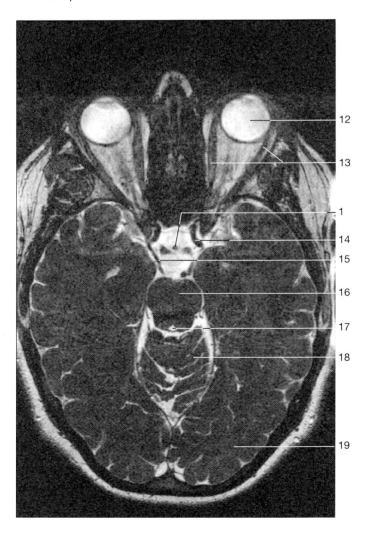

1   Infundibulum
2   Optic chiasma and internal carotid artery
3   Olfactory tract
4   Oculomotor nerve (n. III)
5   Ophthalmic nerve (n. V1)
6   Trigeminal ganglion
7   Falx cerebri
8   Tentorial notch
9   Trochlear nerve (n. IV)
10 Trigeminal nerve (n. V)
11 Cerebellum
12 Eyeball
13 Medial and lateral rectus muscles
14 Internal carotid artery
15 Oculomotor nerve (n. III)
16 Midbrain
17 Cerebral aqueduct
18 Vermis of cerebellum
19 Occipital lobe of the cerebrum
20 Basilar artery

Section through the head at the level of the sella turcica demonstrating cranial nerves (MRI scan, University of Erlangen, Dpt. of Neurosurgery).

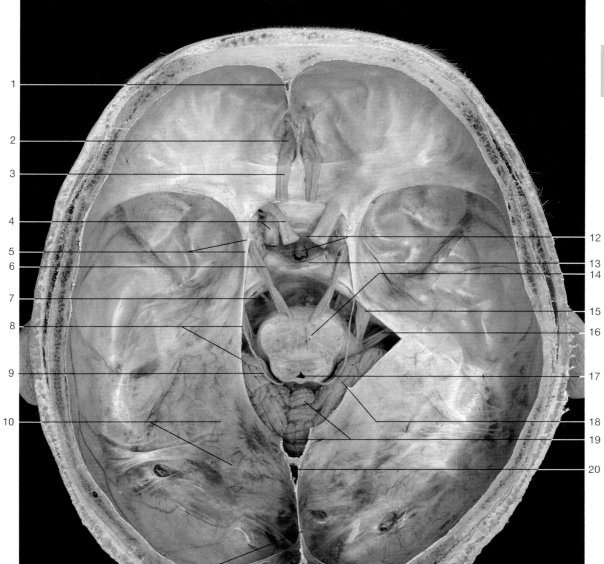

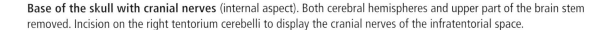

Base of the skull with cranial nerves (internal aspect). Both cerebral hemispheres and upper part of the brain stem removed. Incision on the right tentorium cerebelli to display the cranial nerves of the infratentorial space.

1	Superior sagittal sinus with falx cerebri	12	Hypophysial fossa, infundibulum, and diaphragma sellae
2	Olfactory bulb	13	Dorsum sellae
3	Olfactory tract	14	Midbrain (divided)
4	Optic nerve and internal carotid artery	15	Trigeminal nerve (n. V)
5	Anterior clinoid process and anterior attachment of tentorium cerebelli	16	Facial nerve (n. VII), nervus intermedius, and vestibulocochlear nerve (n. VIII)
6	Oculomotor nerve (n. III)	17	Cerebral aqueduct
7	Abducent nerve (n. VI)	18	Right hemisphere of cerebellum
8	Tentorial notch (incisura tentorii)	19	Vermis of cerebellum
9	Trochlear nerve (n. IV)	20	Straight sinus
10	Tentorium cerebelli		
11	Falx cerebri and confluence of sinuses		

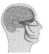

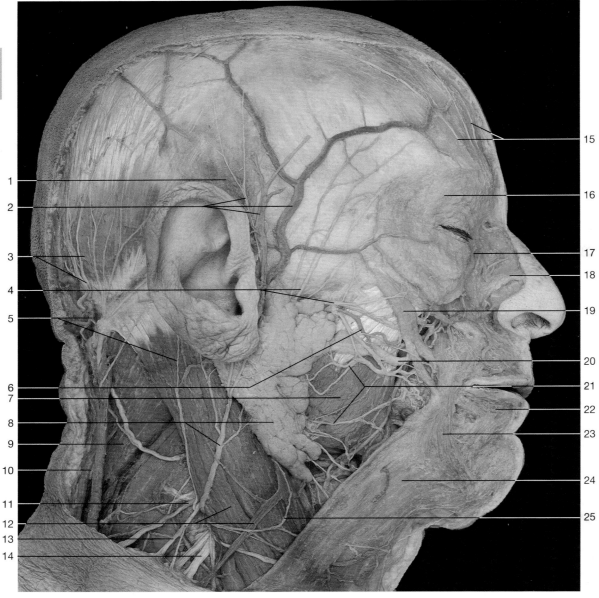

Lateral superficial aspect of the face. Peripheral distribution of facial nerve (n. VII).

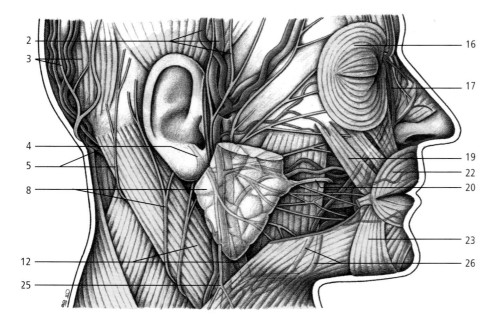

Superficial region of the face. Note the facial plexus within the parotid gland (semischematic drawing).

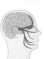

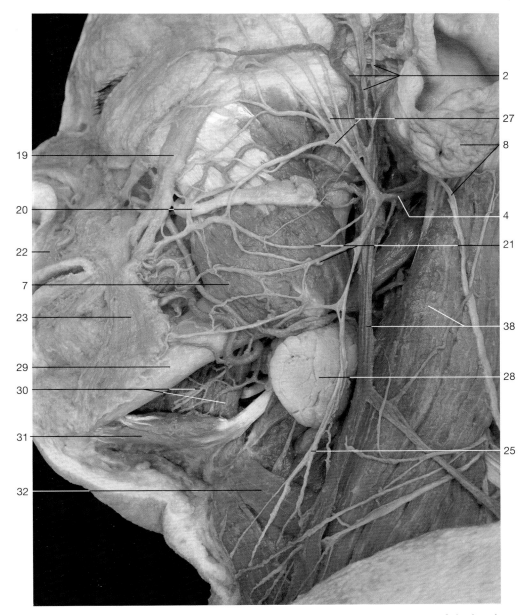

1   Temporoparietalis muscle
2   Superficial temporal artery
    and vein,
    and auriculotemporal nerve
3   Occipital belly of
    occipitofrontalis muscle and
    greater occipital nerve (C$_2$)
4   Facial nerve (n. VII)
5   Lesser occipital nerve and
    occipital artery
6   Transverse facial artery
7   Masseter muscle
8   Parotid gland and great
    auricular nerve
9   Splenius capitis muscle
10 Trapezius muscle
11 Punctum nervosum, point of
    distribution of cutaneous nerves
    of cervical plexus
12 Sternocleidomastoid muscle and
    external jugular vein
13 Supraclavicular nerves
14 Brachial plexus
15 Supra-orbital nerves
16 Orbicularis oculi muscle
17 Angular artery (terminal branch
    of facial artery)
18 Nasalis muscle
19 Zygomaticus major muscle
20 Parotid duct
21 Zygomatic and buccal
    branches of facial nerve
22 Orbicularis oris muscle
23 Depressor anguli oris muscle
24 Platysma muscle
25 Cervical branch of facial nerve
    (anastomosing with transverse
    cervical nerve of cervical plexus)
26 Facial artery and vein
27 Temporal branches of facial
    nerve
28 Submandibular gland
29 Mandible
30 Mylohyoideus muscle and nerve
31 Anterior belly of digastric
    muscle
32 Omohyoid muscle
33 Greater petrosal nerve
34 Geniculate ganglion
35 Chorda tympani
36 Posterior auricular nerve
37 Stylomastoid foramen
38 Sternocleidomastoid muscle
    and retromandibular vein

Deep dissection of facial nerve. Retromandibular and submandibular regions of the head (lateral aspect). The parotid gland has been removed.

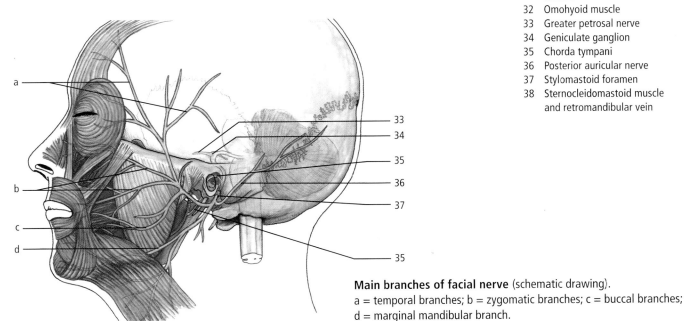

Main branches of facial nerve (schematic drawing).
a = temporal branches; b = zygomatic branches; c = buccal branches;
d = marginal mandibular branch.

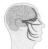

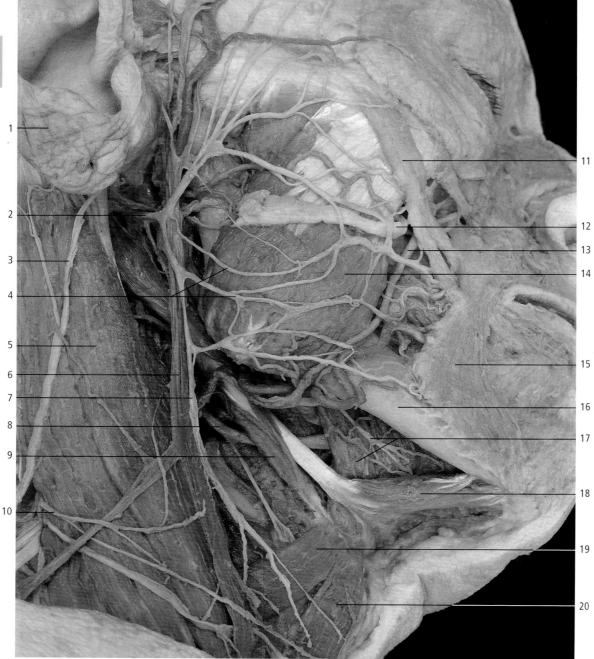

Deep dissection of facial nerve. Retromandibular and submandibular regions of the head (lateral aspect).
The parotid gland and the submandibular gland have been removed. The parotid plexus (4) is formed by anastomosis of the temporal, zygomatic, buccal, marginal mandibular, and cervical branches of the facial nerve, arising in the parotid gland.

1 Parotid gland	8 Hypoglossal nerve (n. XII)	15 Depressor anguli oris muscle
2 Facial nerve (n. VII)	9 Stylohyoid muscle	16 Mandible
3 Great auricular nerve	10 Transverse cervical nerve	17 Mylohyoid muscle and nerve
4 Parotid plexus	11 Zygomaticus major muscle	18 Anterior belly of digastric muscle
5 Sternocleidomastoid muscle	12 Parotid duct	19 Omohyoid muscle
6 Retromandibular vein	13 Facial artery	20 Sternohyoid muscle
7 Cervical branch of facial nerve	14 Masseter muscle	

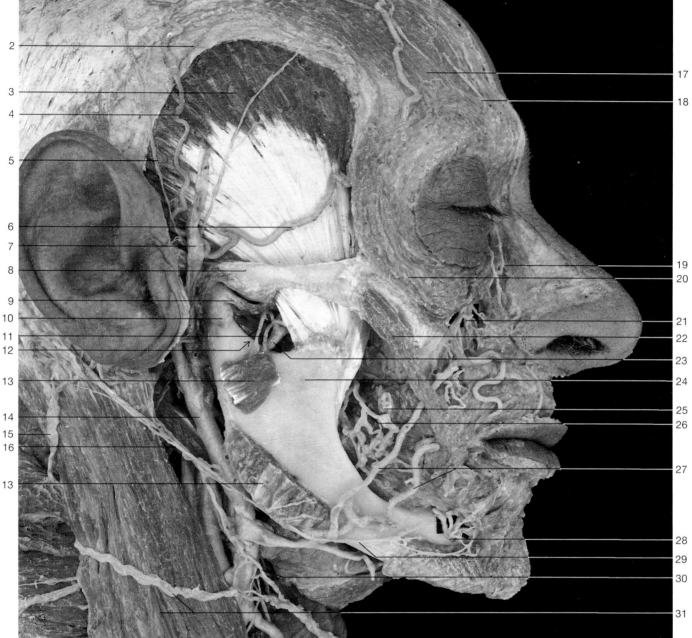

Lateral superficial aspect of the face. Masseter muscle and temporal fascia have been partly removed to display the masseteric artery and nerve.

1	Galea aponeurotica	
2	Temporal fascia	
3	Temporalis muscle	
4	Parietal branch of superficial temporal artery	
5	Auriculotemporal nerve	
6	Frontal branch of superficial temporal artery	
7	Superficial temporal vein	
8	Zygomatic arch	
9	Articular disc of temporomandibular joint	

10	Head of mandible
11	Masseteric artery and nerve
12	Mandibular notch
13	Masseter muscle (divided)
14	External carotid artery
15	Great auricular nerve
16	Facial nerve (reflected)
17	Frontal belly of occipitofrontalis muscle
18	Medial branch of supra-orbital nerve
19	Angular artery
20	Orbicularis oculi muscle
21	Infra-orbital nerve

22	Zygomaticus major muscle
23	Maxillary artery
24	Coronoid process
25	Parotid duct (divided)
26	Buccal nerve
27	Facial artery and vein
28	Mental nerve
29	Mandibular branch of facial nerve
30	Cervical branch of facial nerve
31	Transverse cervical nerve (communicating branch with facial nerve) and sternocleidomastoid muscle

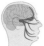

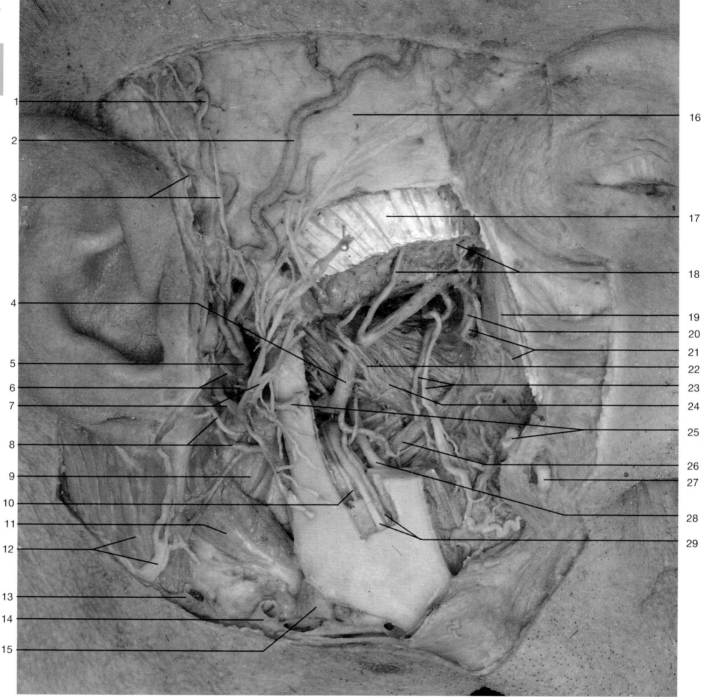

Deep dissection of facial and retromandibular regions. The coronoid process together with the insertions of temporalis muscle have been removed to display the maxillary artery. The upper part of the mandibular canal has been opened.

1 Parietal branch of the superficial temporal artery
2 Frontal branch of the superficial temporal artery
3 Auriculotemporal nerve
4 Maxillary artery
5 Superficial temporal artery
6 Communicating branches between facial and auriculotemporal nerves
7 Facial nerve
8 Posterior auricular artery and anterior auricular branch of superficial temporal artery
9 Internal jugular vein

10 Mylohyoid nerve
11 Posterior belly of digastric muscle
12 Great auricular nerve and sternocleidomastoid muscle
13 External jugular vein
14 Retromandibular vein
15 Submandibular gland
16 Temporal fascia
17 Temporalis tendon
18 Deep temporal arteries
19 Posterior superior alveolar nerve
20 Sphenopalatine artery
21 Posterior superior alveolar arteries

22 Masseteric artery and nerve
23 Buccal nerve and artery
24 Lateral pterygoid
25 Transverse facial artery and parotid duct (divided)
26 Medial pterygoid muscle
27 Facial artery
28 Lingual nerve
29 Inferior alveolar artery and nerve (mandibular canal opened)

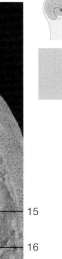

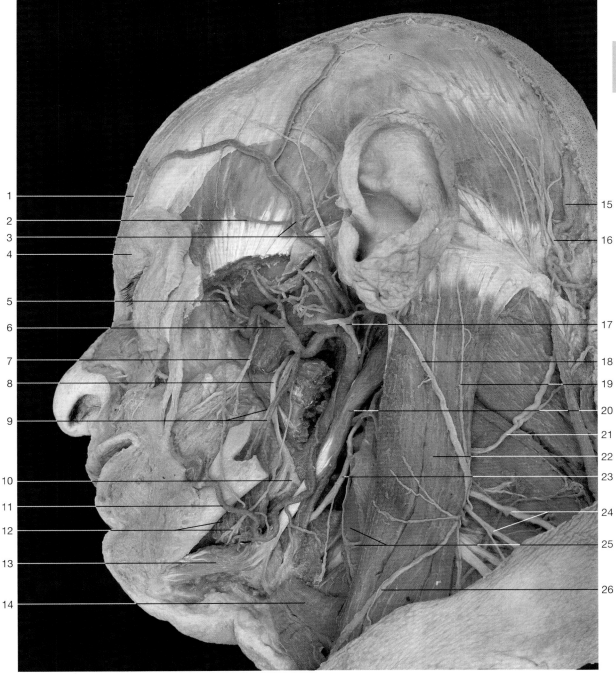

Peripharyngeal and retromandibular regions. The mandible has been partly removed (oblique lateral aspect).

1   Supra-orbital nerve (medial branch)
2   Temporalis muscle
3   Superficial temporal artery and auriculotemporal nerve
4   Orbicularis oculi muscle
5   Anterior deep temporal artery
6   Maxillary artery
7   Buccal nerve
8   Lingual nerve
9   Inferior alveolar nerve and artery
10 Submandibular ganglion
11 Facial artery
12 Mylohyoid muscle and nerve
13 Anterior belly of digastric muscle
14 Omohyoid muscle
15 Occipital artery
16 Greater occipital nerve (C$_2$)
17 Facial nerve (cut) (n. VII)
18 Great auricular nerve
19 Lesser occipital nerve
20 Posterior belly of digastric muscle
21 Accessory nerve (Var.)
22 Sternocleidomastoid muscle
23 Hypoglossus nerve (n. XII)
24 Supraclavicular nerves (lateral and intermedial branches)
25 Internal jugular vein and ansa cervicalis
26 Anterior supraclavicular nerve

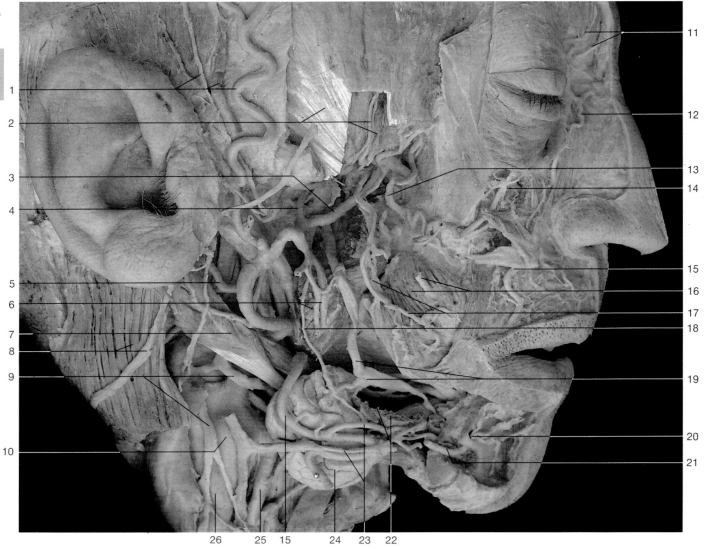

Dissection of deep facial and retromandibular regions after removal of mandible. Pterygoid muscles removed, temporalis muscle fenestrated.

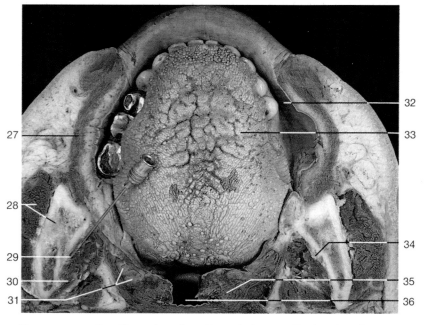

Transverse section through oral cavity and pharynx. The location of inferior alveolar nerve and artery is indicated by a needle.

1   Superficial temporal artery and vein and auriculotemporal nerve
2   Temporalis tendon, deep temporal nerves and artery
3   Maxillary artery
4   Middle meningeal artery
5   Occipital artery
6   Inferior alveolar artery and nerve
7   Posterior belly of digastric muscle
8   Great auricular nerve and sternocleidomastoid muscle
9   Hypoglossal nerve and superior root of ansa cervicalis
10 External carotid artery
11 Supratrochlear nerve and medial branch of supra-orbital artery
12 Angular artery
13 Posterior superior alveolar artery
14 Infra-orbital nerve
15 Facial artery
16 Parotid duct (divided) and buccinator muscle
17 Buccal artery and nerve

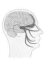

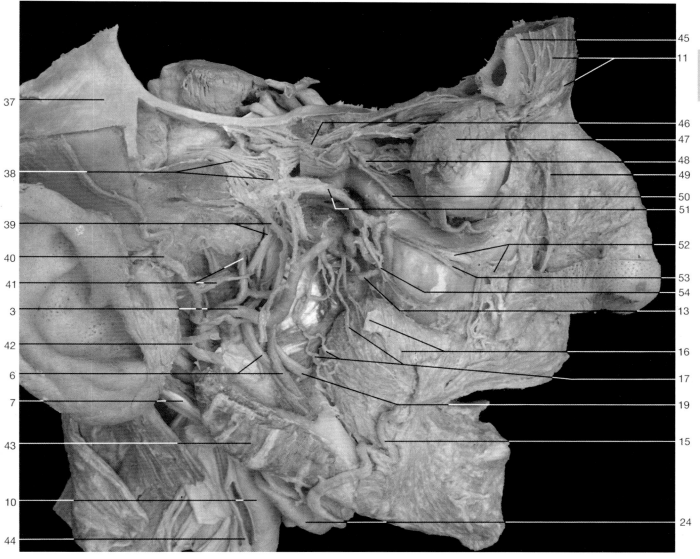

Para- and retropharyngeal regions. The mandible and the lateral wall of the orbit have been removed. The main branches of the trigeminal nerve and its ganglion are displayed.

18	Mylohyoid nerve	36	Pharynx
19	Lingual nerve and submandibular ganglion	37	Tentorium of cerebellum
20	Mental nerve and mental foramen	38	Trigeminal nerve and ganglion
21	Inferior alveolar nerve	39	Mandibular nerve
22	Mylohyoid muscle (divided) and hypoglossal nerve	40	Superficial temporal artery
23	Submental artery and vein	41	Auriculotemporal nerve and middle meningeal artery
24	Submandibular gland	42	Facial nerve (divided)
25	Superior thyroid artery	43	Masseter muscle
26	Common carotid artery	44	Superior root of ansa cervicalis
27	Buccinator muscle	45	Lateral branch of supra-orbital nerve
28	Masseter muscle and mandible	46	Ophthalmic nerve
29	Entrance of mandibular canal	47	Lacrimal gland
30	Medial pterygoid muscle	48	Ciliary ganglion and short ciliary nerves
31	Palatine tonsil	49	Angular artery
32	Oral vestibule	50	Inferior branch of oculomotor nerve
33	Tongue	51	Maxillary nerve
34	Inferior alveolar nerve, artery, and vein	52	Infra-orbital nerve
35	Pharyngeal constrictor muscle	53	Anterior superior alveolar nerve
		54	Posterior superior alveolar nerve

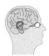

2.3 Brain and Sensory Organs

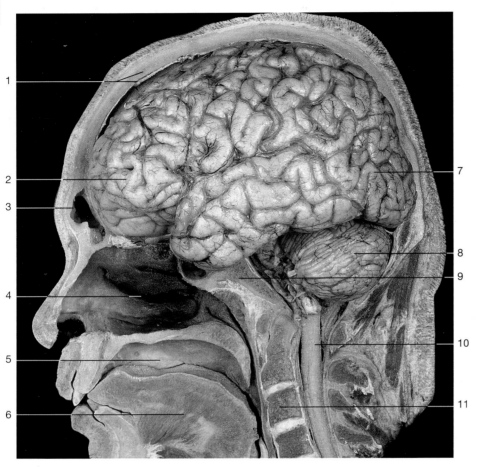

The cranial cavity harbours the brain, the cerebellum, and the brain stem from where the cranial nerves emerge and exit the skull through various openings and fissures. The great sensory organs are located within the orbit (eye), the nasal cavity (olfactory system), and the petrous portion of the temporal bone (vestibulocochlear organ). The brain is enwrapped by the pia mater containing the brain vessels. The dura mater is firmly attached to the skull and provides shelter and stabilization for the brain. Interposed between pia and dura mater lies the arachnoid containing the cerebrospinal fluid.

Dissection of the brain with pia mater and arachnoid in situ. The head is cut in half except for the brain, which is shown in its entirety.

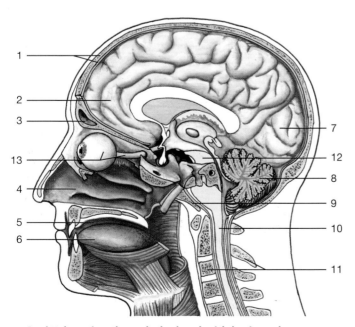

1   Vertex of the skull and dura mater
2   Frontal lobe covered by arachnoid
    and pia mater
3   Frontal sinus
4   Nasal cavity
5   Oral cavity
6   Tongue
7   Occipital lobe
8   Cerebellum
9   Base of skull
10 Spinal cord
11 Vertebral column
12 Brain stem
13 Eye and optic nerve (n. II)

Sagittal section through the head with brain and sensory organs (schematic drawing). The eye with the optic nerve is located within the orbit; the labyrinth organ, within the petrous bone.

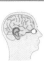

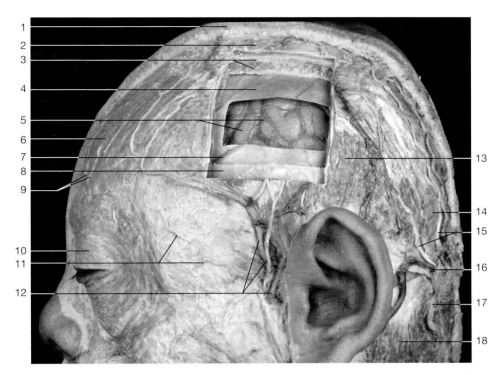

1   Skin
2   Galea aponeurotica
3   Skull diploe
4   Dura mater
5   Arachnoid and pia mater
     with cerebral vessels
6   Frontal belly of occipitofrontalis
     muscle
7   Branch of middle meningeal artery
8   Pericranium (periosteum)
9   Lateral and medial branches of
     supra-orbital nerve
10 Orbicularis oculi muscle
11 Zygomatico-orbital artery
12 Auriculotemporal nerve and
     superficial temporal artery and
     vein
13 Superior auricular muscle
14 Occipital belly of occipitofrontalis
     muscle
15 Occipital nerve
16 Occipital artery and vein
17 Greater occipital nerve
18 Sternocleidomastoid muscle
19 Frontal lobe
20 Chiasmatic cistern
21 Interpeduncular cistern
22 Arachnoid granulations
23 Subarachnoid space
24 Superior sagittal sinus
25 Inferior sagittal sinus
26 Corpus callosum
27 Straight sinus
28 Confluence of sinuses
29 Cerebellum
30 Cerebellomedullar cistern
31 Cerebral cortex

Lateral aspect of the head. Scalp, vertex of the skull, and meninges are demonstrated by a series of window-like openings.

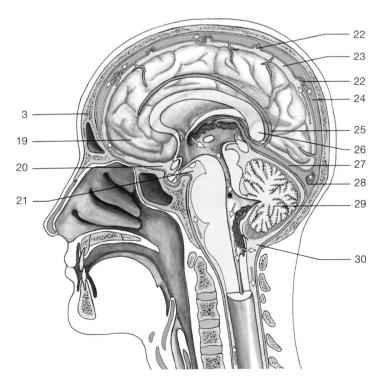

Subarachnoid cisterns of the brain (midsagittal section).
Green = cisterns; blue = dural sinus and ventricles;
red = choroid plexus of third and fourth ventricles; arrows = flow of
cerebrospinal fluid.

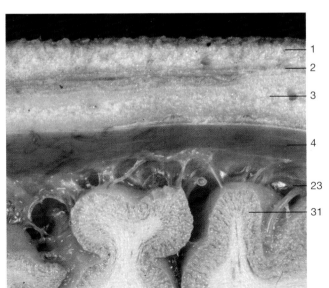

Cross section of the scalp and the meninges.
The subarachnoid space (23) is shown.

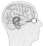

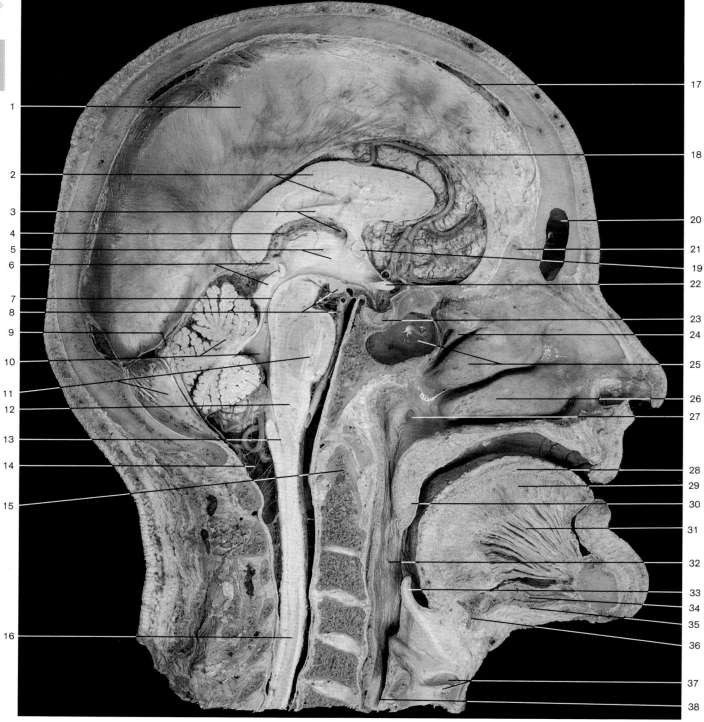

Median sagittal section through the head and neck.

1	Falx cerebri	14	Cerebellomedullary cistern
2	Corpus callosum and septum pellucidum	15	Dens of the axis (odontoid process)
3	Interventricular foramen and fornix	16	Spinal cord
4	Choroid plexus of third ventricle and internal cerebral vein	17	Superior sagittal sinus
5	Third ventricle and interthalamic adhesion	18	Anterior cerebral artery
6	Pineal body and colliculi of the midbrain	19	Anterior commissure
7	Cerebral aqueduct	20	Frontal sinus
8	Mamillary body and basilar artery	21	Crista galli
9	Straight sinus	22	Optic chiasma
10	Fourth ventricle and cerebellum	23	Pituitary gland (hypophysis)
11	Pons and falx cerebelli	24	Superior nasal concha
12	Medulla oblongata	25	Middle nasal concha and sphenoid sinus
13	Central canal	26	Inferior nasal concha

27 Pharyngeal opening of auditory tube
28 Superior longitudinal muscle of tongue
29 Vertical muscle of the tongue
30 Uvula
31 Genioglossus muscle
32 Pharynx
33 Epiglottis
34 Geniohyoid muscle
35 Mylohyoid muscle
36 Hyoid bone
37 Vocal fold and sinus of larynx
38 Esophagus

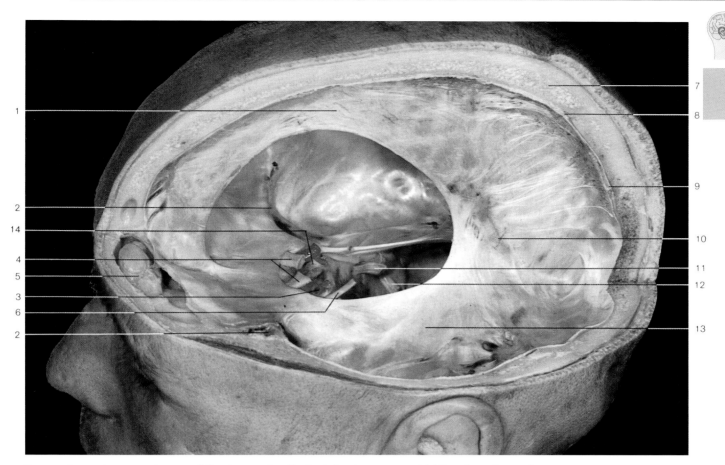

Dura mater and venous sinuses of the dura mater. The brain has been removed (oblique lateral aspect).

1   Falx cerebri
2   Position of middle meningeal
    artery and vein
3   Internal carotid artery
4   Optic nerve (n. II)
5   Frontal sinus
6   Oculomotor nerve (n. III)
7   Diploe
8   Dura mater
9   Superior sagittal sinus
10 Straight sinus
11 Trigeminal nerve (n. V)
12 Facial and vestibulocochlear nerve
    (n. VII and n. VIII)
13 Tentorium cerebelli
14 Pituitary gland (hypophysis)
15 Inferior sagittal sinus
16 Sigmoid sinus
17 Confluence of sinuses
18 Inferior petrosal sinus
19 Transverse sinus
20 Superior petrosal sinus
21 Cavernous and intercavernous sinuses

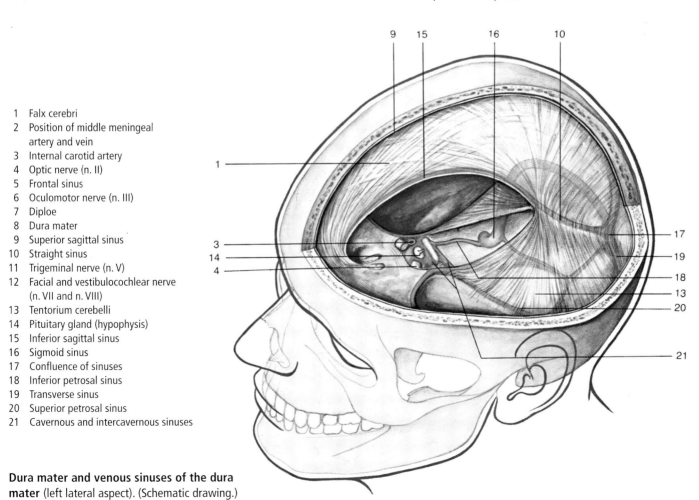

Dura mater and venous sinuses of the dura mater (left lateral aspect). (Schematic drawing.)

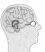

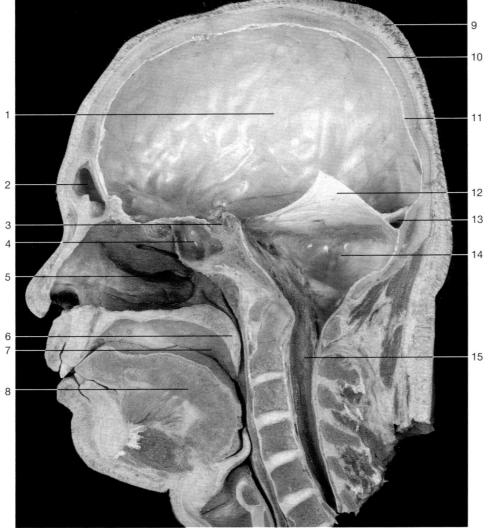

1   Cranial cavity with dura mater (right cerebral hemisphere has been removed)
2   Frontal sinus
3   Hypophysial fossa with pituitary gland
4   Sphenoidal sinus
5   Nasal cavity
6   Soft palate (uvula)
7   Oral cavity
8   Tongue
9   Skin
10 Calvaria
11 Dura mater
12 Tentorium cerebelli
13 Confluence of sinuses
14 Infratentorial space (cerebellum and part of the brain stem have been removed)
15 Vertebral canal
16 Frontal branch of middle meningeal artery and veins
17 Middle meningeal artery
18 Diploe
19 Parietal branch of middle meningeal artery and vein
20 Occipital pole of left hemisphere covered with dura mater

Median section through the head. Demonstration of dura mater covering the cranial cavity. Brain and spinal cord are removed (right half of the head, as seen from medial).

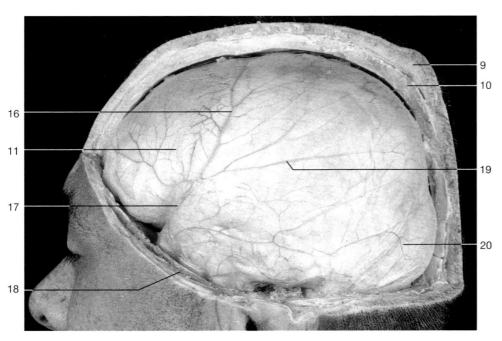

Dissection of dura mater and meningeal vessels. Left half of calvaria removed.

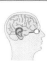

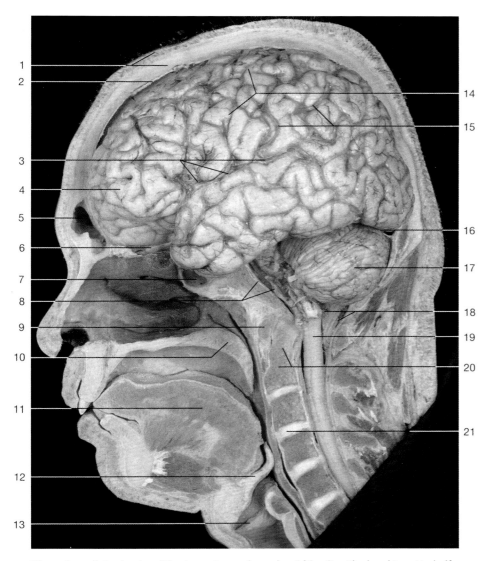

1   Calvaria and skin of the scalp
2   Dura mater (divided)
3   Position of lateral sulcus
4   Frontal lobe covered by arachnoid and pia mater
5   Frontal sinus
6   Olfactory bulb
7   Sphenoidal sinus
8   Dura mater on clivus and basilar artery
9   Atlas (anterior arch, divided)
10 Soft palate
11 Tongue
12 Epiglottis
13 Vocal fold
14 Position of central sulcus
15 Superior cerebral veins
16 Tentorium (divided)
17 Cerebellum
18 Cerebellomedullary cistern
19 Position of foramen magnum and spinal cord
20 Dens of axis
21 Intervertebral disc

Dissection of the brain with pia mater and arachnoid in situ. The head is cut in half except for the brain, which is shown in its entirety.

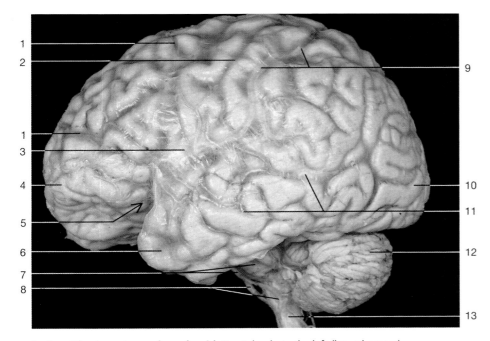

1   Superior cerebral veins
2   Position of central sulcus
3   Position of lateral sulcus and cistern of lateral cerebral fossa
4   Frontal pole
5   Lateral sulcus (arrow)
6   Temporal pole
7   Pons and basilar artery
8   Vertebral arteries
9   Superior anastomotic vein
10 Occipital pole
11 Inferior cerebral veins
12 Hemisphere of cerebellum
13 Medulla oblongata

Brain with pia mater and arachnoid. Frontal pole to the left (lateral aspect).

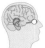

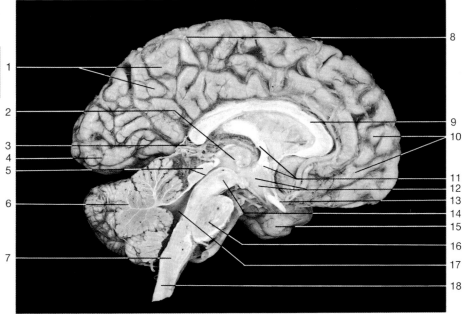

1 Parietal lobe
2 Thalamus, third ventricle, and intermediate mass
3 Great cerebral vein
4 Occipital lobe
5 Colliculi of the midbrain and cerebral aqueduct
6 Cerebellum
7 Medulla oblongata
8 Central sulcus
9 Corpus callosum
10 Frontal lobe
11 Fornix and anterior commissure
12 Hypothalamus
13 Optic chiasma
14 Midbrain
15 Temporal lobe
16 Pons
17 Fourth ventricle
18 Spinal cord
19 Inferior concha and nasal cavity
20 Alveolar process of maxilla
21 Tongue
22 Dens of axis
23 Oral part of pharynx
24 Alveolar process of mandible
25 Epiglottis

Brain and brain stem, median section. Frontal pole to the right.

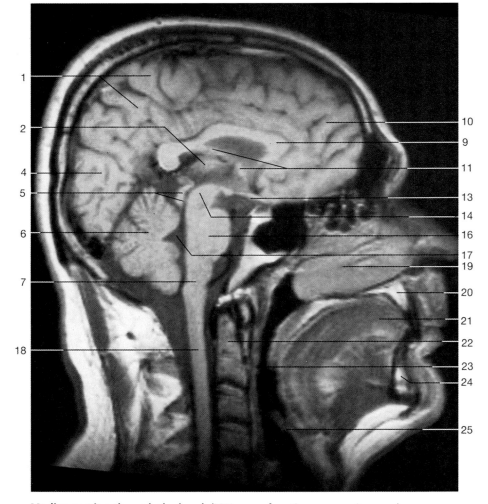

Median section through the head. (MRI scan, cf. section on opposite page.)

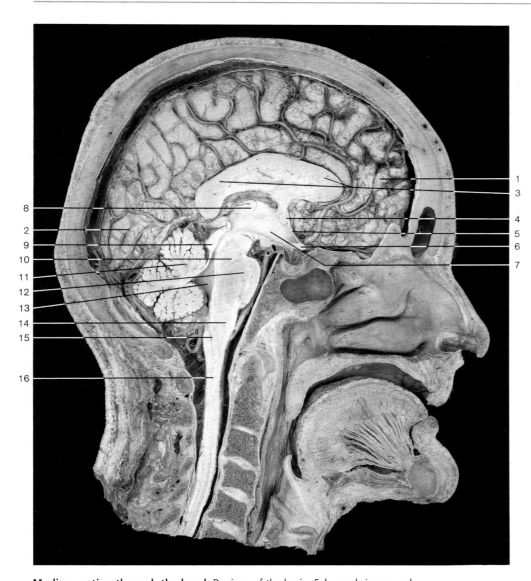

1 Frontal lobe of cerebrum
2 Occipital lobe of cerebrum
3 Corpus callosum
4 Anterior commissure
5 Lamina terminalis
6 Optic chiasma
7 Hypothalamus
8 Thalamus and third ventricle
9 Colliculi of the midbrain
10 Midbrain (inferior portion)
11 Cerebellum
12 Pons
13 Fourth ventricle
14 Medulla oblongata
15 Central canal
16 Spinal cord

Median section through the head. Regions of the brain. Falx cerebri removed.

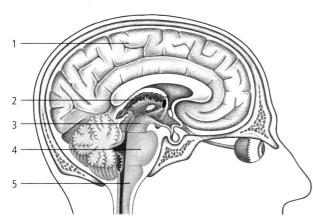

Scheme of brain divisions (cf. table). (Schematic drawing.)
Red = choroidal plexus.

1 Telencephalon (yellow) with lateral ventricles
2 Diencephalon (orange) with third ventricle, optic nerve, and retina
3 Mesencephalon (blue) with cerebral aqueduct
4 Metencephalon (green) with fourth ventricle
5 Myelencephalon (yellow-green)

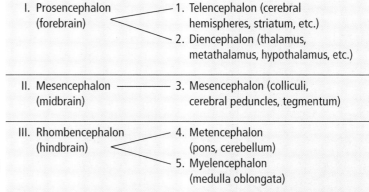

I. Prosencephalon (forebrain)	1. Telencephalon (cerebral hemispheres, striatum, etc.)
	2. Diencephalon (thalamus, metathalamus, hypothalamus, etc.)
II. Mesencephalon (midbrain)	3. Mesencephalon (colliculi, cerebral peduncles, tegmentum)
III. Rhombencephalon (hindbrain)	4. Metencephalon (pons, cerebellum)
	5. Myelencephalon (medulla oblongata)

Main divisions of the brain
I–III = primary brain vesicles; 1–5 = secondary brain vesicles

Diencephalon, midbrain, pons, and medulla oblongata are collectively termed the **brain stem.**

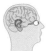

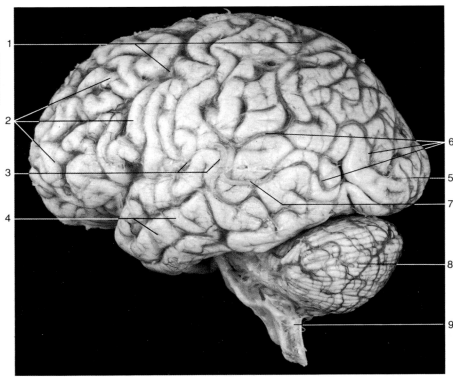

1   Superior cerebral veins and
    parietal lobe
2   Frontal lobe
3   Superficial middle cerebral vein and
    cistern of lateral cerebral fossa
4   Temporal lobe
5   Occipital lobe
6   Inferior cerebral veins and
    transverse occipital sulcus
7   Inferior anastomotic vein
8   Cerebellum
9   Medulla oblongata

Brain with pia mater. Cerebral veins (bluish). In the lateral sulcus the cistern of the
lateral fossa is recognizable. Frontal lobe to the left.

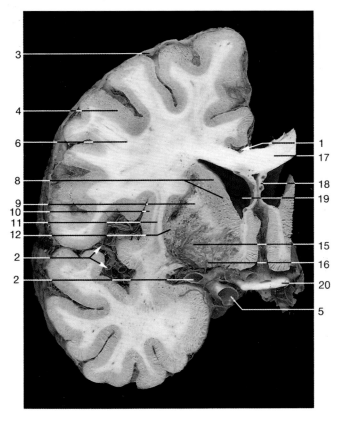

Arteries of the brain. Coronal section. Areas supplied by
cortical and central arteries. Dotted lines indicate boundaries of
arterial supply areas; arrows = direction of blood flow.

◁ **Coronal section through the right hemisphere,** showing
arachnoid, pia mater, and the arterial blood supply (anterior
aspect).

1	Anterior cerebral artery	8	Caudate nucleus	15	Pallidostriate artery
2	Middle cerebral arteries	9	Internal capsule	16	Thalamic artery
3	Arachnoid	10	Insular lobe	17	Corpus callosum
4	Cortex	11	Claustrum	18	Septum pellucidum
5	Internal carotid artery	12	Putamen	19	Lateral ventricle
6	Frontal lobe (white matter)	13	Posterior striate branch	20	Optic chiasma
7	Posterior cerebral artery	14	Insular artery		

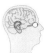

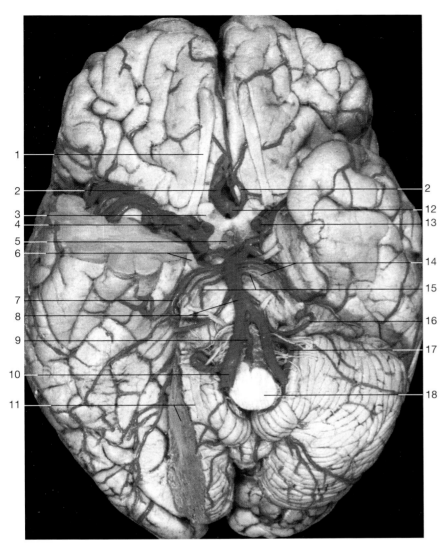

1 Olfactory tract
2 Anterior cerebral artery
3 Optic nerve (n. II)
4 Middle cerebral artery
5 Infundibulum
6 Oculomotor nerve (n. III) and posterior communicating artery
7 Posterior cerebral artery
8 Basilar artery and abducent nerve (n. VI)
9 Anterior spinal artery
10 Vertebral artery
11 Cerebellum
12 Anterior communicating artery
13 Internal carotid artery
14 Superior cerebellar artery and pons
15 Labyrinthine arteries
16 Inferior anterior cerebellar artery
17 Inferior posterior cerebellar artery
18 Medulla oblongata
19 Supratrochlear artery
20 Anterior ciliary arteries
21 Lacrimal artery
22 Posterior ciliary arteries
23 Ophthalmic artery with central retinal artery
24 Trigeminal nerve (n. V)
25 Facial nerve (n. VII) and vestibulocochlear nerve (n. VIII)
26 Glossopharyngeal nerve (n. IX), vagus nerve (n. X), and accessory nerve (n. XI)
27 Olfactory bulb
28 Posterior spinal artery

Arteries of the brain (inferior aspect, frontal pole above). Right temporal lobe and cerebellum partly removed.

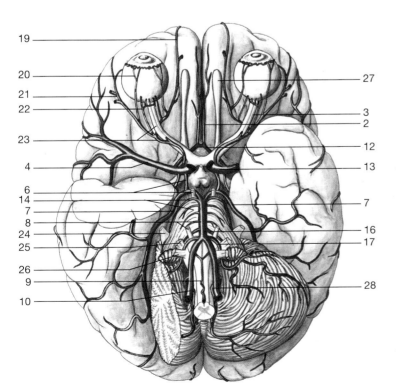

Arteries of the brain (inferior aspect). Right temporal lobe and cerebellum partly removed. Note the arterial circle of Willis around the infundibulum.

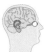

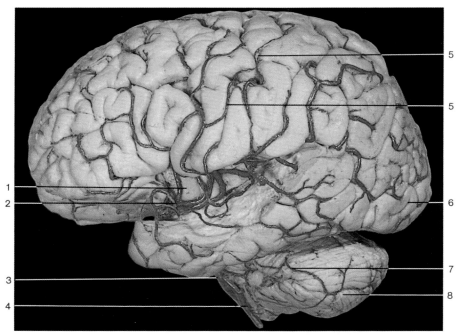

1 Insula
2 Middle cerebral artery (2 branches:
   a Parietal branches,
   b Temporal branches)
3 Basilar artery
4 Vertebral artery
5 Central sulcus
6 Occipital lobe
7 Superior cerebellar artery
8 Cerebellum
9 Anterior cerebral artery
10 Ethmoidal arteries
11 Ophthalmic artery
12 Internal carotid artery
13 Posterior communicating artery
14 Posterior cerebral artery
15 Anterior inferior cerebellar artery
16 Posterior inferior cerebellar artery

Cerebral arteries. Lateral aspect of
the left hemisphere. The upper part of
the temporal lobe has been removed to
display the insula and cerebral arteries.

◁ **Arteries of the brain.**

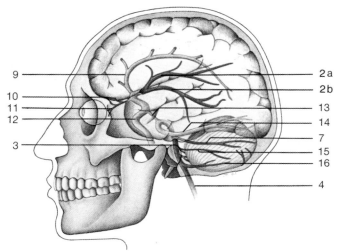

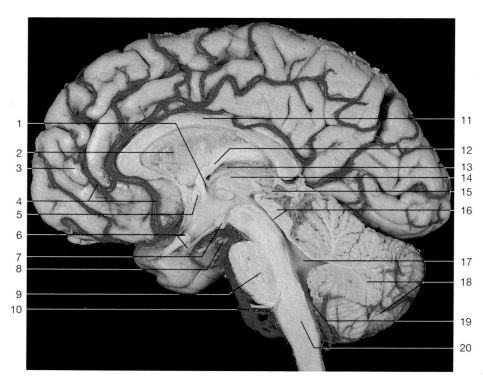

1 Interventricular foramen
2 Septum pellucidum
3 Frontal lobe
4 Anterior cerebral artery
5 Anterior commissure
6 Optic chiasma and infundibulum
7 Mamillary body
8 Oculomotor nerve (n. III)
9 Pons
10 Basilar artery
11 Corpus callosum
12 Fornix
13 Choroid plexus
14 Third ventricle
15 Pineal body
16 Tectum and cerebral aqueduct
17 Fourth ventricle
18 Cerebellum (arbor vitae, vermis)
19 Median aperture of Magendie
20 Medulla oblongata

**Median section through the brain
and brain stem.** Cerebral arteries
injected with red resin.

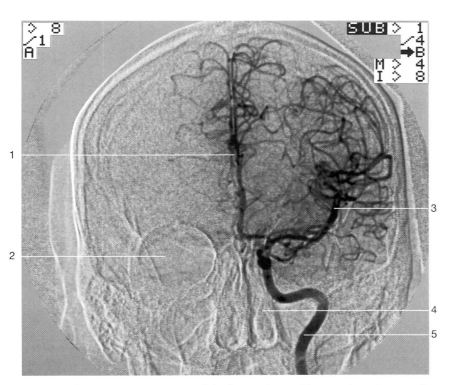

1	Anterior cerebral artery
2	Orbit
3	Middle cerebral artery
4	Nasal cavity
5	Internal carotid artery
6	Arterial circle of Willis
7	Posterior communicating artery
8	Posterior cerebral artery
9	Basilar artery
10	Vertebral artery
11	Subclavian artery
12	Aortic arch
13	Common carotid artery

Arteries of the brain. Angiogram of the internal carotid artery (anterior aspect) (courtesy of Prof. Dr. W. Huk, University of Erlangen-Nürnberg).

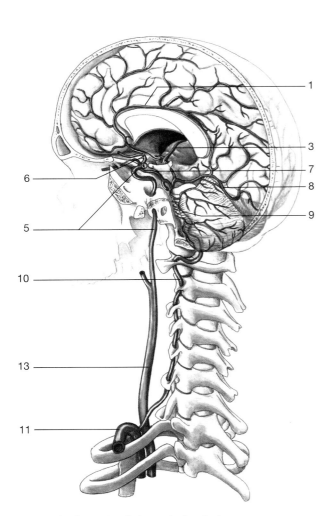

Cerebral arteries (schematic drawing).
Left hemisphere and brain stem have been removed.
Note the arterial circle of Willis around the sella turcica.

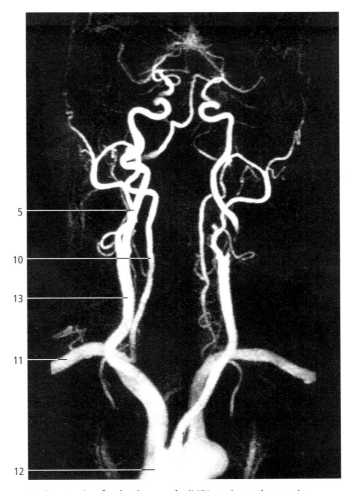

Main arteries for brain supply (MRI angiograph, anterior aspect, courtesy of Prof. Dr. W. Bautz, University of Erlangen-Nürnberg).

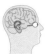

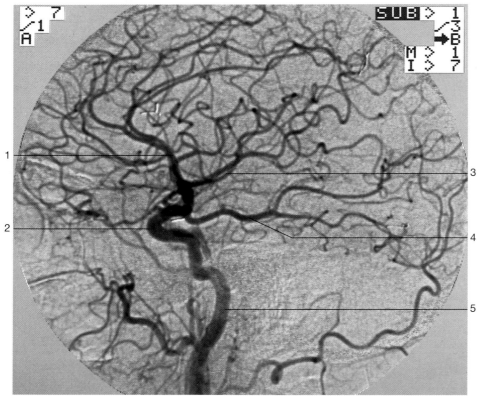

1 Anterior cerebral artery
2 Loop of the internal carotid artery
3 Middle cerebral artery
4 Posterior cerebral artery
5 Internal carotid artery
6 Superior cerebellar artery
7 Anterior inferior cerebellar artery
8 Posterior inferior cerebellar artery
9 Vertebral artery

Arteries of the brain. Angiogram of the internal carotid artery (lateral aspect) (courtesy of Prof. Dr. W. Huk, University of Erlangen-Nürnberg).

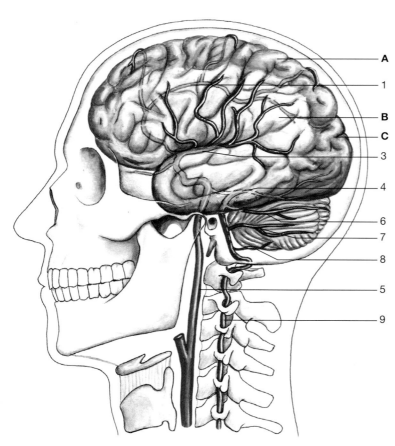

Cerebral arteries. The areas supplied by the main arteries are indicated by different colors (lateral aspect).

Areas of blood supply of the brain (cerebellum = light blue).

A = anterior cerebral artery (upper and medial parts of the cortex) (orange)

B = middle cerebral artery (lateral areas of the frontal, parietal, and temporal lobes) (white)

C = posterior cerebral artery (occipital lobe and inferior parts of the temporal lobe) (blue)

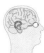

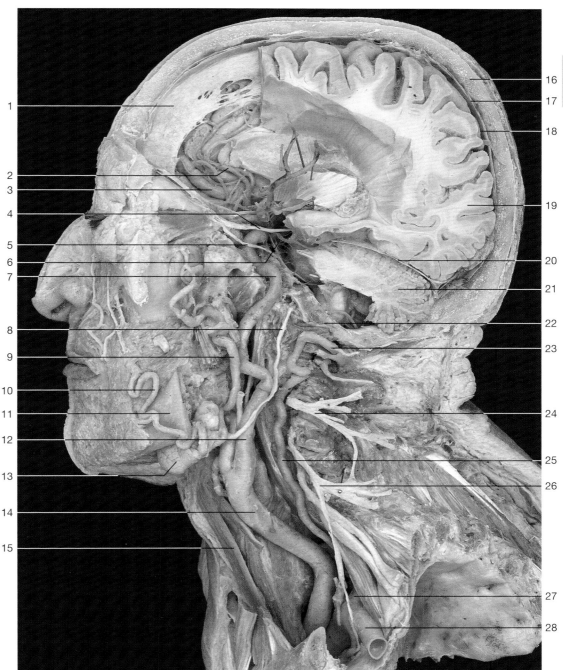

Dissection of the arteries of the brain and head (lateral aspect, superficial layers of facial region and left hemisphere and cerebellum partly removed).

1	Falx cerebri	16	Calvaria
2	Anterior cerebral artery	17	Dura mater
3	Frontal lobe	18	Subarachnoidal space
4	Oculomotor nerve (n. III)	19	Occipital lobe
5	Abducent nerve (n. VI)	20	Tentorium of cerebellum
6	Posterior cerebral artery	21	Cerebellum
7	Internal carotid artery, entering sinus cavernosus	22	Base of skull
		23	Vertebral artery (on the posterior arch of the atlas)
8	Hypoglossus nerve (n. XII)		
9	Maxillary artery	24	Cervical plexus
10	Facial artery	25	Vertebral artery (removed from the cervical vertebrae)
11	Mandible		
12	External carotid artery	26	Brachial plexus
13	Submandibular gland	27	Vertebral artery (branching from the subclavian artery)
14	Common carotid artery		
15	Sternohyoid muscle	28	Subclavian artery

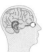

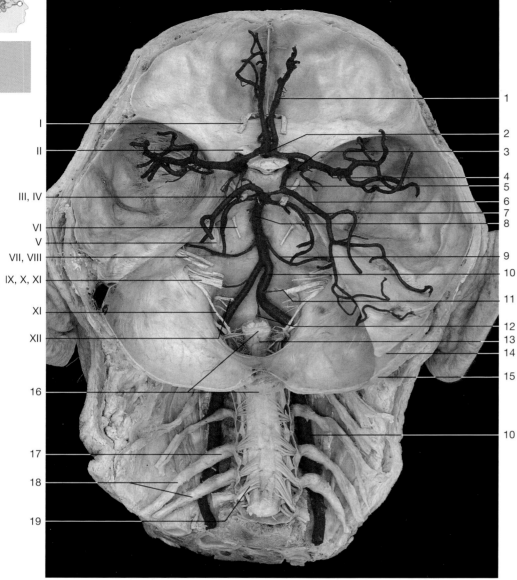

1   Anterior cerebral artery
2   Anterior communicating artery
3   Internal carotid artery
4   Medial cerebral artery
5   Posterior communicating artery
6   Posterior cerebral artery
7   Superior cerebellar artery
8   Basilar artery
9   Anterior inferior cerebellar
    artery with the artery of the   *AICA*
    labyrinth
10 Vertebral artery
11 Posterior inferior cerebellar   *PICA*
    artery
12 Anterior spinal artery
13 Pia mater of spinal cord
14 Tentorium cerebelli
15 Dura mater of the cranial cavity
16 Spinal cord
17 Spinal ganglion
18 Spinal nerves (C₃, C₄)
19 Posterior root filaments
    (fila radicularia post.)
20 Ophthalmic artery
    (within the orbit)
21 Internal carotid artery
    (within carotid canal)
22 Posterior spinal artery

I   Olfactory tract
II   Optic nerve
III   Oculomotor nerve
IV   Trochlear nerve
V   Trigeminal nerve
VI   Abducent nerve
VII   Facial nerve
VIII Vestibulocochlear nerve
IX   Glossopharyngeal nerve
X   Vagus nerve
XI   Accessory nerve
XII   Hypoglossus nerve

Dissection of the arterial circle of the cerebrum at the base of the skull
(from above; calvaria and brain have been removed; arteries are colored in red, cranial nerves
[n. I–XII] in yellow).

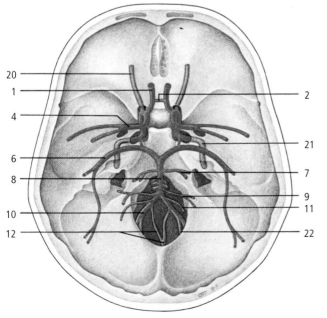

Arterial circle of Willis (superior aspect).
(Schematic drawing.)

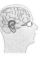

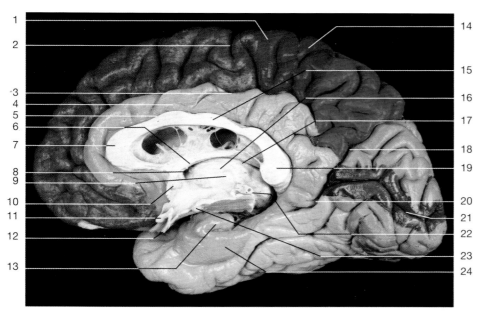

1
2
3
4
5
6
7
8
9
10
11
12
13

14
15
16
17
18
19
20
21
22
23
24

1 Precentral gyrus
2 Precentral sulcus
3 Cingulate sulcus
4 Cingulate gyrus
5 Sulcus of corpus callosum
6 Fornix
7 Genu of corpus callosum
8 Interventricular foramen
9 Intermediate mass
10 Anterior commissure
11 Optic chiasma
12 Infundibulum
13 Uncus hippocampi
14 Postcentral gyrus
15 Body of corpus callosum
16 Third ventricle and thalamus
17 Stria medullaris
18 Parieto-occipital sulcus
19 Splenium of corpus callosum
20 Communication of calcarine and parieto-occipital sulcus
21 Calcarine sulcus
22 Pineal body
23 Mamillary body
24 Parahippocampal gyrus
25 Olfactory bulb
26 Olfactory tract
27 Gyrus rectus
28 Optic nerve
29 Infundibulum and optic chiasma
30 Optic tract
31 Oculomotor nerve
32 Pedunculus cerebri
33 Red nucleus
34 Cerebral aqueduct
35 Corpus callosum
36 Longitudinal fissure
37 Orbital gyri
38 Lateral root of olfactory tract
39 Medial root of olfactory tract
40 Olfactory tubercle and anterior perforated substance
41 Tuber cinereum
42 Interpeduncular fossa
43 Substantia nigra
44 Colliculi of the midbrain
45 Lateral occipitotemporal gyrus
46 Medial occipitotemporal gyrus

Brain, right hemisphere (medial aspect). Frontal pole to the left (midbrain divided, cerebellum and inferior part of brain stem removed).

Red	= Frontal lobe	Dark blue	= Postcentral lobe
Blue	= Parietal lobe	Dark green	= Calcarine sulcus
Green	= Occipital lobe	Dark yellow	= Limbic cortex
Yellow	= Temporal lobe		(cingulate and
Dark red	= Precentral lobe		parahippocampal gyri)

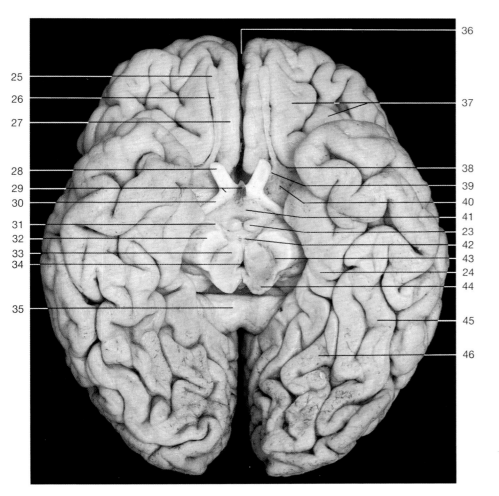

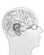

25
26
27
28
29
30
31
32
33
34
35

36
37
38
39
40
41
23
42
43
24
44
45
46

Brain (inferior aspect). Midbrain divided. Cerebellum and inferior part of brain stem removed. Frontal pole at the top.

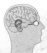

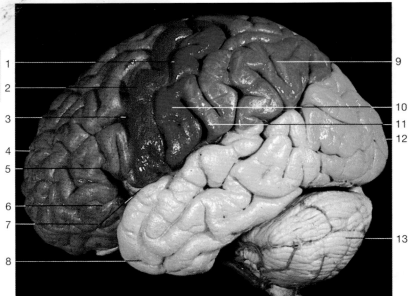

1	Central sulcus
2	Precentral gyrus
3	Precentral sulcus
4	Frontal lobe
5	Anterior ascending ramus of lateral sulcus
6	Anterior horizontal ramus of lateral sulcus
7	Lateral sulcus
8	Temporal lobe
9	Parietal lobe
10	Postcentral gyrus
11	Postcentral sulcus
12	Occipital lobe
13	Cerebellum
14	Superior frontal sulcus
15	Middle frontal gyrus
16	Lunate sulcus
17	Longitudinal fissure
18	Arachnoid granulations

Brain, left hemisphere (lateral aspect). Frontal pole to the left.

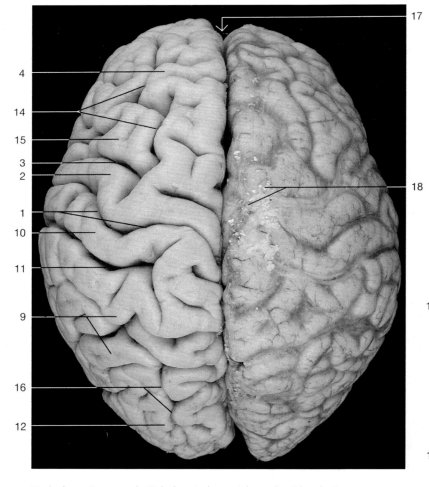

Pink	=	Frontal lobe
Blue	=	Parietal lobe
Green	=	Occipital lobe
Yellow	=	Temporal lobe
Dark red	=	Precentral gyrus
Dark blue	=	Postcentral gyrus

Brain (superior aspect). Right hemisphere with arachnoid and pia mater.

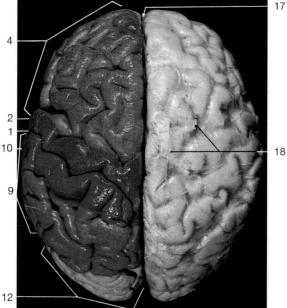

Brain (superior aspect). Lobes of the left hemisphere indicated by color; right hemisphere is covered with arachnoid and pia mater.

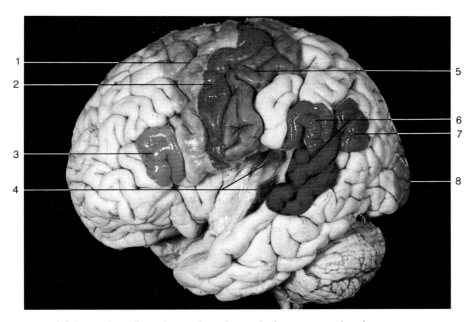

1 Premotor area
2 Somatomotor area
3 Motor speech area of Broca
4 Acoustic area
  (red: high tone, dark green: low tone)
5 Somatosensory area
6 Sensory speech area of Wernicke
7 Reading comprehension area
8 Visuosensory area

Brain, left hemisphere (lateral aspect). **Main cortical areas** are colored.
The lateral sulcus has been opened to display the insula and the inner surface of the temporal lobe.

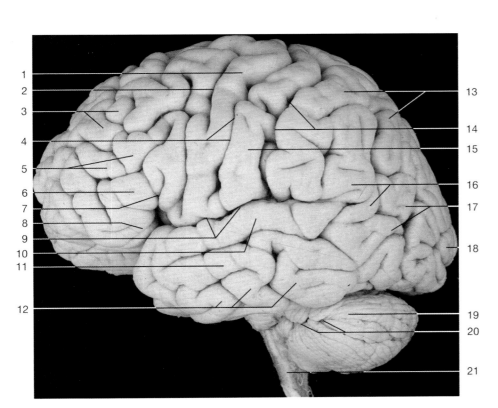

1 Precentral gyrus
2 Precentral sulcus
3 Superior frontal gyrus
4 Central sulcus
5 Middle frontal gyrus
6 Inferior frontal gyrus
7 Ascending ramus ⎤
8 Horizontal ramus ⎬ of lateral sulcus
9 Posterior ramus ⎦
10 Superior temporal gyrus
11 Middle temporal gyrus
12 Inferior temporal gyrus
13 Parietal lobe
14 Postcentral sulcus
15 Postcentral gyrus
16 Supramarginal gyrus
17 Angular gyrus
18 Occipital lobe
19 Cerebellum
20 Horizontal fissure of cerebellum
21 Medulla oblongata

Brain, left hemisphere (lateral aspect). Frontal pole to the left.

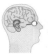

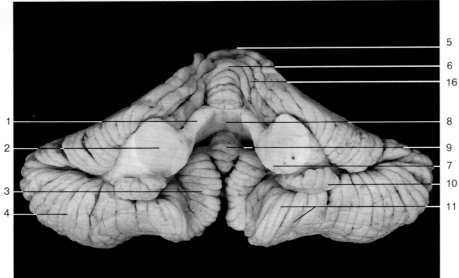

1. Superior cerebellar peduncle
2. Middle cerebellar peduncle
3. Cerebellar tonsil
4. Inferior semilunar lobule
5. Vermis
6. Central lobule of vermis
7. Inferior cerebellar peduncle
8. Superior medullary velum
9. Nodule of vermis
10. Flocculus of cerebellum
11. Biventral lobule
12. Left cerebellar hemisphere
13. Inferior semilunar lobule
14. Biventral lobule
15. Vermis of cerebellum
16. Tuber of vermis
17. Pyramid of vermis
18. Uvula of vermis
19. Tonsil of cerebellum
20. Flocculus of cerebellum
21. Right cerebellar hemisphere
22. Vermis (central lobule)
23. Cerebellar lingula
24. Ala of central lobule
25. Superior cerebellar peduncle
26. Fastigium
27. Fourth ventricle
28. Middle cerebellar peduncle
29. Nodule of vermis
30. Flocculus of cerebellum
31. Cerebellar tonsil
32. Culmen of vermis
33. Declive of vermis
34. Tuber of vermis
35. Inferior semilunar lobule
36. Pyramid of vermis (cut)
37. Uvula of vermis

Cerebellum (inferior anterior aspect). The cerebellar peduncles have been severed.

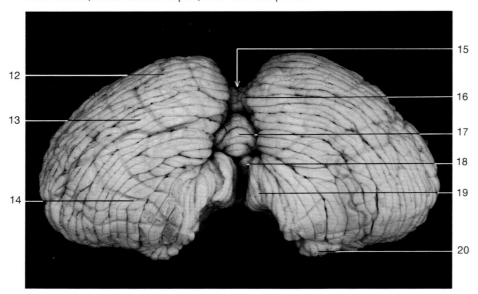

Cerebellum (inferior posterior aspect).

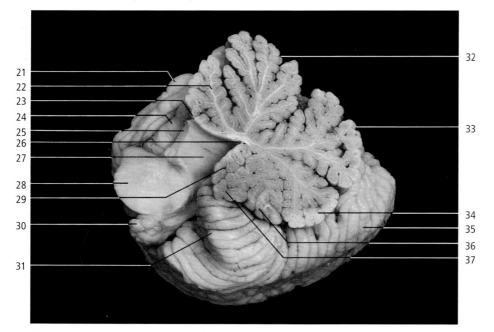

Median section through the cerebellum. Right cerebellar hemisphere and right half of vermis.

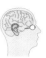

1   Olfactory bulb
2   Olfactory tract
3   Lateral olfactory stria
4   Anterior perforated substance
5   Infundibulum (divided)
6   Mamillary body
7   Substantia nigra
8   Cerebral peduncle (cut)
9   Red nucleus
10 Decussation of superior cerebellar peduncle
11 Cerebellar hemisphere
12 Medial olfactory stria
13 Optic nerve
14 Optic chiasma
15 Optic tract
16 Posterior perforated substance
17 Interpeduncular fossa
18 Superior cerebellar peduncle and cerebellorubral tract
19 Dentate nucleus
20 Vermis of cerebellum
21 Cingulate gyrus
22 Corpus callosum
23 Stria terminalis
24 Septum pellucidum
25 Columna fornicis
26 Cerebral peduncle at midbrain level
27 Pons
28 Inferior olive
29 Medulla oblongata with lateral pyramidal tract
30 Occipital lobe
31 Calcarine sulcus
32 Thalamus
33 Inferior colliculus with brachium
34 Medial lemniscus
35 Superior cerebellar peduncle
36 Inferior cerebellar peduncle
37 Middle cerebellar peduncle
38 Cerebellar hemisphere

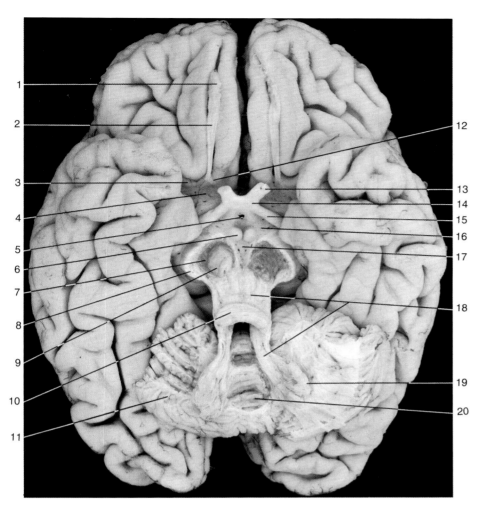

Brain and cerebellum (inferior aspect). Parts of the cerebellum have been removed to display the dentate nucleus and the main pathway to the midbrain (cerebellorubral tract).

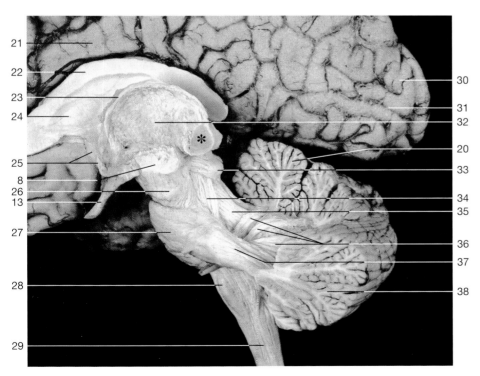

Dissection of the cerebellar peduncles and their connection with midbrain and diencephalon. A small part of pulvinar thalami (✳) has been cut to show inferior brachium.

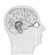

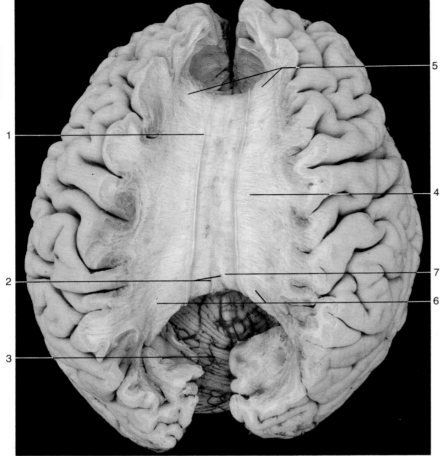

1 Lateral longitudinal stria
   of indusium griseum
2 Medial longitudinal stria
   of indusium griseum
3 Cerebellum
4 Radiating fibers of the corpus callosum
5 Forceps minor of corpus callosum
6 Forceps major of corpus callosum
7 Splenium of corpus callosum

Dissection of the brain I. The fiber system of the corpus callosum has been displayed by removing the cortex lying above it. Frontal pole at the top.

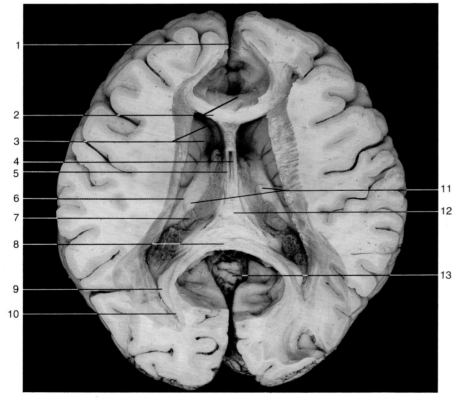

1 Longitudinal cerebral fissure
2 Genu of corpus callosum
3 Head of caudate nucleus and
   anterior horn of lateral ventricle
4 Cavum of septum pellucidum
5 Septum pellucidum
6 Stria terminalis
7 Choroid plexus of lateral ventricle
8 Splenium of corpus callosum
9 Calcar avis
10 Posterior horn of lateral ventricle
11 Thalamus (lamina affixa)
12 Commissure of fornix
13 Vermis of cerebellum

Dissection of the brain II. The lateral ventricles and subcortical nuclei of the brain are dissected. The corpus callosum has been partly removed. Frontal pole at the top.

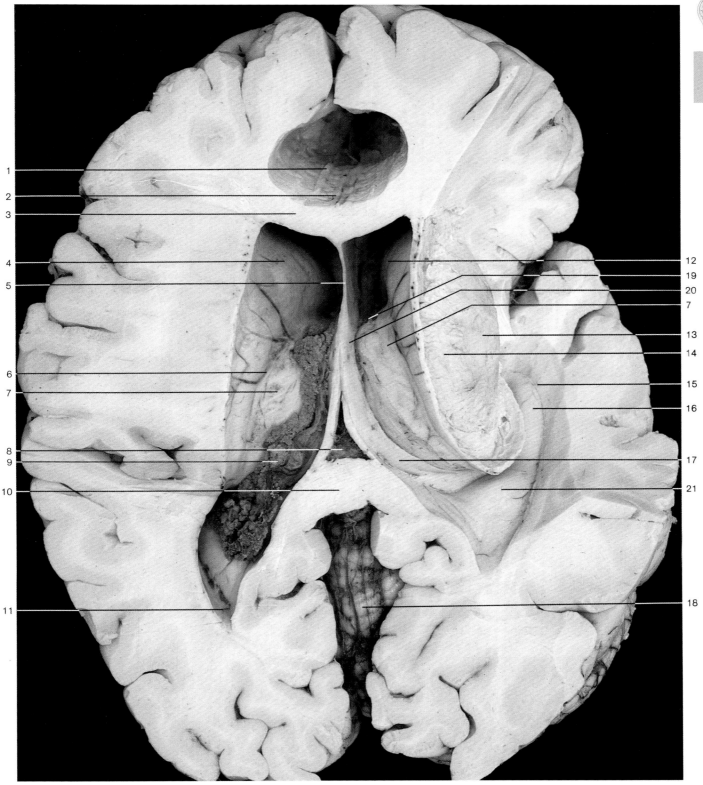
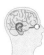

Dissection of the brain III (superior view of lateral ventricle and subcortical nuclei of the brain). Corpus callosum partly removed. At right, the entire lateral ventricle has been opened, the insula with claustrum and the extreme and external capsules have been removed, exposing the lentiform nucleus and the internal capsule.

1	Lateral longitudinal stria	9	Choroid plexus of lateral ventricle
2	Medial longitudinal stria	10	Splenium of corpus callosum
3	Genu of corpus callosum	11	Posterior horn of lateral ventricle
4	Head of caudate nucleus	12	Anterior horn of lateral ventricle
5	Septum pellucidum		(head of caudate nucleus)
6	Stria terminalis	13	Putamen of lentiform nucleus
7	Thalamus (lamina affixa)	14	Internal capsule
8	Choroid plexus of third ventricle	15	Inferior horn of lateral ventricle

16	Pes hippocampi
17	Crus of fornix
18	Vermis of cerebellum with arachnoid and pia mater
19	Interventricular foramen
20	Right column of fornix
21	Collateral eminence

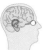

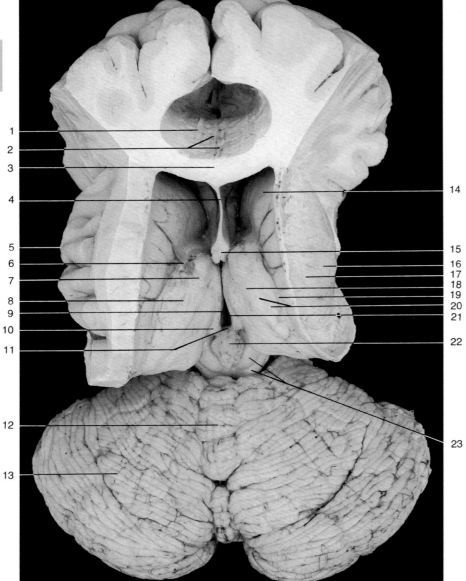

1   Lateral longitudinal stria
2   Medial longitudinal stria
3   Corpus callosum
4   Septum pellucidum
5   Insular gyri
6   Thalamostriate vein
7   Anterior tubercle of thalamus
8   Thalamus
9   Stria medullaris of thalamus
10 Habenular trigone
11 Habenular commissure
12 Vermis of cerebellum
13 Left hemisphere of cerebellum
14 Head of caudate nucleus
15 Columns of fornix
16 Putamen of lentiform nucleus
17 Internal capsule
18 Taenia of choroid plexus
19 Stria terminalis and thalamostriate vein
20 Lamina affixa
21 Third ventricle
22 Pineal body
23 Superior and inferior colliculus of midbrain

Dissection of the brain IVa. Temporal lobe, fornix, and the posterior corpus callosum have been removed (this part of the specimen is depicted below). Frontal pole at top (superior aspect).

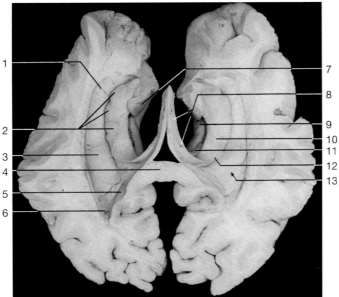

1   Inferior horn of lateral ventricle
2   Hippocampal digitations
3   Collateral eminence
4   Splenium of corpus callosum
5   Calcar avis
6   Posterior horn of lateral ventricle
7   Uncus of parahippocampal gyrus
8   Body and crus of fornix
9   Parahippocampal gyrus
10 Pes hippocampi
11 Dentate gyrus
12 Hippocampal fimbria
13 Lateral ventricle

Dissection of the brain IVb. Depicted is the portion of the brain removed from the specimen above. **Temporal lobe and limbic system** (superior aspect). Columns of fornix are cut.

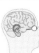

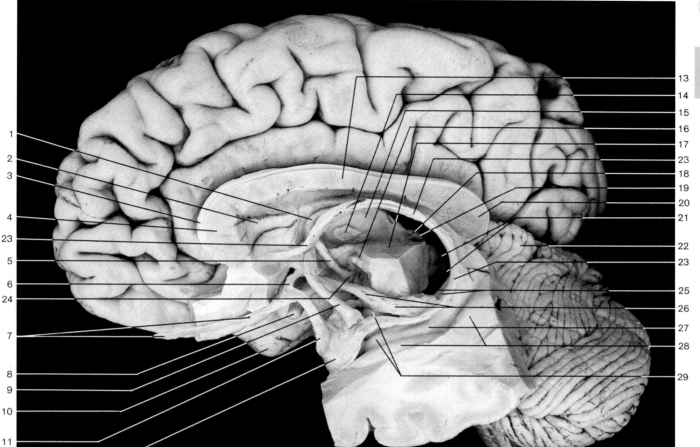

Dissection of the limbic system. Left side, lateral aspect. Corpus callosum has been cut in the median plane. The left thalamus and the left hemisphere have been partly removed.

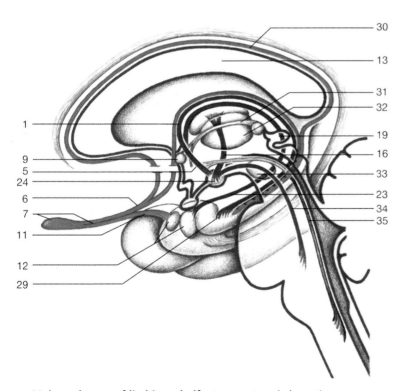

1	Body of fornix	21	Colliculi of midbrain
2	Septum pellucidum	22	Vermis of cerebellum
3	Lateral longitudinal stria	23	Stria terminalis
4	Genu of corpus callosum	24	Mamillary body
5	Column of fornix	25	Fimbria of hippocampus
6	Medial olfactory stria		and pes hippocampi
7	Olfactory bulb and	26	Left optic tract and
	olfactory tract		lateral geniculate body
8	Optic nerve	27	Lateral ventricle and
9	Anterior commissure		parahippocampal gyrus
	(left half)	28	Collateral eminence
10	Right temporal lobe	29	Hippocampal digitations
11	Lateral olfactory stria	30	Supracallosal gyrus
12	Amygdala		(longitudinal stria)
13	Body of corpus callosum	31	Stria medullaris of
14	Interthalamic adhesion		thalamus
15	Third ventricle and right	32	Thalamus
	thalamus	33	Red nucleus
16	Mamillothalamic fasciculus	34	Mamillotegmental
17	Part of the thalamus		fasciculus
18	Habenular commissure	35	Dorsal longitudinal
19	Pineal body		fasciculus (Schütz)
20	Splenium of corpus		
	callosum		

Main pathways of limbic and olfactory system (schematic drawing). Blue = afferent pathways; red = efferent pathways.

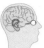

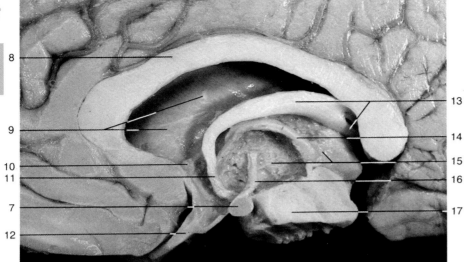

1   Paraventricular nucleus ⎫
2   Pre-optic nucleus   ⎪
3   Ventromedial nucleus   ⎬ Hypothalamic
4   Supra-optic nucleus   ⎪ nuclei
5   Posterior nucleus   ⎪
6   Dorsomedial nucleus   ⎭
7   Mamillary body
8   Corpus callosum
9   Lateral ventricle (showing caudate nucleus)
10 Anterior commissure
11 Column of fornix
12 Optic chiasma
13 Crus of fornix
14 Stria medullaris of thalamus
15 Thalamus and interthalamic adhesion
16 Mamillothalamic fasciculus of Vicq d'Azyr
17 Cerebral peduncle
18 Pineal body
19 Tectum of midbrain
20 Lamina terminalis

Median section through the diencephalon. Medial part of the thalamus and septum pellucidum have been removed to show the fornix and mamillothalamic fasciculus.

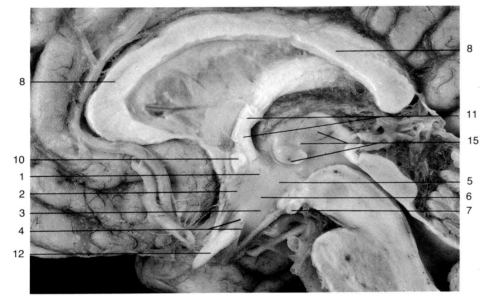

Median section through the diencephalon and midbrain; location of hypothalamic nuclei.

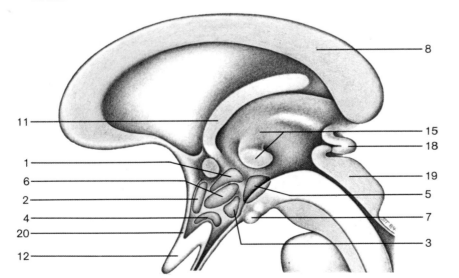

Position of main hypothalamic nuclei (schematic drawing).

1 Circular sulcus of insula
2 Long gyrus of insula
3 Short gyri of insula
4 Limen insulae
5 Opercula (cut)
   a Frontal operculum
   b Frontoparietal operculum
   c Temporal operculum
6 Corona radiata
7 Lentiform nucleus
8 Anterior commissure
9 Olfactory tract
10 Cerebral arcuate fibers
11 Optic radiation
12 Cerebral peduncle
13 Trigeminal nerve (n. V)
14 Flocculus of cerebellum
15 Pyramidal tract
16 Decussation of pyramidal tract
17 Internal capsule
18 Optic tract
19 Optic nerve (n. II)
20 Infundibulum
21 Temporal lobe (right side)
22 Mamillary bodies
23 Oculomotor nerve (n. III)
24 Transverse fibers of pons

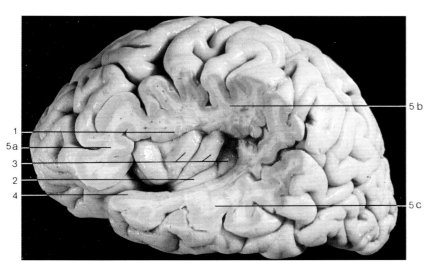

Insula (Reili). The opercula of the frontal, parietal, and temporal lobes have been removed to display the insular gyri. Left hemisphere.

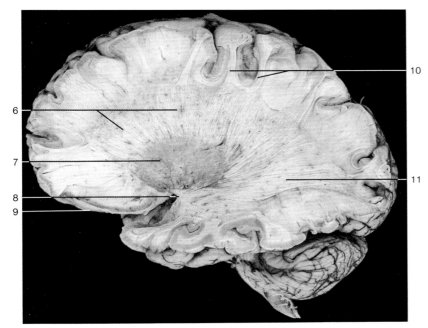

Dissection of the corona radiata, left hemisphere. Frontal pole on the left.

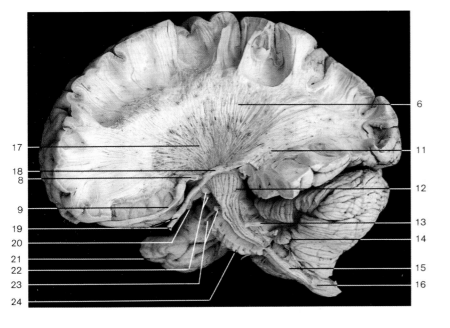

◁ **Corona radiata and internal capsule,** left hemisphere. Lentiform nucleus removed (frontal pole to the left).

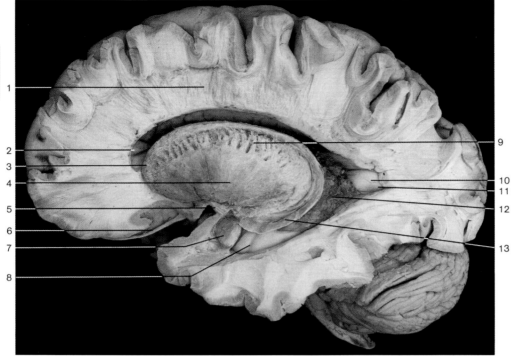

1   Corona radiata
2   Anterior horn of lateral ventricle
3   Head of caudate nucleus
4   Putamen
5   Anterior commissure
6   Olfactory tract
7   Amygdala
8   Hippocampal digitations
9   Internal capsule
10   Calcar avis
11   Posterior horn of lateral ventricle
12   Choroid plexus of lateral ventricle
13   Caudal extremity of caudate nucleus
14   Pulvinar of thalamus
15   Mamillary body
16   Optic tract
17   Anterior commissure
18   Fornix
19   Longitudinal stria
20   Dentate gyrus
21   Hippocampal fimbria
22   Pes hippocampi

Dissection of the subcortical nuclei and internal capsule, left hemisphere (lateral aspect). Frontal pole to the left. The lateral ventricle has been opened, and the insular gyri and claustrum have been removed, revealing the lentiform nucleus and the internal capsule.

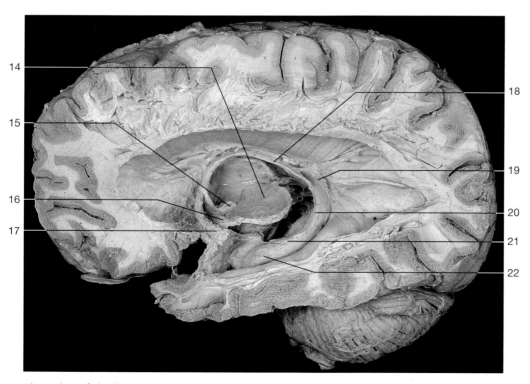

Dissection of the limbic system and the fornix (lateral aspect). Frontal pole to the left.

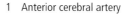

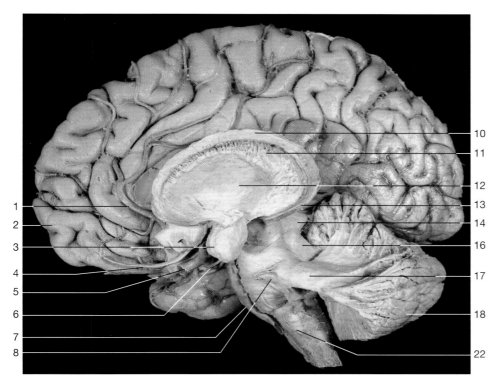

1   Anterior cerebral artery
2   Frontal lobe
3   Amygdala (amygdaloid body)
4   Olfactory tract
5   Internal carotid artery
6   Oculomotor nerve (n. III)
7   Basilar artery
8   Trigeminal nerve (n. V)
9   Hypoglossal nerve (n. XII)
10 Caudate nucleus
11 Internal capsule
12 Lentiform nucleus
13 Caudal extremity of caudate
    nucleus
14 Inferior colliculus of midbrain
15 Trochlear nerve (n. IV)
16 Superior cerebellar peduncle
17 Middle cerebellar peduncle
18 Cerebellum
19 Facial nerve (n. VII) and
    vestibulocochlear nerve
    (n. VIII)
20 Abducent nerve (n. VI)
21 Glossopharyngeal nerve (n. IX),
    vagus nerve (n. X), and
    accessory nerve (n. XI)
22 Inferior olive

Right hemisphere together with brain stem and cerebellum (lateral aspect).
The connections of the brain stem with the cerebellum are dissected. The amygdala of the left
hemisphere is shown. The corpus callosum has been partly removed.

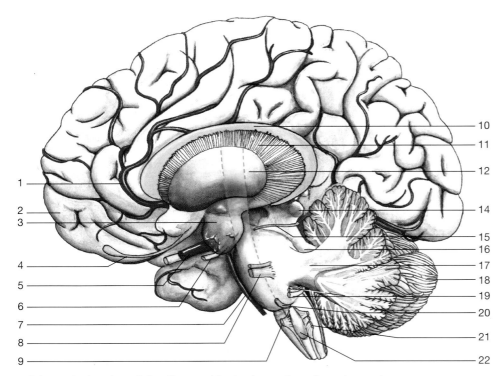

Schematic drawing of the dissected brain shown above (lateral aspect).
The course of the pyramidal tracts is indicated in red. Cranial nerves = yellow.

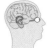

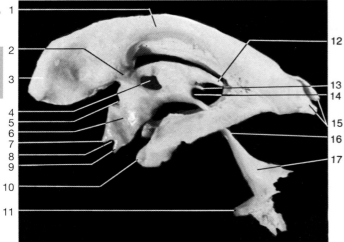

Cast of ventricular cavities of the brain (lateral aspect), frontal pole to the left.

1   Central part of the lateral ventricle
2   Interventricular foramen of Monro
3   Anterior horn of the lateral ventricle
4   Site of interthalamic adhesion
5   Notch for anterior commissure
6   Third ventricle
7   Optic recess
8   Notch for optic chiasma
9   Infundibular recess
10 Inferior horn of lateral ventricle with indentation
    of amygdaloid body
11 Lateral recess and lateral aperture of Luschka
12 Suprapineal recess
13 Pineal recess
14 Notch for posterior commissure
15 Posterior horn of lateral ventricle
16 Cerebral aqueduct

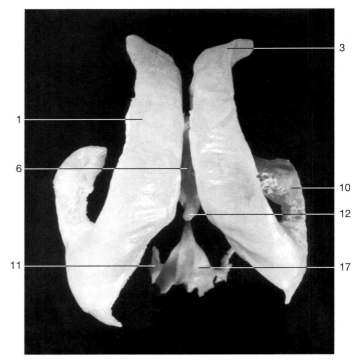

Cast of ventricular cavities of the brain (superior aspect), frontal pole at top.

17 Fourth ventricle
18 Median aperture of Magendie
19 Cerebellomedullary cistern
20 Superior sagittal sinus
21 Inferior sagittal sinus
22 Intervaginal space of optic nerve
23 Arachnoid granulations of Pacchioni
24 Straight sinus

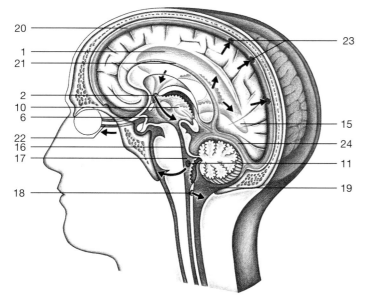

Position of ventricular cavities (schematic drawing).
The direction of flow of cerebrospinal fluid is indicated by arrows. Green = right lateral ventricle; red = choroidal plexus with cerebrospinal fluid.

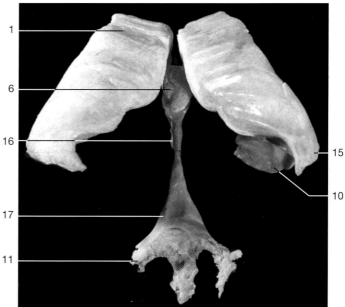

Cast of ventricular cavities of the brain (posterior aspect).

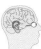

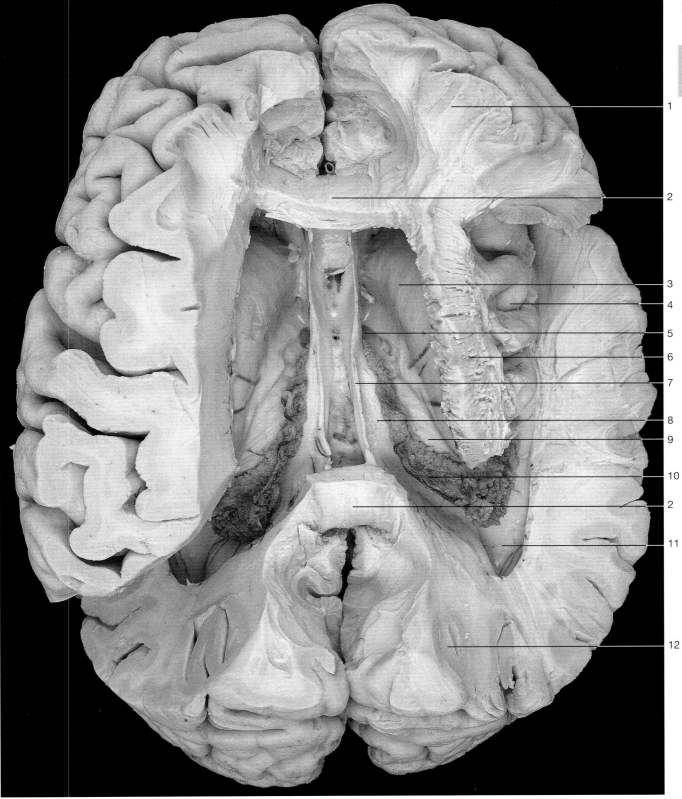

Dissection of the brain (superior view of the lateral ventricle and of the subcortical nuclei of the brain). Corpus callosum partly removed. Fornix and choroid plexus of the left lateral ventricle are shown.

1	Frontal lobe of brain
2	Corpus callosum
3	Caudate nucleus (head)
4	Insular cortex
5	Interventricular foramen
6	Internal capsule
7	Lateral longitudinal stria
8	Body of fornix
9	Thalamus
10	Choroid plexus
11	Lateral ventricle (occipital horn)
12	Occipital lobe of brain

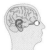

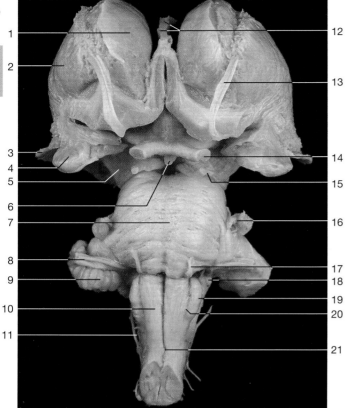

Brain stem (ventral aspect).

1 Caudate nucleus
2 Lentiform nucleus
3 Caudal extremity of caudate nucleus
4 Amygdaloid body
5 Cerebral peduncle
6 Infundibulum
7 Pons
8 Facial nerve (n. VII) and vestibulocochlear nerve (n. VIII)
9 Cerebellar flocculus
10 Medulla oblongata
11 Accessory nerve (n. XI)
12 Fornix and column of fornix
13 Olfactory tract
14 Optic nerve (n. II)
15 Oculomotor nerve (n. III)
16 Trigeminal nerve (n. V)
17 Abducent nerve (n. VI)
18 Glossopharyngeal nerve (n. IX) and vagus nerve (n. X)
19 Inferior olive
20 Hypoglossal nerve (n. XII)
21 Decussation of the pyramids
22 Thalamus
23 Epiphysis
24 Tectum of midbrain (superior and inferior colliculus)
25 Motor nucleus of trigeminal nerve (n. V)
26 Facial nucleus (n. VII)
27 Middle cerebellar peduncle
28 Visceral nucleus of glossopharyngeal and vagus nerves (n. IX and n. X), salivatory nucleus
29 Vestibular nucleus (n. VIII)
30 Ambiguus nucleus (n. IX, n. X, n. XI)
31 Spinal nucleus of accessory nerve (n. XI)
32 Motor nucleus of oculomotor nerve (n. III)
33 Trochlear nucleus and nerve (n. IV)
34 Sensory nucleus of trigeminal nerve (n. V)
35 Abducent nucleus (n. VI)
36 Hypoglossal nucleus (n. XII)

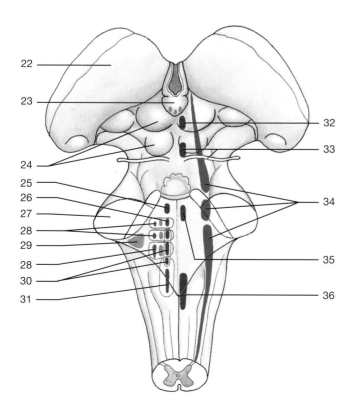

Brain stem (dorsal aspect, schematic drawing).
Location of cranial nerve nuclei.

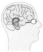

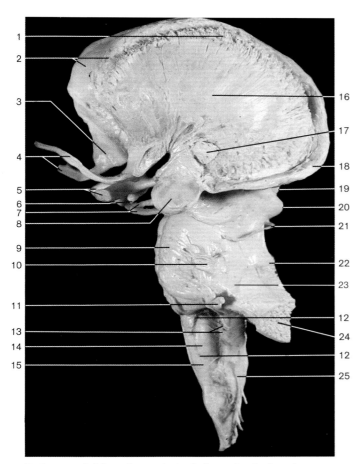

Brain stem (left lateral aspect). Cerebellar peduncles have been severed, cerebellum and cerebral cortex have been removed.

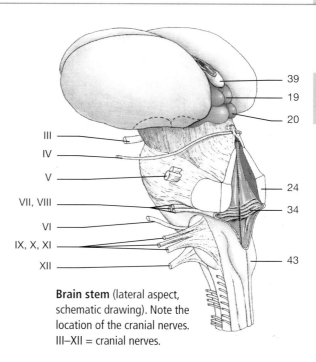

Brain stem (lateral aspect, schematic drawing). Note the location of the cranial nerves. III–XII = cranial nerves.

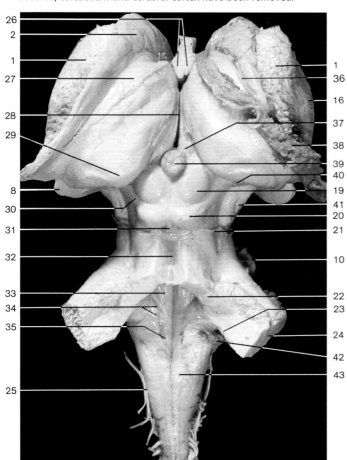

Brain stem (dorsal aspect). Cerebellum removed.

1 Internal capsule
2 Head of the caudate nucleus
3 Olfactory trigone
4 Olfactory tracts
5 Optic nerves (n. II)
6 Infundibulum
7 Oculomotor nerve (n. III)
8 Amygdaloid body
9 Pons
10 Trigeminal nerve (n. V)
11 Facial and vestibulocochlear nerves (n. VII, n. VIII)
12 Hypoglossal nerve (n. XII)
13 Glossopharyngeal and vagus nerves (n. IX, n. X)
14 Inferior olive
15 Medulla oblongata
16 Lentiform nucleus
17 Anterior commissure
18 Tail of caudate nucleus
19 Superior colliculus
20 Inferior colliculus
21 Trochlear nerve (n. IV)
22 Superior cerebellar peduncle
23 Inferior cerebellar peduncle
24 Middle cerebellar peduncle
25 Accessory nerve (n. XI)
26 Columns of fornix (divided)
27 Lamina affixa
28 Third ventricle
29 Pulvinar of thalamus
30 Inferior brachium
31 Frenulum veli
32 Superior medullary velum
33 Facial colliculus
34 Striae medullares and rhomboid fossa
35 Hypoglossal trigone
36 Stria terminalis and thalamostriate vein
37 Habenular trigone
38 Choroid plexus of lateral ventricle
39 Pineal body
40 Medial geniculate body
41 Cerebral peduncle
42 Choroid plexus of fourth ventricle
43 Clava

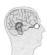

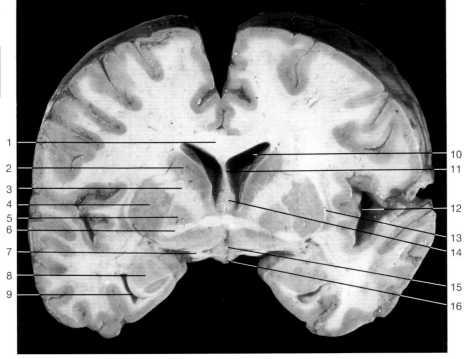

1   Corpus callosum
2   Head of caudate nucleus
3   Internal capsule
4   Putamen
5   Globus pallidus
6   Anterior commissure
7   Optic tract
8   Amygdaloid body
9   Inferior horn of lateral ventricle
10   Lateral ventricle
11   Septum pellucidum
12   Lobus insularis (insula)
13   External capsule
14   Column of fornix
15   Optic recess
16   Infundibulum
17   Thalamus
18   Claustrum
19   Lenticular ansa
20   Third ventricle and hypothalamus
21   Basilar artery and pons
22   Cortex of temporal lobe
23   Inferior colliculus
24   Superior colliculus
25   Cerebral aqueduct
26   Red nucleus
27   Substantia nigra
28   Cerebral peduncle
29   Trochlear nerve (n. IV)
30   Gray matter
31   Nucleus of oculomotor nerve
32   Fibers of oculomotor nerve (n. III)
33   Vermis of cerebellum
34   Fourth ventricle
35   Reticular formation
36   Pons and transverse pontine fibers
37   Emboliform nucleus
38   Dentate nucleus
39   Middle cerebellar peduncle
40   Choroid plexus
41   Hypoglossal nucleus at rhomboid fossa
42   Medial longitudinal fasciculus
43   Trigeminal nerve (n. V.)
44   Inferior olivary nucleus
45   Corticospinal fibers and arcuate fibers
46   Fourth ventricle with choroid plexus
47   Vestibular nuclei
48   Nucleus and tractus solitarius
49   Inferior cerebellar peduncle (restiform body)
50   Reticular formation
51   Medial lemniscus
52   Cuneate nucleus of Burdach
53   Central canal
54   Pyramidal tract
55   Flocculus of cerebellum
56   Cerebellar hemisphere with pia mater
57   "Arbor vitae" of cerebellum
58   Nucleus gracilis of Goll
59   Lateral recess of choroid plexus of fourth ventricle
60   Posterior inferior cerebellar artery
61   Choroid plexus of lateral ventricle

Coronal section through the brain at the level of the anterior commissure. Section 1.

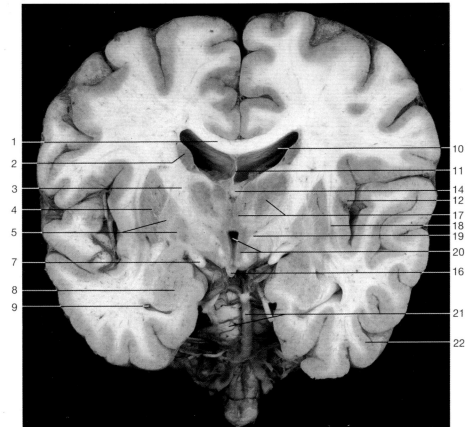

Coronal section through the brain at the level of the third ventricle and the interthalamic adhesion. Section 2.

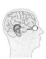

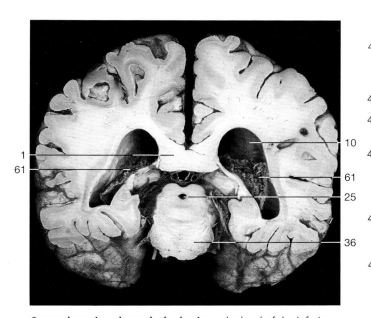

Coronal section through the brain at the level of the inferior colliculus (posterior aspect). Section 3.

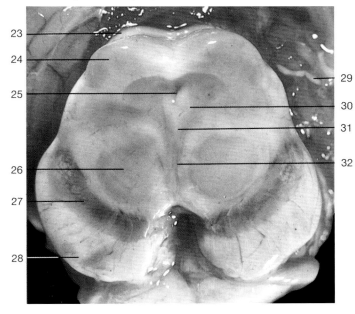

Cross section of the midbrain (mesencephalon) at the level of the superior colliculus (superior aspect). Section 4.

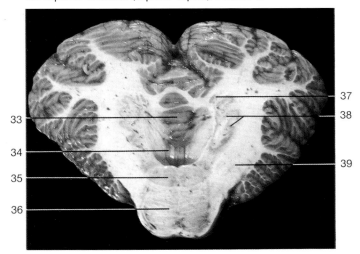

Cross section through the rhombencephalon at the level of the pons (inferior aspect). Section 5.

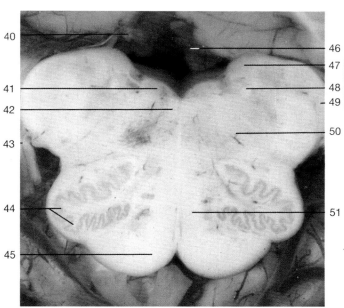

Cross section of the rhombencephalon at the level of the olive (inferior aspect). Section 6.

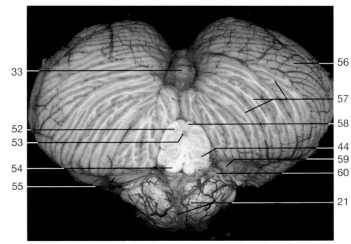

Cross section through medulla oblongata and cerebellum (inferior aspect). Section 7.

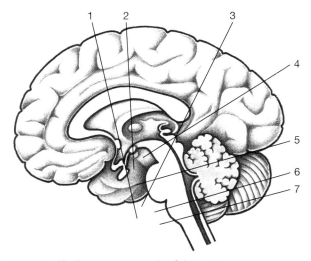

Right half of the brain. Levels of the sections are indicated.

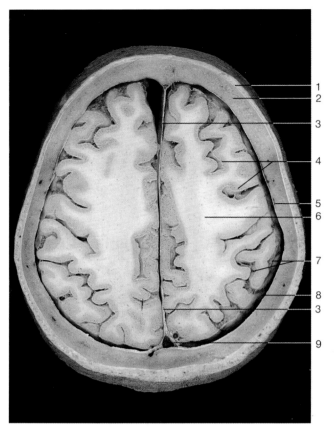

Horizontal section through the head.
Section 1.

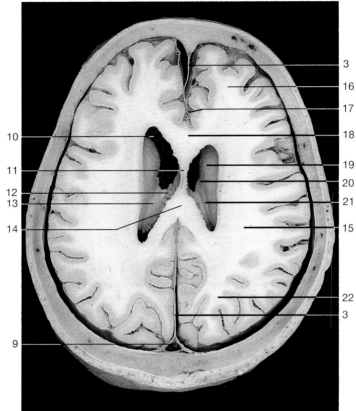

Horizontal section through the head.
Section 2.

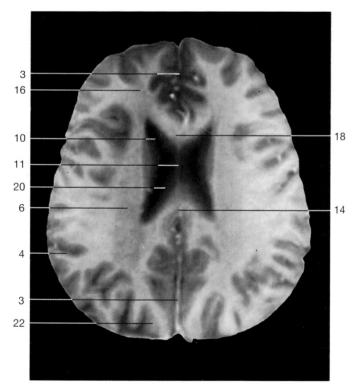

MRI scan of the human head at the level of section 2.

1 Skin of scalp
2 Calvaria (diploe of the skull)
3 Falx cerebri
4 Gray matter of brain (cortex)
5 Dura mater
6 White matter of brain
7 Arachnoid and pia mater with vessels
8 Subdural space (slightly expanded due to shrinkage of the brain)
9 Superior sagittal sinus
10 Anterior horn of lateral ventricle
11 Septum pellucidum
12 Choroid plexus
13 Thalamus
14 Splenium of corpus callosum
15 Parietal lobe
16 Frontal lobe
17 Anterior cerebral artery
18 Genu of corpus callosum
19 Caudate nucleus
20 Central part of lateral ventricle
21 Stria terminalis
22 Occipital lobe

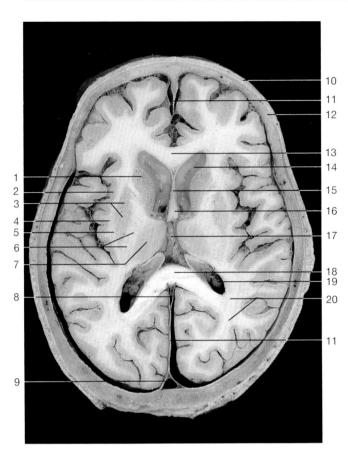

1 Caudate nucleus
2 Lobus insularis (insula)
3 Lentiform nucleus
4 Claustrum
5 External capsule
6 Internal capsule
7 Thalamus
8 Inferior sagittal sinus
9 Superior sagittal sinus
10 Skin of scalp
11 Falx cerebri
12 Calvaria (diploe of skull)
13 Genu of corpus callosum
14 Anterior horn of lateral ventricle
15 Septum pellucidum
16 Column of fornix
17 Choroid plexus of third ventricle
18 Splenium of corpus callosum
19 Entrance to inferior horn of lateral ventricle with choroid plexus
20 Optic radiation
21 Third ventricle

Horizontal section through the head at the level of third ventricle of internal capsule and neighboring nuclei.
Section 3.

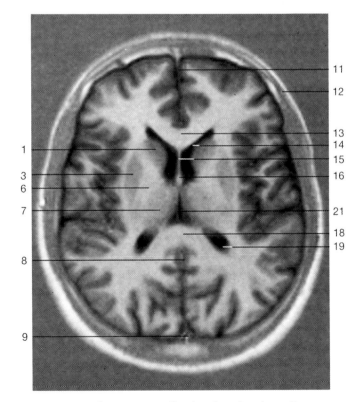

MRI scan at the corresponding level to the above figure.
Section 3.

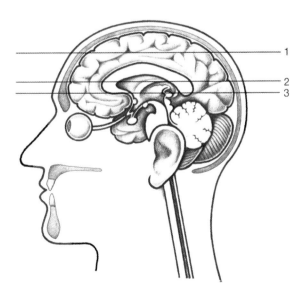

Sagittal section through the head.
Levels of the horizontal sections are indicated.

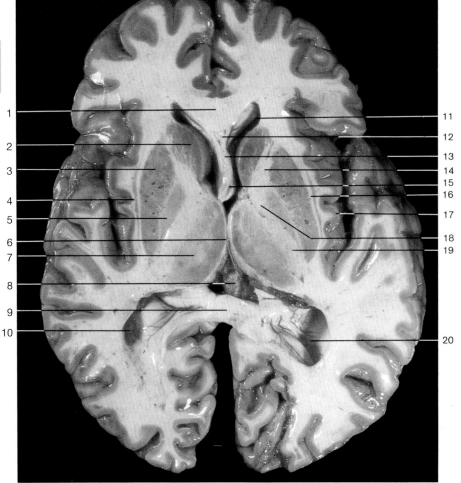

1   Genu of corpus callosum
2   Head of caudate nucleus
3   Putamen
4   Claustrum
5   Globus pallidus
6   Third ventricle
7   Thalamus
8   Pineal body
9   Splenium of corpus callosum
10 Choroid plexus of the lateral ventricle
11 Anterior horn of lateral ventricle
12 Cavity of septum pellucidum
13 Septum pellucidum
14 Anterior limb of internal capsule
15 Column of fornix
16 External capsule
17 Lobus insularis (insula)
18 Genu of internal capsule
19 Posterior limb of internal capsule
20 Posterior horn of lateral ventricle
21 Anterior commissure
22 Optic radiation
23 Falx cerebri
24 Maxillary sinus
25 Position of auditory tube
26 Tympanic cavity
27 External acoustic meatus
28 Medulla oblongata
29 Fourth ventricle
30 Cerebellum (left hemisphere)
31 Temporomandibular joint
32 Tympanic membrane
33 Base of cochlea
34 Mastoid air cells
35 Sigmoid sinus
36 Vermis of cerebellum
37 Intermediate mass

Horizontal section through the brain, showing the subcortical nuclei and internal capsule. Section 1.

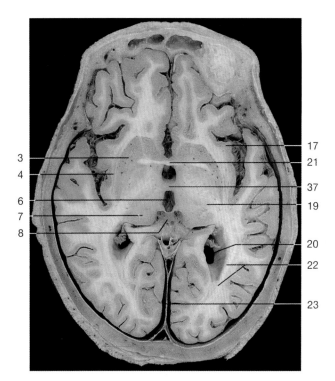

Horizontal section through the head. Section 2.

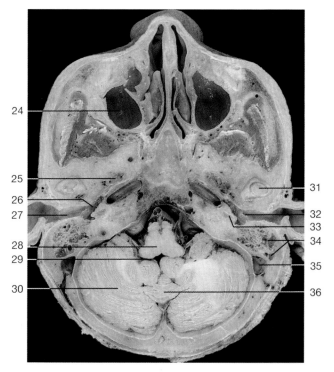

Horizontal section through the head. Section 4.

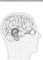

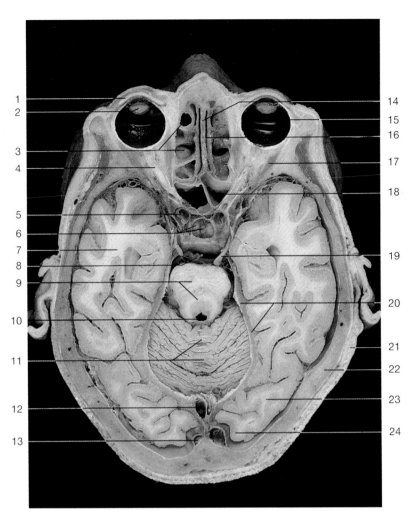

Horizontal section through the head. Section 3.

1   Upper lid (tarsal plate)
2   Lens
3   Ethmoidal sinus
4   Optic nerve (n. II)
5   Internal carotid artery
6   Infundibulum and pituitary gland
7   Temporal lobe
8   Basilar artery
9   Pons (cross section of brain stem)
10 Cerebral aqueduct (beginning of fourth ventricle)
11 Vermis of cerebellum
12 Straight sinus
13 Transverse sinus
14 Nasal septum
15 Eyeball (sclera)
16 Nasal cavity
17 Lateral rectus muscle
18 Sphenoidal sinus
19 Oculomotor nerve (n. III)
20 Tentorium of cerebellum
21 Skin of scalp
22 Calvaria
23 Occipital lobe
24 Striate cortex (visual cortex)

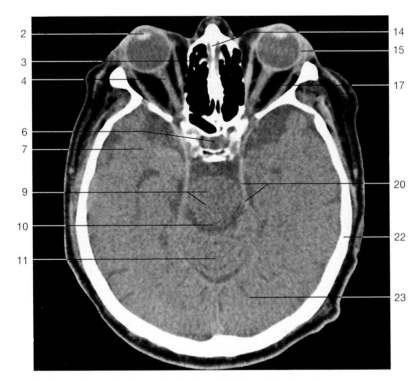

Horizontal section through the head. (CT scan.) Section 3.

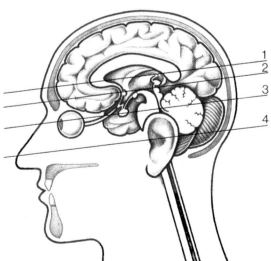

Sagittal section through the head.
Levels of the horizontal sections are indicated.

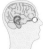

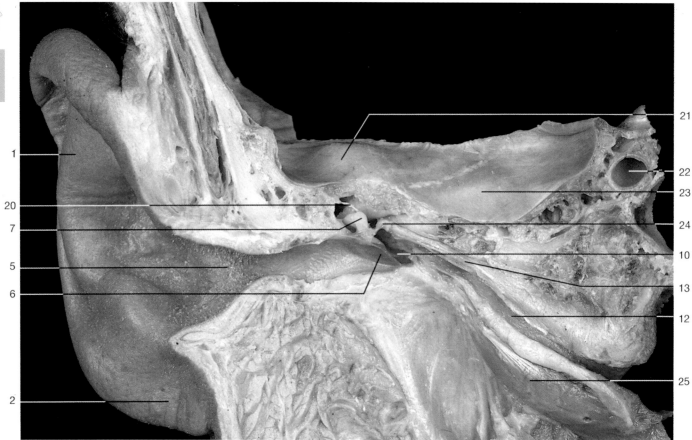

Longitudinal section through the right temporal bone. The outer and middle ear and auditory ossicles and tube are shown (anterior aspect).

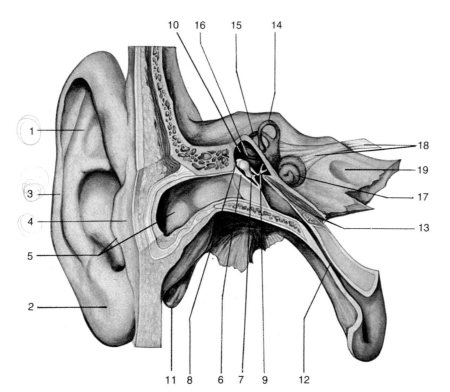

Right auditory and vestibular apparatus (anterior aspect).
(Schematic drawing.)

Outer ear

1 Auricle
2 Lobule of auricle
3 Helix
4 Tragus
5 External acoustic meatus

Middle ear

6 Tympanic membrane
7 Malleus
8 Incus
9 Stapes
10 Tympanic cavity
11 Mastoid process
12 Auditory tube
13 Tensor tympani muscle

Inner ear

14 Anterior semicircular duct
15 Posterior semicircular duct
16 Lateral semicircular duct
17 Cochlea
18 Vestibulocochlear nerve
19 Petrous part of the temporal bone

Additional structures

20 Superior ligament of malleus
21 Arcuate eminence
22 Internal carotid artery
23 Anterior surface of pyramid with dura mater
24 Stapes
25 Levator veli palatini muscle

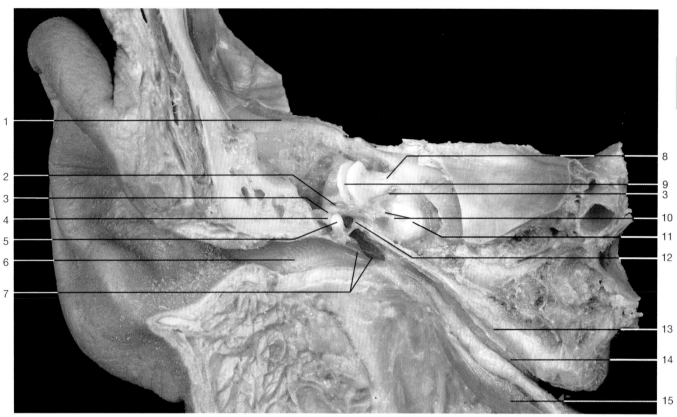

Longitudinal section through the right outer, middle, and inner ear. The cochlea and semicircular canals have been further dissected (anterior aspect).

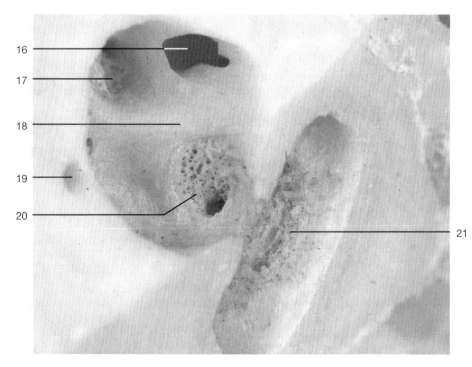

Internal acoustic meatus, left side. The bone was partly removed to show the bottom of the meatus.

1 Roof of tympanic cavity
2 Lateral osseous semicircular canal
3 Facial nerve
4 Incus
5 Malleus
6 External acoustic meatus
7 Tympanic cavity and tympanic membrane
8 Vestibulocochlear nerve
9 Anterior osseous semicircular canal
10 Geniculate ganglion and greater petrosal nerve
11 Cochlea
12 Stapes
13 Tensor tympani muscle
14 Auditory tube
15 Levator veli palatini muscle
16 Area of facial nerve
17 Superior vestibular area
18 Transverse crest
19 Foramen singulare
20 Foraminous spiral tract (outlet of cochlear part of vestibulocochlear nerve)
21 Base of cochlea

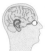

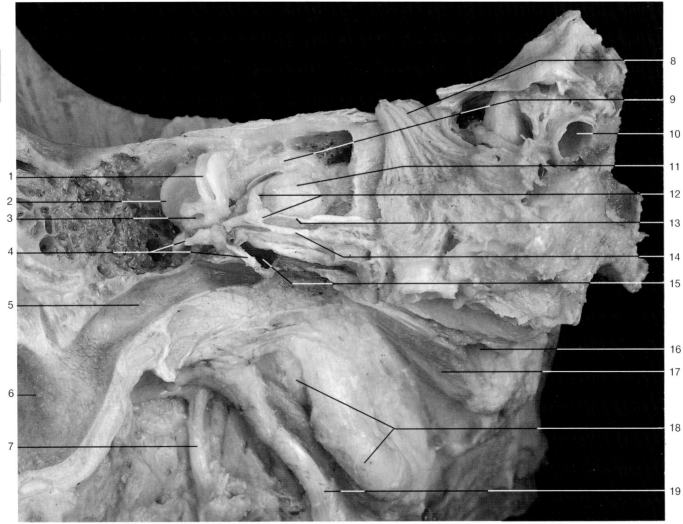

Longitudinal section through the outer, middle, and inner ear. Deeper dissection to display facial nerve and lesser and greater petrosal nerves (anterior aspect).

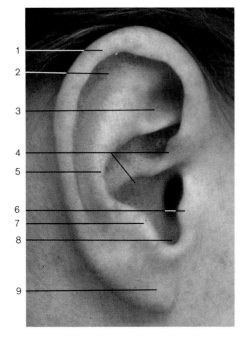

Right auricle (lateral aspect).

1 Helix
2 Scaphoid fossa
3 Triangular fossa
4 Concha
5 Antihelix
6 Tragus
7 Antitragus
8 Intertragic notch
9 Lobule

1 Anterior osseous semicircular canal (opened)
2 Posterior osseous semicircular canal
3 Lateral osseous semicircular canal (opened)
4 Facial nerve and chorda tympani
5 External acoustic meatus
6 Auricle
7 Facial nerve
8 Trigeminal nerve
9 Bony base of internal acoustic meatus
10 Internal carotid artery within cavernous sinus
11 Cochlea
12 Facial nerve with geniculate ganglion
13 Greater petrosal nerve
14 Lesser petrosal nerve
15 Tympanic cavity
16 Auditory tube
17 Levator veli palatini muscle
18 Internal carotid artery and internal jugular vein
19 Styloid process

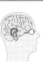

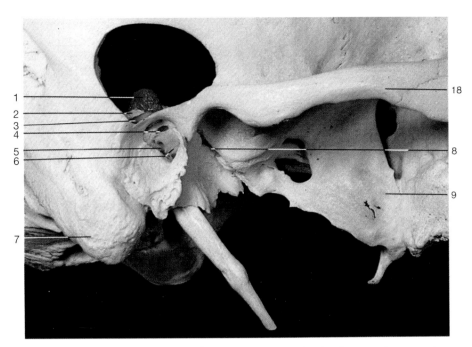

1   Anterior semicircular canal (red)
2   Posterior semicircular canal (yellow)
3   Lateral or horizontal semicircular canal (green)
4   Fenestra vestibuli
5   Fenestra cochleae
6   Tympanic cavity
7   Mastoid process
8   Petrotympanic fissure (red probe: chorda tympani)
9   Lateral pterygoid plate
10 Mastoid air cells
11 Facial canal (blue)
12 Foramen ovale
13 Carotid canal (red)
14 Tympanic ring
15 Petromastoid part of temporal bone
16 Squamous part of temporal bone
17 Squamomastoid suture
18 Zygomatic process of temporal bone
19 Incisure of tympanic ring
20 Promontory
21 Apex of cochlea (cupula)
22 Spiral canal of cochlea at base of cochlea
23 Epitympanic recess
24 Auditory ossicles and tympanic cavity
25 Hypotympanic recess
26 Canaliculus chordae tympani (green probe)
27 Mastoid process
28 Canaliculus for stapedius nerve (red)
29 Cochlea
30 Canaliculus mastoideus (red probe)

Right temporal bone (lateral aspect). Petrosquamous portion has been partly removed to display the semicircular canals.

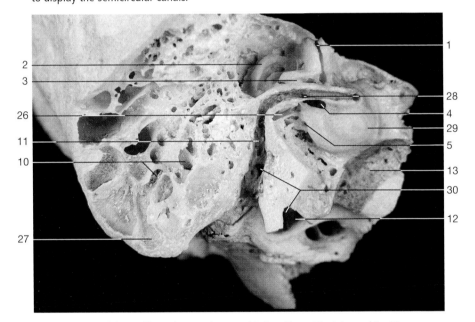

Right temporal bone (lateral aspect). Mastoid air cells and facial canal had been opened. The three semicircular canals were dissected.

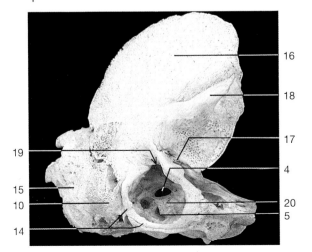

Right temporal bone of the newborn (lateral aspect).

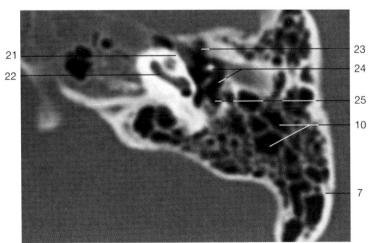

Frontal section through petrous part. (CT scan.)

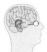

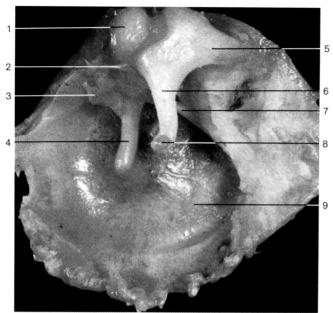

1 Head of malleus
2 Anterior ligament of malleus
3 Tendon of tensor tympani muscle
4 Handle of malleus
5 Short crus of incus
6 Long crus of incus
7 Chorda tympani
8 Lenticular process
9 Tympanic membrane

Tympanic membrane with malleus and incus (internal aspect; right side).

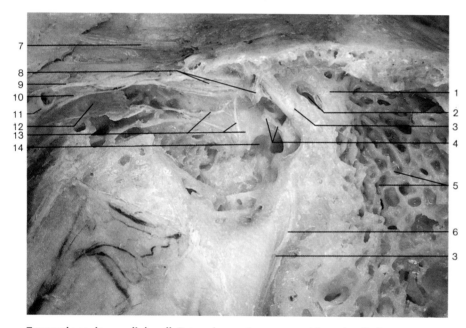

1 Tympanic antrum
2 Lateral semicircular canal (opened)
3 Facial canal
4 Stapes with tendon of stapedius
5 Mastoid air cells
6 Chorda tympani (intracranial part)
7 Greater petrosal nerve
8 Tensor tympani muscle (processus cochleariformis)
9 Lesser petrosal nerve
10 Anterior tympanic artery
11 Middle meningeal artery
12 Auditory tube
13 Promontory with tympanic plexus
14 Fenestra cochleae

Tympanic cavity, medial wall. External acoustic meatus and lateral wall of tympanic cavity together with incus. Malleus and tympanic membrane have been removed; mastoid air cells are opened (left side).

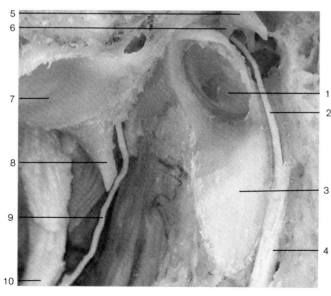

1 Tympanic membrane
2 Chorda tympani (intracranial part)
3 Floor of the external acoustic meatus
4 Facial nerve and facial canal
5 Incus
6 Head of malleus
7 Mandibular fossa
8 Spine of sphenoid
9 Chorda tympani (extracranial part)
10 Styloid process

Tympanic membrane (lateral aspect). External acoustic meatus and facial canal have been opened to expose the chorda tympani (magn. ~1.5×) (left side).

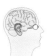

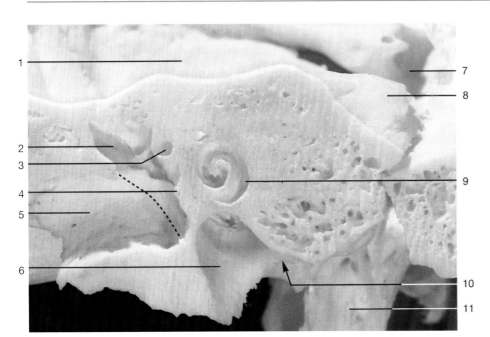

Frontal section through the petrous part of the left temporal bone at the level of the cochlea (posterior aspect). Position of tympanic membrane indicated by dotted line.

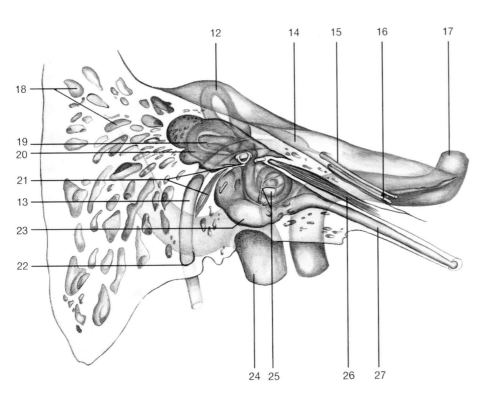

Medial wall of tympanic cavity and its relation to neighboring structures of the inner ear, facial nerve, and blood vessels (schematic drawing). Frontal section through the right temporal bone (anterior aspect).

1 Anterior surface of the pyramid	10 Carotid canal	20 Posterior semicircular duct
2 Mastoid antrum	11 Pterygoid process	21 Stapes with stapedius muscle
3 Lateral semicircular canal	12 Anterior semicircular duct	22 Stylomastoid foramen
4 Cochleariform process	13 Facial nerve	23 Inferior recess of tympanic cavity
5 External acoustic meatus	14 Geniculate ganglion	(hypotympanon)
6 Jugular fossa	15 Greater petrosal nerve	24 Internal jugular vein
7 Foramen lacerum	16 Lesser petrosal nerve	25 Promontory with tympanic plexus
8 Apex of petrous part	17 Internal carotid artery	(position of cochlea)
9 Position of cochlea (modiolus with	18 Mastoid air cells	26 Tensor muscle of tympanum
crista spiralis ossea)	19 Lateral semicircular duct	27 Auditory tube

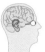

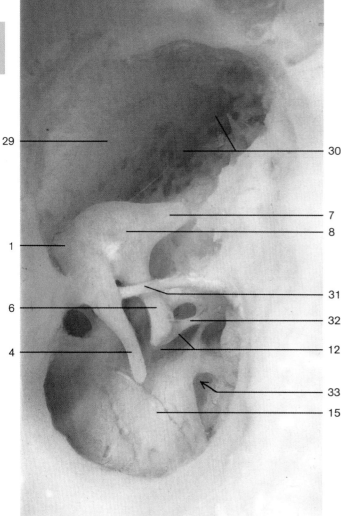

29

30

1

7
8

6

31

32

4

12

33

15

Tympanic cavity with malleus, incus, and stapes, left side (lateral aspect). Tympanic membrane removed, mastoid antrum opened.

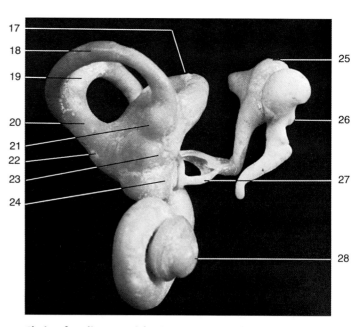

17
18
19
20
21
22
23
24

25

26

27

28

Chain of auditory ossicles in connection with the inner ear, left side (antero-lateral aspect).

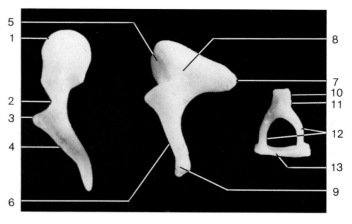

5
1

8

2

7
10
11

3

4

12

13

6

9

Auditory ossicles (isolated).

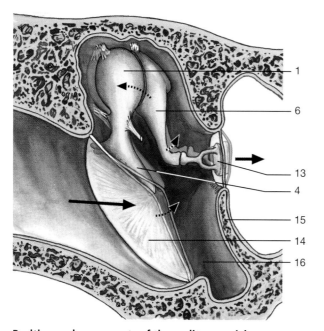

1

6

13
4

15

14

16

Position and movements of the auditory ossicles (schematic drawing).

Malleus
1 Head
2 Neck
3 Lateral process
4 Handle

Incus
5 Articular facet for malleus
6 Long crus
7 Short crus
8 Body
9 Lenticular process

Stapes
10 Head
11 Neck
12 Anterior and posterior crura
13 Base

Walls of tympanic cavity
14 Tympanic membrane
15 Promontory
16 Hypotympanic recess of tympanic cavity

Internal ear (labyrinth)
17 Lateral semicircular duct
18 Anterior semicircular duct
19 Posterior semicircular duct
20 Common crus
21 Ampulla
22 Beginning of endolymphatic duct
23 Utricular prominence
24 Saccular prominence
25 Incus
26 Malleus
27 Stapes
28 Cochlea

Tympanic cavity
29 Epitympanic recess
30 Mastoid antrum
31 Chorda tympani
32 Tendon of stapedius muscle
33 Round window (fenestra cochleae)

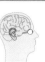

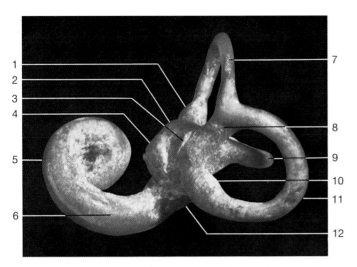

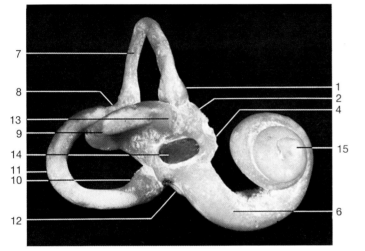

1	Ampulla (anterior semicircular canal)
2	Elliptical recess
3	Aqueduct of the vestibule
4	Spherical recess
5	Cochlea
6	Base of cochlea
7	Anterior semicircular canal
8	Crus commune or common limb
9	Lateral semicircular canal
10	Posterior bony ampulla
11	Posterior semicircular canal (posterior canal)
12	Fenestra cochleae
13	Bony ampulla
14	Fenestra vestibuli
15	Cupula of cochlea
16	External acoustic meatus
17	Mastoid air cells
18	Tympanic cavity and fenestra cochleae (probe)
19	External acoustic meatus
20	Facial canal
21	Base of cochlea and musculotubal canal
22	Malleus and incus
23	Stapes
24	Tympanic membrane
25	Tympanic cavity
26	Aqueduct of cochlea
27	Endolymphatic sac
28	Endolymphatic duct
29	Macula of utricle
30	Macula of saccule

Cast of the right labyrinth (postero-medial aspect).

Cast of the right labyrinth (lateral aspect).

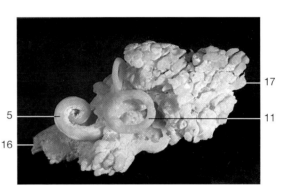

Cast of the labyrinth and mastoid cells.
Life size (posterior aspect).

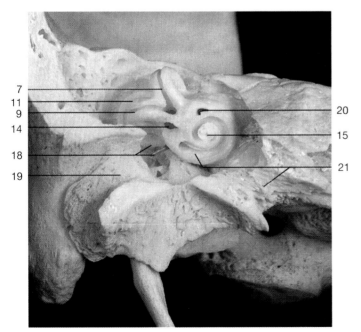

Dissection of bony labyrinth in situ. Semicircular canals and cochlear duct opened.

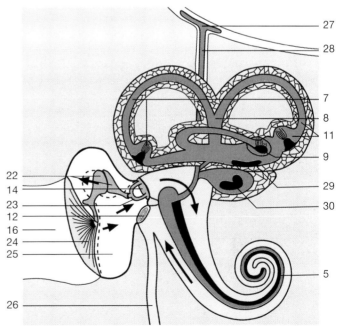

Auditory and vestibular apparatus. Arrows = direction of sound waves; blue = perilymphatic ducts (schematic drawing; from Lütjen-Drecoll, Rohen, Innenansichten des menschlichen Körpers, 2010).

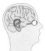

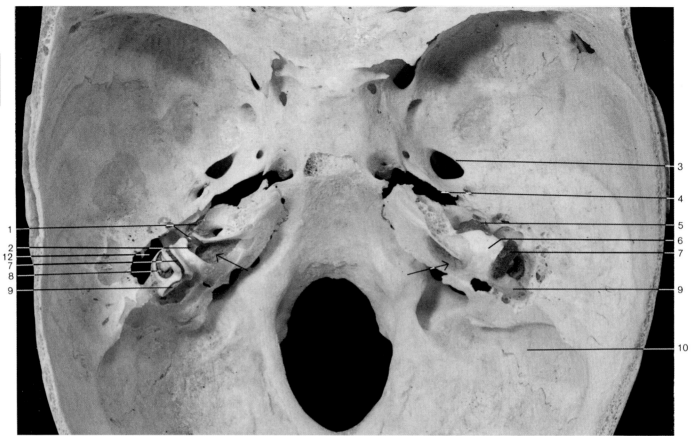

Bony labyrinth, petrous part of the temporal bone (from above). At left: semicircular canals opened; at right: closed. Arrows: internal acoustic meatus.

1	Facial canal and semicanal of auditory tube	9	Posterior semicircular canal	17	Fenestra vestibuli
2	Superior vestibular area	10	Groove for sigmoid sinus	18	Promontory
3	Foramen ovale	11	Sigmoid sinus	19	Zygomatic process
4	Foramen lacerum	12	Tympanic cavity	20	Fenestra cochleae
5	Cochlea	13	Auditory tube	21	Mastoid process
6	Vestibule	14	Mastoid air cells		
7	Anterior semicircular canal	15	Facial and vestibulocochlear nerves		
8	Lateral semicircular canal	16	Temporal fossa		

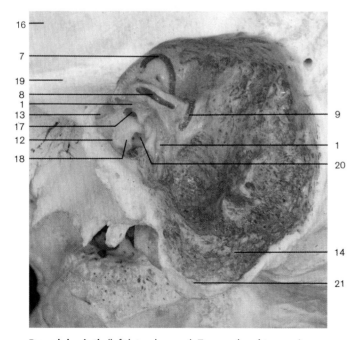

Bony labyrinth (left lateral aspect). Temporal and tympanic bone partly removed, semicircular canals opened.

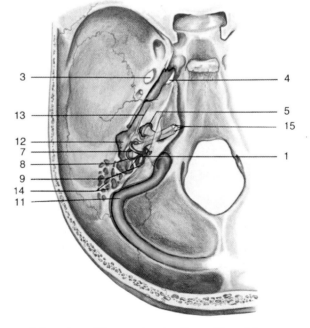

Internal ear. Diagram showing the position of the membranous labyrinth and the tympanic cavity.

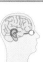

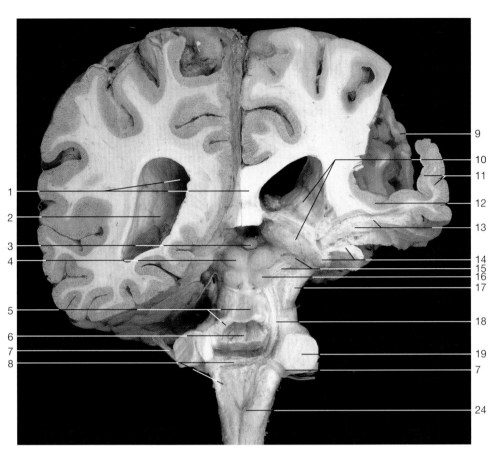

1   Left lateral ventricle
     and corpus callosum
2   Thalamus
3   Pineal gland (epiphysis)
4   Superior colliculus
5   Superior medullary velum and
     superior cerebellar peduncle
6   Rhomboid fossa
7   Vestibulocochlear nerve (n. VIII)
8   Dorsal acoustic striae and
     inferior cerebellar peduncle
9   Insular lobe
10   Caudate nucleus and thalamus
11   Temporal lobe (superior temporal
     gyrus) (area of acoustic centers)
12   Transverse temporal gyri of
     Heschl (area of primary
     acoustic centers)
13   Acoustic radiation of internal
     capsule
14   Lateral geniculate body and
     optic radiation (cut)
15   Medial geniculate body and
     brachium of inferior colliculus
16   Inferior colliculus
17   Cerebral peduncle
18   Lateral lemniscus
19   Middle cerebellar peduncle
20   Dorsal (posterior) cochlear
     nucleus
21   Ventral (anterior) cochlear
     nucleus
22   Inferior olive with olivo-
     cochlear tract of Rasmussen (red)
23   Ganglion spirale
24   Obex
25   Frontal lobe
26   Temporal lobe
27   Middle temporal gyrus (area of
     tertiary acoustic centers)
28   Trapezoid body

Dissection of the brain stem showing the auditory pathway. Cerebellum and posterior part of the two hemispheres have been removed (dorsal aspect).

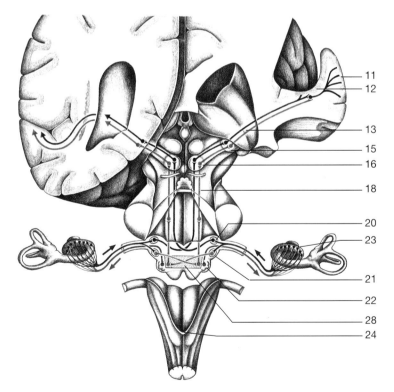

Auditory pathway (schematic drawing, compare with figure above). Red = descending (efferent) pathway (olivocochlear tract of Rasmussen); green and blue = ascending (afferent) pathways.

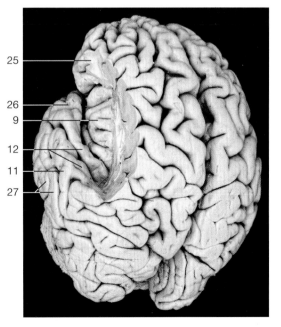

Auditory areas in the left hemisphere (supero-lateral aspect). Parts of the frontal and parietal lobes have been removed.

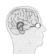

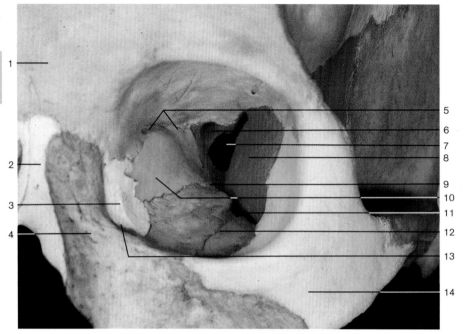

1 Frontal bone
2 Nasal bone
3 Lacrimal bone
4 Maxilla (frontal process)
5 Ethmoidal foramina
6 Lesser wing of sphenoid bone and optic canal
7 Superior orbital fissure
8 Greater wing of sphenoid bone
9 Orbital process of palatine bone
10 Orbital plate of ethmoid bone
11 Inferior orbital fissure
12 Infra-orbital sulcus
13 Nasolacrimal canal
14 Zygomatic bone
15 Frontal sinus
16 Superior rectus muscle
17 Orbital fatty tissue
18 Optic nerve
19 Sclera
20 Inferior rectus muscle
21 Periorbita and maxilla
22 Maxillary sinus
23 Levator palpebrae superioris muscle
24 Superior conjunctival fornix
25 Superior tarsal plate
26 Inferior tarsal plate
27 Inferior conjunctival fornix
28 Inferior oblique muscle
29 Lateral rectus muscle
30 Medial rectus muscle
31 Superior oblique muscle
32 Nasal septum
33 Middle nasal concha
34 Inferior nasal concha
35 Tenon's space
36 Ophthalmic artery
37 Cornea
38 Lens

Bones of the left orbit (indicated by different colors).

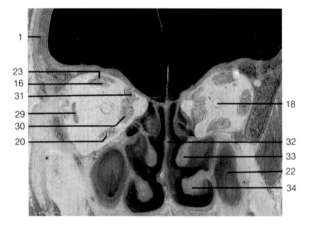

Frontal section through the posterior part of the orbit.

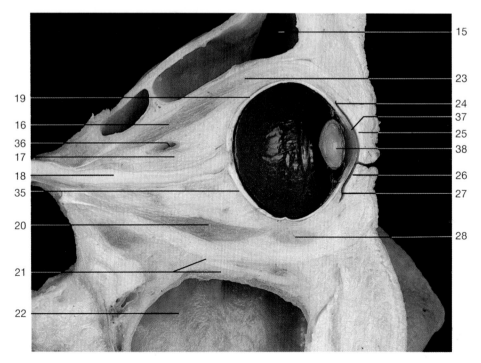

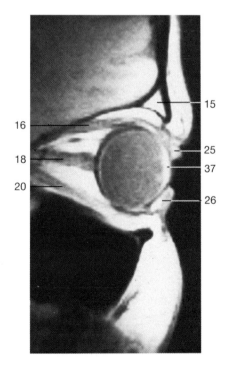

Sagittal section through orbit and eyeball. (Right: MRI scan.)

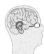

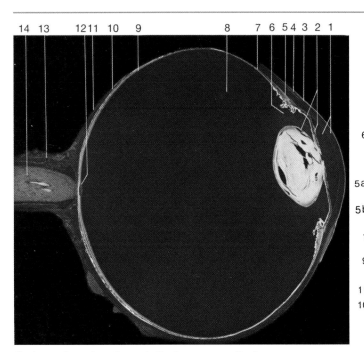

Horizontal section through the human eye (2×).

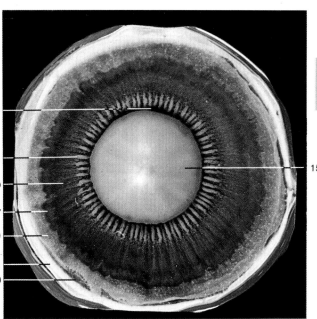

Anterior segment of the eyeball (posterior aspect).
The opacity of the lens is an artifact.

◁

Organization of the eyeball.
Demonstration of vascular tunic of bulb
(schematic drawing).

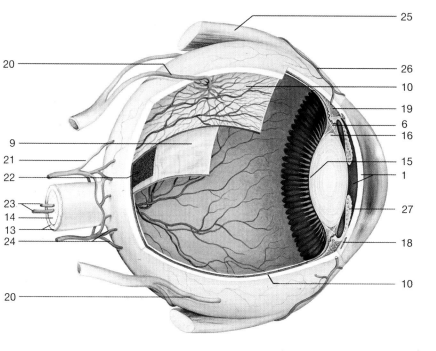

1   Cornea and anterior chamber
2   Iris and lens
3   Transitional zone between corneal
    and conjunctival epithelium
4   Conjunctiva of the eyeball
5   Ciliary body
    a   Ciliary processes (pars plicata)
    b   Ciliary ring (pars plana)
6   Zonular fibers
7   Ora serrata
8   Vitreous body
9   Retina
10 Choroid
11 Sclera
12 Optic disc
13 Dura mater and subarachnoid space
14 Optic nerve (n. II)
15 Lens (posterior pole)
16 Equator of lens
17 Lens (anterior pole)
18 Canal of Schlemm
19 Ciliary muscle
20 Vena vorticosa
21 Long posterior ciliary artery
22 Retinal pigmented epithelium
23 Central retinal artery and vein
24 Short posterior ciliary arteries
25 External ocular muscle
26 Anterior ciliary artery
27 Iris

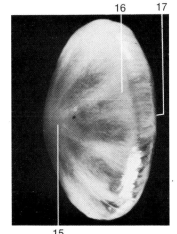

Lens (equatorial aspect),
anterior pole to the right.

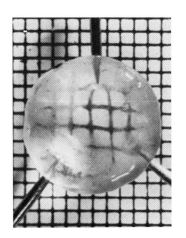

Lens (frontal aspect). Note the
magnification effect.

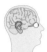

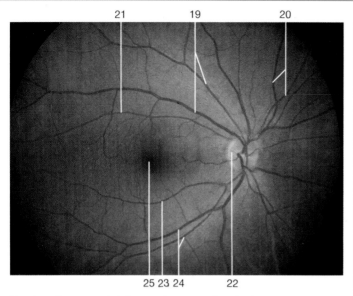

Fundus of a normal right eye (courtesy of Prof. Okamura, Univ. Eye Dept., Kumamoto, Japan). Notice, the arteries are smaller and lighter than the veins.

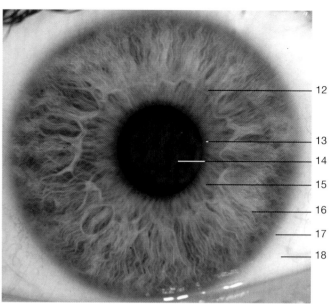

Anterior segment of the human eye (courtesy of Prof. Naumann, Eye Dept., University of Erlangen, Germany). Note the colored iris (16) and the location of the lens behind the iris (14).

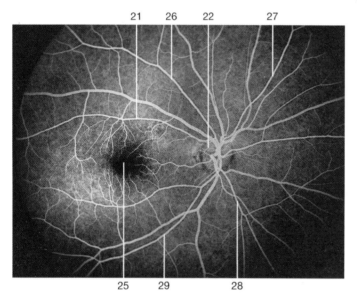

Fluorescent angiography of the right eye; retinal vessels. The same eye as above (courtesy of Prof. Okamura, Univ. Eye Dept., Kumamoto, Japan).

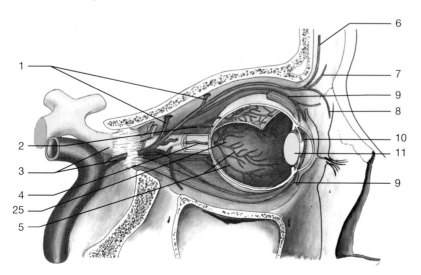

Diagram of the ophthalmic artery and its branches.

1	Posterior and anterior ethmoidal arteries
2	Long and short posterior ciliary arteries
3	Optic nerve and ophthalmic artery
4	Central retinal artery
5	Retinal arteries
6	Supratrochlear artery
7	Supra-orbital artery
8	Dorsal nasal artery
9	Anterior ciliary artery
10	Iridial arteries
11	Lens
12	Iridial fold
13	Pupillary margin of iris
14	Anterior pole of lens
15	Lesser circle of iris
16	Greater circle of iris
17	Margin of cornea or limbus
18	Sclera
19	Superior temporal artery and vein of retina
20	Superior nasal artery and vein of retina
21	Superior macular artery
22	Optic disc
23	Inferior macular artery
24	Inferior temporal artery and vein
25	Fovea centralis and macula lutea
26	Superior temporal artery ⎫
27	Superior nasal artery ⎬ of retina
28	Inferior nasal artery ⎪
29	Inferior temporal artery ⎭

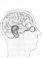

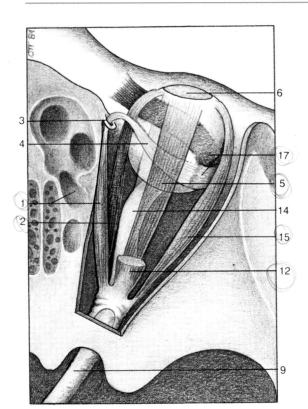

Schematic diagram of the extra-ocular muscles.
Right orbit (from above). Levator palpebrae superioris
muscle has been severed.

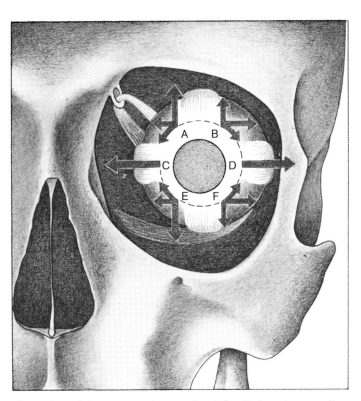

The action of the extra-ocular muscles. Left orbit (anterior aspect).

A = Superior rectus muscle
B = Inferior oblique muscle
C = Medial rectus muscle

D = Lateral rectus muscle
E = Inferior rectus muscle
F = Superior oblique muscle

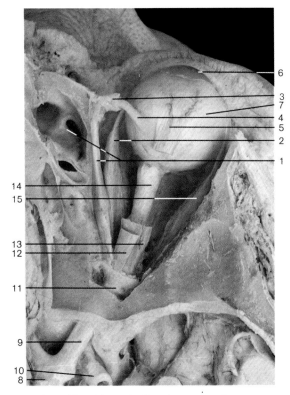

**Right orbit with eyeball and extra-ocular
muscles** (from above). The roof of the orbit has been
removed, the superior rectus muscle and the levator
palpebrae superioris muscle have been severed.

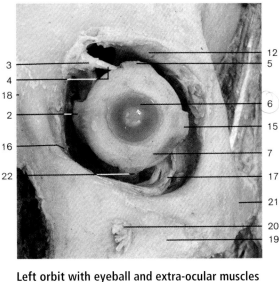

Left orbit with eyeball and extra-ocular muscles
(anterior aspect). Lids, conjunctiva, and lacrimal apparatus have been removed.

1	Superior oblique muscle and ethmoid air cells	12	Levator palpebrae superioris muscle
2	Medial rectus muscle	13	Superior rectus muscle
3	Trochlea	14	Optic nerve (extracranial part)
4	Tendon of superior oblique muscle	15	Lateral rectus muscle
5	Superior rectus muscle	16	Nasolacrimal duct
6	Cornea	17	Inferior oblique muscle
7	Eyeball	18	Nasal bone
8	Optic chiasma	19	Maxilla
9	Optic nerve (intracranial part)	20	Infra-orbital foramen and nerves
10	Internal carotid artery	21	Zygomatic bone
11	Common annular tendon	22	Inferior rectus muscle

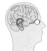

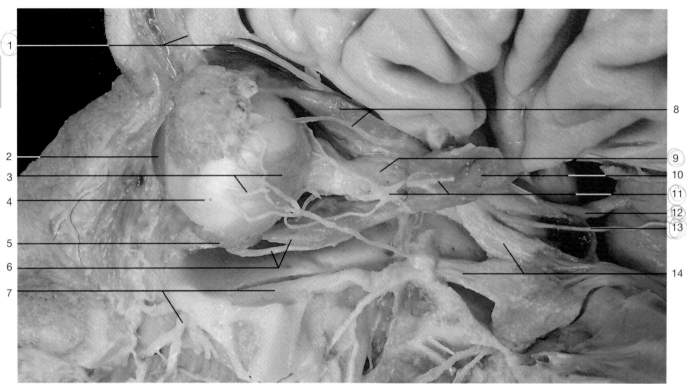

Extra-ocular muscles and their nerves (lateral aspect of left eye). Lateral rectus divided and reflected.

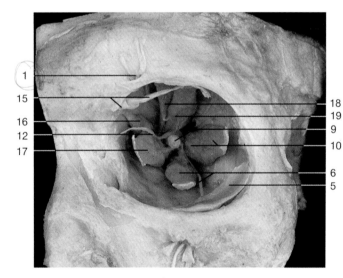

Left orbit with extra-ocular muscles (anterior aspect). Eyeball removed.

Extra-ocular eye muscles (antero-lateral aspect).

1	Supra-orbital nerve
2	Cornea
3	Insertion of lateral rectus muscle
4	Eyeball (sclera)
5	Inferior oblique muscle
6	Inferior rectus muscle and inferior branch of oculomotor nerve
7	Infra-orbital nerve
8	Superior rectus muscle and lacrimal nerve
9	Optic nerve
10	Lateral rectus muscle
11	Ciliary ganglion and abducens nerve (n. VI)

12	Oculomotor nerve (n. III)
13	Trochlear nerve (n. IV)
14	Ophthalmic nerve (n. V$_1$) and maxillary nerve (n. V$_2$)
15	Trochlea and tendon of superior oblique muscle
16	Superior oblique muscle
17	Medial rectus muscle
18	Levator palpebrae superioris muscle
19	Superior rectus muscle
20	Inferior rectus muscle
21	Greater alar cartilage
22	Supra-orbital nerve and levator palpebrae superioris muscle
23	Levator labii superioris muscle

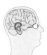

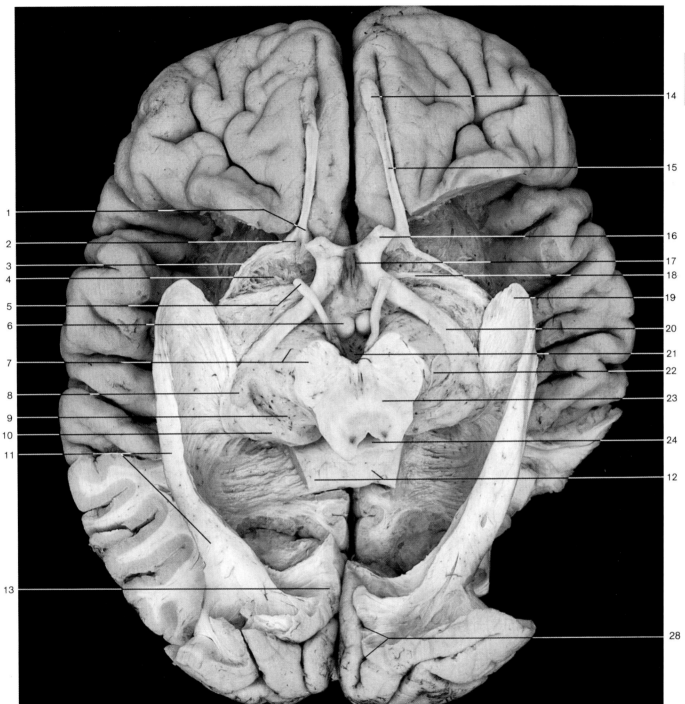

Dissection of the visual pathway (inferior aspect). Frontal pole at top, midbrain divided.

1 Medial olfactory stria
2 Olfactory trigone
3 Lateral olfactory stria
4 Anterior perforated substance
5 Oculomotor nerve (n. III)
6 Mamillary body
7 Cerebral peduncle
8 Lateral geniculate body
9 Medial geniculate body
10 Pulvinar of thalamus
11 Optic radiation
12 Splenium of the corpus callosum (commissural fibers)
13 Cuneus
14 Olfactory bulb

15 Olfactory tract
16 Optic nerve (n. II)
17 Infundibulum
18 Anterior commissure
19 Genu of optic radiation
20 Optic tract
21 Interpeduncular fossa and posterior perforated substance
22 Trochlear nerve (n. IV)
23 Substantia nigra
24 Cerebral aqueduct
25 Visual cortex
26 Line of Gennari
27 Gyrus of striate cortex
28 Calcarine sulcus

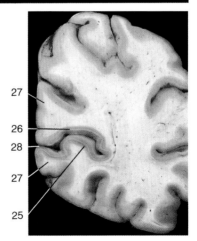

Frontal section of the striate cortex at the level of the striate area in the occipital lobe.

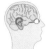

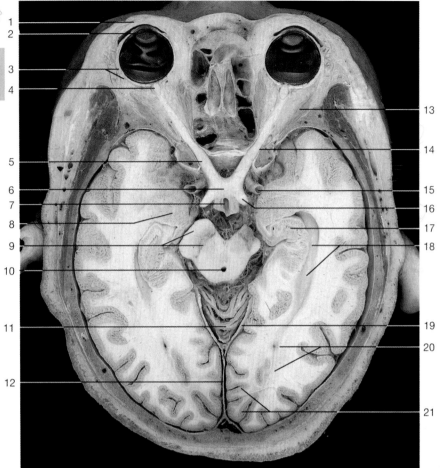

1   Upper lid
2   Cornea
3   Eyeball (sclera, retina)
4   Head of optic nerve
5   Optic nerve
6   Optic chiasma
7   Infundibular recess of hypothalamus
8   Amygdaloid body
9   Substantia nigra and crus cerebri
10 Cerebral aqueduct
11 Vermis of cerebellum
12 Falx cerebri
13 Lateral rectus muscle
14 Optic canal
15 Internal carotid artery
16 Optic tract
17 Hippocampus
18 Inferior horn of lateral ventricle
19 Tentorium cerebelli
20 Optic radiation of Gratiolet
21 Visual cortex (area calcarina, striate cortex)
22 Lens
23 Eyeball
24 Ethmoidal cells
25 Optic nerve with dura sheath
26 Cerebral peduncle
27 Aqueduct of mesencephalon
28 Vermis of cerebellum

Horizontal section through the head at the level of optic chiasma and striate cortex (superior aspect). Note the relationship of hypothalamic infundibulum to optic chiasma.

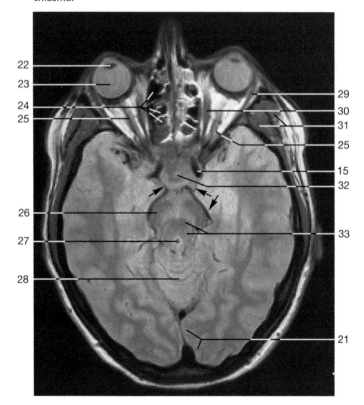

Horizontal section through the human head
(MRI scan, courtesy of Prof. W. J. Huk, Erlangen, Germany).
Arrows = branches of arterial circle of Willis.

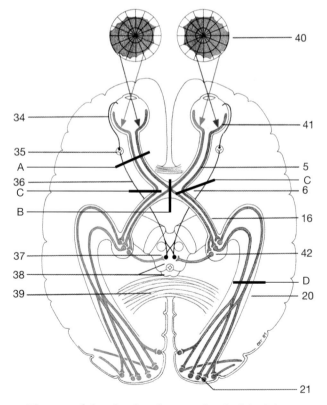

Diagram of the visual pathway and path of the light reflex.

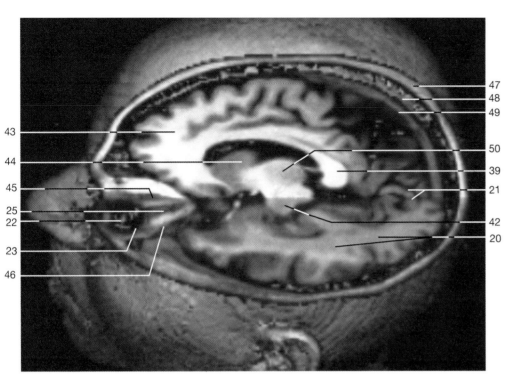

29	Lateral rectus muscle
30	Medial rectus muscle
31	Temporalis muscle
32	Hypophysis (pituitary gland)
33	Midbrain
34	Ciliary nerves (long and short)
35	Ciliary ganglion
36	Oculomotor nerve
37	Accessory oculomotor nucleus
38	Colliculi of midbrain
39	Corpus callosum
40	Visual field
41	Retina
42	Lateral geniculate body
43	Frontal lobe
44	Caudate nucleus
45	Medial rectus muscle
46	Lateral rectus muscle
47	Skin
48	Diploe (skull)
49	Dura mater
50	Thalamus
51	Anterior cerebral artery
52	Caudate nucleus
53	Frontal sinus
54	Internal capsule
55	Lentiform nucleus (putamen)
56	Hippocampus
57	Temporal lobe of left hemisphere

3-D reconstruction of the human visual system (MRI scan flash 40°, courtesy of Prof. Huk, University of Erlangen, Germany).

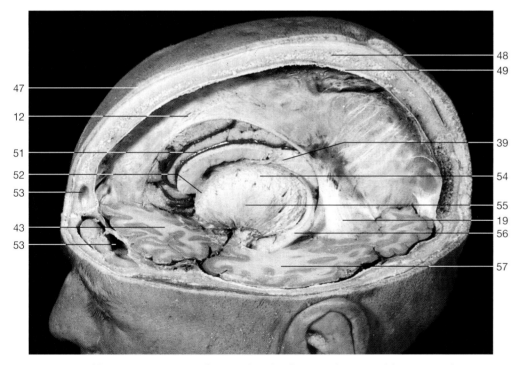

Dissection of brain stem in situ. Left hemisphere has been partly removed (compare with MRI scan above).

In **binocular vision** the visual field (40) is projected upon portions of both retinae (blue and red in the drawing). In the chiasma the fibers from the two retinal portions are combined to form the left optic tract. The fibers of the two eyes remain separated from each other throughout the entire visual pathway up to their final termination in the calcarine cortex (21). **Injuries on the optic pathway** produce visual defects whose nature depends on the location of the injury. Destruction of one optic nerve (A) produces **blindness in the corresponding eye** with loss of pupillary light reflex. If **lesions of the chiasma** destroy the crossing fibers of the nasal portions of the retina (B), both temporal fields of vision are lost **(bitemporal hemianopsia)**. If both lateral angles of the chiasma are compressed (C), the nondecussating fibers from the temporal retinae are affected, resulting in loss of nasal visual fields **(binasal hemianopsia)**. Lesions posterior to the chiasma (D) (i.e., optic tract, lateral geniculate body, optic radiation, or visual cortex) result in a loss of the entire opposite field of vision **(homonymous hemianopsia)**.

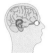

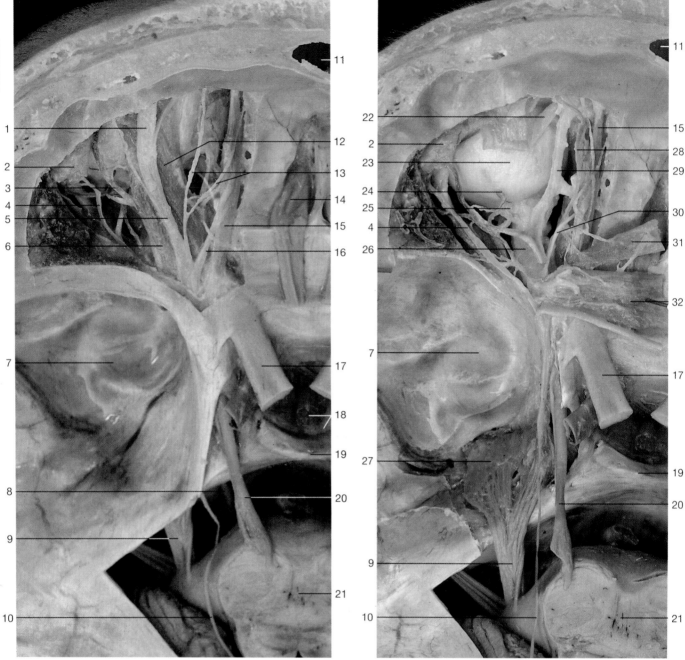

Superficial layer of the left orbit (superior aspect). The roof of the orbit and a portion of the left tentorium have been removed.

Middle layer of the left orbit (superior aspect). The roof of the orbit has been removed and the superior extra-ocular muscles have been divided and reflected.

1	Lateral branch of frontal nerve	10	Trochlear nerve (intracranial part) (n. IV)
2	Lacrimal gland	11	Frontal sinus
3	Lacrimal vein	12	Levator palpebrae superioris muscle
4	Lacrimal nerve	13	Branches of supratrochlear nerve
5	Frontal nerve	14	Olfactory bulb
6	Superior rectus	15	Superior oblique muscle
7	Middle cranial fossa	16	Trochlear nerve (intra-orbital part) (n. IV)
8	Abducent nerve (n. VI)	17	Optic nerve (intracranial part)
9	Trigeminal nerve (n. V)	18	Pituitary gland and infundibulum

19	Dorsum sellae		
20	Oculomotor nerve (n. III)		
21	Midbrain		
22	Tendon of superior oblique muscle		
23	Eyeball		
24	Vena vorticosa		
25	Short ciliary nerves		
26	Optic nerve (extracranial part)		
27	Trigeminal ganglion		

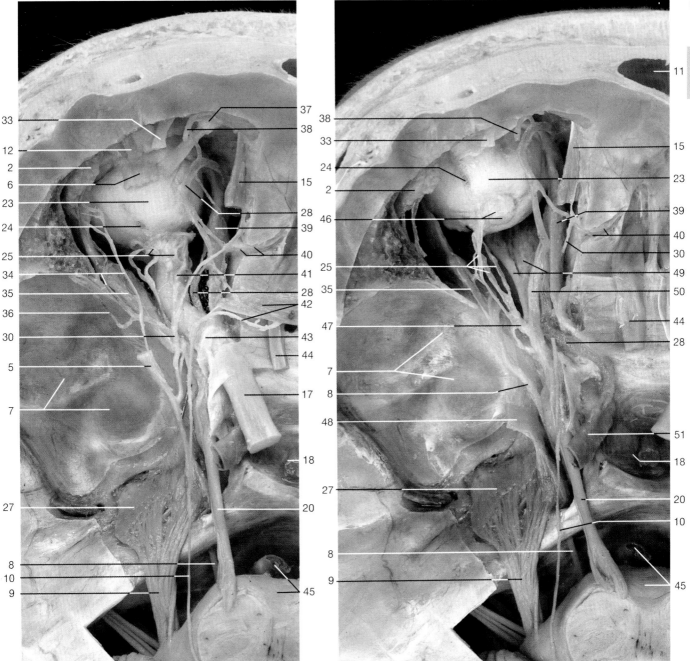

Middle layer of the left orbit (superior aspect). The roof of the orbit and the superior extra-ocular muscles have been removed.

Deeper layer of the left orbit (superior aspect). The optic nerve has now been removed.

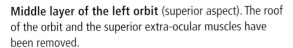

28 Ophthalmic artery
29 Superior ophthalmic vein
30 Nasociliary nerve
31 Levator palpebrae superioris muscle (reflected)
32 Superior rectus muscle (reflected)
33 Lateral branch of supra-orbital nerve
34 Lacrimal nerve and artery
35 Lateral rectus muscle
36 Meningolacrimal artery (anastomosing with middle meningeal artery)

37 Trochlea
38 Medial branch of supra-orbital nerve
39 Medial rectus muscle
40 Anterior ethmoidal artery and nerve
41 Long ciliary nerve
42 Superior oblique muscle and trochlear nerve
43 Common tendinous ring
44 Olfactory tract

45 Basilar artery and pons
46 Optic nerve (external sheath of optic nerve, divided)
47 Ciliary ganglion
48 Ophthalmic nerve (divided, reflected)
49 Inferior branch of oculomotor nerve and inferior rectus muscle
50 Superior branch of oculomotor nerve
51 Internal carotid artery

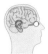

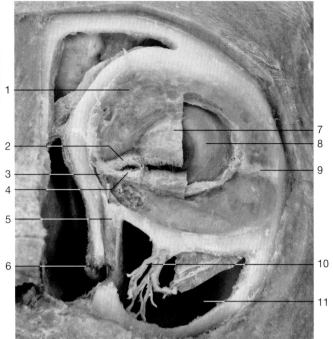

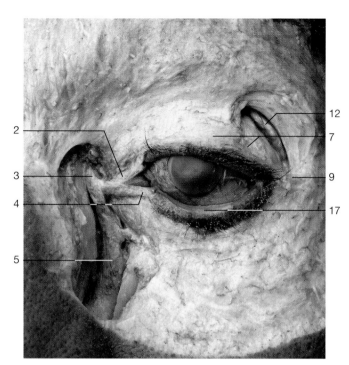

Lids and lacrimal apparatus of the left eye. Parts of the eyelids have been removed to reveal the underlying eyeball. The maxillary sinus has been opened.

Lacrimal apparatus of the left eye.

1 Orbicularis oculi muscle	10 Infra-orbital artery and nerve
2 Superior lacrimal canaliculus	11 Maxillary sinus
3 Lacrimal sac	12 Lacrimal gland
4 Inferior lacrimal canaliculus	13 Medial palpebral ligament
5 Nasolacrimal duct	14 Aponeurosis of levator palpebrae superioris muscle
6 Inferior nasal concha	15 Palpebral portion of the orbicularis oculi muscle
7 Upper eyelid	16 Infra-orbital foramen
8 Eyeball	17 Palpebral conjunctiva of lower lid
9 Lateral palpebral ligament	

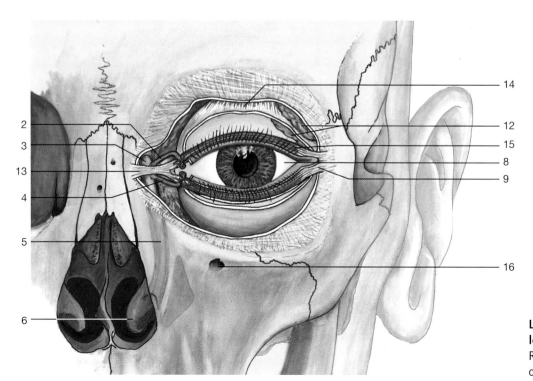

Lacrimal apparatus of the left eye (schematic drawing). Red = Palpebral portion of the orbicularis oculi muscle.

2.4 Oral and Nasal Cavities

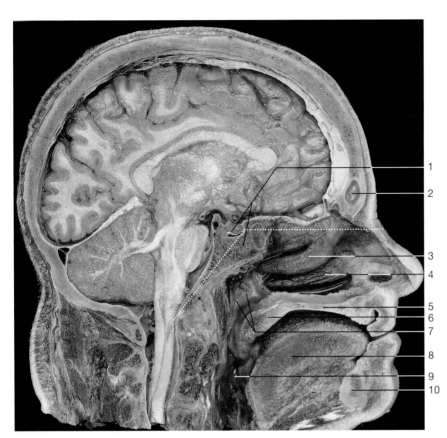

During evolution, the oral and nasal cavities of the human head were situated upon each other, so the human face developed in the frontal plane. The **nasal cavities** are separated by the nasal septum. They contain three conchae, where openings to the ethmoidal and maxillary sinus are located. Posteriorly the two nasal cavities open into the nasopharynx through the choanae.

The **oral cavity** is separated from the nasal cavity by the palate. When the mouth is closed, the oral cavity is fully occupied by the tongue, which is characterized by its high mobility, necessary for the development of speech and song. Specific lymphatic organs (tonsils) are located at the entrance of the nasopharynx in both the nasal and oval cavities to protect the digestive tract from infection. The respiratory and digestory tracts cross each other within the nasopharynx, the most important requirement for the development of speech.

Median sagittal section through the head. The palate separates nasal and oral cavities. The base of the skull forms an angle of about 150° at the sella turcica (dotted line).

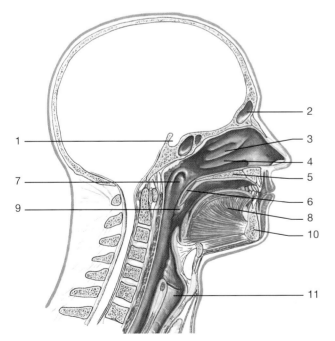

1   Hypophysis within hypophysial fossa
2   Frontal sinus
3   Middle nasal concha
4   Inferior nasal concha
5   Hard palate
6   Soft palate
7   Pharynx with auditory tube
8   Tongue
9   Pharynx with palatine tonsil
10 Mandible
11 Larynx

Median sagittal section through the head (schematic drawing). The tongue has been disposed to show the connection of the oral cavity with the pharynx and the position of the palatine tonsil.

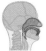

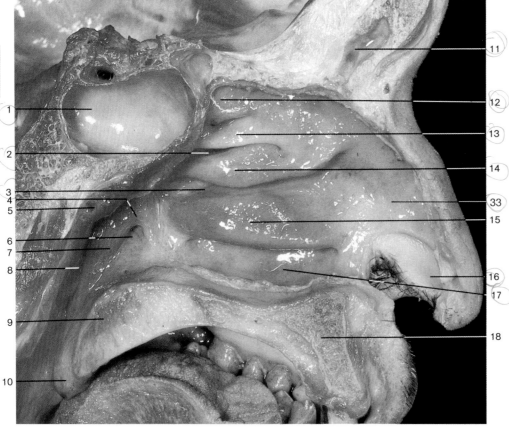

Lateral wall of the nasal cavity. Septum removed.

1　Sphenoidal sinus
2　Superior meatus
3　Middle meatus
4　Tubal elevation
5　Pharyngeal tonsil
6　Pharyngeal orifice of auditory tube
7　Salpingopharyngeal fold
8　Pharyngeal recess
9　Soft palate
10　Uvula
11　Frontal sinus
12　Spheno-ethmoidal recess
13　Superior nasal concha
14　Middle nasal concha
15　Inferior nasal concha
16　Vestibule
17　Inferior meatus
18　Hard palate
19　Grooves for the middle meningeal artery and parietal bone (yellow)
20　Maxillary hiatus
21　Perpendicular process of palatine bone
22　Openings of ethmoidal air cells
23　Opening of frontal sinus
24　Medial pterygoid plate (red)
25　Horizontal plate of palatine process
26　Ethmoidal air cells
27　Maxillary sinus
28　Nasal septum
29　Pterygoid hamulus
30　Nasal bone (white)
31　Frontal process of maxilla (violet)
32　Palatine process of maxilla (violet)
33　Nasal atrium

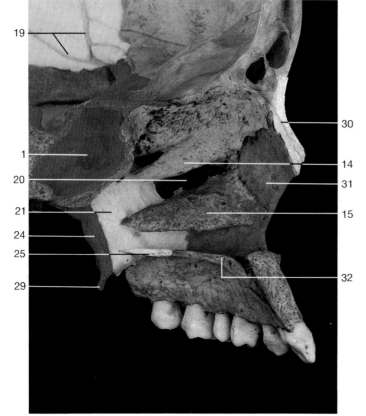

Bones of left nasal cavity (medial aspect).

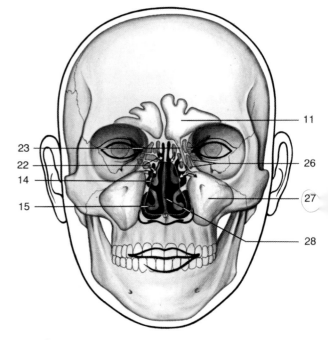

Schematic diagram showing the position of paranasal sinuses. Openings indicated by arrows.

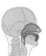

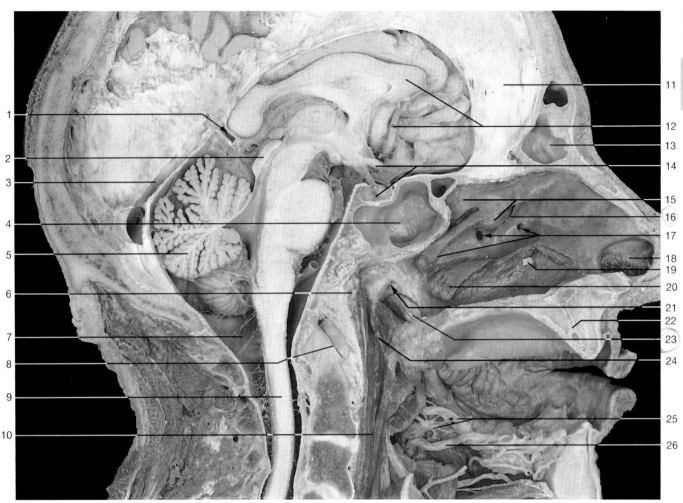

Median section through the head with nasal and oral cavities. The middle and inferior nasal conchae have been partly removed to show the openings of paranasal sinuses.

1	Great cerebral vein (Galen's vein)
2	Tectum of midbrain
3	Straight sinus
4	Sphenoidal sinus
5	Cerebellum
6	Pharyngeal tonsil
7	Cerebellomedullary cistern
8	Median atlanto-axial joint
9	Spinal cord
10	Oral part of pharynx
11	Falx cerebri
12	Corpus callosum and anterior cerebral artery
13	Frontal sinus
14	Optic chiasm and pituitary gland
15	Superior nasal concha and ethmoidal bulla
16	Semilunar hiatus
17	Accessory openings to maxillary sinus and cut edge of middle nasal concha
18	Vestibule
19	Opening of nasolacrimal duct
20	Inferior nasal concha (cut)
21	Opening of auditory tube
22	Incisive canal
23	Levator veli palatini muscle
24	Salpingopharyngeal fold
25	Lingual nerve and submandibular ganglion
26	Submandibular duct
27	Nasofrontal duct
28	Nasolacrimal duct
29	Spheno-ethmoidal recess (of Rosenmüller)
30	Salpingopalatine fold

Lateral wall of nasal cavity. Openings indicated by red arrows (schematic drawing).

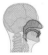

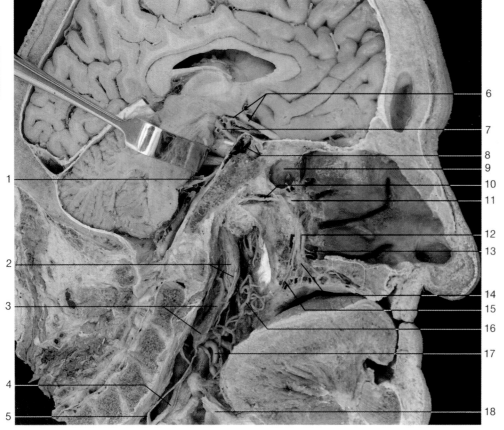

Nerves of the lateral wall of nasal cavity. Sagittal section through the head.
Mucous membranes partly removed, pterygoid canal opened.

1   Facial nerve
2   Internal carotid artery and
    internal carotid plexus
3   Superior cervical ganglion
4   Vagus nerve
5   Sympathetic trunk
6   Optic nerve and ophthalmic
    artery
7   Oculomotor nerve
8   Internal carotid artery and
    cavernous sinus
9   Sphenoidal sinus
10 Nerve of the pterygoid canal
11 Pterygopalatine ganglion
12 Descending palatine artery
13 Lateral inferior posterior
    nasal branches and lateral
    posterior nasal and septal
    arteries
14 Greater palatine nerves and
    artery
15 Lesser palatine nerves and
    arteries
16 Branches of ascending
    pharyngeal artery
17 Lingual artery
18 Epiglottis
19 Anterior ethmoidal artery
20 Olfactory bulb
21 Olfactory tract
22 Nasopalatine nerve
23 Choanae
24 Frontal sinus
25 Crista galli
26 Anterior ethmoidal artery
    and nerve, and nasal branch
    of anterior ethmoidal artery
27 Nasal septum
28 Septal artery
29 Crest of nasal septum
30 Hard palate
31 Tentorium cerebelli
32 Trochlear nerve
33 Trigeminal nerve with
    motor root
34 Internal carotid plexus
35 Lingual nerve with chorda
    tympani
36 Medial pterygoid muscle and
    medial pterygoid plate
37 Inferior alveolar nerve
38 Sympathetic trunk
39 Oculomotor nerve
40 Palatine nerves
41 Tongue
42 Trigeminal ganglion
43 Trigeminal nerve (n. V)
44 Facial nerve (n. VII)
45 Geniculate ganglion
46 Stylomastoid foramen
47 Medial pterygoid muscle

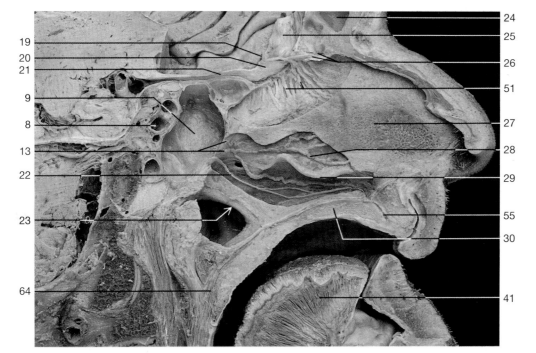

Nasal septum. Dissection of nerves and vessels.

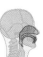

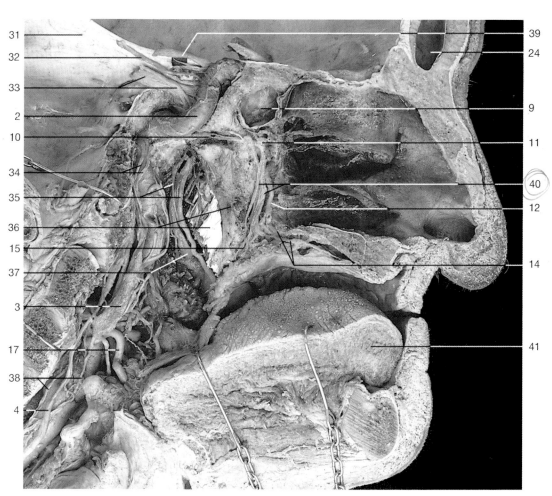

48 Greater petrosal nerve
49 Maxillary nerve
50 Olfactory bulb
51 Olfactory nerves
52 Internal nasal branches of anterior ethmoidal nerve
53 Lateral superior posterior nasal branches
54 Lateral inferior posterior nasal branches
55 Incisive canal with nasopalatine nerve
56 Greater palatine nerve
57 Deep petrosal nerve
58 Mandibular nerve
59 Nasal cavity and inferior nasal concha
60 Opening of auditory tube
61 Tensor veli palatini muscle
62 Levator veli palatini muscle
63 Pharyngeal recess in the nasopharynx
64 Uvula
65 Palatoglossal arch
66 Tonsillar branch of ascending palatine artery
67 Palatine tonsil
68 Palatopharyngeal arch

Nerves of the lateral wall of nasal cavity. Carotid canal opened, mucous membranes of pharynx and nasal cavity partly removed.

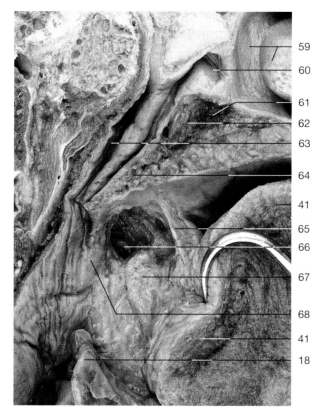

Dissection of palatine tonsil located in the lateral wall of the nasopharynx (left side). Root of tongue reflected.

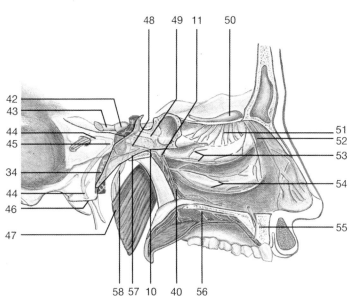

Nerves of the lateral wall of nasal cavity. Body of sphenoid bone appears transparent (schematic drawing).

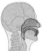

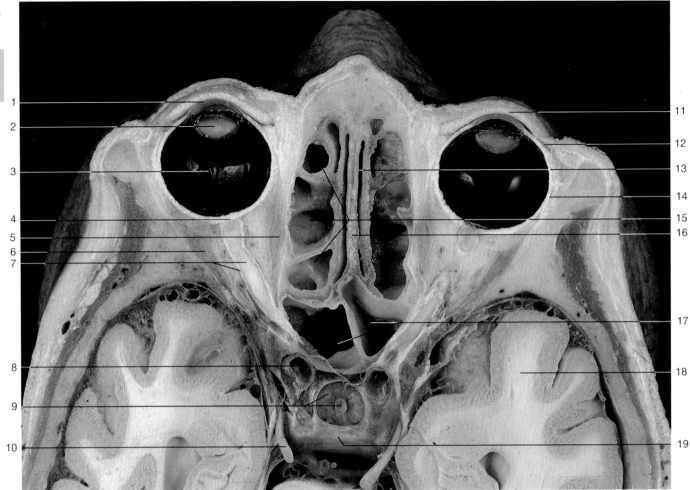

Horizontal section through the nasal cavity, the orbits, and temporal lobes of the brain at the level of pituitary gland.

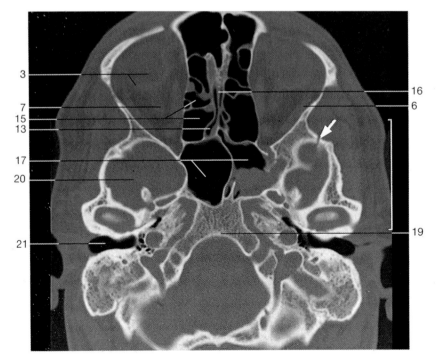

Horizontal section through the head. CT scan. Bar = 2 cm.
Arrow: fracture.

1 Cornea
2 Lens
3 Vitreous body (eyeball)
4 Head of optic nerve
5 Medial rectus muscle
6 Lateral rectus muscle
7 Optic nerve with dural sheath
8 Internal carotid artery
9 Pituitary gland and infundibulum
10 Oculomotor nerve
11 Superior tarsal plate of eyelid
12 Fornix of conjunctiva
13 Nasal cavity
14 Sclera
15 Ethmoidal sinus
16 Nasal septum
17 Sphenoidal sinus
18 Temporal lobe
19 Clivus
20 Middle cranial fossa
21 External acoustic meatus
22 Superior sagittal sinus
23 Falx cerebri
24 Superior rectus and levator
   palpebrae superioris muscles
25 Eyeball and lacrimal gland
26 Inferior rectus and inferior oblique muscles
27 Zygomatic bone
28 Maxillary sinus
29 Inferior nasal concha
30 Hard palate

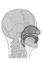

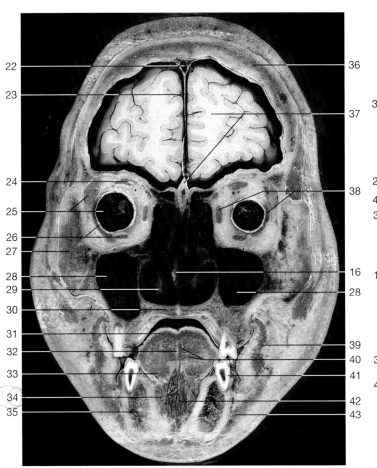

22
23
24
25
26
27
28
29
30
31
32
33
34
35

36
37
38
16
28
39
40
41
42
43

Coronal section through the head at the level of the second premolar of the mandible.

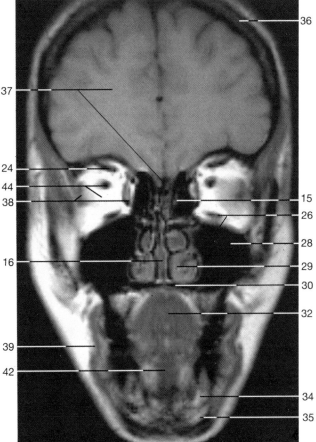

36
37
24
44
38
16
39
42

36
15
26
28
29
30
32
34
35

Coronal section through the head (MRI scan, courtesy of Prof. Heuck, Munich, Germany). Note the situation of the head cavities.

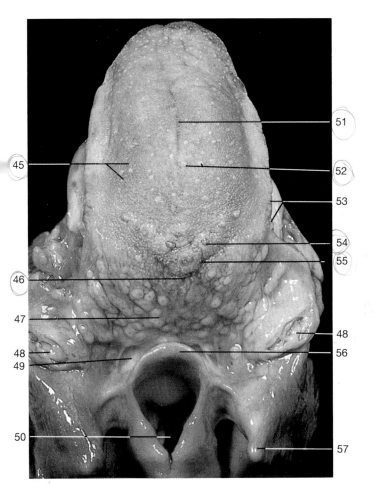

45
46
47
48
49
50

51
52
53
54
55
48
56
57

31   Superior longitudinal muscle of tongue
32   Lingual septum
33   Inferior longitudinal muscle of tongue
34   Sublingual gland
35   Mandible
36   Calvaria
37   Frontal lobe of brain and crista galli
38   Lateral and medial rectus muscles
39   Buccinator muscle
40   Vertical and transverse muscles of tongue
41   Second premolar of mandible
42   Genioglossus muscle
43   Platysma muscle
44   Orbit and optic nerve
45   Filiform papillae
46   Foramen cecum
47   Root of tongue (lingual tonsil)
48   Palatine tonsil
49   Vallecula of epiglottis
50   Vestibule of larynx
51   Median sulcus of tongue
52   Fungiform papillae
53   Foliate papillae
54   Circumvallate papilla
55   Sulcus terminalis
56   Epiglottis
57   Greater cornu of hyoid bone

◁ **Dorsal surface of the tongue and laryngeal inlet.**

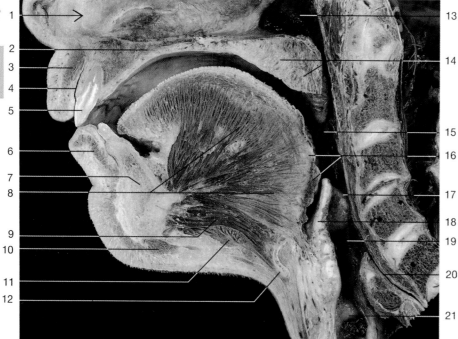

1	Nasal cavity
2	Hard palate
3	Upper lip and orbicularis oris muscle
4	Vestibule of oral cavity
5	First incisor
6	Lower lip and orbicularis oris muscle
7	Mandible
8	Genioglossus muscle
9	Geniohyoid muscle
10	Anterior belly of diagastric muscle
11	Mylohyoid muscle
12	Hyoid bone
13	Nasopharynx
14	Soft palate and uvula
15	Oropharynx
16	Root of tongue and lingual tonsil
17	Laryngopharynx
18	Epiglottis
19	Ary-epiglottic fold
20	Laryngopharynx continuous with esophagus
21	Larynx

Median sagittal section through the oral cavity and pharynx.

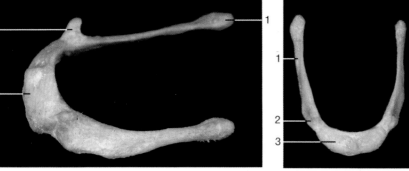

1	Greater cornu	
2	Lesser cornu	} of hyoid bone
3	Body	

Hyoid bone (oblique lateral aspect).   **Hyoid bone** (anterior aspect).

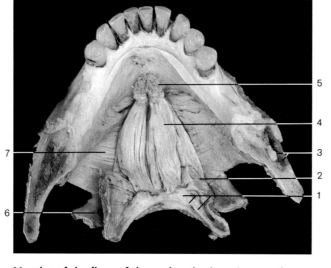

Muscles of the floor of the oral cavity (superior aspect).

1   Lesser cornu and body of hyoid bone
2   Hyoglossus muscle (divided)
3   Ramus of mandible and inferior alveolar nerve
4   Geniohyoid muscle
5   Genioglossus muscle (divided)
6   Stylohyoid muscle (divided)

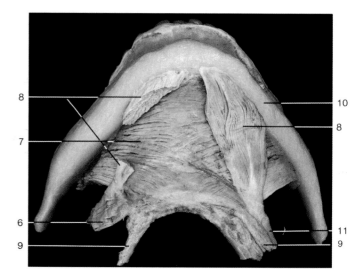

Oral diaphragm, muscles (inferior aspect). Cut on the base.

7   Mylohyoid muscle
8   Anterior belly of digastric muscle
9   Hyoid bone
10 Mandible
11 Intermediate tendon of digastric muscle

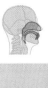

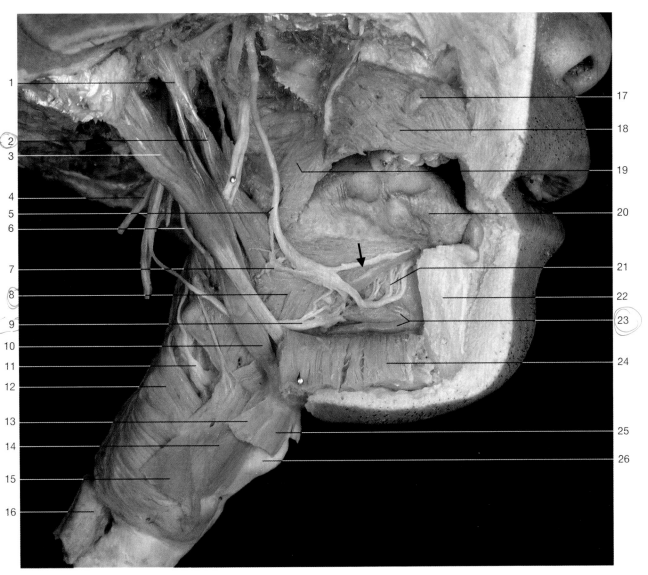

Parapharyngeal and sublingual regions. Innervation of the tongue. Lateral part of face and mandible removed, oral cavity opened. Arrow: submandibular duct.

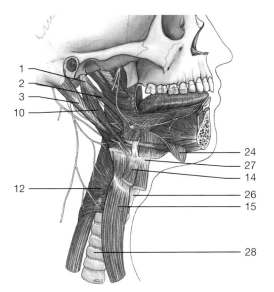

Supra- and infrahyoid muscles and pharynx (schematic drawing).

1	Styloid process	14	Thyrohyoid muscle
2	Styloglossus muscle	15	Sternothyroid muscle
3	Digastric muscle (posterior belly)	16	Esophagus
4	Vagus nerve (n. X)	17	Parotid duct (divided)
5	Lingual nerve (n. V₃)	18	Buccinator
6	Glossopharyngeal nerve (n. IX)	19	Superior constrictor muscle of pharynx
7	Submandibular ganglion	20	Tongue
8	Hyoglossus muscle	21	Terminal branches of lingual nerve
9	Hypoglossal nerve (n. XII)	22	Mandible (divided)
10	Stylohyoid muscle	23	Genioglossus and geniohyoid muscles
11	Internal branch of superior laryngeal nerve (branch of vagus nerve, not visible)	24	Mylohyoid muscle (divided and reflected)
12	Middle constrictor muscle of pharynx	25	Sternohyoid muscle (divided)
13	Omohyoid muscle (divided)	26	Thyroid cartilage
		27	Hyoid bone
		28	Trachea

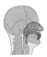

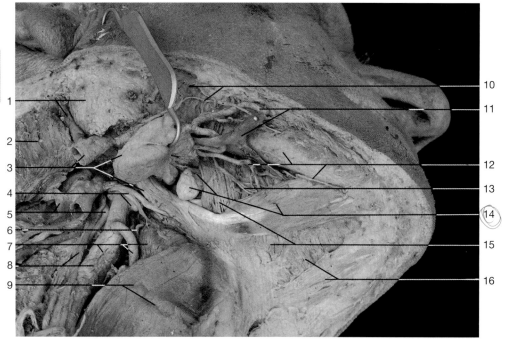

1   Parotid gland and
    retromandibular vein
2   Sternocleidomastoid muscle
3   Retromandibular vein,
    submandibular gland, and
    stylohyoid muscle
4   Hypoglossal nerve and lingual
    artery
5   Vagus nerve and internal
    jugular vein
6   Superior laryngeal artery
7   External carotid artery,
    thyrohyoid muscle, and
    superior thyroid artery
8   Common carotid artery and
    superior root of ansa cervicalis
9   Omohyoid and sternohyoid
    muscles
10 Masseter muscle and marginal
    mandibular branch of facial
    nerve
11 Facial artery and vein
12 Mandible and submental
    artery and vein
13 Mylohyoid nerve
14 Submandibular duct, sublingual
    gland, and anterior belly of
    digastric muscle
15 Mylohyoid muscle
16 Mylohyoid muscle and anterior
    belly of left digastric muscle
17 Hyoglossus muscle and lingual
    artery
18 Lingual nerve
19 Hypoglossal nerve
20 Geniohyoid muscle
21 Anterior belly of right digastric
    muscle
22 Submandibular gland and duct

Submandibular triangle, superficial dissection. Right side (inferior aspect). Submandibular gland has been reflected.

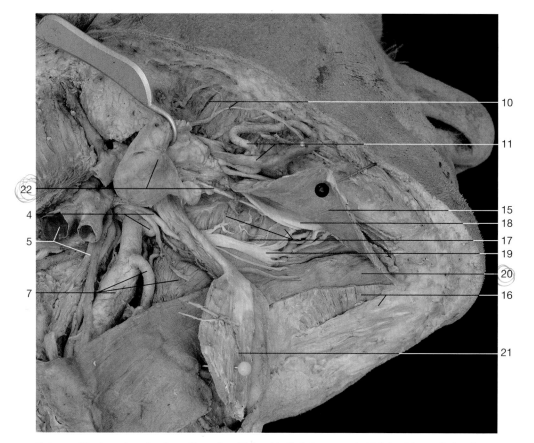

Submandibular triangle, deep dissection. Right side (inferior aspect). Mylohyoid muscle has been severed and reflected to display the lingual and hypoglossal nerves.

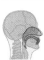

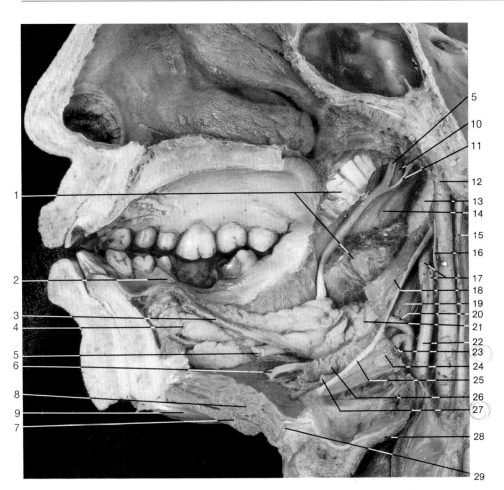

1 Medial pterygoid muscle
2 Sublingual papilla
3 Submandibular duct
4 Sublingual gland
5 Lingual nerve
6 Hypoglossal nerve
7 Mylohyoid muscle
8 Geniohyoid muscle
9 Anterior belly of digastric muscle
10 Inferior alveolar nerve
11 Chorda tympani
12 Internal carotid artery
13 Parotid gland
14 Sphenomandibular ligament
15 Vagus nerve
16 Glossopharyngeal nerve
17 Superficial temporal artery and ascending pharyngeal artery
18 Styloglossus muscle
19 Posterior belly of digastric muscle
20 Facial artery
21 Submandibular gland
22 External carotid artery
23 Lingual artery
24 Middle pharyngeal constrictor muscle
25 Stylohyoid ligament
26 Hyoglossus muscle
27 Deep lingual artery
28 Epiglottis
29 Hyoid bone
30 Buccinator muscle
31 Tongue
32 Mandible (divided)
33 Parotid duct
34 Masseter muscle
35 Right and left sublingual papillae

Oral cavity (internal aspect). Tongue and pharyngeal wall removed.

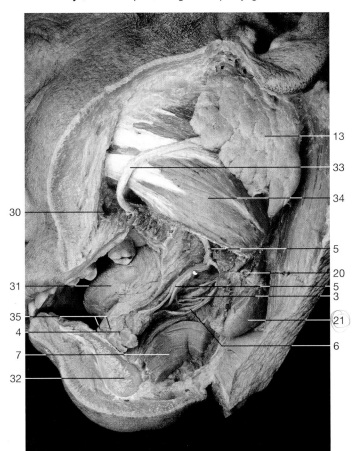

Dissection of major salivary glands. Left mandible and buccinator muscle partly removed to view the oral cavity (infero-lateral aspect).

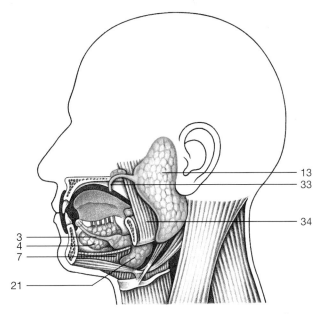

Location of the major salivary glands in relation to the oral cavity.

2.5 Neck and Organs of the Neck

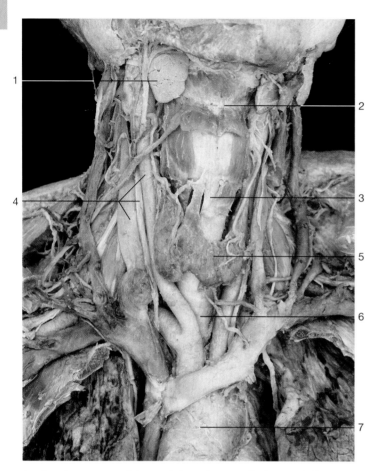

Regional anatomy of the neck (anterior aspect). The anteriorly located muscles and the thoracic wall have been removed.

The anterior aspect of the neck contains the trachea and larynx, which are connected to the nasal cavity via the pharynx. Behind the trachea lies the esophagus, which is connected to the oral cavity, again via the pharynx.

The thyroid gland is located anterior to the trachea, whereas the carotid artery and jugular vein together with the vagus nerve are situated laterally, conjoining the head with the thoracic organs and upper limb.

Underneath the sternocleidomastoid muscle, the cervical portion of the spinal nerves forms the cervical and brachial nervous plexuses that give rise to the innervations of neck and upper limb respectively.

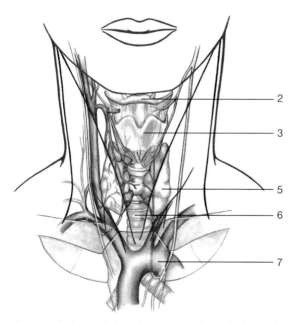

Organs of the neck (anterior aspect, schematic drawing). The main arterial trunks are indicated in red.

1   Submandibular gland
2   Hyoid bone
3   Larynx (thyroid cartilage)
4   Nerves and vessels of the neck
    (carotid artery, internal jugular vein, and vagus nerve)
5   Thyroid gland
6   Trachea
7   Aortic arch

1 Nasal septum
2 Uvula
3 Genioglossus muscle
4 Mandible
5 Geniohyoid muscle
6 Mylohyoid muscle
7 Hyoid bone
8 Thyroid cartilage
9 Manubrium sterni
10 Sphenoidal sinus
11 Nasopharynx
12 Oropharynx
13 Epiglottis
14 Laryngopharynx
15 Arytenoid muscle
16 Vocal fold
17 Cricoid cartilage
18 Trachea
19 Left brachiocephalic vein
20 Thymus
21 Esophagus

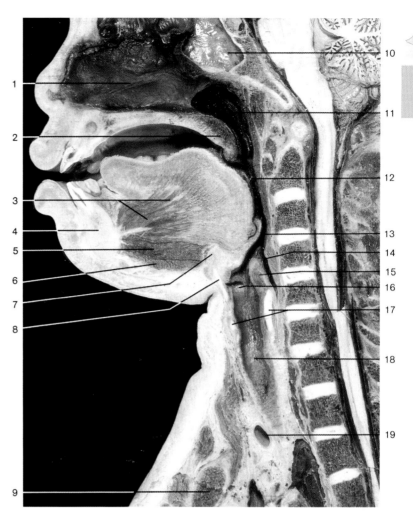

Median section through adult head and neck. Note the low position of the adult larynx when compared with that of the neonate (cf. with the figure below).

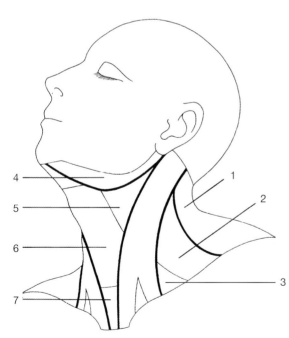

Regions and triangles of the neck (schematic drawing).

1 Posterior cervical region
2 Lateral cervical region
3 Supraclavicular triangle
4 Submandibular triangle
5 Carotid triangle
6 Anterior cervical region
7 Jugular fossa

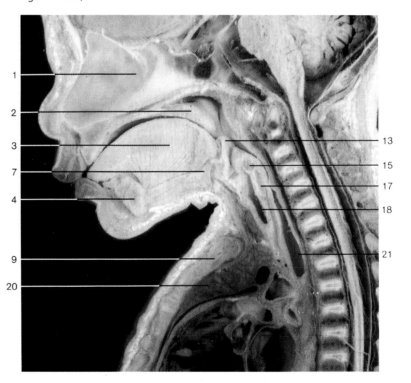

Median section through neonate head and neck. Note the high position of the larynx permitting the epiglottis to nearly reach the uvula (cf. with the figure above).

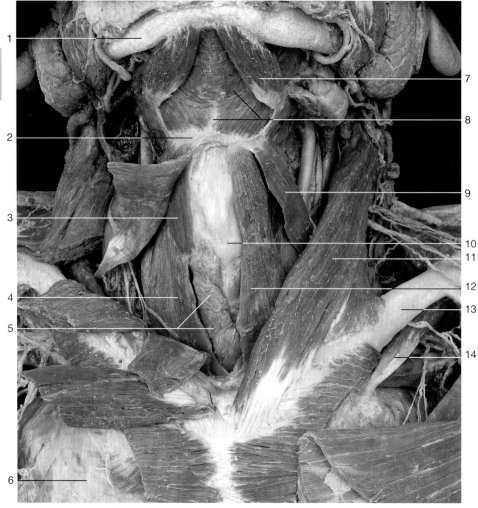

1   Mandible
2   Hyoid bone
3   Thyrohyoid muscle
4   Sternothyroid muscle
5   Thyroid gland
6   Second rib
7   Anterior belly of digastric muscle
8   Mylohyoid muscle
     (and mylohyoid raphe)
9   Omohyoid muscle
10   Thyroid cartilage
11   Sternocleidomastoid muscle
12   Sternohyoid muscle
13   Clavicle
14   Subclavius muscle
15   Posterior belly of digastric muscle
16   Stylohyoid muscle
17   Scalenus muscles
18   Trapezius muscle
19   First rib
20   Scapula
21   Trachea
22   Manubrium sterni

Muscles of the neck (anterior aspect). Sternocleidomastoid and sternohyoid muscles on the right have been divided and reflected.

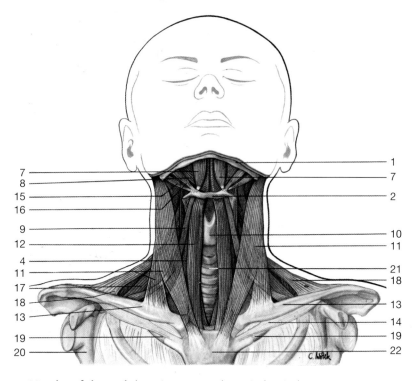

Muscles of the neck (anterior aspect, schematic drawing).

The muscles of the neck are complex and highly sophisticated. There are two major groups of muscles to be distinguished according to their functional aspects. One group is constituted by muscles connecting head to the hyoid bone and the larynx. The second category of muscles links the head and the ribcage.

The sternocleidomastoid muscle represents the border between the anterior and posterior cervical triangle.

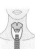

1   Sternohyoid and thyrohyoid
    muscles
2   Larynx
3   Cricoid cartilage
4   Internal jugular vein, common
    carotid artery, and vagus nerve
5   Esophagus
6   Body of cervical vertebra
7   Vertebral artery
8   Spinal cord
9   Scalenus posterior muscle
10 Deep muscles of the neck
11 Trapezius muscle
12 Omohyoid muscle
13 Thyroid gland
14 Sternocleidomastoid muscle
15 Longus colli and longus capitis
    muscles
16 Cervical spinal nerve
17 Vertebral artery and vein,
    and foramen transversarium
18 Ventral and dorsal root of cervical
    spinal nerve
19 Trachea
20 Sympathetic trunk
21 Anterior tubercle of transverse
    process and origin of scalenus
    anterior and medius muscles
22 Superior facet of articular process
23 Spinous process

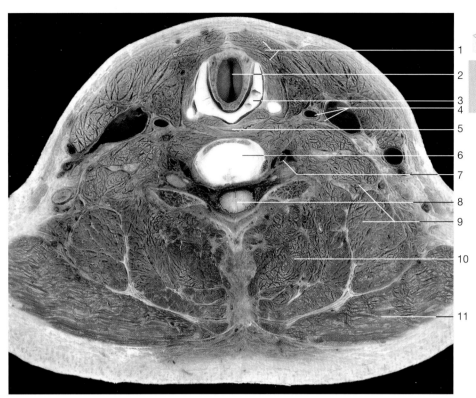

Axial section of the neck at the level of the intervertebral disc between the 5th and 6th cervical vertebra (inferior aspect).

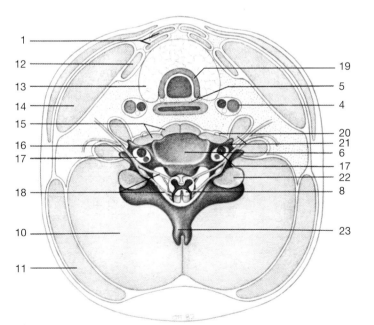

Organization of the neck (axial section at the level of the thyroid gland; schematic drawing).

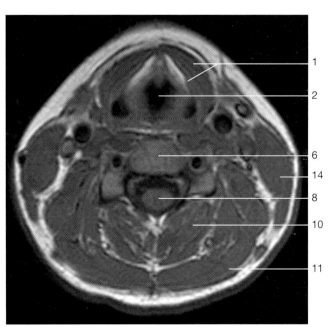

Axial section of the neck at the level of the 4th cervical vertebra (MRI scan; from Heuck et al., MRT-Atlas, 2009).

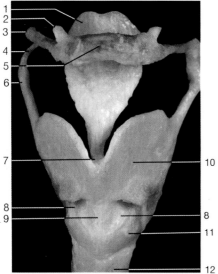

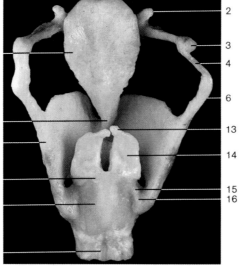

1   Epiglottis
2   Lesser cornu of hyoid bone
3   Greater cornu of hyoid bone
4   Lateral thyrohyoid ligament
5   Body of hyoid bone
6   Superior cornu of thyroid cartilage
7   Thyro-epiglottic ligament
8   Conus elasticus
9   Cricothyroid ligament
10   Thyroid cartilage
11   Cricoid cartilage
12   Trachea
13   Corniculate cartilage
14   Arytenoid cartilage
15   Posterior crico-arytenoid ligament
16   Cricothyroid joint
17   Crico-arytenoid joint

Cartilages of the larynx and the hyoid bone (anterior aspect).

Cartilages of the larynx and the hyoid bone (posterior aspect).

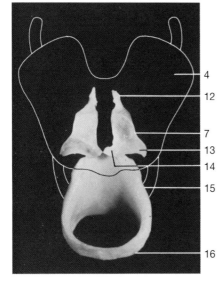

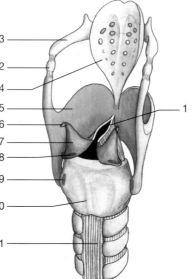

1   Hyoid bone
2   Epiglottis
3   Thyrohyoid membrane
4   Thyroid cartilage
5   Vocal ligament
6   Conus elasticus
7   Arytenoid cartilage
8   Cricoid cartilage
9   Crico-arytenoid joint
10   Cricothyroid joint
11   Tracheal cartilages
12   Corniculate cartilage
13   Muscular process of arytenoid cartilage
14   Vocal process of arytenoid cartilage
15   Lamina of cricoid cartilage
16   Arch of cricoid cartilage

Cartilages of the larynx (anterior aspect). Thyroid cartilage is indicated by the outline.

Cartilages and ligaments of the larynx (lateral aspect).

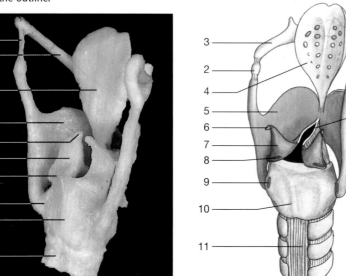

1   Vocal ligament
2   Lateral thyrohyoid ligament
3   Greater cornu of hyoid bone
4   Epiglottis
5   Thyroid cartilage
6   Corniculate cartilage
7   Arytenoid cartilage
8   Crico-arytenoid joint
9   Cricothyroid joint
10   Cricoid cartilage
11   Trachea

Cartilages of the larynx (oblique-posterior aspect).

Cartilages of the larynx (oblique-posterior aspect).

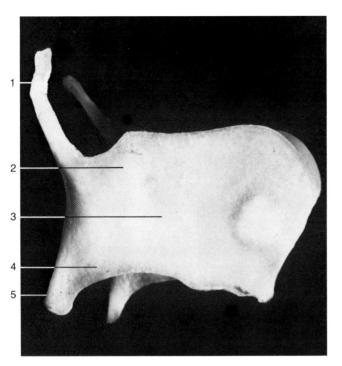

Thyroid cartilage (lateral aspect).

1   Superior cornu
2   Superior thyroid tubercle
3   Lamina of thyroid cartilage

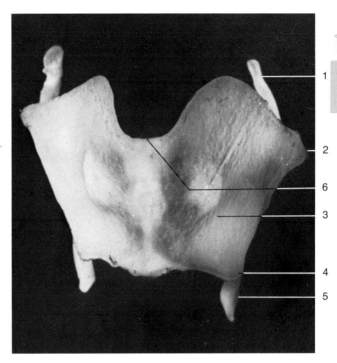

Thyroid cartilage (anterior aspect).

4   Inferior thyroid tubercle
5   Inferior cornu
6   Superior thyroid notch

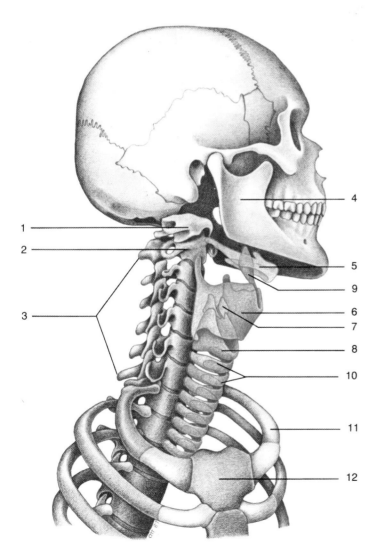

1   Atlas
2   Axis
3   Cervical vertebrae (C₂–C₇)
4   Mandible
5   Hyoid bone
6   Thyroid cartilage
7   Arytenoid cartilage
8   Cricoid cartilage
9   Epiglottis
10 Tracheal cartilages
11 First rib
12 Manubrium sterni

Position of the larynx in the neck (oblique-lateral aspect).
(Schematic drawing.)

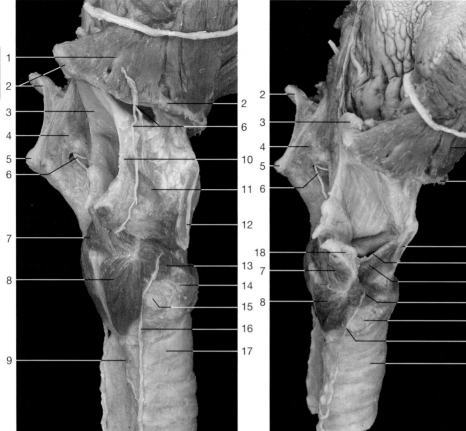

1   Hyoglossus muscle
2   Hyoid bone
3   Epiglottis
4   Thyrohyoid membrane
5   Superior cornu of thyroid
    cartilage
6   Superior laryngeal nerve
7   Transverse arytenoid
    muscle
8   Posterior crico-arytenoid
    muscle
9   Transverse muscle of
    trachea
10 Ary-epiglottic fold
11 Thyro-epiglottic muscle
12 Thyroid cartilage
13 Lateral crico-arytenoid
    muscle
14 Cricoid cartilage
15 Articular facet for thyroid
    cartilage
16 Inferior laryngeal nerve
    (branch of recurrent nerve)
17 Trachea
18 Arytenoid cartilage
19 Vocal ligament
20 Vocalis muscle (part of
    thyro-arytenoid muscle)
21 Thyrohyoideus muscle
22 Cricothyroideus muscle
23 Root of tongue
24 Cuneiform tubercle
25 Corniculate tubercle
26 Ary-epiglottic muscle

Laryngeal muscles (lateral aspect).
Thyroid cartilage (12) and thyro-arytenoid
muscle have been partly removed.

Laryngeal muscles (lateral aspect).
Half of the thyroid cartilage (12) has been
removed. Dissection of the vocal ligament (19).

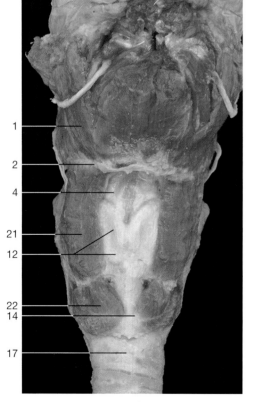

Laryngeal muscles and larynx
(anterior aspect).

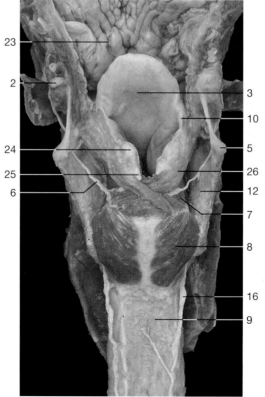

Laryngeal muscles and larynx
(posterior aspect).

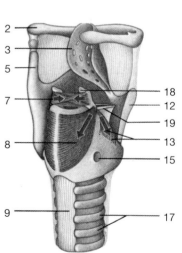

**Action of internal muscles of
the larynx** (schematic drawing).

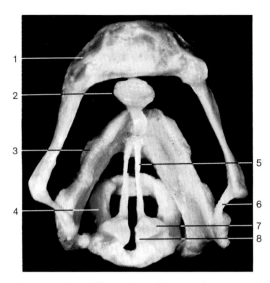

Laryngeal cartilages (superior aspect).

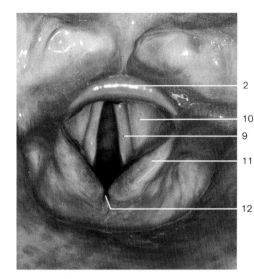

Glottis in vivo (superior aspect).

1 Hyoid bone
2 Epiglottis
3 Thyroid cartilage
4 Cricoid cartilage
5 Vocal ligament
6 Thyrohyoid ligament
7 Arytenoid cartilage
8 Corniculate cartilage
9 Vocal fold
10 Vestibular fold
11 Ary-epiglottic fold
12 Interarytenoid notch
13 Mandible
14 Anterior belly of digastric muscle
15 Mylohyoid muscle
16 Pyramidal lobe of thyroid gland
17 Sternohyoid and sternothyroid muscles
18 Common carotid artery
19 Internal jugular vein
20 Rima glottidis
21 Sternocleidomastoid muscle
22 Transverse arytenoid muscle
23 Pharynx and inferior constrictor muscle
24 Ventricle of larynx
25 Vocalis muscle
26 Trachea
27 Superior cornu of thyroid cartilage
28 Root of tongue (lingual tonsil)
29 Piriform recess
30 Vocalis muscle
31 Lateral crico-arytenoid muscle
32 Thyroid gland

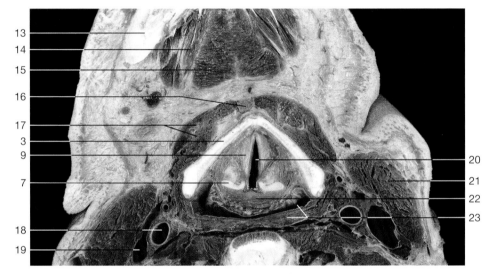

Horizontal section through the larynx at the level of the vocal folds (superior aspect).

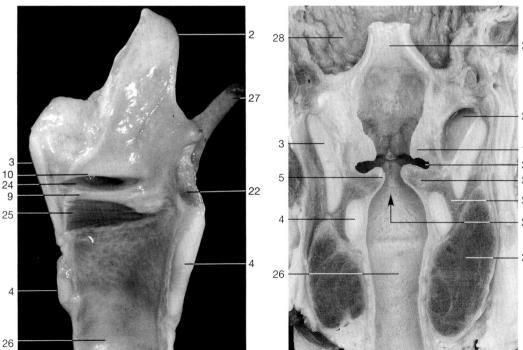

Sagittal section through the larynx.

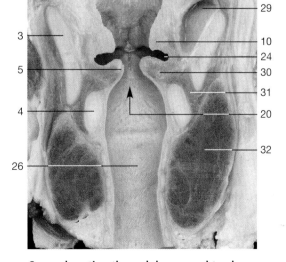

Coronal section through larynx and trachea.

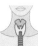

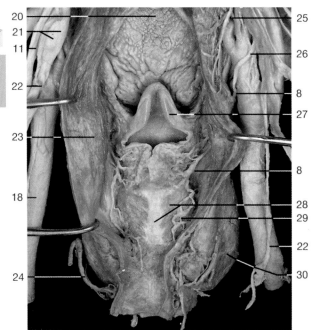

Larynx and its innervation (posterior aspect). Dissection of superior and inferior laryngeal nerves. Pharynx has been opened.

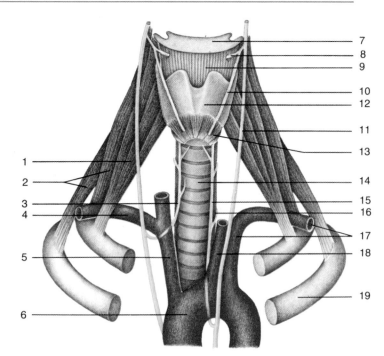

Innervation of the larynx (schematic drawing).

1   Scalenus anterior muscle
2   Scalenus medius and posterior muscles
3   Right recurrent laryngeal nerve
4   Right subclavian artery
5   Brachiocephalic trunk
6   Aortic arch
7   Hyoid bone
8   Internal branch of superior laryngeal nerve
9   Thyrohyoid membrane
10 External branch of superior laryngeal nerve
11 Vagus nerve
12 Thyroid cartilage
13 Cricothyroid muscle
14 Trachea
15 Left recurrent laryngeal nerve
16 Esophagus
17 Left subclavian artery
18 Left common carotid artery
19 Second rib
20 Tongue
21 Superior cervical ganglion
22 Sympathetic trunk
23 Inferior constrictor muscle of pharynx
24 Inferior thyroid artery
25 Glossopharyngeal nerve
26 Superior laryngeal nerve
27 Epiglottis
28 Posterior crico-arytenoid muscle and cricoid cartilage
29 Inferior laryngeal branch of recurrent laryngeal nerve
30 Thyroid gland
31 Superior thyroid artery
32 Thyrocervical trunk
33 Internal thoracic artery
34 Phrenic nerve
35 Hypoglossal nerve
36 Transverse cervical artery
37 Middle cervical ganglion
38 Middle cervical cardiac nerves (branches of sympathetic trunk)
39 Ligamentum arteriosum

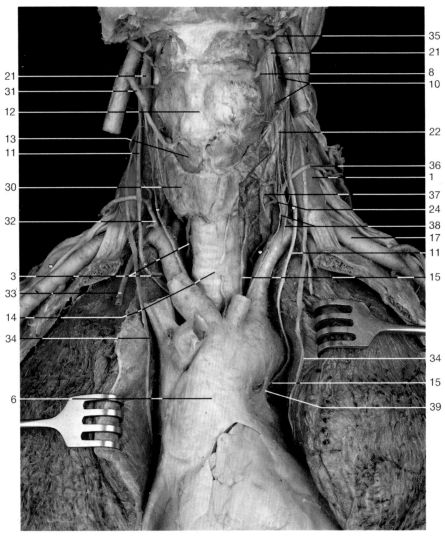

Larynx and thoracic organs (anterior aspect). Dissection of vagus and recurrent laryngeal nerves.

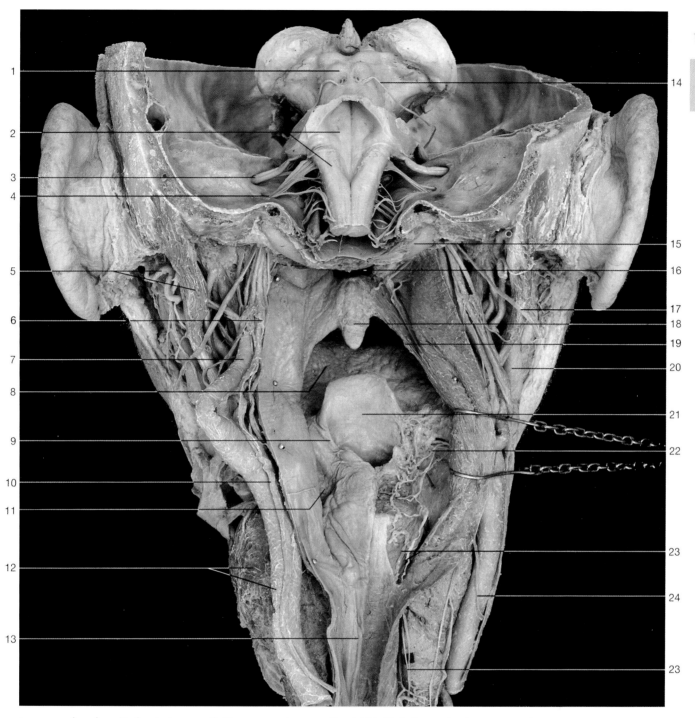

Larynx and oral cavity (posterior aspect). Mucous membrane on the right half of pharynx has been removed.

1 Midbrain (inferior colliculus)	9 Ary-epiglottic fold	18 Uvula and soft palate
2 Rhomboid fossa and medulla oblongata	10 Vagus nerve	19 Palatopharyngeus muscle
3 Vestibulocochlear and facial nerve	11 Piriform recess	20 External carotid artery
4 Glossopharyngeal, vagus, and accessory nerves	12 Thyroid gland and common carotid artery	21 Epiglottis
5 Occipital artery and posterior belly of digastric muscle	13 Esophagus	22 Internal branch of superior laryngeal nerve
6 Superior cervical ganglion	14 Trochlear nerve	23 Inferior laryngeal nerve
7 Internal carotid artery	15 Occipital condyle	24 Ansa cervicalis
8 Oral cavity (tongue)	16 Nasal cavity (choana)	
	17 Accessory nerve	

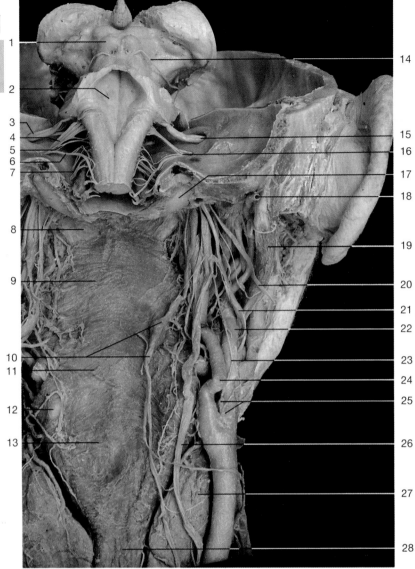

1　Inferior colliculus of midbrain
2　Facial colliculus in floor of rhomboid fossa
3　Vestibulocochlear and facial nerves
4　Glossopharyngeal nerve
5　Vagus nerve
6　Accessory nerve
7　Hypoglossal nerve
8　Pharyngobasilar fascia
9　Superior constrictor muscle of pharynx
10　Sympathetic trunk and superior cervical
　　ganglion (medially displaced)
11　Middle constrictor muscle of pharynx
12　Greater cornu of hyoid bone
13　Inferior constrictor muscle of pharynx
14　Trochlear nerve
15　Internal acoustic meatus with facial and
　　vestibulocochlear nerves
16　Jugular foramen with glossopharyngeal,
　　vagus, and assessory nerves
17　Occipital condyle
18　Occipital artery
19　Posterior belly of digastric muscle
20　Accessory nerve (extracranial part)
21　Hypoglossal nerve (extracranial part)
22　External carotid artery
23　Carotid sinus nerve
24　Internal carotid artery
25　Carotid sinus and carotid body
26　Vagus nerve
27　Thyroid gland
28　Esophagus
29　Choanae
30　Medial pterygoid plate
31　Foramen lacerum
32　Pharyngeal tubercle
33　Hard palate
34　Greater and lesser palatine foramen
35　Pterygoid hamulus
36　Lateral pterygoid plate
37　Pterygoid canal
38　Foramen ovale
39　Mandibular fossa
40　Carotid canal
41　Styloid process and stylomastoid
　　foramen

Pharynx and parapharyngeal nerves in connection with brain stem (posterior aspect).

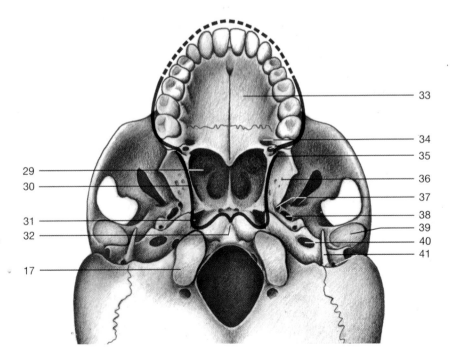

Inferior aspect of the skull.
Red line = outline of superior constrictor muscle in continuation with buccinator muscle and orbicularis oris muscle (semischematic drawing).

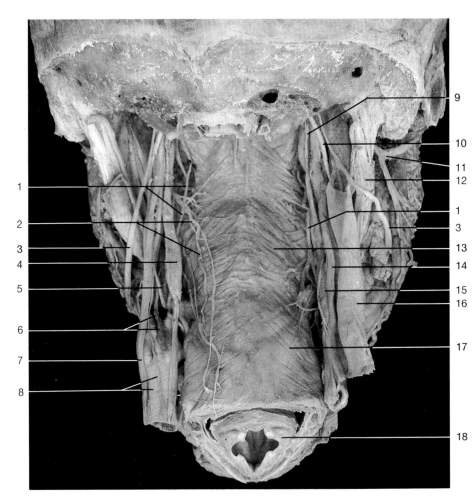

1 Ascending pharyngeal artery
2 Pharyngeal plexus
3 Accessory nerve
4 Superior cervical ganglion of sympathetic trunk
5 Superior laryngeal nerve
6 Carotid body and carotid sinus nerve
7 Left vagus nerve
8 Common carotid artery and cardiac branch of vagus nerve
9 Glossopharyngeal nerve
10 Hypoglossal nerve
11 Facial nerve
12 Posterior belly of digastric muscle
13 Middle constrictor muscle of pharynx
14 Right vagus nerve
15 Sympathetic trunk
16 Internal jugular vein
17 Inferior constrictor muscle of pharynx
18 Larynx
19 Buccinator muscle
20 Soft palate and palatine glands
21 Palatine tonsil
22 Uvula of palate
23 Pharynx (oral part)
24 Parotid gland
25 Longus capitis muscle
26 Median atlanto-axial joint and anterior arch of atlas
27 Dens of axis
28 Spinal cord
29 Dura mater
30 Incisive papilla
31 Oral vestibule
32 Masseter muscle
33 Mandible
34 Mandibular canal with vessels and nerve
35 Medial pterygoid muscle
36 External carotid artery
37 Internal carotid artery
38 Atlas
39 Vertebral artery
40 Splenius capitis muscle
41 Semispinalis capitis muscle

Parapharyngeal nerves and vessels. Dorsal aspect of the pharynx.

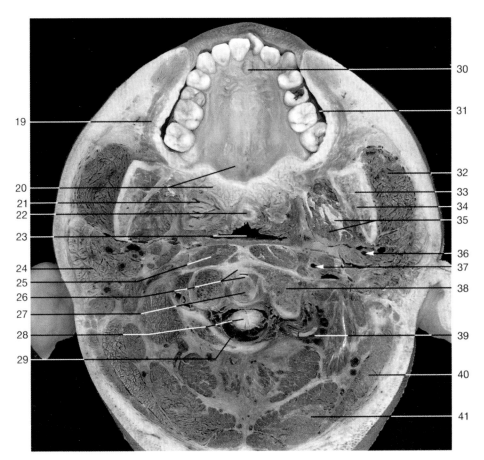

Cross section of head and neck at the level of the atlas (inferior aspect).

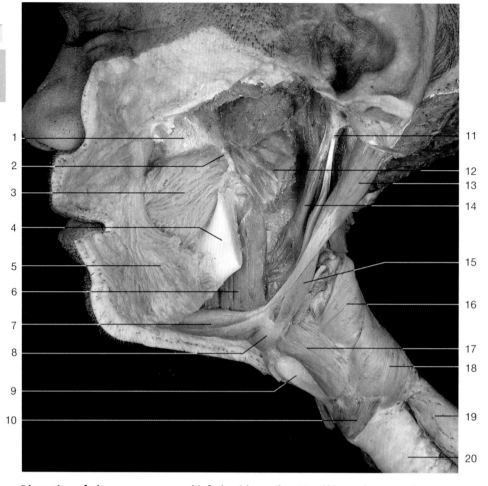

Dissection of pharynx, supra-, and infrahyoid muscles. Mandible partly removed (lateral aspect).

1 Maxilla
2 Pterygomandibular raphe
3 Buccinator muscle
4 Mandible (divided)
5 Depressor anguli oris muscle
6 Mylohyoid muscle
7 Anterior belly of digastric muscle
8 Hyoid bone
9 Thyroid cartilage
10 Cricothyroid muscle
11 Styloid process
12 Medial pterygoid muscle (divided)
13 Posterior belly of digastric muscle
14 Styloglossus muscle
15 Stylohyoid muscle
16 Thyropharyngeal part of inferior constrictor muscle of pharynx
17 Thyrohyoid muscle
18 Cricopharyngeal part of inferior constrictor muscle of pharynx
19 Esophagus
20 Trachea
21 First molar of maxilla
22 Tongue
23 Inferior longitudinal muscle of tongue
24 Genioglossus muscle
25 Superior constrictor muscle of pharynx
26 Hypoglossal nerve
27 Hyoglossus muscle
28 Superior laryngeal nerve and superior laryngeal artery

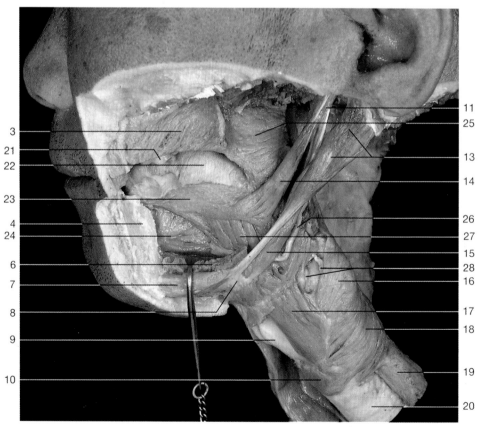

Dissection of pharynx, supra-, and infrahyoid muscles. Oral cavity opened (lateral aspect).

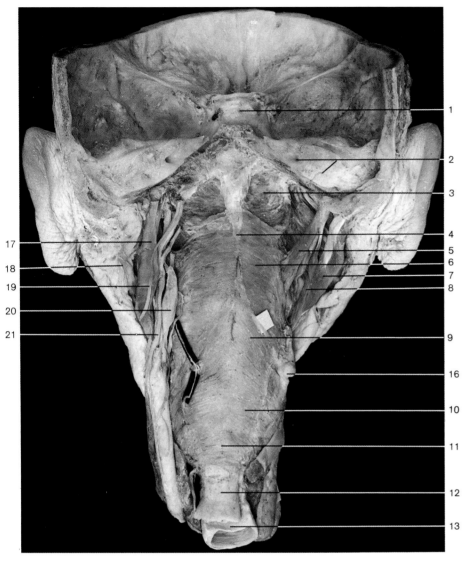

Muscles of the pharynx (posterior aspect).

1 Sella turcica
2 Internal acoustic meatus and petrous part of temporal bone
3 Pharyngobasilar fascia
4 Fibrous raphe of pharynx
5 Stylopharyngeal muscle
6 Superior constrictor muscle of pharynx
7 Posterior belly of digastric muscle
8 Stylohyoid muscle
9 Middle constrictor muscle of pharynx
10 Inferior constrictor muscle of pharynx
11 Muscle-free area (Killian's triangle)
12 Esophagus
13 Trachea
14 Thyroid and parathyroid glands
15 Medial pterygoid muscle
16 Greater horn of hyoid bone
17 Internal jugular vein
18 Parotid gland
19 Accessory nerve
20 Superior cervical ganglion of sympathetic trunk
21 Vagus nerve
22 Laimer's triangle (area prone to developing diverticula)
23 Orbicularis oculi muscle
24 Nasalis muscle
25 Levator labii superioris and levator labii alaeque nasi muscles
26 Levator anguli oris muscle
27 Orbicularis oris muscle
28 Buccinator muscle
29 Depressor labii inferioris muscle
30 Hyoglossus muscle
31 Thyrohyoid muscle
32 Thyroid cartilage
33 Cricothyroid muscle
34 Pterygomandibular raphe
35 Tensor veli palatini muscle
36 Levator veli palatini muscle
37 Depressor anguli oris muscle
38 Mentalis muscle
39 Styloglossus muscle

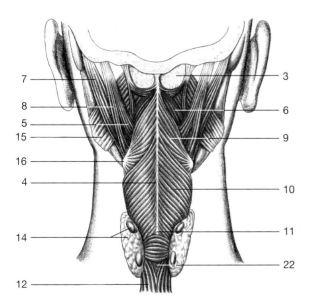

Muscles of the pharynx (posterior aspect). (Schematic drawing.)

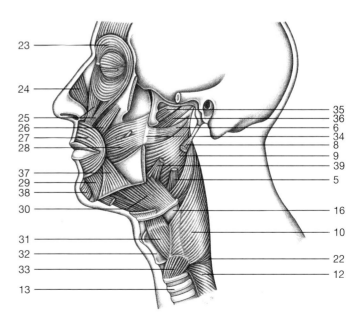

Muscles of the pharynx (lateral aspect). (Schematic drawing.)

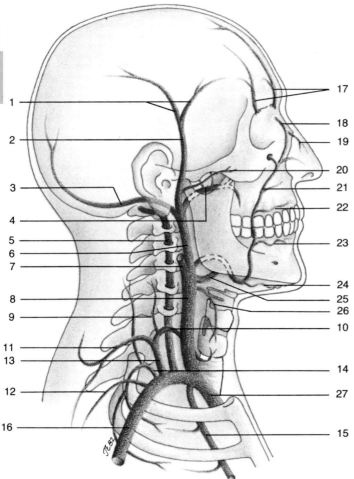

1   Frontal and parietal branches of superficial temporal artery
2   Superficial temporal artery
3   Occipital artery
4   Maxillary artery
5   Vertebral artery
6   External carotid artery
7   Internal carotid artery
8   Common carotid artery (divided)
9   Ascending cervical artery
10 Inferior thyroid artery
11 Transverse cervical artery with two branches (superficial cervical artery and descending scapular artery)
12 Suprascapular artery
13 Thyrocervical trunk
14 Costocervical trunk with two branches (deep cervical artery and superior intercostal artery)
15 Internal thoracic artery
16 Axillary artery
17 Supra-orbital and supratrochlear arteries
18 Angular artery
19 Dorsal nasal artery
20 Transverse facial artery
21 Facial artery
22 Superior labial artery
23 Inferior labial artery
24 Submental artery
25 Lingual artery
26 Superior thyroid artery
27 Brachiocephalic trunk

Arteries of head and neck. Diagram of the main branches of external carotid and subclavian arteries.

▷   **To page 169:**

1   Galea aponeurotica
2   Frontal branch ⎤ of superficial
3   Parietal branch ⎦ temporal artery
4   Superior auricular muscle
5   Superficial temporal artery and vein
6   Middle temporal artery
7   Auriculotemporal nerve
8   Branches of facial nerve
9   Facial nerve
10 External carotid artery within the retromandibular fossa
11 Posterior belly of digastric muscle
12 Sternocleidomastoid artery
13 Sympathetic trunk and superior cervical ganglion
14 Sternocleidomastoid muscle (divided and reflected)
15 Clavicle (divided)
16 Transverse cervical artery
17 Ascending cervical artery and phrenic nerve
18 Scalenus anterior muscle
19 Suprascapular artery

20 Dorsal scapular artery
21 Brachial plexus and axillary artery
22 Thoraco-acromial artery
23 Lateral thoracic artery
24 Median nerve (displaced) and pectoralis minor muscle (reflected)
25 Frontal belly of occipitofrontalis muscle
26 Orbital part of orbicularis oculi muscle
27 Angular artery and vein
28 Facial artery
29 Superior labial artery
30 Zygomaticus major muscle
31 Inferior labial artery
32 Parotid duct
33 Buccal fat pad
34 Maxillary artery
35 Masseter muscle
36 Facial artery and mandible
37 Submental artery
38 Anterior belly of digastric muscle

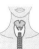

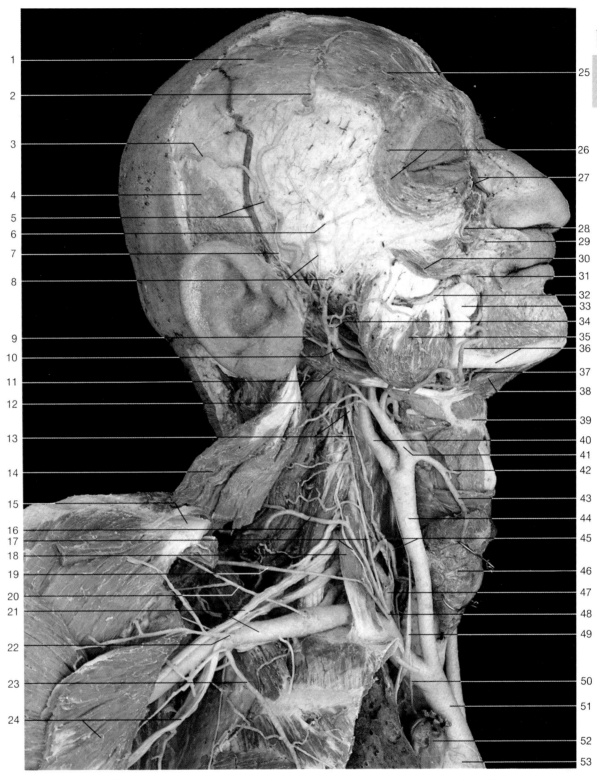

Main branches of head and neck arteries (lateral aspect). Anterior thoracic wall and clavicle partly removed; pectoralis muscles have been reflected to display the subclavian and axillary arteries.

39	Hyoid bone	46	Thyroid gland (right lobe)
40	Internal carotid artery	47	Vertebral artery
41	External carotid artery	48	Thyrocervical trunk
42	Superior laryngeal artery	49	Vagus nerve
43	Superior thyroid artery	50	Ansa subclavia of sympathetic trunk
44	Common carotid artery	51	Brachiocephalic trunk
45	Thyroid ansa of sympathetic trunk and inferior thyroid artery	52	Superior vena cava (divided)
		53	Aortic arch

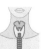

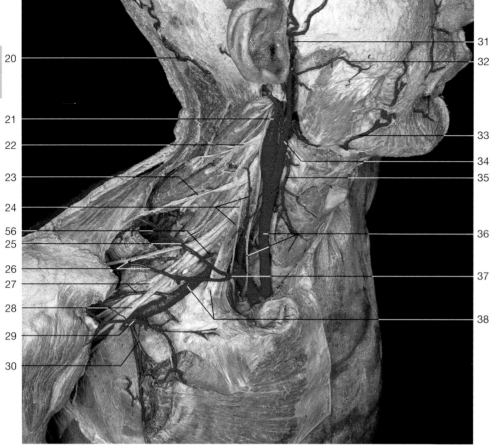

Arteries of head and neck (antero-lateral aspect). Clavicle, sternocleidomastoid muscle, and veins have been partly removed; the arteries have been colored.

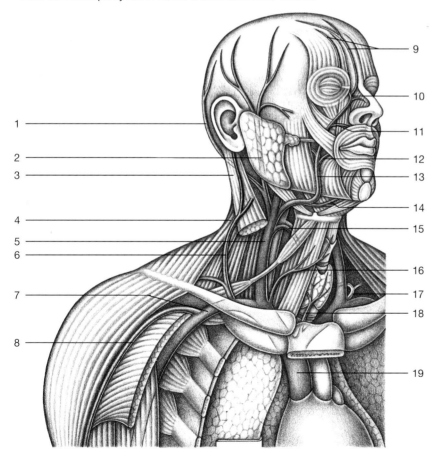

Veins of head and neck. Sternocleidomastoid muscle and anterior thoracic wall partly removed. Note the venous connection with the superior vena cava.

1   Occipital vein
2   Superficial temporal vein
3   Sternocleidomastoid muscle
4   Trapezius muscle
5   Internal jugular vein
6   External jugular vein
7   Subclavian vein
8   Cephalic vein
9   Supra-orbital veins
10 Angular vein
11 Superior labial vein
12 Inferior labial vein
13 Facial vein
14 Submental vein
15 Superior thyroid vein
16 Anterior jugular vein
17 Thoracic duct
18 Inferior thyroid vein
19 Superior vena cava
20 Occipital branch of occipital artery
21 Internal carotid artery
22 Cervical plexus
23 Supraclavicular nerve
24 Phrenic nerve and ascending cervical artery on scalenus anterior muscle
25 Superficial cervical artery
26 Suprascapular artery and nerve
27 Brachial plexus and anterior circumflex humeral artery
28 Lateral cord of brachial plexus
29 Thoraco-acromial artery
30 Lateral thoracic artery
31 Superficial temporal artery
32 Transverse facial artery
33 Facial artery
34 External carotid artery
35 Superior thyroid artery
36 Common carotid artery, vagus nerve, and thyroid gland
37 Thyrocervical trunk
38 Subclavian artery and scalenus anterior muscle
39 Parotid gland and facial nerve
40 Great auricular nerve
41 External jugular vein
42 Brachial plexus
43 Cephalic vein in deltopectoral groove
44 Axillary vein and artery
45 Right brachiocephalic vein
46 Superior vena cava
47 Right lung (reflected)
48 Superficial temporal artery and vein
49 Facial artery and vein
50 Cervical branch of facial nerve and submandibular gland
51 Internal jugular vein, common carotid artery, and omohyoid muscle
52 Anterior jugular vein and thyroid gland
53 Jugular venous arch
54 Left brachiocephalic vein
55 Pericardium of heart (location of right atrium)
56 Transverse cervical artery

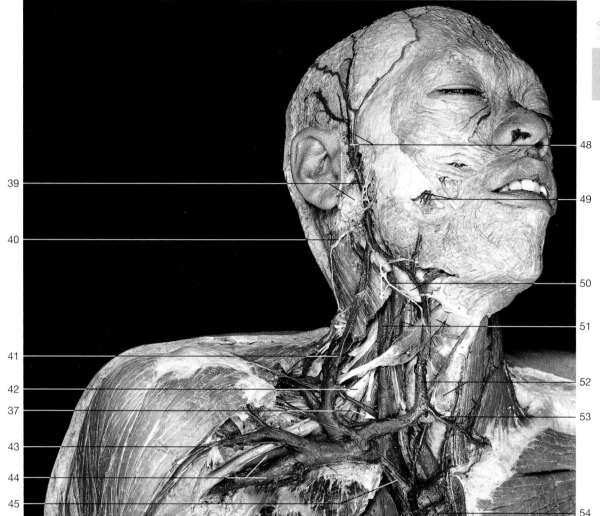

Veins of head and neck (anterior aspect). Part of the thoracic wall, clavicle, and sternocleidomastoid muscle have been removed. Veins are colored blue; arteries, red.

The **internal jugular vein** is the continuation of the sigmoid sinus, which drains most of the venous blood from the brain together with the external cerebrospinal fluid. By joining the subclavian vein, it forms the right brachiocephalic vein, which continues on the right side directly into the superior vena cava. The common way to introduce the lead from a pacemaker device into the heart is by way of the cephalic vein. On the left side, the thoracic duct joins the internal jugular vein at the point where the subclavian vein and the internal jugular vein form the left brachiocephalic vein. Note that the subclavian vein lies in front of the scalenus anterior muscle, whereas the subclavian artery and the brachial plexus lie posterior to that muscle. The **cephalic vein** joins the axillary vein by passing into the deltopectoral triangle. **The subclavian vein** is strongly fixed to the first rib, so it can be punctured with a needle at that point (underneath the sternal end of the clavicle) to introduce a catheter (subclavian line).

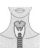

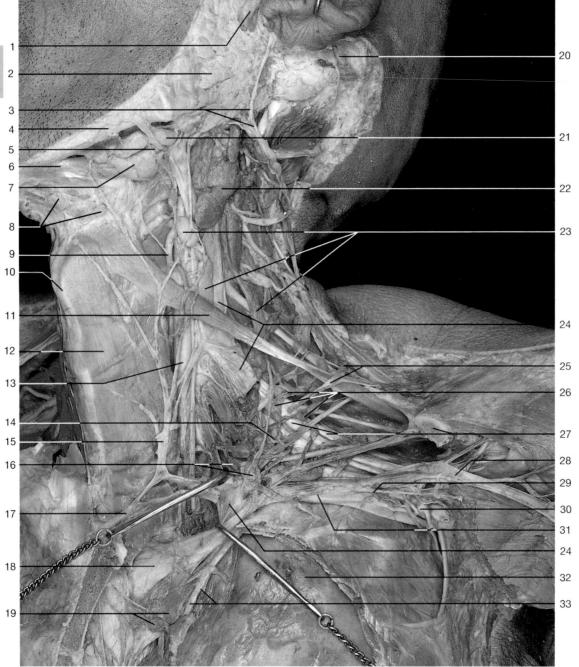

Lymph nodes and lymph vessels of the neck, left side oblique (oblique-lateral aspect). The sternocleidomastoid muscle and the left half of the thoracic wall have been removed. Lower part of the internal jugular vein has been cut and laterally displaced to show the thoracic duct.

1 Superficial parotid lymph node	13 Common carotid artery	24 Internal jugular vein
2 Parotid gland	14 Supraclavicular lymph nodes	25 External jugular vein
3 Great auricular nerve	15 Anterior jugular vein	26 Jugulo-omohyoid lymph nodes
4 Mandible	16 Thoracic duct and internal jugular vein	27 Brachial plexus
5 Facial vein	17 Jugular venous arch	28 Cephalic vein
6 Anterior belly of digastric muscle	18 Left brachiocephalic vein	29 Subclavian trunk
7 Submandibular gland	19 Superior mediastinal lymph nodes	30 Infraclavicular lymph nodes
8 Submental lymph nodes	20 Retro-auricular lymph nodes	31 Subclavian vein
9 Superior thyroid artery	21 Submandibular nodes	32 Lung
10 Thyroid cartilage	22 Superficial cervical lymph nodes	33 Internal thoracic artery and vein
11 Omohyoid muscle	23 Jugulodigastric lymph nodes and jugular trunk	
12 Sternohyoid muscle		

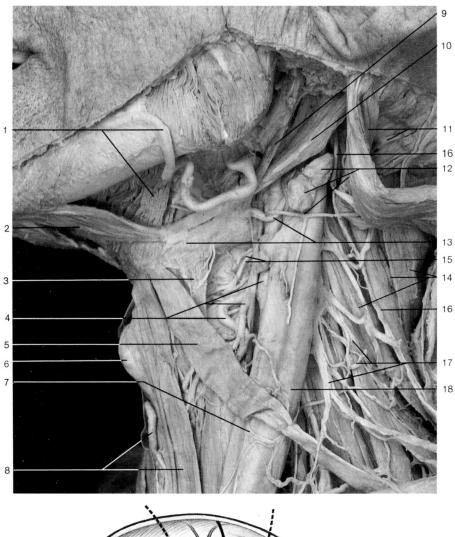

Carotid triangle, left side (lateral aspect). Sternocleidomastoid muscle reflected.

1   Mylohyoid muscle and facial artery
2   Anterior belly of digastric muscle
3   Thyrohyoid
4   External carotid artery, superior thyroid artery, and vein
5   Omohyoid muscle
6   Thyroid cartilage
7   Ansa cervicalis
8   Sternohyoid muscle and superior thyroid artery
9   Stylohyoid muscle
10 Posterior belly of digastric muscle
11 Sternocleidomastoid muscle (reflected)
12 Superior cervical lymph nodes and sternocleidomastoid artery
13 Hyoid bone and hypoglossal nerve (n. XII)
14 Splenius capitis and levator scapulae muscles
15 Superior laryngeal artery and internal branch of superior laryngeal nerve
16 Accessory nerve
17 Cervical plexus
18 Internal jugular vein
19 Facial vein
20 Submental nodes
21 Thoracic duct
22 Retro-auricular nodes
23 Parotid nodes
24 Occipital nodes
25 Submandibular nodes
26 Jugulodigastric nodes } deep cervical
27 Jugulo-omohyoid nodes } nodes
28 Jugular trunk
29 Subclavian trunk
30 Infraclavicular nodes
31 External jugular vein

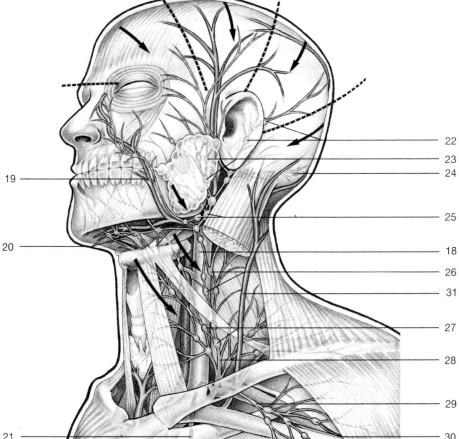

Lymph nodes and veins of head and neck. Dotted lines = border between irrigation areas; arrows: direction of lymph flow.

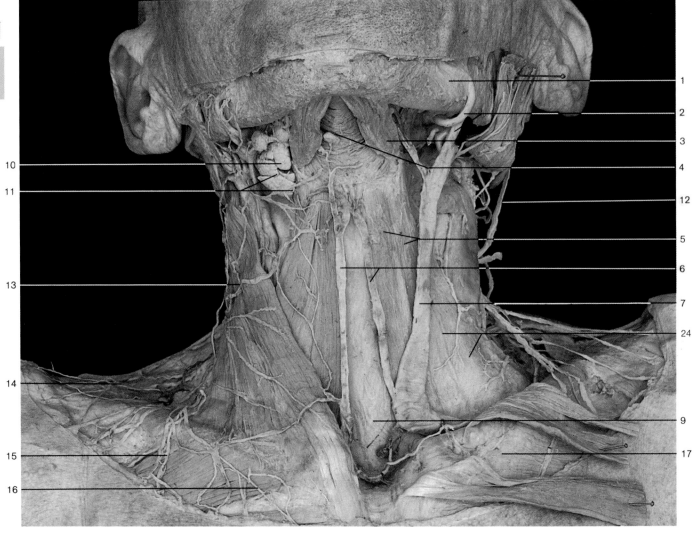

Anterior region of the neck. The superficial fascia has been removed.

1   Mandible
2   Facial artery and vein
3   Anterior belly of digastric muscle
4   Mylohyoid muscle
5   Infrahyoid muscles (sternohyoid, sternothyroid, and omohyoid muscles)
6   Anterior jugular veins
7   External jugular vein
8   Sternocleidomastoid muscle
9   Thyroid gland
10 Submandibular gland
11 Cervical branch of facial nerve
12 Great auricular nerve   ⎫ Cutaneous
13 Transverse cervical nerves   ⎬ branches
14 Lateral supraclavicular nerves   ⎬ of cervical
15 Middle supraclavicular nerves   ⎬ plexus
16 Medial supraclavicular nerves   ⎭
17 Clavicle
18 Platysma muscle
19 Prevertebral lamina of cervical fascia, covering longus colli muscle
20 Vertebral artery and vein
21 Scalenus muscles
22 Trapezius muscle
23 Superficial lamina of cervical fascia
24 Pretracheal lamina of cervical fascia
25 Prevertebral lamina of cervical fascia
26 Carotid sheath with common carotid artery, internal jugular vein, and vagus nerve
27 Cervical part of sympathetic trunk
28 Carotid sheath

◁ **Cross section of the neck** at the level of the thyroid gland. Notice the position of the three laminae of cervical fascia (23, 24, 25).

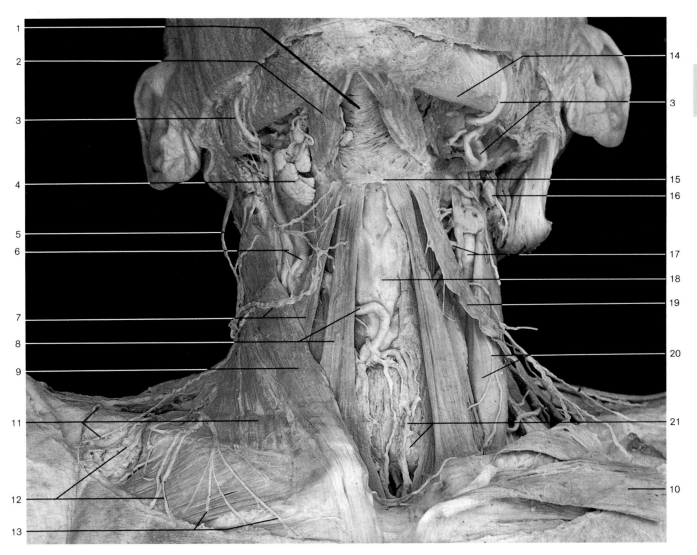

Anterior region of the neck with anterior triangle. The pretracheal lamina of cervical fascia and left sternocleidomastoid muscle have been removed.

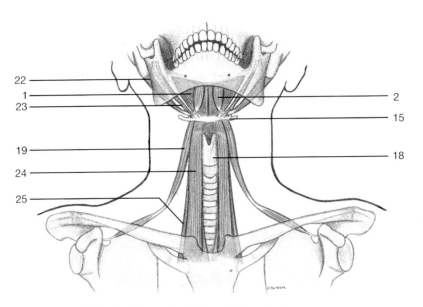

Supra- and infrahyoid muscles (schematic drawing).

1   Mylohyoid muscle
2   Anterior belly of digastric muscle
3   Facial artery
4   Submandibular gland
5   Great auricular nerve
6   Internal jugular vein and common carotid artery
7   Transverse cervical nerve and omohyoid muscle
8   Sternohyoid muscle and superior thyroid artery
9   Sternocleidomastoid muscle (sternal head)
10 Left sternocleidomastoid muscle (reflected)
11 Sternocleidomastoid muscle (clavicular head)
    and lateral supraclavicular nerves
12 Middle supraclavicular nerves
13 Medial supraclavicular nerves
14 Mandible
15 Hyoid bone
16 Superficial cervical lymph nodes
17 Left superior thyroid artery and external carotid
    artery
18 Thyroid cartilage
19 Omohyoid muscle (superior belly)
20 Internal jugular vein and branches of ansa
    cervicalis
21 Thyroid gland and unpaired inferior thyroid vein
22 Posterior belly of digastric muscle
23 Stylohyoid muscle
24 Sternohyoid muscle
25 Sternothyroid muscle

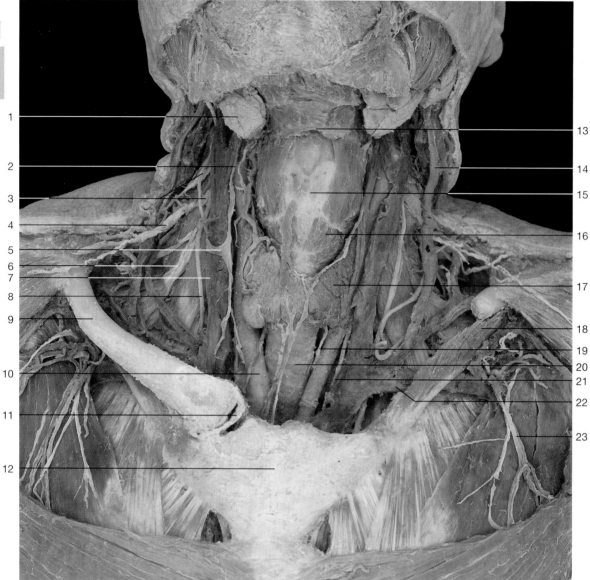

Anterior region of the neck. Sternocleidomastoid muscles and left clavicle have been removed. Thyroid gland in relation to trachea, larynx, and vessels of the neck is shown.

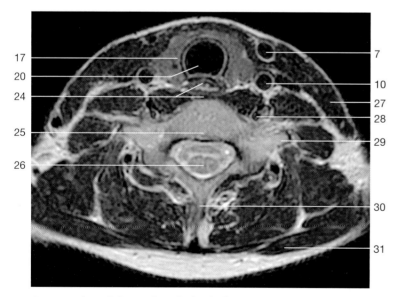

Cross section of the neck at the level of the thyroid gland (MRI scan, courtesy of Prof. Heuck, Munich).

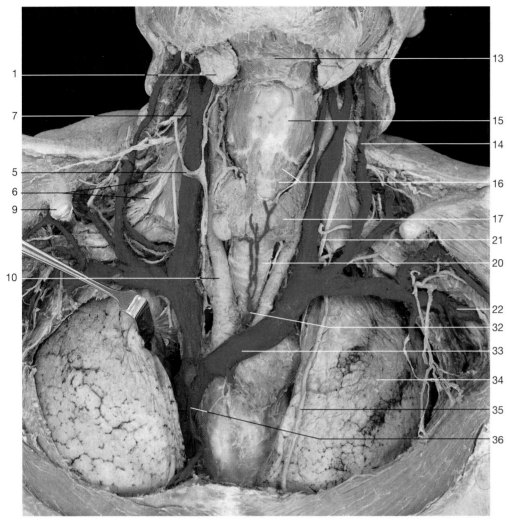

1   Submandibular gland
2   Cervical branch of facial
    nerve (n. VII)
3   Cervical plexus
4   Middle supraclavicular
    nerves
5   Ansa cervicalis
6   Brachial plexus
7   Internal jugular vein
8   Phrenic nerve
9   Clavicle
10 Common carotid artery
11 Sternoclavicular articulation
    with articular disc
12 Manubrium of sternum
13 Hyoid bone
14 External jugular vein
15 Thyroid cartilage
16 Cricothyroid muscle
17 Thyroid gland
18 Subclavius muscle
19 Recurrent laryngeal nerve
20 Trachea
21 Vagus nerve (n. X)
22 Subclavian vein
23 Middle pectoral nerve
24 Esophagus
25 Body of cervical vertebra
26 Spinal cord
27 Sternocleidomastoid muscle
28 Vertebral artery
29 Transverse process of
    cervical vertebra
30 Spinous process of
    cervical vertebra
31 Trapezius muscle
32 Inferior thyroid vein
33 Left brachiocephalic vein
34 Superior lobe of left lung
35 Internal thoracic artery
36 Superior vena cava
37 Superior thyroid artery
38 Inferior thyroid artery
39 Thyrocervical trunk
40 Subclavian artery
41 Aortic arch

Anterior region of the neck and thoracic cavity. Both clavicles, sternum, and ribs have been removed. Main veins are colored in blue.

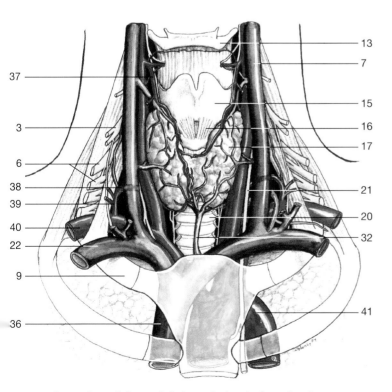

Anterior region of the neck (schematic drawing). Regional anatomy of the thyroid gland with related blood vessels.

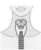

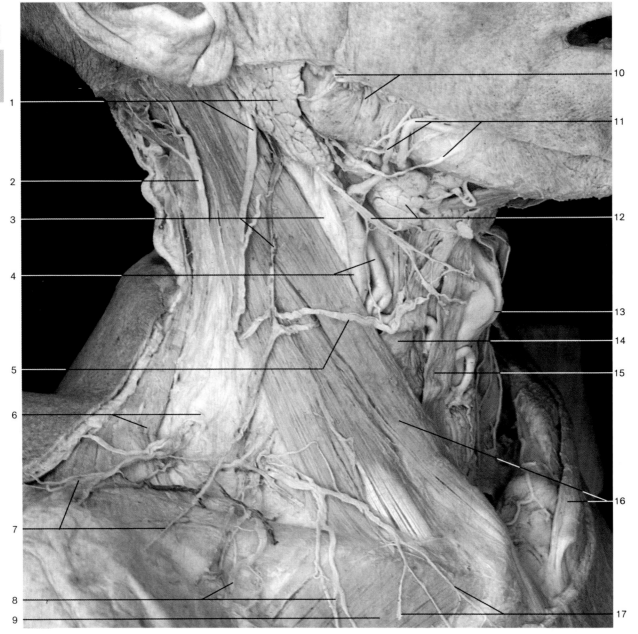

Lateral region of the neck with posterior and carotid triangles. Superficial dissection.

1 Parotid gland and great
auricular nerve
2 Lesser occipital nerve
3 Internal and external
jugular veins
4 Retromandibular vein and
external carotid artery
5 Transverse cervical nerve
with communicating branch
to cervical branch
of facial nerve
6 Trapezius muscle and
superficial lamina of
cervical fascia
7 Lateral supraclavicular nerves
8 Middle supraclavicular nerves
9 Pectoralis major muscle
10 Buccal branch of facial
nerve and masseter muscle

11 Facial artery and vein
and mandibular branch
of facial nerve
12 Cervical branch of facial
nerve and submandibular
gland
13 Thyroid cartilage
14 Omohyoid muscle
15 Sternohyoid muscle
16 Sternocleidomastoid
muscle
17 Medial supraclavicular
nerves
18 Mandibular branch
of facial nerve
19 Cervical branch of facial
nerve with communicating
branch to transverse
cervical nerve

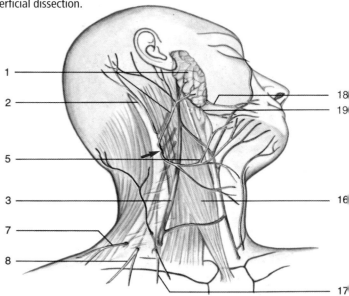

Cutaneous branches of cervical plexus. Erb's point is indicated
by an arrowhead (schematic drawing).

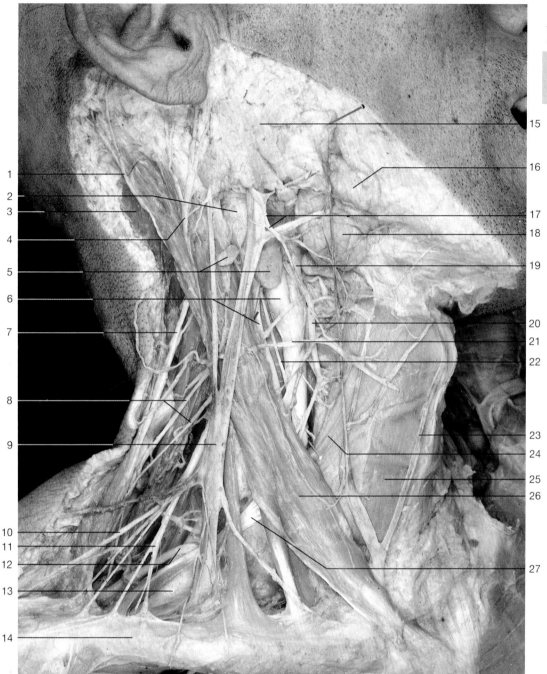

Lateral region of the neck with posterior and carotid triangles. Superficial dissection. The superficial lamina of cervical fascia has been removed to display the cutaneous branches of the cervical plexus and subcutaneous veins.

1 Lesser occipital nerve
2 Internal jugular vein
3 Splenius capitis muscle
4 Great auricular nerve
5 Submandibular nodes
6 Internal carotid artery and vagus nerve
7 Accessory nerve
8 Muscular branches of cervical plexus
9 External jugular vein
10 Posterior supraclavicular nerves
11 Middle supraclavicular nerves
12 Suprascapular artery
13 Pretracheal lamina of fascia of neck
14 Clavicle

15 Parotid gland
16 Mandible
17 Cervical branch of facial nerve
18 Submandibular gland
19 External carotid artery
20 Superior thyroid artery
21 Transverse cervical nerve
22 Superior root of ansa cervicalis
23 Anterior jugular vein
24 Omohyoid muscle
25 Sternohyoid muscle
26 Sternocleidomastoid muscle
27 Intermediate tendon of omohyoid muscle

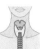

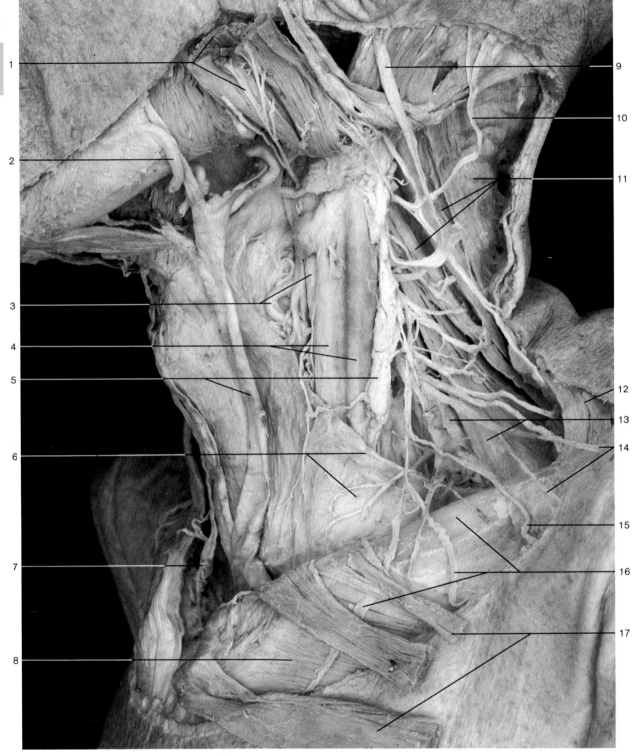

Neck, superficial dissection (lateral aspect). Sternocleidomastoid muscle has been cut and reflected to display the pretracheal lamina of the cervical fascia.

1 Sternocleidomastoid muscle (reflected) and branch of accessory nerve
2 Facial artery
3 External carotid artery and superior thyroid artery
4 Internal jugular vein
5 Deep cervical lymph nodes and external jugular vein
6 Omohyoid muscle and pretracheal lamina of cervical fascia
7 Anterior jugular vein
8 Pectoralis major muscle

9 Great auricular nerve
10 Lesser occipital nerve
11 Splenius capitis and levator scapulae muscles
12 Trapezius muscle
13 Scalenus medius muscle and brachial plexus
14 Posterior supraclavicular nerves
15 Middle supraclavicular nerve
16 Clavicle and anterior supraclavicular nerves
17 Sternocleidomastoid muscle (reflected)

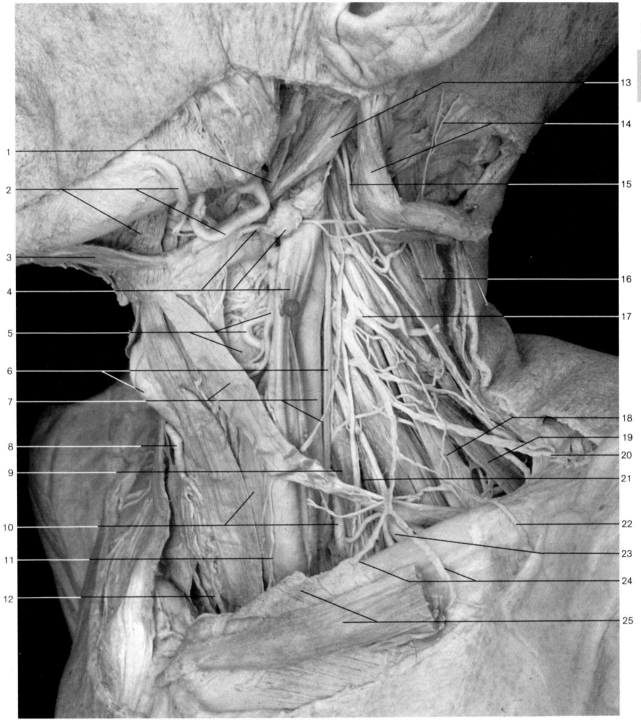
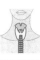

Neck, deep dissection (lateral aspect). The internal jugular vein has been reflected to expose the carotid artery and vagus nerve.

1   Stylohyoid muscle
2   Facial artery and mylohyoid muscle
3   Anterior belly of digastric muscle
4   Internal jugular vein, hypoglossal nerve,
    and superficial cervical lymph nodes
5   Superior thyroid artery and vein and inferior pharyngeal
    constrictor muscle
6   Thyroid cartilage and vagus nerve
7   Ansa cervicalis, omohyoid muscle, and common carotid artery
8   Right superior thyroid artery
9   Scalenus anterior muscle
10 Sternothyroid muscle and inferior thyroid artery
11 Muscular branches of ansa cervicalis to the infrahyoid muscles
12 Inferior thyroid vein

13 Posterior belly of digastric muscle
14 Sternocleidomastoid muscle and lesser occipital nerve
15 Accessory nerve
16 Splenius capitis muscle
17 Cervical plexus
18 Scalenus posterior muscle
19 Levator scapulae muscle
20 Posterior supraclavicular nerves
21 Phrenic nerve
22 Middle supraclavicular nerve
23 Brachial plexus
24 Anterior supraclavicular nerves
25 Sternocleidomastoid muscle

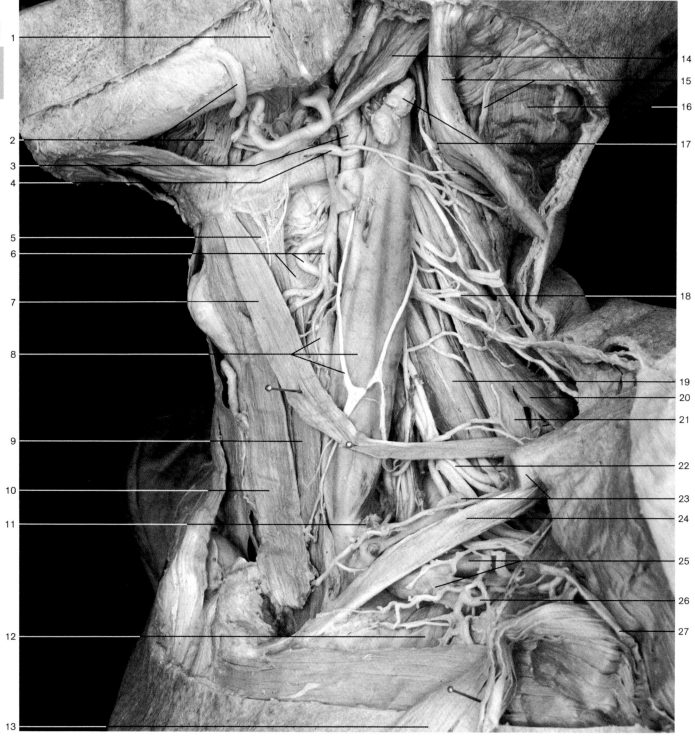

Neck, deeper dissection (lateral aspect). **Ansa cervicalis.** The cervical fascia and the clavicle are partly removed. Ansa cervicalis and infrahyoid muscles are displayed.

1	Masseter muscle
2	Mylohyoid muscle and facial artery
3	External carotid artery and anterior belly of digastric muscle
4	Hypoglossal nerve
5	Thyrohyoid muscle
6	Superior thyroid artery and vein and inferior pharyngeal constrictor muscle
7	Omohyoid muscle (superior belly)
8	Ansa cervicalis, thyroid gland, and internal jugular vein
9	Sternothyroid muscle
10	Sternohyoid muscle
11	Thoracic duct
12	Pectoralis minor muscle
13	Pectoralis major muscle
14	Posterior belly of digastric muscle
15	Sternocleidomastoid muscle and lesser occipital nerve
16	Splenius capitis muscle
17	Superficial cervical lymph nodes and accessory nerve
18	Cervical plexus
19	Scalenus medius muscle
20	Levator scapulae muscle
21	Scalenus posterior muscle
22	Brachial plexus
23	Transverse cervical artery and clavicle
24	Subclavius muscle
25	Subclavian artery and vein
26	Thoraco-acromial artery
27	Cephalic vein

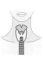

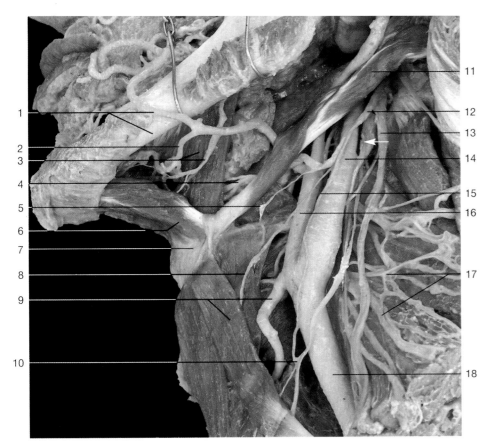

1 Facial artery and mandible
2 Submental artery
3 Mylohyoid muscle and nerve
4 Hypoglossal nerve
(lingual branches)
5 Thyrohyoid branch of hypoglossal
nerve (n. XII)
6 Anterior belly of digastric muscle
7 Hyoid bone
8 Omohyoid branch of hypoglossal
nerve (n. XII)
9 Omohyoid muscle and superior
thyroid artery
10 Ansa cervicalis
11 Posterior belly of digastric muscle
12 Hypoglossal nerve (n. XII)
13 Vagus nerve (n. X)
14 Internal carotid artery
15 Superior root of ansa cervicalis
16 External carotid artery
17 Cervical plexus
18 Common carotid artery
19 Facial artery and vein
20 Omohyoid muscle
21 Internal jugular vein
22 Sternohyoid and sternothyroid
muscles
23 Clavicle
24 Superficial temporal artery and vein
25 Occipital artery
26 Spinal nerves (C_3 and C_4)
27 Spinal processes of cervical
vertebrae (C_4 and C_5)
28 Scapula

Neck with submandibular region (lateral aspect). **Hypoglossal nerve** (n. XII). Mandible slightly elevated. Arrow = superior cervical ganglion.

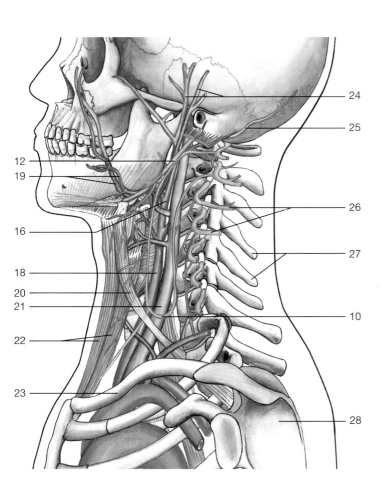

Nerves and vessels of the neck (lateral aspect).
The ansa cervicalis with connection to the spinal nerves is depicted.

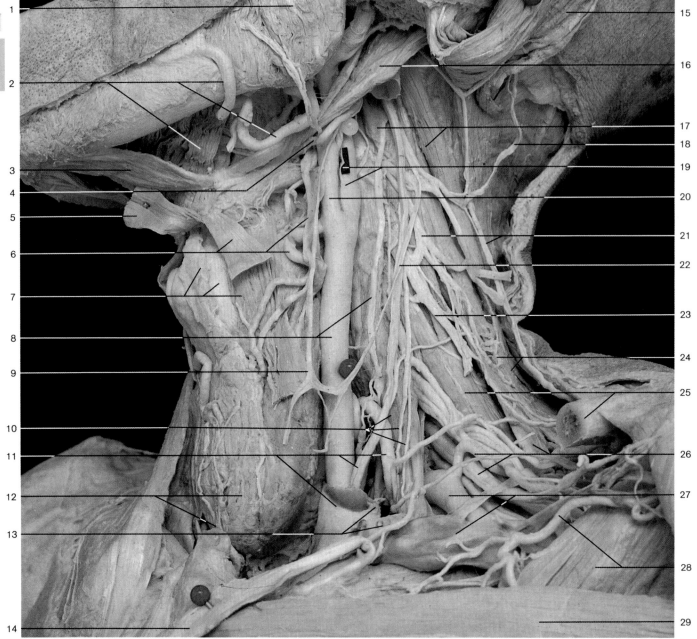

Neck, deeper dissection (lateral aspect). Clavicle partly removed to show the slit between the scalenus muscles. Internal jugular vein removed.

1 Masseter muscle
2 Mylohyoid muscle and facial artery
3 Anterior belly of digastric muscle
4 Hypoglossal nerve
5 Sternohyoid muscle
6 Omohyoid muscle, superior thyroid artery and vein
7 Sternothyroid muscle, thyroid cartilage, and pyramidal lobe of thyroid gland
8 Common carotid artery and sympathetic trunk
9 Ansa cervicalis
10 Phrenic nerve, ascending cervical artery, and anterior scalenus muscle

11 Inferior thyroid artery, vagus nerve, and internal jugular vein (cut)
12 Thyroid gland and unpaired inferior thyroid venous plexus
13 Thoracic duct and left subclavian trunk
14 Subclavius muscle (reflected)
15 Sternocleidomastoid muscle (reflected)
16 Posterior belly of digastric muscle
17 Superior cervical ganglion and splenius muscle
18 Lesser occipital nerve
19 Internal carotid artery and branch of the glossopharyngeal nerve to the carotid body
20 External carotid artery

21 Cervical plexus and accessory nerve
22 Inferior root of ansa cervicalis
23 Supraclavicular nerve
24 Levator scapulae muscle
25 Scalenus medius muscle and clavicle
26 Transverse cervical artery, brachial plexus, and scalenus posterior muscle
27 Subclavian artery and vein
28 Thoraco-acromial artery and pectoralis minor muscle
29 Pectoralis major muscle

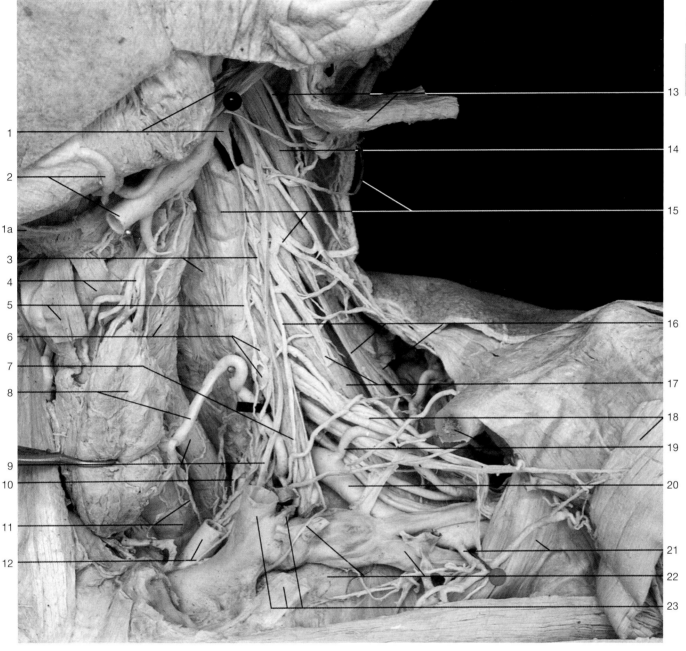

Neck, deepest dissection (antero-lateral aspect). Thyroid gland reflected to expose the esophagus and the recurrent laryngeal nerve.

1 Superior cervical ganglion of sympathetic trunk and posterior belly of digastric muscle
1a Anterior belly of digastric muscle
2 Facial artery and common carotid artery (reflected anteriorly)
3 Ascending cervical artery and longus colli muscle
4 Omohyoid muscle and superior thyroid artery
5 Sympathetic trunk and sternohyoid muscle
6 Middle cervical ganglion and inferior pharyngeal constrictor muscle
7 Scalenus anterior muscle and phrenic nerve
8 Thyroid gland and inferior thyroid artery
9 Vagus nerve and esophagus
10 Stellate ganglion
11 Recurrent laryngeal nerve and trachea

12 Common carotid artery and cervical cardiac branch of vagus nerve
13 Sternocleidomastoid muscle and accessory nerve
14 Splenius capitis muscle
15 Lesser occipital nerve, longus capitis muscle, and cervical plexus
16 Phrenic nerve, scalenus posterior muscle, and levator scapulae muscle
17 Supraclavicular nerves and scalenus medius muscle
18 Brachial plexus and pectoralis major muscle (clavicular head)
19 Transverse cervical artery and clavicle
20 Subclavian artery
21 Thoraco-acromial artery and pectoralis minor muscle
22 First rib, accessory phrenic nerve, and subclavian vein
23 Internal jugular vein, thoracic duct, and subclavius muscle

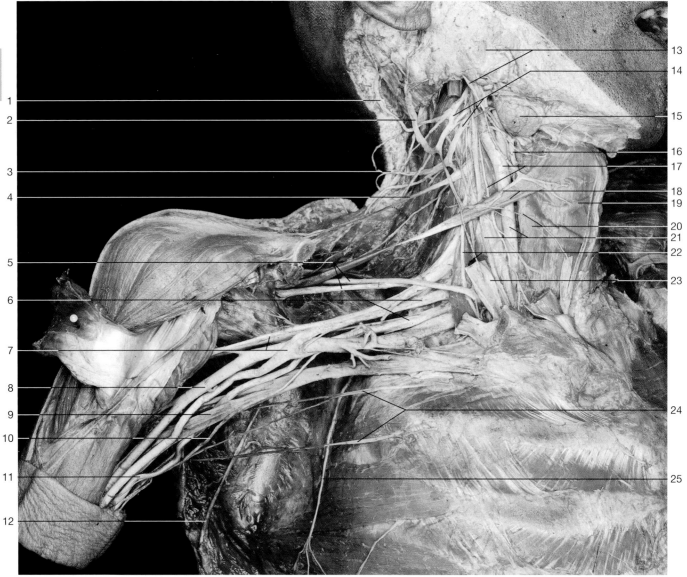

Neck and arm, deepest dissection (antero-lateral aspect). **Cervical and brachial plexuses** and their relation to the blood vessels are shown. Note the location and content of scalene triangle. Sternocleidomastoid muscle and clavicle have been removed; the internal jugular vein was divided to display the roots of cervical and brachial plexuses.

1 Lesser occipital nerve	15 Submandibular gland
2 Great auricular nerve	16 Superior thyroid artery
3 Cutaneous branches of cervical plexus	17 Common carotid artery dividing in internal and external
4 Supraclavicular nerve	carotid artery and superior root of ansa cervicalis
5 Suprascapular nerve and artery	18 Omohyoid muscle and cervical branch of facial nerve
6 Brachial plexus	joining the transverse cervical nerve (C₂, C₃)
7 Median nerve (with two roots) and musculocutaneous nerve	19 Sternohyoid muscle
8 Axillary artery	20 Transverse cervical nerve and sternothyroid muscle
9 Axillary vein	21 Common carotid artery and vagus nerve
10 Medial brachial cutaneous nerve	22 Phrenic nerve and scalenus anterior muscle
11 Ulnar nerve	23 Internal jugular vein
12 Thoracodorsal nerve	24 Intercostobrachial nerves
13 Parotid gland and facial nerve (cervical branch)	25 Long thoracic nerve
14 Cervical plexus	

3 Trunk

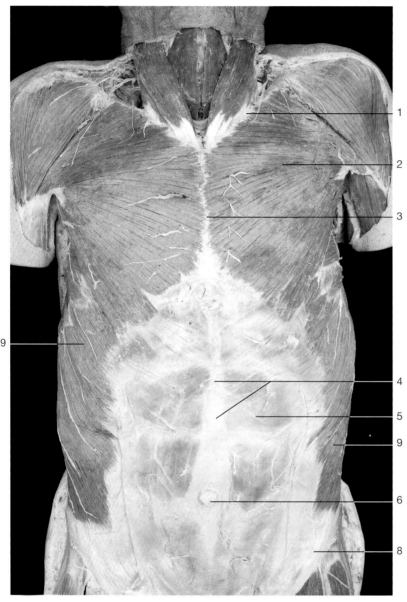

The anterior abdominal and thoracic walls reveal a segmental structure. The ribs are connected by intercostal muscles forming defined skeleto-motoric and neuro-vascular segments.

At the abdominal wall, the segments form great flat muscles, that end anteriorly in strong sheet-like aponeuroses. The aponeurosis interlace at the linea alba with their counterparts from the opposite side to form the tough tendinous sheath of the rectus muscle. Movements of the abdominal wall also support the process of respiration functionally related to the diaphragm.

Anterior thoracic and abdominal walls with superficial musculature.
The fascia of pectoralis major muscle and the abdominal wall have been removed; the anterior layer of the sheath of the rectus abdominis muscle is displayed.

1 Clavicle
2 Pectoralis major muscle
3 Sternum
4 Linea alba
5 Anterior layer of rectus sheath
6 Umbilicus
7 Internal abdominal oblique muscle
8 Inguinal ligament
9 External abdominal oblique muscle

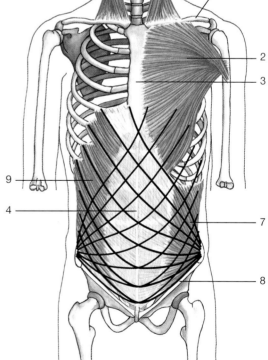

Organization of the thoracic and abdominal walls.
The architecture of tendon fibers of the two abdominal oblique muscles in the rectus sheath is shown.

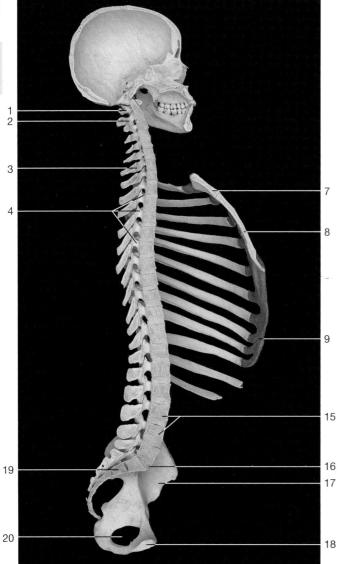

Median sagittal section through the vertebral column, head, and thorax of the adult.

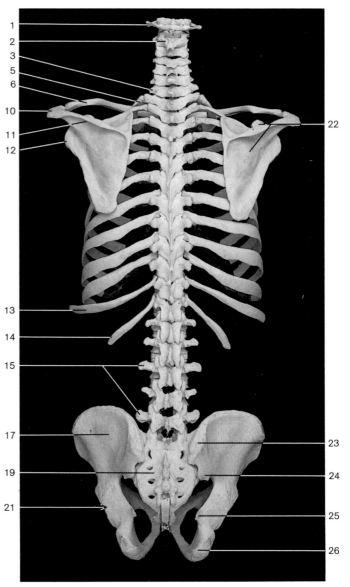

Skeleton of the trunk, vertebral column, thorax, and pelvis (posterior aspect).

1	Atlas	14	Twelfth rib
2	Axis	15	Lumbar vertebrae
3	Seventh cervical vertebra (vertebra prominens)	16	Sacral promontory
4	Vertebral canal	17	Hip bone
5	First rib	18	Pubic symphysis
6	Clavicle	19	Sacrum
7	Manubrium sterni	20	Obturator foramen
8	Body of sternum	21	Acetabulum
9	Costal arch	22	Scapula with coracoid process
10	Acromion	23	Posterior superior iliac spine
11	Spine of scapula	24	Posterior inferior iliac spine
12	Glenoid cavity (lateral angle of scapula)	25	Ischial spine
13	Eleventh rib	26	Ischial tuberosity

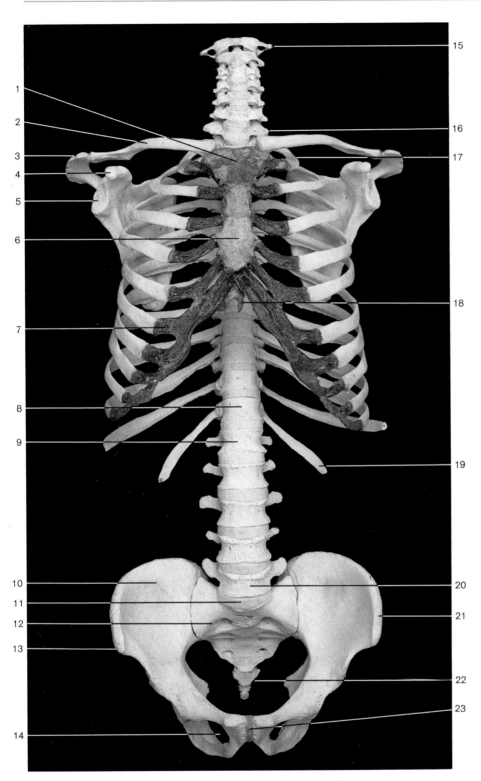

Skeleton of the trunk, vertebral column, pelvis, thorax, and shoulder girdle (anterior aspect).

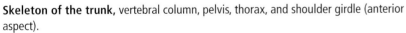

1 Manubrium sterni	13 Anterior superior iliac spine
2 Clavicle	14 Obturator foramen
3 Acromion	15 Atlas
4 Coracoid process	16 Seventh cervical vertebra
5 Glenoid cavity	17 First rib
6 Body of sternum	18 Xiphoid process
7 Costal cartilage	19 Twelfth rib
8 Body of the twelfth thoracic vertebra	20 Body of the fifth lumbar vertebra
9 Body of the first lumbar vertebra	21 Iliac crest
10 Hip bone	22 Coccyx
11 Sacral promontory	23 Pubic symphysis
12 Sacrum	

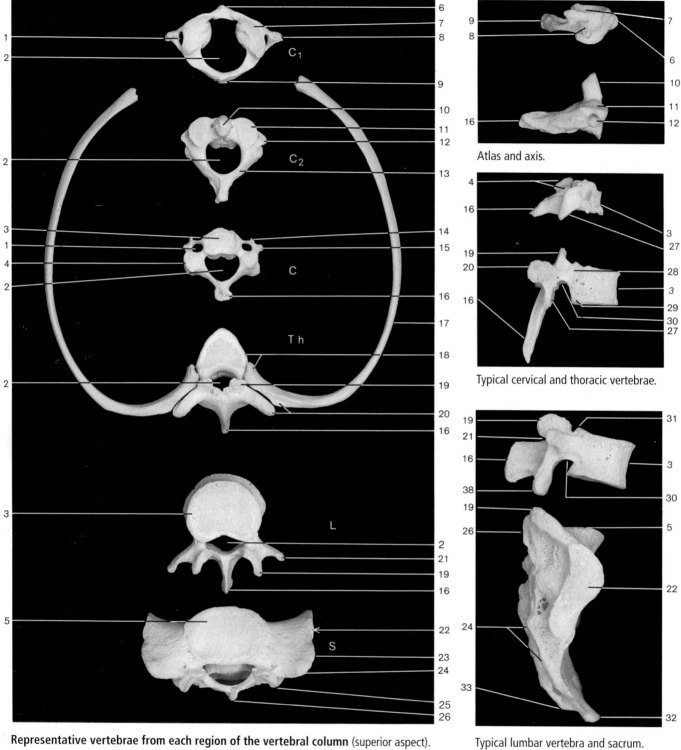

Representative vertebrae from each region of the vertebral column (superior aspect). From top to bottom: atlas (C₁), axis (C₂), cervical vertebra (C), thoracic vertebra (Th), lumbar vertebra (L), and sacrum (S).

Atlas and axis.

Typical cervical and thoracic vertebrae.

Typical lumbar vertebra and sacrum.

△

Representative vertebrae from each region of the vertebral column (lateral aspect, ventral surface on the right).

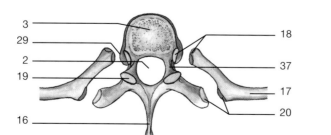

General organization of ribs and vertebrae (schematic drawing).

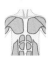

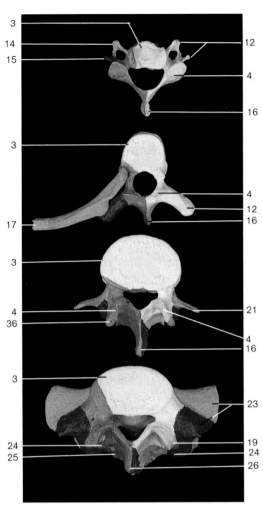

General characteristics of the vertebrae.
Typical cervical, thoracic, and lumbar vertebrae
and sacrum.

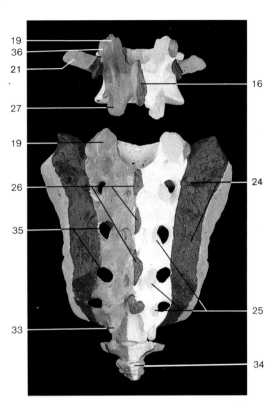

**General characteristics of lumbar vertebrae
and sacrum** (posterior aspect).

Green   = ribs or homologous processes
Red   = muscular processes
        (transverse and spinous processes)
Orange = laminae and articular processes
Yellow   = articular facets
and blue

1	Foramen transversarium
2	Vertebral foramen
3	Body of vertebra
4	Superior articular facet
5	Base of sacrum
6	Anterior tubercle of atlas
7	Superior articular facet of atlas
8	Transverse process
9	Posterior tubercle of atlas
10	Dens of axis
11	Superior articular surface
12	Transverse process
13	Arch of vertebra
14	Anterior tubercle of transverse process
15	Posterior tubercle of transverse process
16	Spinous process
17	Shaft of rib
18	Body of vertebra and head of rib articulating with each other (costovertebral joint)
19	Superior articular process

20	Transverse process and tubercle of rib articulating with each other (costotransverse joint)
21	Costal process
22	Auricular surface
23	Lateral part of sacrum
24	Lateral sacral crest
25	Intermediate sacral crest
26	Median sacral crest
27	Inferior articular facet
28	Superior demifacet for head of rib
29	Inferior demifacet for head of rib
30	Inferior vertebral notch
31	Superior vertebral notch
32	Apex of the sacrum
33	Sacral cornu
34	Coccyx
35	Dorsal sacral foramina
36	Mamillary process
37	Pedicle
38	Inferior articular process

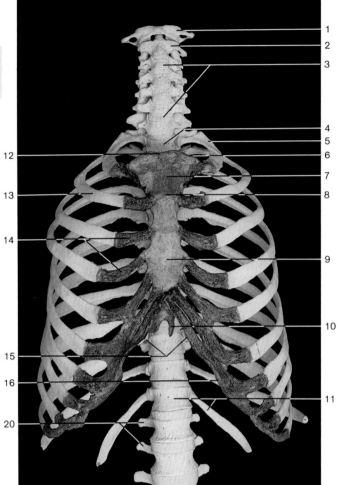

Skeleton of the thorax (anterior aspect).

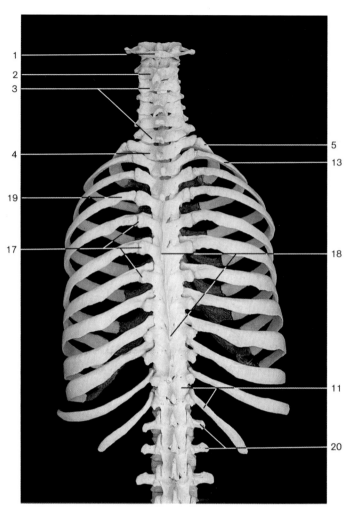

Skeleton of the thorax (posterior aspect).

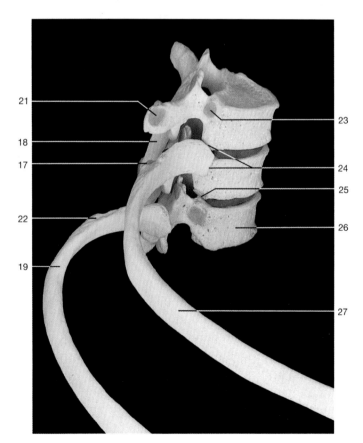

Costovertebral articulation (right lateral aspect).

1 Atlas
2 Axis
3 Cervical vertebrae
4 First thoracic vertebra
5 First rib
6 Facet for clavicle and clavicular notch
7 Manubrium sterni
8 Sternal angle
9 Body of sternum
10 Xiphoid process
11 Twelfth thoracic vertebra and rib
12 Jugular notch
13 Second rib
14 Costal cartilages
15 Infrasternal angle
16 Costal arch
17 Costotransverse joints between the transverse processes of thoracic vertebra and the tubercles of the ribs
18 Spinous processes
19 Costal angle
20 Costal processes of lumbar vertebrae
21 Facet for articulation with rib
22 Tubercle of rib
23 Superior facet for articulation with head of rib
24 Articulation of head of rib with two vertebrae
25 Inferior facet for articulation with head of rib
26 Body of thoracic vertebra
27 Body or shaft of rib

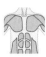

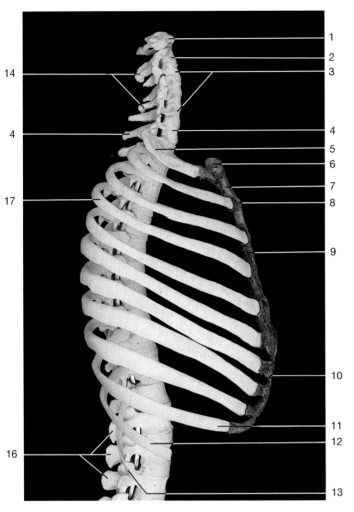

Skeleton of the thorax (right lateral aspect).

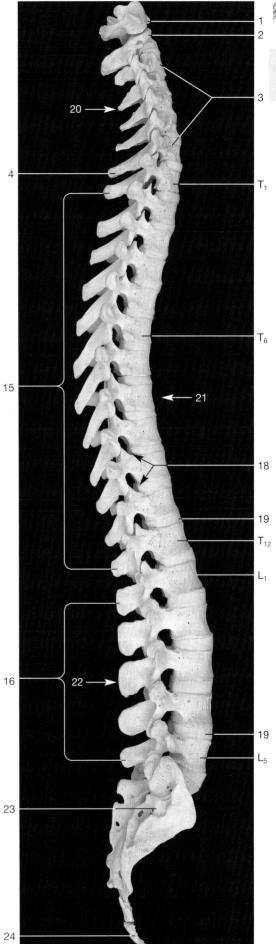

1   Atlas
2   Axis
3   Cervical vertebrae
4   Seventh cervical vertebra (vertebra prominens)
5   First rib
6   Facet for clavicle
7   Manubrium sterni
8   Sternal angle
9   Body of sternum
10 Costal arch
11 Tenth rib
12 Eleventh rib
13 Twelfth rib
14 Spinous processes of cervical vertebrae
15 Spinous processes of thoracic vertebrae
16 Spinous processes of lumbar vertebrae
17 Costal angle
18 Intervertebral foramina
19 Intervertebral discs
20 Cervical curvature
21 Thoracic curvature
22 Lumbar curvature
23 Sacrum
24 Coccyx

Vertebral column
(right lateral aspect).

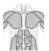

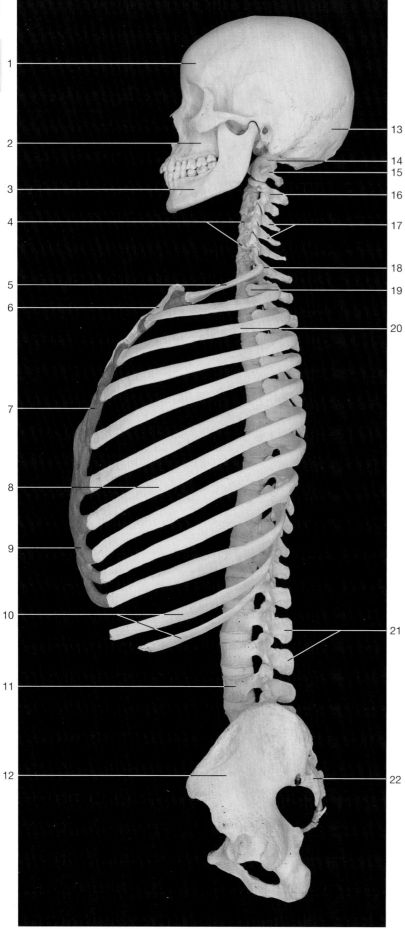

1   Frontal bone
2   Maxilla
3   Mandible
4   Bodies of cervical vertebrae
5   First rib
6   Manubrium of sternum
7   Sternum (corpus sterni)
8   Seventh rib (last of the true ribs)
9   Costal arch (arcus costalis)
10 Floating ribs (costae fluctuantes)
11 Body of fourth lumbar vertebra
12 Pelvis
13 Occipital bone
14 Atlanto-occipital joint
15 Atlas
16 Axis
17 Spinous processes of cervical vertebrae (C_4, C_5)
18 Costotransverse joint of first rib
19 Head of second rib
20 Third rib
21 Spinous processes of lumbar vertebrae (L_2, L_3)
22 Sacrum

Vertebral column and thorax in connection with head and pelvis (lateral aspect).

1 Atlas
2 Dens of axis
3 Axis
4 Body of cervical vertebra
5 Intervertebral discs
6 Sternocleidomastoid muscle
7 Scalenus muscles
8 Body of vertebra
9 Superior articular facet
10 Vertebral arch
11 Transverse process of vertebra
12 Zygapophysial joint
13 Spinous process
14 Articular facet
     of costovertebral joint
15 Transverse process
     with articular facet
     of costotransverse joint
16 Costal process of lumbar
     vertebra
17 Sacrum
18 Median sacral crest
19 Dorsal sacral foramina
20 Coccyx

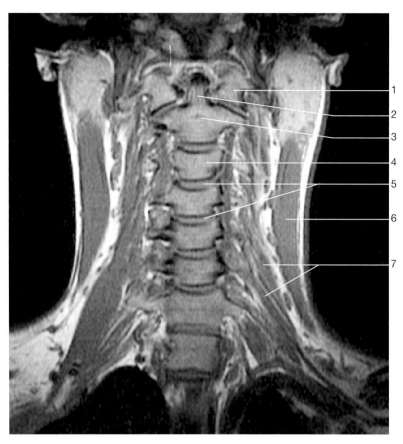

Coronal section through the neck at the level of the cervical vertebrae (MRI scan, courtesy of Prof. Heuck, Munich).

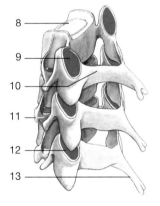

Cervical vertebrae (lateral aspect, articular facets = blue).

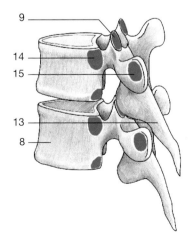

Thoracic vertebrae (lateral aspect, articular facets = blue).

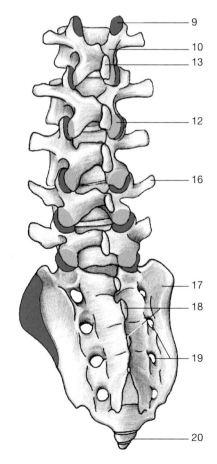

Lumbar vertebrae with sacrum and coccyx (posterior aspect, articular facets = blue).

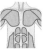

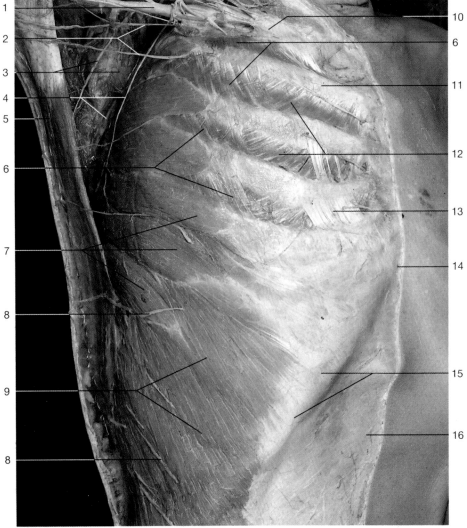

1   Axillary vein
2   Intercostobrachial nerves
3   Subscapularis muscle and thoracodorsal nerve
4   Long thoracic nerve, lateral thoracic artery and vein
5   Latissimus dorsi muscle
6   External intercostal muscles
7   Serratus anterior muscle
8   Lateral cutaneous branches of intercostal nerves
9   External abdominal oblique muscle
10   Clavicle (divided)
11   Second rib (costochondral junction)
12   Internal intercostal muscles
13   External intercostal membrane
14   Position of xiphoid process
15   Costal arch or margin
16   Anterior layer of rectus sheath

Muscles of the thorax, superficial layer (lateral aspect). Upper limb elevated. Pectoralis major and minor muscles have been removed.

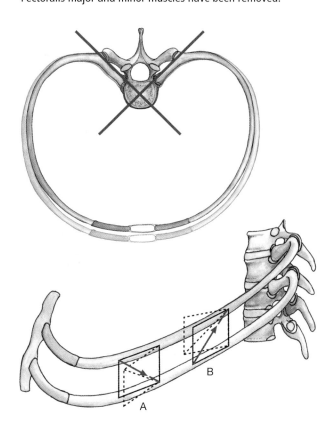

Effect of intercostal muscles on the costovertebral and costotransverse joints. Axes of movement indicated by red lines; direction of movements indicated by red arrows.
A = action of internal intercostal muscles (expiration);
B = action of external intercostal muscles (inspiration).

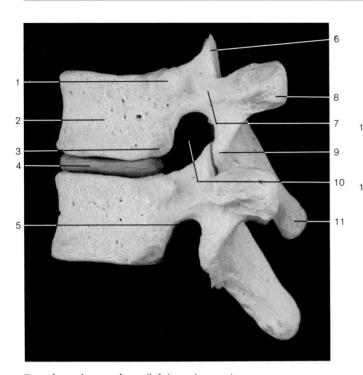

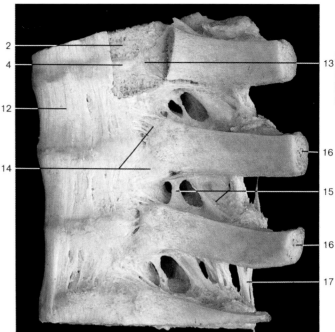

Two thoracic vertebrae (left lateral aspect).

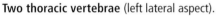

1 Superior demifacet for head of rib	8 Transverse process and facet
2 Body of vertebra	for tubercle of rib
3 Inferior demifacet for head of rib	9 Inferior articular process
4 Intervertebral disc	10 Intervertebral foramen
5 Inferior vertebral notch	11 Spinous process
6 Superior articular facet and	12 Anterior longitudinal ligament
superior articular process	13 Intra-articular ligament
7 Pedicle	14 Radiate ligament

Ligaments of thoracic vertebrae and costovertebral joints (left antero-lateral aspect). In the upper joint, most of the radiate ligament and the anterior part of the head of the rib have been removed to expose the two joint cavities and the interposed intra-articular ligament.

15 Superior costotransverse ligament	
16 Body of rib	
17 Intertransverse ligament	

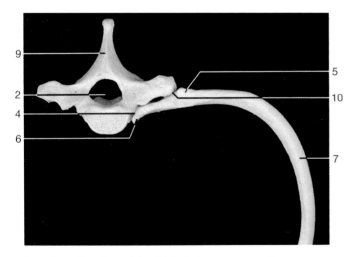

Location of costovertebral joints (superior aspect).

1 Superior articular process	7 Shaft or body of rib
2 Vertebral canal	8 Transverse process
3 Body of thoracic vertebra	with articular facet
4 Costovertebral joint	9 Spinous process
(articular facets)	10 Costotransverse joint
5 Tubercle of rib	(articular facets)
6 Head of rib	

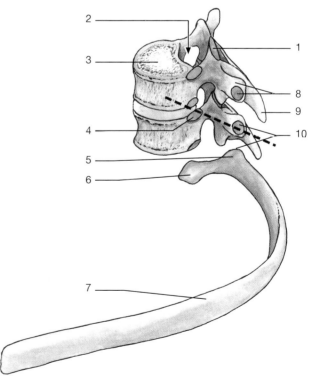

Costovertebral joints (schematic drawing). Two thoracic vertebrae with an articulating rib (separated). Axis of movement indicated by dashed line. Blue = articular facets.

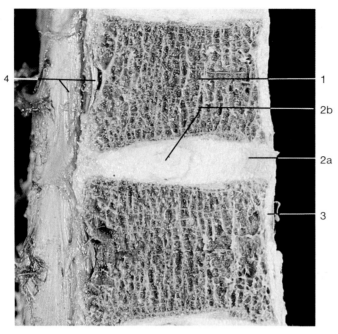

4

1

2b

2a

3

Median-sagittal section of the bodies of the vertebrae,
showing the **intervertebral discs,** each of which consists
of an outer laminated portion and an inner core.

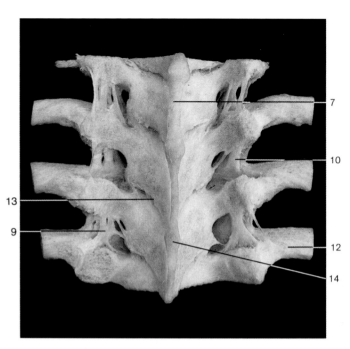

7

10

13

9

12

14

Ligaments of the vertebral column (dorsal aspect).

1	Body of vertebra	8 Interspinous ligament
2	Intervertebral disc	9 Intertransverse ligament
	a Outer portion (anulus fibrosus)	10 Superior costotransverse ligament
	b Inner core (nucleus pulposus)	11 Transverse process of thoracic
3	Anterior longitudinal ligament	vertebra
4	Posterior longitudinal ligament and spinal dura mater	12 Rib
5	Costal process of lumbar vertebra	13 Ligamentum flavum
6	Sacrum	14 Spinous process
7	Supraspinous ligament	15 Intervertebral foramen

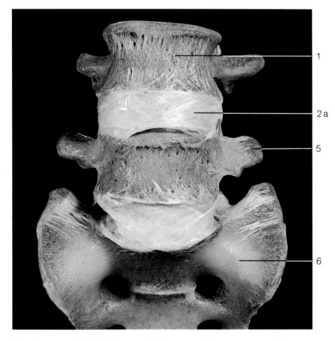

1

2a

5

6

**The two caudal lumbar vertebrae and the sacrum with
their intervertebral discs** (anterior aspect). Anterior longitudinal
ligament removed.

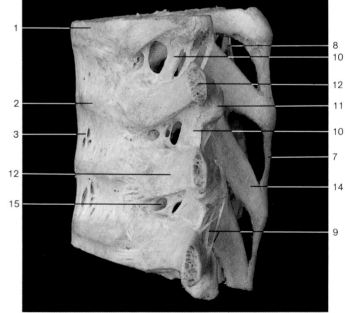

1

8
10

12
11

2

3

10

12

7

15

14

9

Ligaments of the vertebral column, thoracic part (left lateral
aspect).

Disarticulated thorax skeleton. ▷
The twelve ribs (I–XII) are arranged
in a craniocaudal direction.

1   Anterior longitudinal ligament
2   Body of vertebra
3   Intervertebral disc
4   Intra-articular ligament
5   Radiate ligament
6   Posterior longitudinal ligament
7   Superior articular facet
8   Articular facets of
     costovertebral joints
9   Superior costotransverse ligament
10   Costovertebral joint
11   Rib
12   Interspinal ligament
13   Costotransverse joint
14   Lateral costotransverse ligament
15   Spinous process
16   Supraspinal ligament
17   Nucleus pulposus
18   Costal process
19   Vertebral arch
20   Intervertebral foramen
21   Intertransverse ligament   ▽

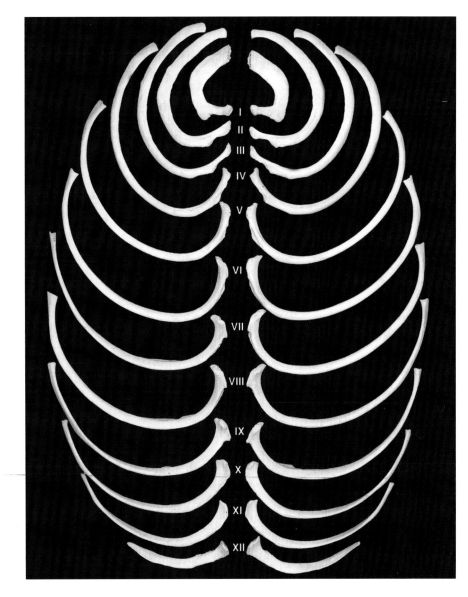

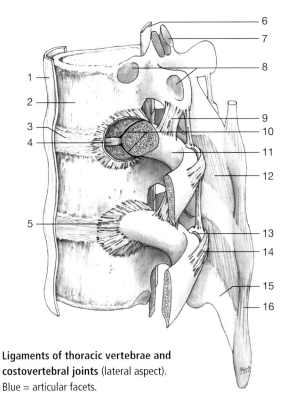

**Ligaments of thoracic vertebrae and
costovertebral joints** (lateral aspect).
Blue = articular facets.

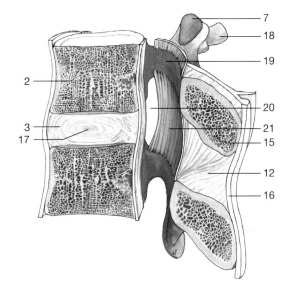

Median-sagittal section of two lumbar vertebrae showing
ligaments and vertebral discs.

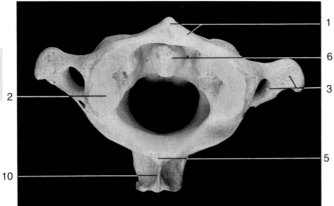

Atlas and axis (from above).

Median atlanto-axial joint and transverse ligament of atlas (from above). Dens of axis partly severed.

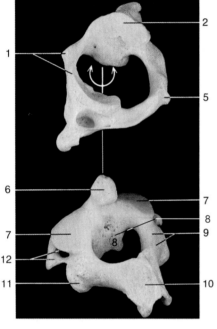

1 Anterior arch of atlas with anterior tubercle
2 Superior articular facet of atlas
3 Foramen transversarium and transverse process
4 Posterior arch of atlas and vertebral artery
5 Posterior tubercle of atlas
6 Dens of axis
7 Superior articular surface of axis
8 Body of axis
9 Pedicle and lamina of axis
10 Spinous process
11 Inferior articular process
12 Transverse process and foramen transversarium of axis
13 Median atlanto-axial joint (anterior part)

14 Articular capsule of atlanto-occipital joint
15 Transverse ligament of atlas
16 Occipital bone
17 Atlanto-occipital joint
18 Lateral atlanto-axial joint
19 Third cervical vertebra
20 Superior longitudinal band of cruciform ligament
21 Alar ligaments
22 Transverse ligament of atlas
23 Inferior longitudinal band of cruciform ligament
24 Spinous process of axis
25 Dura mater
26 Occipital bone

Atlas and axis. Left oblique postero-lateral aspect, demonstrating the articulation of the dens of axis with atlas (cf. arrows).

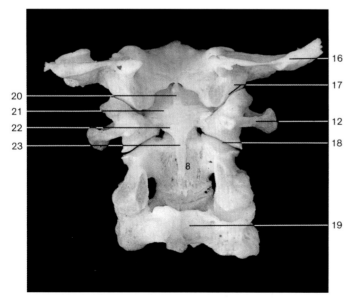

Atlanto-occipital and atlanto-axial joints (posterior aspect). Posterior part of occipital bone, posterior arch of atlas, and axis have been removed to show the cruciform ligament.

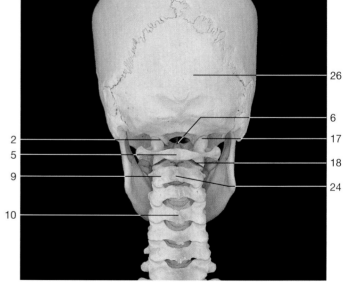

Head and cervical spine (posterior aspect). Bones of atlanto-occipital and atlanto-axial joints.

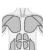

1   Cerebellum
2   Occipital condyle
3   Atlanto-occipital joint
4   Atlas
5   Lateral atlanto-axial joint
6   Intervertebral disc
7   Cistern of pons
8   Head of mandible
9   Dens of axis
10 Axis
11 Body of cervical vertebra (C$_3$)
12 External occipital protuberance
13 Foramen magnum
14 Transverse process of atlas
15 Posterior longitudinal ligament
16 Spinous process of cervical vertebra
17 Occipital bone
18 Membrana tectoria
19 Dorsum sellae
20 Clivus
21 Sella turcica
22 Superior orbital fissure
23 Internal acoustic meatus
24 Jugular foramen
25 Hypoglossal canal
26 Superior longitudinal
     band of cruciform ligament
27 Alar ligaments
28 Transverse ligament of atlas
29 Inferior longitudinal band of
     cruciform ligament

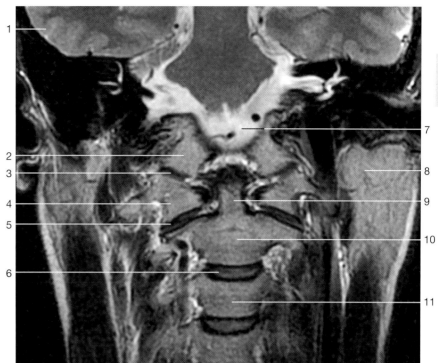

Coronal section of the neck at the level of dens of axis (MRI scan, courtesy of Prof. Heuck, Munich).

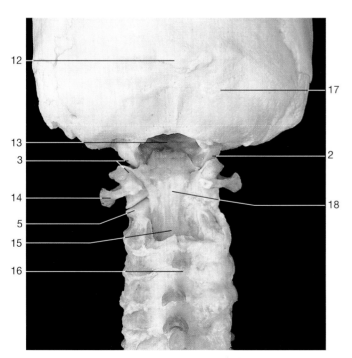

Cervical vertebral column and skull with ligaments (posterior aspect). Posterior arches of atlas and axis removed to show the membrana tectoria.

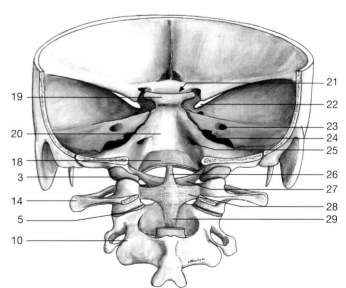

Atlanto-occipital and atlanto-axial joints with ligaments (posterior aspect). Posterior part of occipital bone and posterior arch of atlas have been removed to show the cruciform ligament.

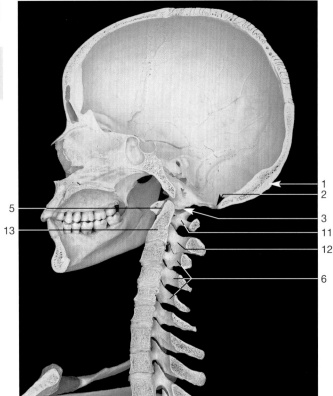

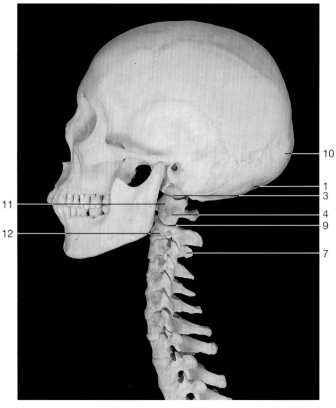

Cervical vertebral column in relation to the head (midsagittal section, medial aspect).

Atlas and axis in relation to the head (lateral aspect).

1	External occipital protuberance	9	Lateral atlanto-axial joint
2	Foramen magnum	10	Occipital bone
3	Atlanto-occipital joint	11	Atlas
4	Transverse process of atlas	12	Axis
5	Median atlanto-axial joint	13	Dens of axis
6	Vertebral canal	14	Hypoglossal canal
7	Spinous process of third cervical vertebra	15	Spinous process of axis
8	Occipital condyle		

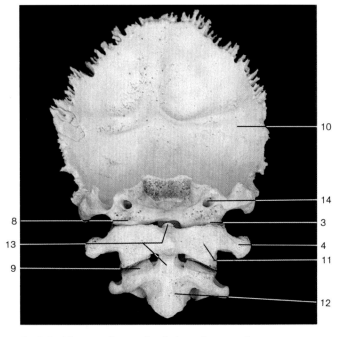

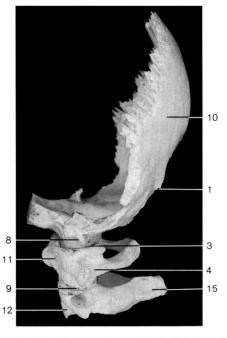

Occipital bone, atlas, and axis (anterior aspect).

Occipital bone, atlas, and axis (left lateral aspect).

1   Pons
2   Base of skull (clivus)
3   Medulla oblongata
4   Atlas (anterior arch)
5   Dens of axis
6   Intervertebral disc
7   Body of cervical vertebra (C$_4$)
8   Site of larynx
9   Trachea
10 Cerebellum
11 Cerebellomedullary cistern
12 Spinal cord
13 Trapezius muscle
14 Muscles of the neck
15 Spinous process of cervical
    vertebra (C$_7$)
16 Internal jugular vein
17 Common carotid artery
18 Vagus nerve (n. X)
19 Larynx
20 Body of cervical vertebra
21 Vertebral artery
22 Spinal nerve with spinal ganglion
23 Transverse process of cervical vertebra
24 Spinous process of cervical vertebra

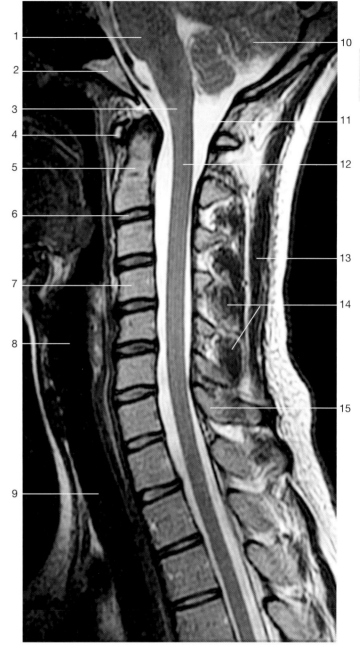

Midsagittal section of the neck showing the spinal cord in connection with medulla oblongata (MRI scan, courtesy of Prof. Heuck, Munich).

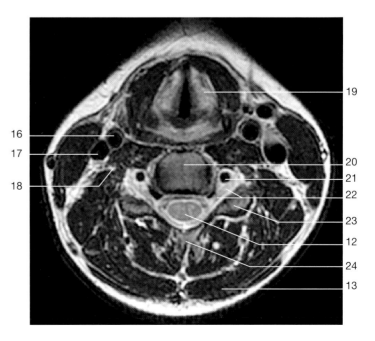

Horizontal section of the neck at the level of the larynx (MRI scan, courtesy of Prof. Heuck, Munich).

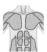

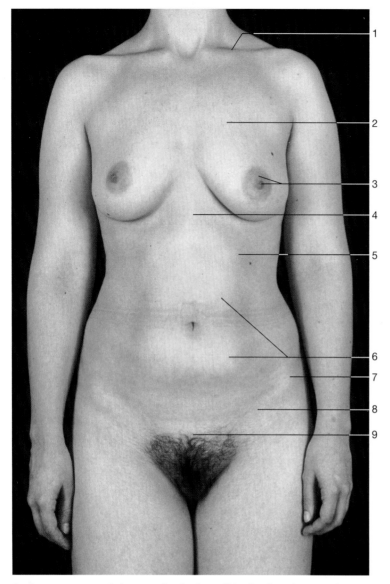

1	Clavicle
2	Pectoralis major muscle
3	Areola and nipple
4	Infrasternal angle
5	Costal arch
6	Rectus abdominis muscle
7	Anterior superior iliac spine
8	Inguinal ligament
9	Mons pubis
10	Epidermis
11	Subcutaneous layer
12	Muscles of the back
13	Kidney
14	Body of lumbar vertebra
15	External abdominal oblique muscle
16	Small intestine
17	Deltoid muscle
18	Anterior serratus muscle
19	External intercostal muscle
20	Internal abdominal oblique muscle
21	Transverse abdominal muscle
22	Rectus sheath
23	Spermatic cord
24	Pectoralis minor muscle
25	Linea alba

Surface anatomy of the anterior body wall in the female. Note the differences in thickness and structure of skin and hairs (compare with the section below).

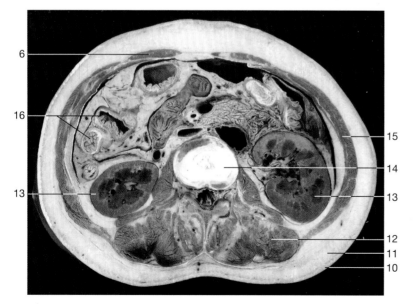

Cross section of the body at the first lumbar vertebra. Note the differences in thickness of the subcutaneous layers.

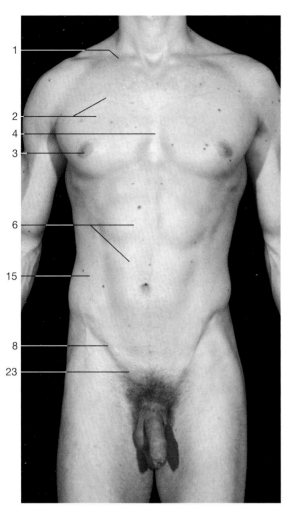

Surface anatomy of the anterior body wall in the male. Localization and structure of the muscles can be identified.

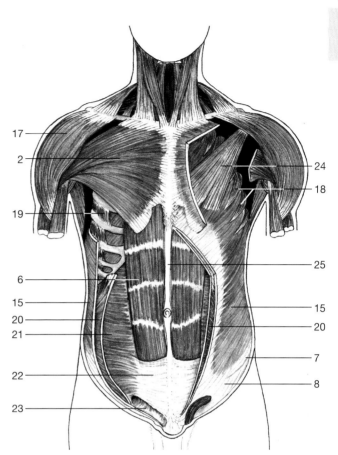

Muscles of the anterior body wall (schematic drawing).

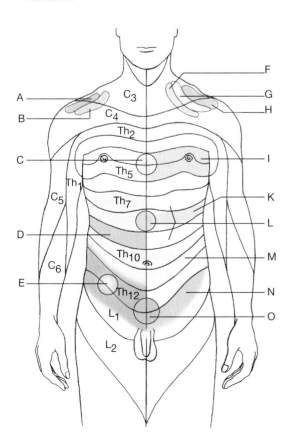

Head's areas

A = duodenum
B = gallbladder, liver (C_3–C_4)
C = esophagus (Th_4, Th_5)
D = liver, gallbladder (Th_6–Th_{11})
E = colon, vermiform appendix ($Th_{11–12}$, L_1)
F = heart
G = pancreas
H = stomach (C_3, C_4)
I = heart (Th_3, Th_4)
K = pancreas (Th_8)
L = stomach (Th_6–Th_9)
M = small intestine (Th_{10}–L_1)
N = kidney, ureter, testis (Th_{10}–L_1)
O = urinary bladder (Th_{11}–L_1)

◁ **Segments of anterior body wall.**
Head's areas are indicated.

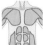

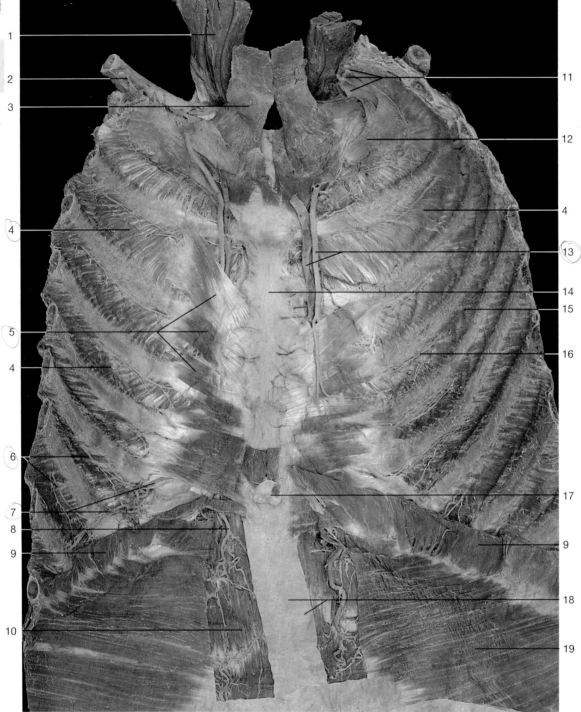

Anterior thoracic wall (posterior aspect). Diaphragm partly removed, posterior layer of rectus sheath fenestrated on both sides.

1 Sternocleidomastoid muscle (divided)
2 Clavicle
3 Sternothyroid muscle
4 Internal intercostal muscle
5 Transversus thoracic muscle
6 Intercostal arteries and nerves
7 Musculophrenic artery
8 Superior epigastric artery and vein
9 Diaphragm (divided)
10 Rectus abdominis muscle

11 Subclavian artery and brachial plexus
12 First rib
13 Internal thoracic artery and vein
14 Sternum
15 Innermost intercostal muscle
16 Intercostal artery and vein
17 Xiphoid process
18 Linea alba and posterior layer of rectus sheath
19 Transversus abdominis muscle

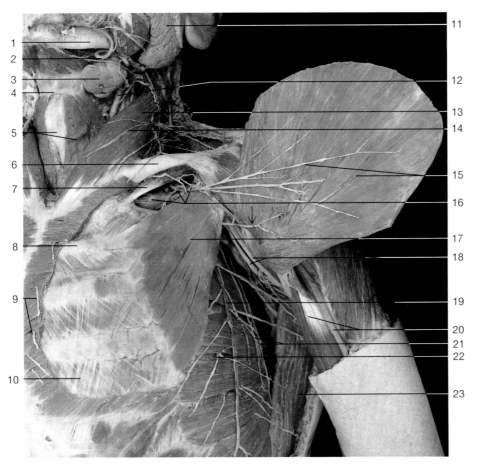

Thoracic wall (anterior aspect). Left pectoralis major muscle has been divided and reflected.
Note the connection of the cephalic vein with the subclavian vein.
Arrow: medial pectoral nerve.

1	Mandible
2	Facial artery
3	Submandibular gland
4	Hyoid bone
5	Thyroid cartilage and sternohyoid muscle
6	Clavicle
7	Subclavius muscle
8	Second rib
9	Anterior cutaneous branches of intercostal nerves
10	External intercostal membrane
11	Parotid gland
12	External carotid artery
13	Sternocleidomastoid muscle and cutaneous branches of cervical plexus
14	Supraclavicular nerves
15	Pectoralis major muscle and lateral pectoral nerves
16	Thoraco-acromial artery and subclavian vein
17	Pectoralis minor muscle
18	Median and ulnar nerve
19	Thoraco-epigastric vein
20	Cephalic vein and long head of biceps brachii muscle
21	Lateral thoracic artery and long thoracic nerve
22	Lateral cutaneous branches of intercostal nerve
23	Latissimus dorsi muscle
24	Median nerve
25	Axillary artery
26	Intercostobrachial nerves
27	Thoracodorsal nerve
28	Long thoracic nerve
29	Latissimus dorsi muscle
30	Serratus anterior muscle
31	Thoraco-acromial artery
32	Clavicle
33	External intercostal muscle
34	Third rib
35	Internal intercostal muscle
36	Anterior intercostal artery and vein, and intercostal nerve
37	Costal arch or margin

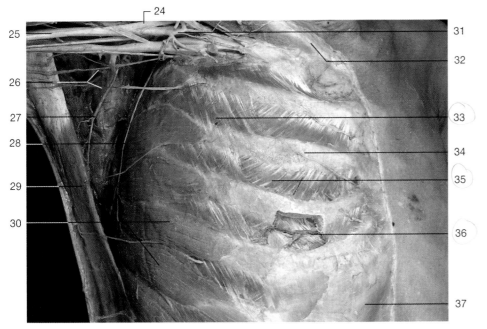

Thoracic wall (lateral aspect). Pectoralis major and minor muscles have been removed.
A section of the fourth rib has been cut and removed to display the intercostal vessels and
nerve.

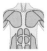

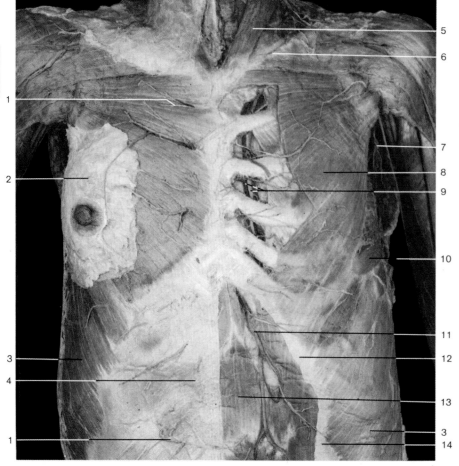

1 Anterior perforating branches of intercostal nerve
2 Mammary gland
3 External abdominal oblique muscle
4 Rectus sheath (anterior layer)
5 Sternocleidomastoid muscle
6 Clavicle
7 Lateral thoracic artery and vein
8 Pectoralis major muscle
9 Internal thoracic artery and vein
10 Serratus anterior muscle
11 Superior epigastric artery and vein
12 Costal margin
13 Rectus abdominis muscle
14 Cut edge of the anterior layer of the rectus sheath
15 Subclavian artery
16 Highest intercostal artery
17 Internal thoracic artery
18 Musculophrenic artery
19 Superficial epigastric artery
20 Deep circumflex iliac artery
21 Superior epigastric artery
22 Inferior epigastric artery
23 Superficial circumflex iliac artery

Thoracic wall (anterior aspect). Dissection of the **internal thoracic artery and vein.** Left pectoralis major muscle partly removed. Anterior lamina of the rectus sheath on the left side has been removed.

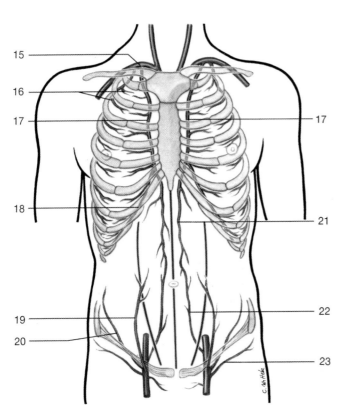

Main arteries of thoracic and abdominal walls.

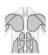

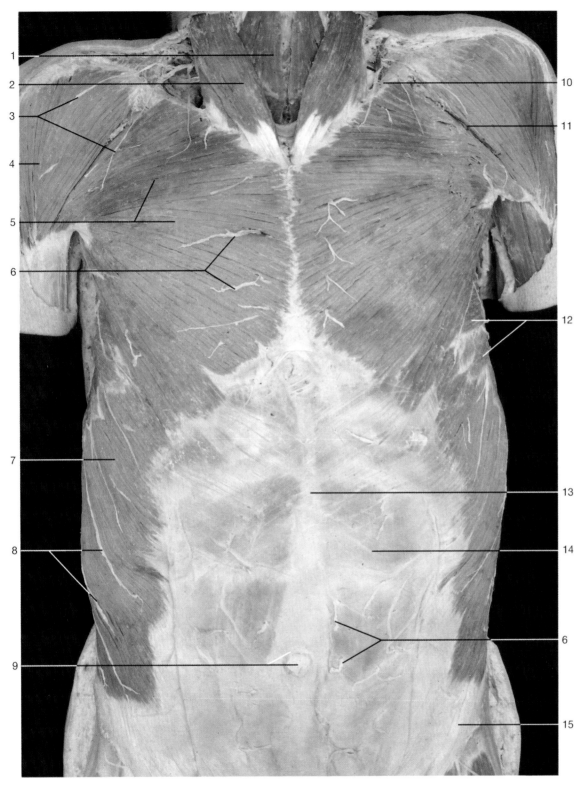

Anterior thoracic and abdominal walls with superficial muscles. The fascia of pectoralis major muscle and the abdominal wall have been removed; the anterior layer of the sheath of the rectus abdominis muscle is displayed.

1 Sternohyoid muscle	9 Umbilicus and umbilical ring
2 Sternocleidomastoid muscle	10 Clavicle
3 Supraclavicular nerves (branches of cervical plexus)	11 Cephalic vein
4 Deltoid muscle	12 Serratus anterior muscle
5 Pectoralis major muscle	13 Linea alba
6 Anterior cutaneous branches of intercostal nerves	14 Sheath of rectus abdominis muscle
7 External abdominal oblique muscle	(anterior layer)
8 Lateral cutaneous branches of intercostal nerves	15 Inguinal ligament

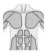

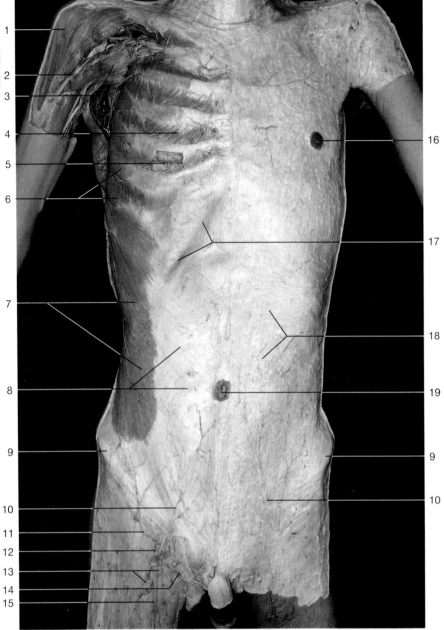

1 Deltoid muscle
2 Cephalic vein
3 Pectoralis major muscle (divided)
4 Internal intercostal muscle
5 Intercostal artery and vein (intercostal space, fenestrated)
6 Serratus anterior muscle
7 External abdominal oblique muscle
8 Anterior layer of rectus sheath
9 Iliac crest
10 Superficial epigastric vein
11 Superficial circumflex iliac vein
12 Saphenous opening
13 Superficial inguinal lymph nodes
14 Superficial external pudendal veins
15 Great saphenous vein
16 Nipple
17 Costal margin
18 Subcutaneous fatty tissue
19 Umbilicus
20 Anterior layer of rectus sheath
21 Rectus abdominis muscle
22 Posterior layer of rectus sheath
23 Internal abdominal oblique muscle
24 External abdominal oblique muscle (cut)
25 Transversus abdominis muscle
26 Transversalis fascia and peritoneum
27 Psoas major muscle
28 Body of lumbar vertebra (L$_4$)
29 Quadratus lumborum muscle
30 Medial tract of erector spinae muscle
31 Lateral tract of erector spinae muscle (longissimus and iliocostalis muscles)
32 Small intestine
33 Left ureter
34 Abdominal aorta
35 Inferior vena cava
36 Descending colon
37 Spinous process

Thoracic and abdominal walls. Right pectoralis major and minor muscles are divided. Muscles of thoracic and abdominal walls on right side are displayed.

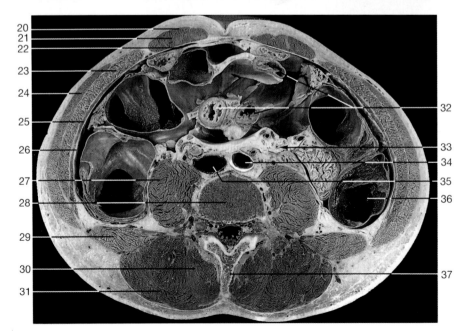

Horizontal section of the trunk at the level of the umbilicus, superior to arcuate line (inferior aspect).

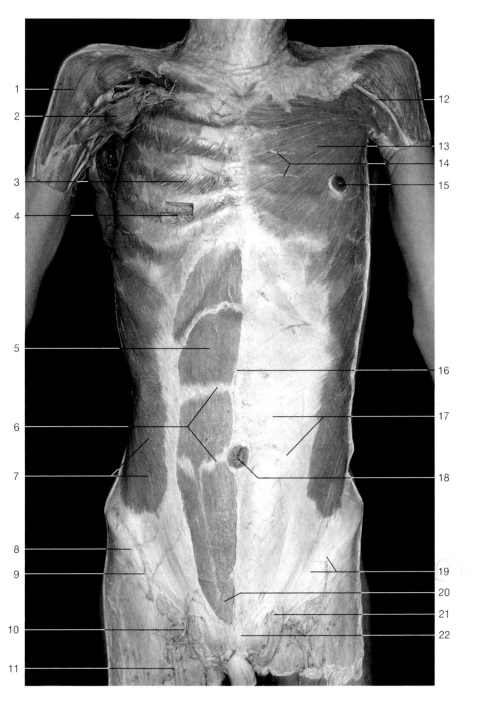

1 Deltoid muscle
2 Pectoralis major muscle (divided)
3 Internal intercostal muscle
4 Intercostal artery and vein
5 Rectus abdominis muscle
6 Tendinous intersections
7 External abdominal oblique muscle
8 Anterior superior iliac spine
9 Superficial circumflex iliac vein
10 Superficial epigastric vein
11 Great saphenous vein
12 Cephalic vein
13 Pectoralis major muscle
14 Anterior cutaneous branches of
    intercostal nerves
15 Nipple
16 Linea alba
17 Anterior layer of rectus sheath
18 Umbilicus
19 Inguinal ligament
20 Pyramidal muscle
21 Superficial inguinal ring and spermatic
    cord
22 Suspensory ligament of penis
23 Longissimus and iliocostalis muscles
24 Multifidus muscle
25 Quadratus lumborum muscle
26 Latissimus dorsi muscle
27 Psoas major muscle
28 Spinous process
29 Body of first lumbar vertebra
30 Transversus abdominis muscle
31 Internal abdominal oblique muscle

Thoracic and abdominal walls. Right
pectoralis major and minor muscles and
anterior layer of rectus sheath have been
removed on the right side.

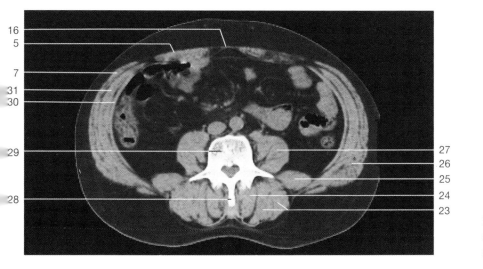

Horizontal section through the body
at the level of fourth lumbar vertebra;
seen from below. (CT scan.)

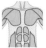

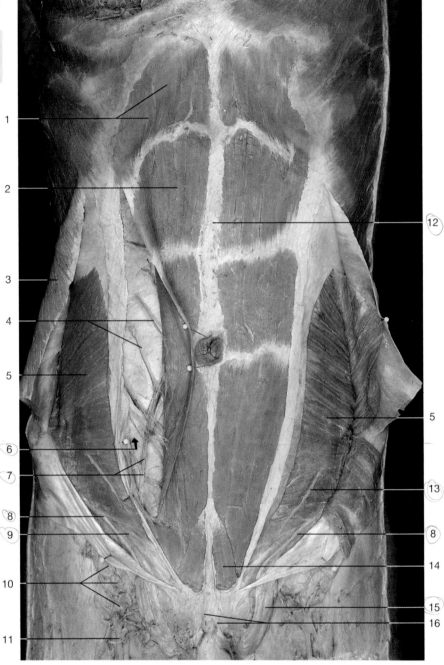

1   Costal margin
2   Rectus abdominis muscle
3   External abdominal oblique muscle
    (reflected)
4   Thoraco-abdominal (intercostal) nerves
    with accompanying vessels
5   Internal abdominal oblique muscle
6   Arcuate line (arrow)
7   Inferior epigastric artery and vein
8   Ilio-inguinal nerve
9   Position of deep inguinal ring
10 Superficial inguinal lymph nodes
11 Great saphenous vein
12 Linea alba
13 Iliohypogastric nerve
14 Pyramidal muscle
15 Spermatic cord
16 Fundiform ligament of penis

Thoracic and abdominal walls.
External abdominal oblique muscle has been
divided and reflected on both sides. The right
rectus muscle has been reflected medially
to display the posterior layer of rectus sheath.
Arrow: location of arcuate line.

1   Anterior layer of rectus sheath
2   Rectus abdominis muscle
3   Posterior layer of rectus sheath
4   Transversalis fascia
5   Transversus abdominis muscle
6   Internal oblique muscle
7   External oblique muscle
8   Thoracolumbar fascia with
    superficial and deep layer
9   Lateral column of erector spinae muscle
10 Medial column of intrinsic muscles
    of the back

Horizontal section of the trunk superior
to arcuate line (schematic drawing).

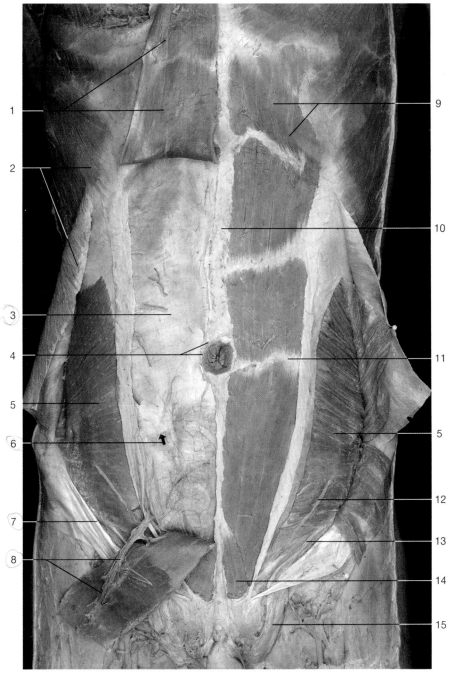

1   Rectus abdominis muscle (reflected)
2   External abdominal oblique muscle
    (divided)
3   Posterior layer of rectus sheath
4   Umbilical ring
5   Internal abdominal oblique muscle
6   Arcuate line (arrow)
7   Inguinal ligament
8   Inferior epigastric artery and vein
    and rectus abdominis muscle
    (divided and reflected)
9   Costal margin
10 Linea alba
11 Tendinous intersection
12 Iliohypogastric nerve
13 Ilio-inguinal nerve
14 Pyramidal muscle
15 Spermatic cord

Thoracic and abdominal walls.
External abdominal oblique muscle has been
divided and reflected on both sides. The right
rectus muscle has been cut and reflected
to display the posterior layer of rectus sheath.
Arrow: location of arcuate line.

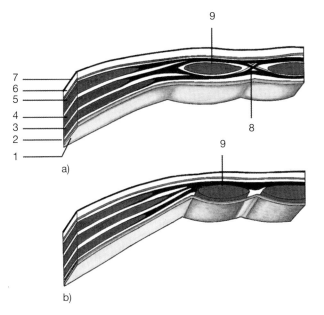

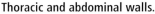

1   Peritoneum
2   Transversalis fascia (green)
3   Transversus abdominis muscle
4   Internal abdominal oblique muscle
5   External abdominal oblique muscle
6   Fascia of external abdominal oblique
    muscle (green)
7   Skin
8   Linea alba
9   Rectus abdominis muscle

**Transverse sections through the
abdominal wall** superior (a) and inferior (b)
to arcuate line.

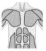

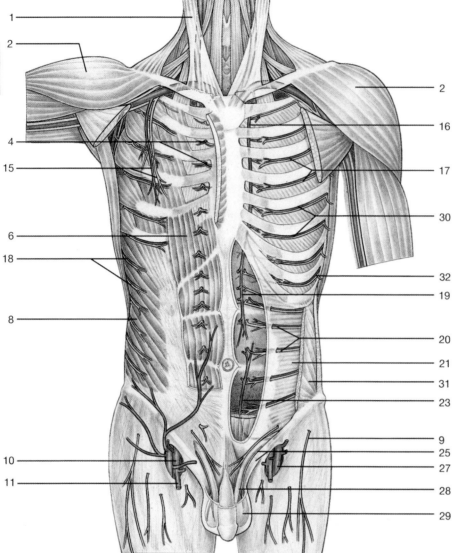

1   Sternocleidomastoid muscle
2   Deltoid muscle
3   Pectoralis major muscle
4   Anterior cutaneous branches of intercostal nerves
5   Cut edge of anterior layer of rectus sheath
6   Rectus abdominis muscle
7   Tendinous intersection
8   External abdominal oblique muscle
9   Lateral femoral cutaneous nerve
10   Femoral vein
11   Great saphenous vein
12   Medial supraclavicular nerves
13   Pectoralis minor muscle (reflected) and medial pectoral nerves
14   Axillary vein
15   Long thoracic nerve and lateral thoracic artery
16   Internal thoracic artery
17   Intercostal nerves
18   Lateral cutaneous branches of intercostal nerves
19   Superior epigastric artery
20   Thoraco-abdominal (intercostal) nerves
21   Transversus abdominis muscle
22   Posterior layer of rectus sheath
23   Inferior epigastric artery
24   Lateral femoral cutaneous nerve
25   Inguinal ligament and ilio-inguinal nerve
26   Femoral nerve
27   Femoral artery
28   Spermatic cord
29   Testis
30   Posterior intercostal arteries
31   Internal abdominal oblique muscle
32   Lateral cutaneous branch of intercostal nerve
33   Dorsal branch of spinal nerve
34   Latissimus dorsi muscle
35   Deep muscles of the back (medial and lateral tract)
36   Anterior layer of rectus sheath
37   Posterior layer of rectus sheath
38   Thoracolumbar fascia
39   Spinal cord
40   Aorta
41   Ventral root ⎫ of spinal
42   Dorsal root ⎬ nerve

Thoracic and abdominal walls (schematic drawing). Note the segmental organization of the blood vessels and nerves. Right side: superficial layers; left side: deeper layers.

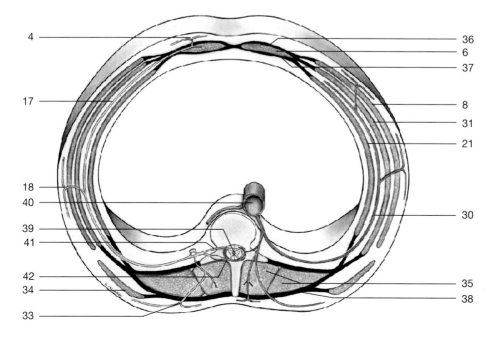

Horizontal section of the abdominal wall (from below) showing the location of the intercostal arteries (left side) and nerves (right side).

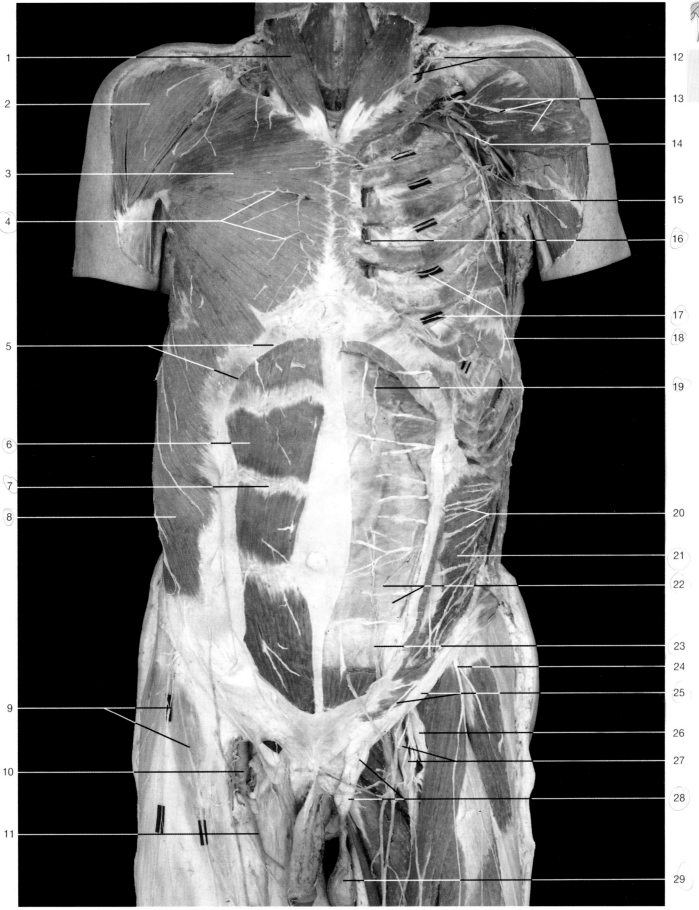

Thoracic and abdominal walls with vessels and nerves (anterior aspect). Right side: superficial layers; left side: deeper layers. Pectoralis major and minor muscles, the external and internal intercostal muscles on the left side have been removed to display the intercostal nerves. The anterior layer of rectus sheath, the left rectus abdominis muscle, and the external and internal abdominal oblique muscles have been removed to show the thoraco-abdominal nerves within the abdominal wall.

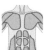

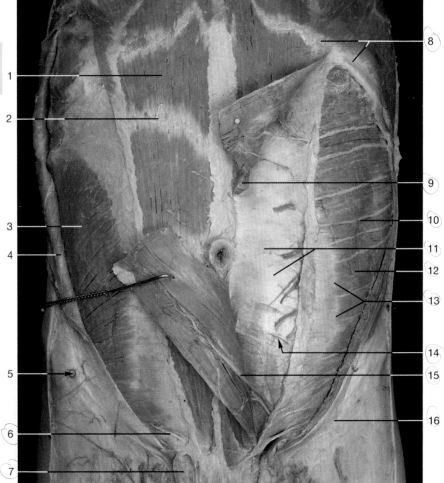

1   Rectus abdominis muscle
2   Tendinous intersection
3   Internal abdominal oblique muscle
4   External abdominal oblique muscle
    (reflected)
5   Anterior superior iliac spine
6   Ilio-inguinal nerve
7   Spermatic cord
8   Costal margin
9   Superior epigastric artery
10 Thoraco-abdominal (intercostal)
    nerves
11 Posterior layer of rectus sheath
12 Transversus abdominis muscle
13 Semilunar line
14 Arcuate line
15 Inferior epigastric artery
16 Inguinal ligament

Abdominal wall with vessels and nerves. The left rectus abdominis muscle has been divided and reflected to display the inferior epigastric vessels. The left internal abdominal oblique muscle has been removed to show the thoraco-abdominal nerves.

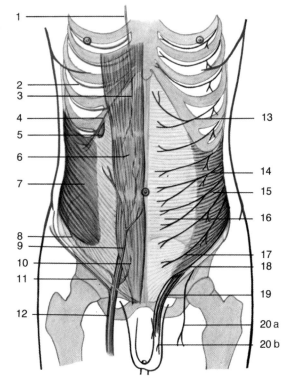

1   Internal thoracic artery
2   Intercostal artery
3   Superior epigastric artery
4   Musculophrenic artery
5   Gallbladder
6   Rectus abdominis muscle
7   External abdominal oblique muscle
8   Deep circumflex iliac artery
9   Superficial epigastric artery
10 Inferior epigastric artery
11 Superficial circumflex iliac artery
12 Femoral artery
13 Intercostal nerve
14 Thoraco-abdominal nerve (T$_{10}$)
15 Transversus abdominis muscle
16 Posterior layer of the rectus sheath
17 Iliohypogastric nerve (L$_1$)
18 Ilio-inguinal nerve (L$_1$)
19 Spermatic cord
20 Genitofemoral nerve (L$_1$, L$_2$)
    a Femoral branch
    b Genital branch

Arteries and nerves that supply the thoracic and abdominal walls.
Note their segmental arrangement (schematic drawing).

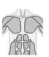

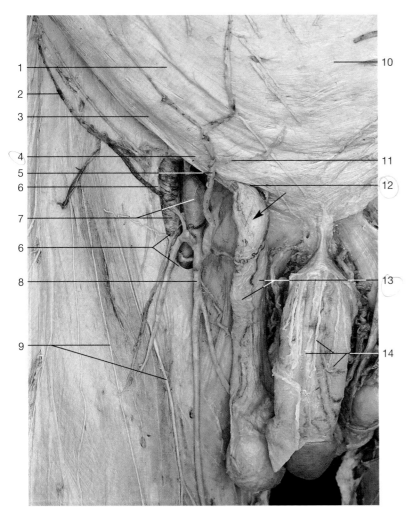

1 Aponeurosis of external abdominal oblique muscle
2 Superficial circumflex iliac vein
3 Inguinal ligament
4 Lateral crus of inguinal ring
5 Superficial epigastric vein
6 Saphenous opening
7 Femoral artery and vein
8 Great saphenous vein
9 Anterior cutaneous branches of femoral nerve
10 Anterior layer of rectus sheath
11 Intercrural fibers
12 Superficial inguinal ring
13 Spermatic cord and genital branch
   of genitofemoral nerve
14 Penis with dorsal nerves and deep dorsal vein
   of penis
15 Aponeurosis of external abdominal oblique
   muscle (divided and reflected)
16 Internal abdominal oblique muscle
17 Ilio-inguinal nerve
18 Anterior cutaneous branches of iliohypogastric
   nerve
19 Superficial external pudendal veins

Inguinal canal in the male, right side (superficial layer, anterior aspect).
There is a small inguinal hernia (arrow).

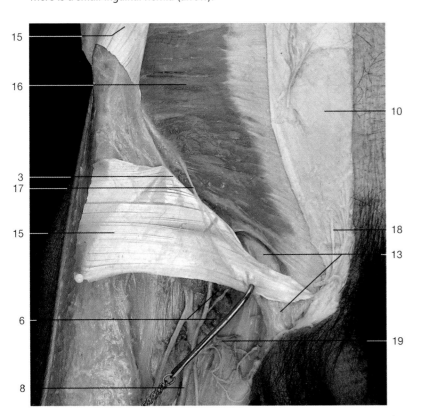

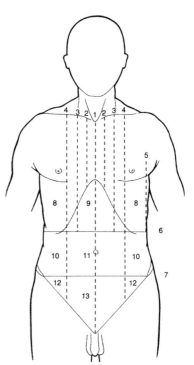

Regions and reference lines
for delineating surface projections.
1 Median line
2 Lateral sternal line
3 Parasternal line
4 Midclavicular line
5 Axillary line
6 Transpyloric plane
7 Transtubercular plane
8 Hypochondriac region
9 Epigastric region
10 Lumbar region
11 Umbilical region
12 Iliac region
13 Hypogastric region

Inguinal canal in the male, right side (anterior aspect). The external
abdominal oblique muscle has been divided to display the inguinal canal.

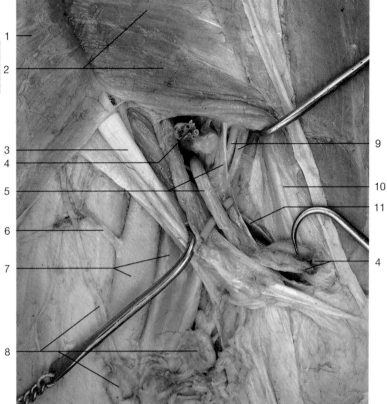

1. Internal abdominal oblique muscle (reflected)
2. Transversus abdominis muscle
3. Inguinal ligament
4. Spermatic cord with the exception of the ductus deferens (divided and reflected)
5. Ductus deferens and interfoveolar ligament
6. Superficial circumflex iliac artery
7. Femoral artery and vein
8. Superficial inguinal lymph nodes and inguinal lymph vessel
9. Inferior epigastric artery and vein
10. Falx inguinalis or conjoint tendon (cut)
11. Pubic branch of inferior epigastric artery
12. Superficial inguinal ring
13. Penis
14. External abdominal oblique muscle
15. Anterior superior iliac spine
16. Intercrural fibers
17. Fascia lata and sartorius muscle
18. Saphenous opening and great saphenous vein
19. Deep inguinal ring
20. Skin of scrotum and dartos muscle
21. Cremaster muscle
22. Internal spermatic fascia
23. Ductus deferens
24. Epididymis
25. Peritoneum (blue)
26. Remnant of processus vaginalis
27. Tunica vaginalis testis
28. Rectus abdominis muscle
29. Spermatic cord with ductus deferens covered by external spermatic fascia
30. Anterior layer of rectus sheath
31. Suspensory ligament of penis
32. Testis and epididymis
33. Ductus deferens
34. Pampiniform venous plexus and testicular artery
35. Inferior epigastric artery
36. Lateral femoral cutaneous nerve
37. Ilio-inguinal nerve
38. Femoral nerve
39. Sartorius muscle
40. Deep dorsal vein of penis

Inguinal canal in the male, right side (deep layer, anterior aspect). Spermatic cord with exception of ductus deferens (probe) has been divided and reflected.

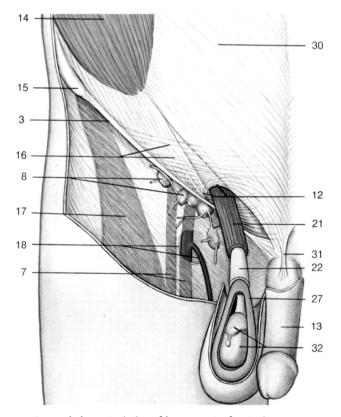

General characteristics of lower part of anterior abdominal wall and inguinal canal (schematic drawing).

Inguinal hernias may either pass through the inguinal canal lateral to the inferior epigastric artery (indirect or lateral inguinal hernias, A and C) or directly penetrate the abdominal wall through the inguinal triangle located medial to the inferior epigastric artery (direct or medial inguinal hernias, B). The lateral hernias can be congenital if the vaginal process remains open (C) or acquired (A) if the hernia develops independently of a patent processus vaginalis.

Femoral hernias generally protrude through the femoral ring below the inguinal ligament. Proper assessment of the site of herniation requires the identification of both the inguinal ligament and the epigastric artery.

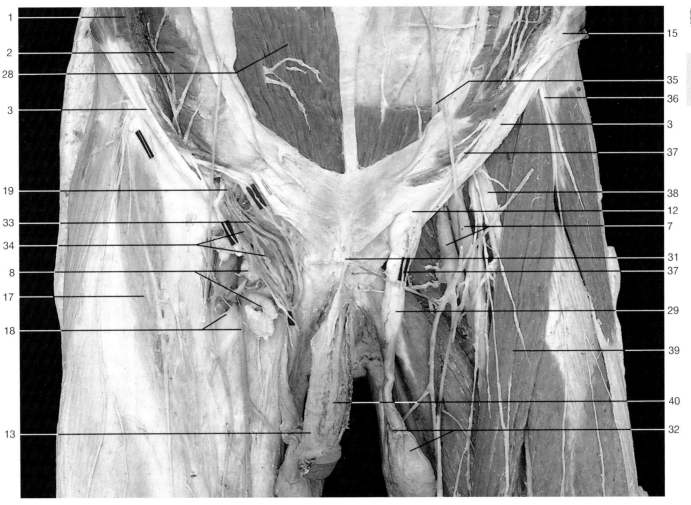

Inguinal and femoral regions in the male (anterior aspect). On the right, the spermatic cord was dissected to display the ductus deferens and the accompanying vessels and nerves. The fascia lata on the left side has been removed.

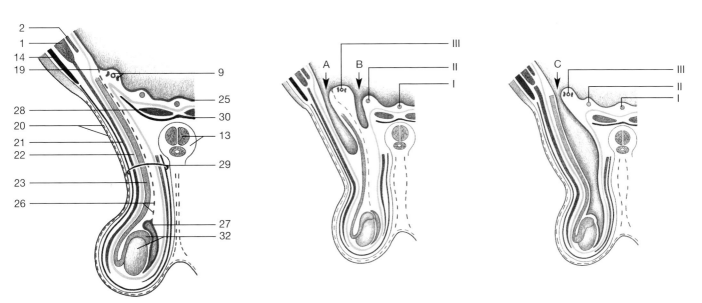

Layers of spermatic cord and types of hernias. Left: normal situation. Middle: location of acquired inguinal hernias:
A = indirect; B = direct inguinal hernia. Right: congenital indirect inguinal hernia (C); the vaginal process remained open.
I   = median umbilical fold containing urachus chord.
II = medial umbilical fold with remnants of umbilical artery.
III = lateral umbilical fold with inferior epigastric artery and vein.

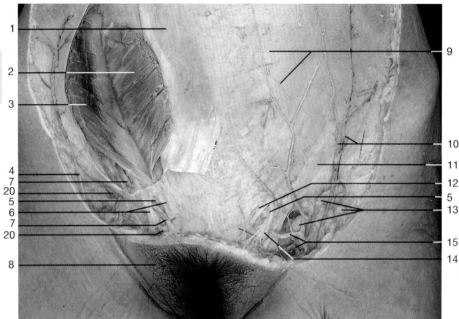

1   Aponeurosis of external abdominal
    oblique muscle
2   Internal abdominal oblique muscle
    (divided and reflected)
3   Transversus abdominis muscle
4   Superficial circumflex iliac artery and
    vein
5   Superficial inguinal ring with fat pad
6   Medial and lateral crural fibers
7   Round ligament (ligamentum teres uteri)
8   Labium majus pudendi
9   Anterior layer of rectus sheath
10 Superficial epigastric artery and vein
11 Inguinal ligament
12 Cutaneous branch of ilio-inguinal nerve
13 Superficial inguinal lymph nodes
14 Entrance of round ligament into the
    labium majus
15 External pudendal artery and vein
16 Position of deep inguinal ring
17 Ilio-inguinal nerve
18 Internal abdominal oblique muscle
19 Pubic branch of inferior epigastric
    artery
20 Genital branch of genitofemoral nerve
21 Fat pad of inguinal canal
22 Ilio-inguinal nerve
23 Sheath of round ligament
    (inguinal canal)
24 Transversalis fascia

Inguinal region in the female (anterior aspect). Left side: superficial layer;
right side: external and internal abdominal oblique muscle divided and reflected.

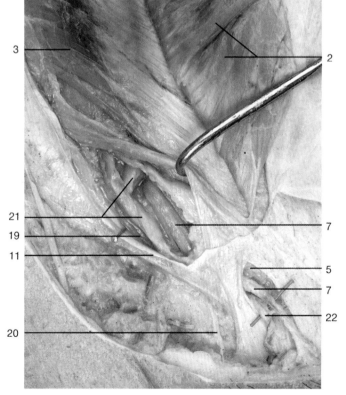

Inguinal canal of the female (anterior aspect, right side).
The external abdominal oblique muscle has been divided and
reflected, to display the ilio-inguinal nerve and the round
ligament.

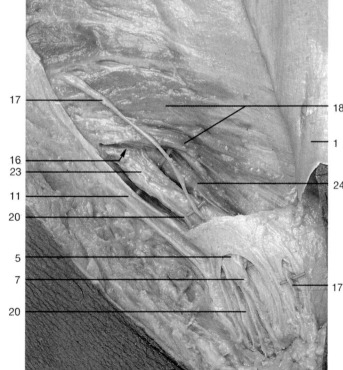

Inguinal canal of the female (anterior aspect, right side).
The external and internal abdominal oblique muscle have been
divided and reflected to show the content of the inguinal canal.

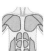

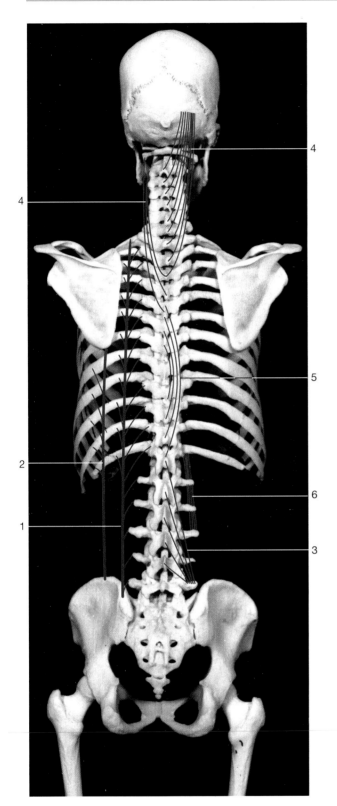

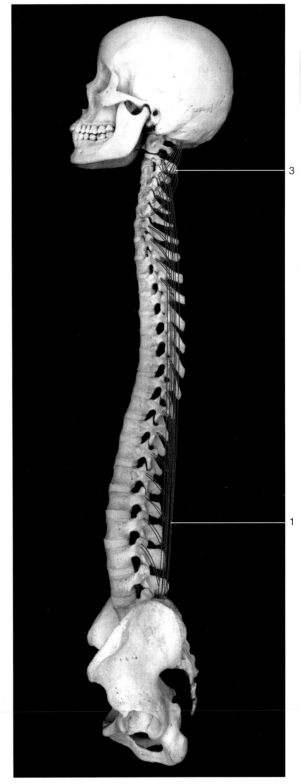

Skeleton of the trunk (dorsal and lateral aspect).
The long muscles of the back [longissimus (1) and iliocostalis (2) muscles] originate at the sacrum and pelvis and insert at the spinous or transverse processes of the vertebrae or at the ribs. There are also muscles that insert at the occipital bone.
The long muscles form the lateral tract, whereas muscles of the medial tract are situated within the groove between the spinous and transverse processes of the vertebrae [transversospinal (3) and spinotransversal (4) muscles] or between the spinous processes [spinalis muscles (5)] or between the transverse processes [intertransversarii muscles (6)] of the vertebrae.

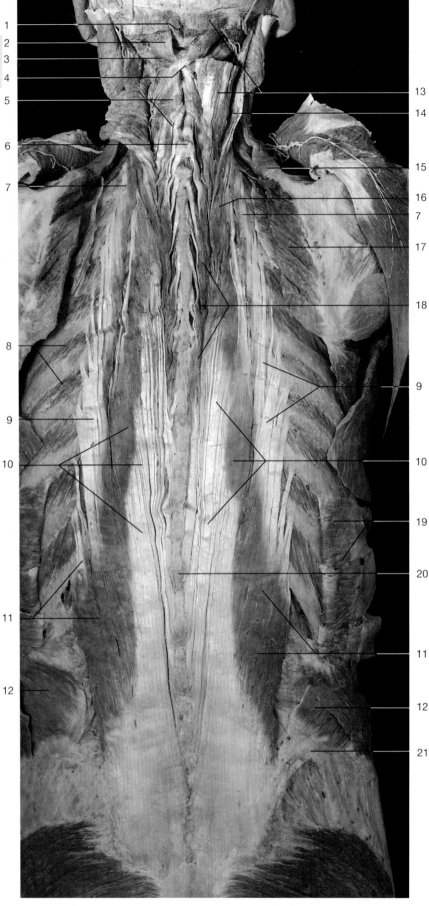

Muscles of the back. Dissection of the erector spinae muscle (lateral column of the intrinsic back muscles).

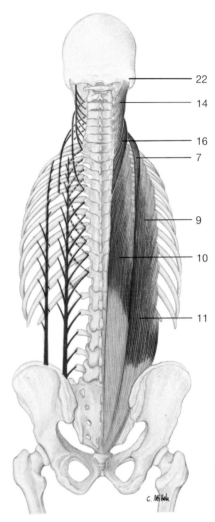

Origin and insertion of iliocostalis and longissimus muscles (schematic drawing).

1 Rectus capitis posterior minor muscle
2 Rectus capitis posterior major muscle
3 Obliquus capitis inferior muscle
4 Spinous process of axis
5 Semispinalis cervicis muscle
6 Spinous process of seventh vertebra
7 Iliocostalis cervicis muscle
8 External intercostal muscles
9 Iliocostalis thoracis muscle
10 Longissimus thoracis muscle
11 Iliocostalis lumborum muscle
12 Internal abdominal oblique muscle
13 Semispinalis capitis muscle (divided)
14 Longissimus capitis muscle
15 Levator scapulae muscle
16 Longissimus cervicis muscle
17 Rhomboid major muscle
18 Spinalis thoracis muscle
19 Serratus posterior inferior muscle (reflected)
20 Spinous process of second lumbar vertebra
21 Iliac crest
22 Mastoid process

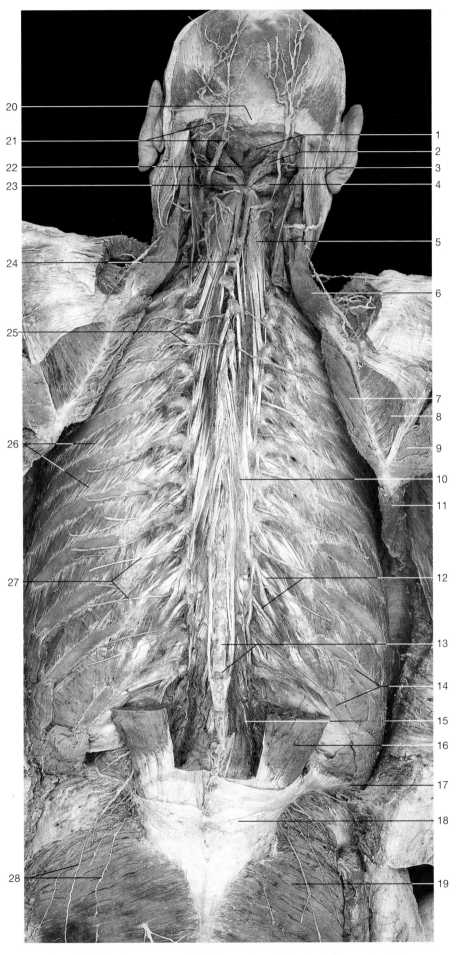

1   Rectus capitis posterior minor muscle
2   Rectus capitis posterior major muscle
3   Obliquus capitis superior muscle
4   Obliquus capitis inferior muscle
5   Semispinalis cervicis muscle
6   Levator scapulae muscle
7   Rhomboideus major muscle
8   Scapula with infraspinatus muscle
9   Teres major muscle
10 Spinalis muscle
11 Latissimus dorsi muscle
12 Levatores costarum muscles
13 Spinous processes of lumbar vertebrae
14 Ribs (Th$_{11}$, Th$_{12}$)
15 Multifidus muscle
16 Longissimus and iliocostalis
     muscles (cut)
17 Iliac crest (lumbar triangle)
18 Thoracolumbar fascia
19 Gluteus maximus muscle
20 Protuberantia occipitalis externa
21 Occipital artery and greater occipital
     nerve (C$_2$)
22 Posterior tubercle of atlas
23 Spinous process of axis
24 Spinous process of seventh cervical
     vertebra (vertebra prominens)
25 Medial branches of dorsal branches
     of spinal nerves
26 External intercostal muscles
27 Lateral branches of dorsal branches
     of spinal nerves
28 Superior cluneal nerves

Muscles of the back. Dissection of the deeper layer of the intrinsic muscles of the back (longissimus and iliocostalis muscles are cut).

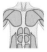

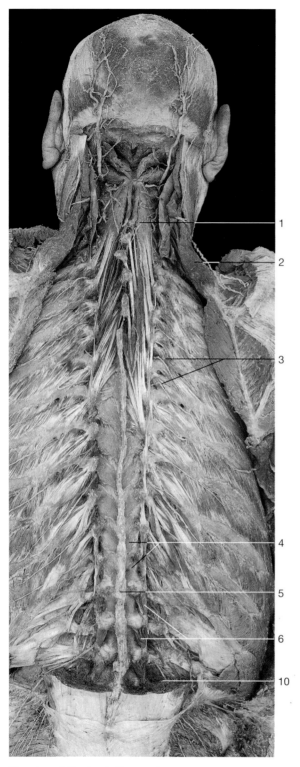

Muscles of the back. Deepest layer.

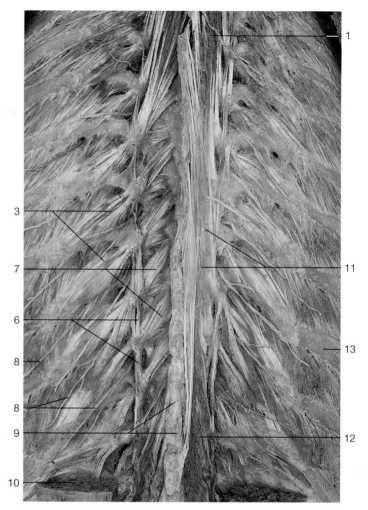

Muscles of the back. Deepest layer. Lumbar region (higher magnification).

1 Semispinalis cervicis muscle
2 Levator scapulae muscle
3 Levatores costarum muscles
4 Vertebral arches of lumbar vertebrae
5 Supraspinal ligaments
6 Intertransverse lumbar muscles
7 Lumbar rotator muscles
8 Cutaneous branches of spinal nerves
9 Lumbar interspinal muscles
10 Longissimus and iliocostalis muscle (cut)
11 Spinal muscle of the back
12 Multifidus muscle
13 Tenth rib (T_{10})

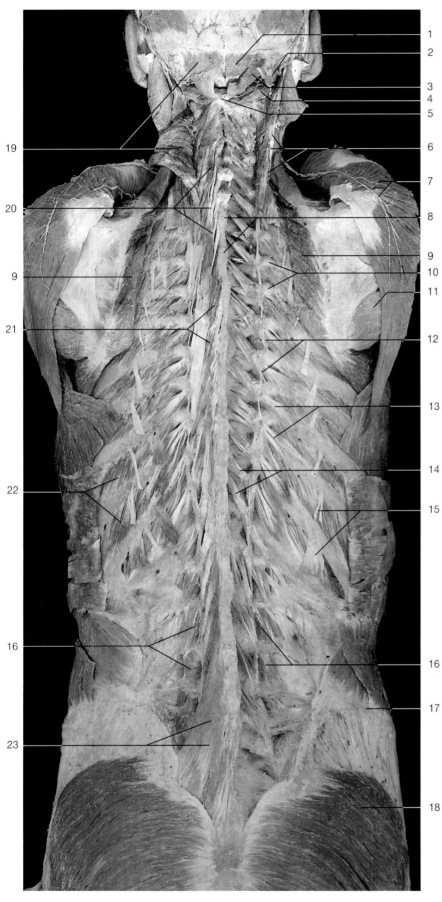

Muscles of the back. Transversospinal muscles, deepest layer on the right, where all parts of semispinalis and multifidus muscles have been removed.

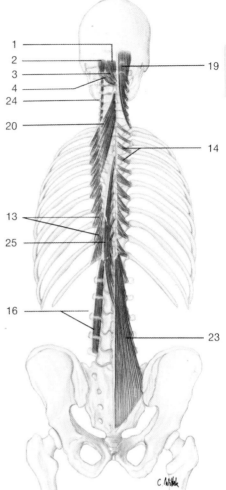

Medial column of intrinsic muscles of the back. Transversospinal and intertransversal system (schematic drawing).

1 Rectus capitis posterior minor muscle
2 Obliquus capitis superior muscle
3 Rectus capitis posterior major muscle
4 Obliquus capitis inferior muscle
5 Spinous process of axis
6 Longissimus capitis muscle
7 Trapezius muscle (reflected) and accessory nerve (n. XI)
8 Spinous processes
9 Rhomboid major muscle
10 Transverse processes of thoracic vertebrae
11 Teres major muscle
12 Intertransverse ligaments
13 Levatores costarum muscles
14 Rotatores muscles
15 Tendons of iliocostalis muscle
16 Intertransversarii lumborum muscles (lateral)
17 Iliac crest
18 Gluteus maximus muscle
19 Semispinalis capitis muscle
20 Semispinalis cervicis muscle
21 Semispinalis thoracis muscle
22 External intercostal muscles
23 Multifidus muscle
24 Posterior cervical intertransversarii muscles
25 Spinalis thoracis muscle

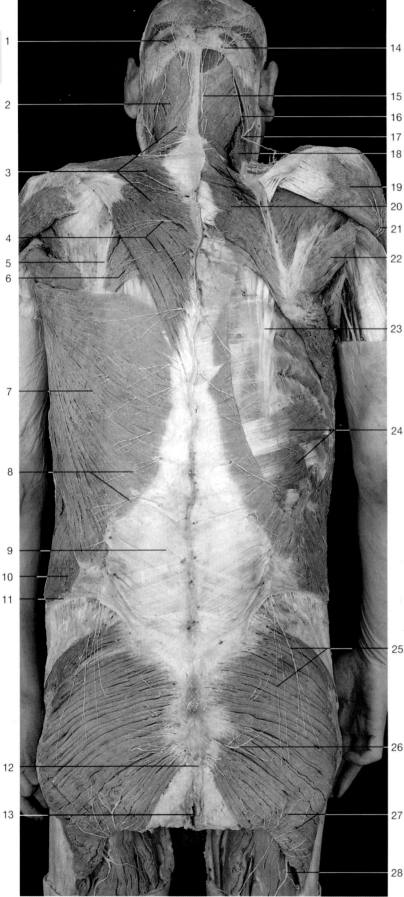

1 Occipital belly of occipitofrontalis muscle
2 Splenius capitis muscle
3 Trapezius muscle
4 Medial cutaneous branches of dorsal rami of spinal nerves
5 Medial margin of scapula
6 Rhomboid major muscle
7 Latissimus dorsi muscle
8 Lateral cutaneous branches of dorsal rami of spinal nerves
9 Thoracolumbar fascia
10 External abdominal oblique muscle
11 Iliac crest
12 Last coccygeal vertebra
13 Anus
14 Greater occipital nerve
15 Third occipital nerve
16 Lesser occipital nerve
17 Cutaneous branches of cervical plexus
18 Levator scapulae muscle
19 Deltoid muscle
20 Rhomboid major and minor muscles
21 Upper lateral cutaneous nerve of arm (branch of axillary nerve)
22 Teres major muscle
23 Iliocostalis thoracis muscle
24 Serratus posterior inferior muscle
25 Superior cluneal nerves
26 Middle cluneal nerves
27 Inferior cluneal nerves
28 Posterior femoral cutaneous nerve

Innervation of the back. Superficial (left) and deeper (right) layers. Right trapezius and latissimus dorsi muscles removed.

▷ **To page 227:**

1 Trapezius muscle
2 Infraspinatus muscle
3 Left latissimus dorsi muscle
4 Thoracolumbar fascia
5 Splenius cervicis muscle
6 Serratus posterior superior muscle
7 Medial branches of dorsal rami of thoracic spinal nerves
8 Lateral branches of dorsal rami of thoracic spinal nerves
9 Iliocostalis muscle
10 Serratus posterior inferior muscle
11 Latissimus dorsi muscle (reflected)

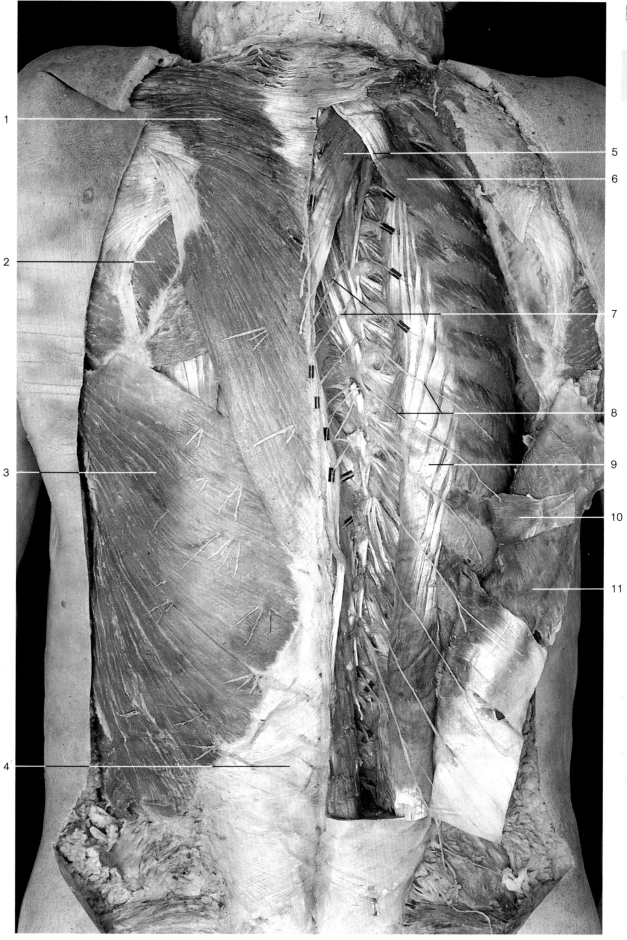

Innervation of the back. Dissection of the dorsal branches of spinal nerves. On the right, longissimus thoracis muscle has been removed and iliocostalis muscle laterally reflected.

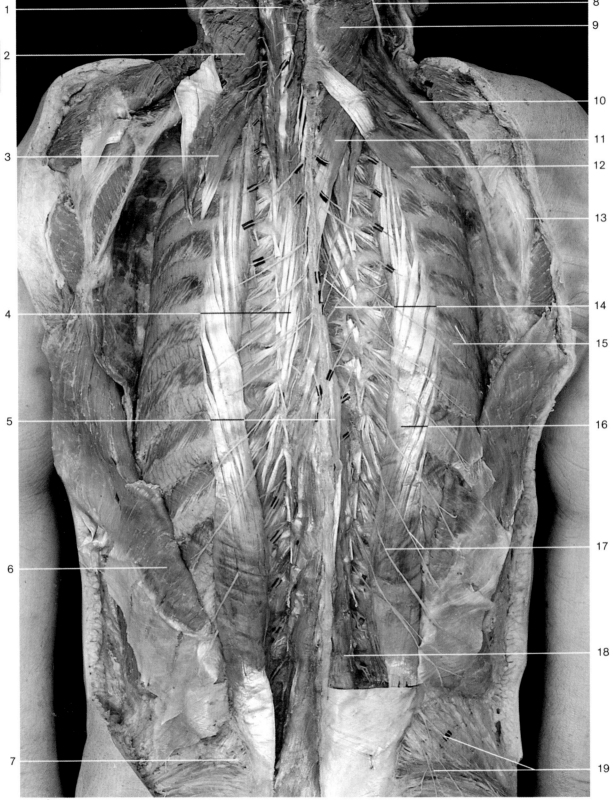

Innervation of the back. Deeper layer (dorsal aspect).

1 Semispinalis capitis muscle	7 Iliac crest	14 Medial branches of dorsal rami of spinal nerves
2 Left splenius capitis muscle (cut and reflected)	8 Lesser occipital nerve	15 Rib and external intercostal muscle
3 Left splenius cervicis muscle (cut and reflected)	9 Splenius capitis muscle	16 Iliocostalis thoracis muscle
4 Semispinalis thoracis muscle	10 Levator scapulae muscle	17 Lateral branches of dorsal rami of spinal nerves
5 Spinalis thoracis muscle	11 Splenius cervicis muscle	18 Multifidus muscle
6 Latissimus dorsi muscle (reflected)	12 Serratus posterior superior muscle	19 Superior cluneal nerves
	13 Scapula	

1   Greater occipital nerve (C$_2$)
2   Suboccipital nerve (C$_1$)
3   Medial branches of dorsal rami of spinal nerves
4   Lateral branches of dorsal rami of spinal nerves
5   Superior cluneal nerves (L$_1$–L$_3$)
6   Middle cluneal nerves (S$_1$–S$_3$)
7   Inferior cluneal nerves (derived from branches
    of the sacral plexus, ventral rami)
8   Lesser occipital nerve
9   Great auricular nerve
10 Trapezius muscle
11 Deltoid muscle
12 Latissimus dorsi muscle
13 Gluteus maximus muscle
14 External intercostal muscle
15 Internal intercostal muscle
16 Innermost intercostal muscle
17 Dorsal ramus of spinal nerve
18 Spinal nerve and spinal ganglion
19 Sympathetic trunk with ganglion
20 Intercostal nerve
21 Lateral cutaneous branch ⎫
22 Anterior cutaneous branch ⎭ of intercostal nerve
23 Longissimus thoracis muscle
24 Spinal cord
25 Aorta
26 Esophagus
27 Body of rib
28 Thoracic rib
29 Thoracic duct
30 Azygos vein

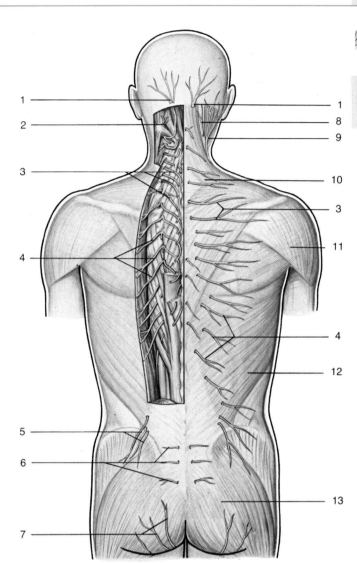

General characteristics of the innervation of the back.
Distribution of dorsal branches of spinal nerves. Note the
segmental arrangement of the innervation of the dorsal part
of the trunk (schematic drawing).

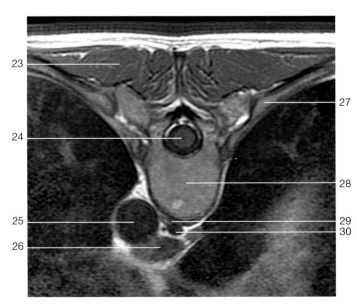

Posterior part of the thoracic wall (MRI scan, coronal section;
from Heuck et al., MRT-Atlas, 2009).

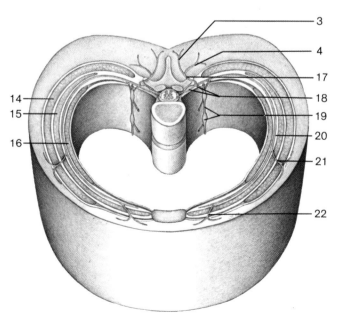

**Position and branches of spinal nerves in one segment of
thoracic wall** (schematic drawing).

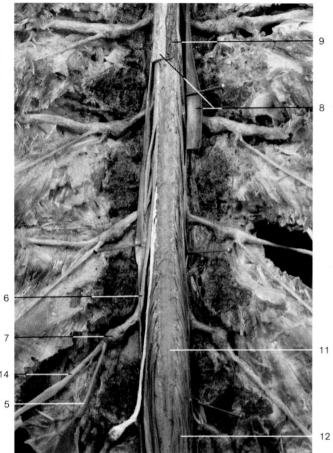

Lumbar portion of spinal cord. Note the relation between the nervous and muscular segments.

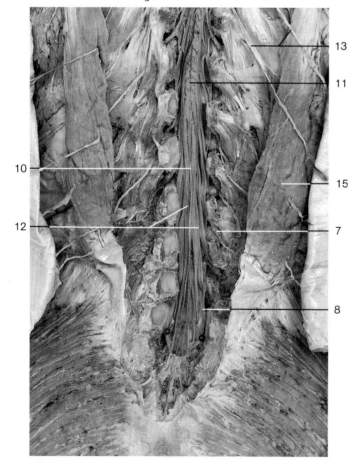

Terminal part of spinal cord. Dura removed.

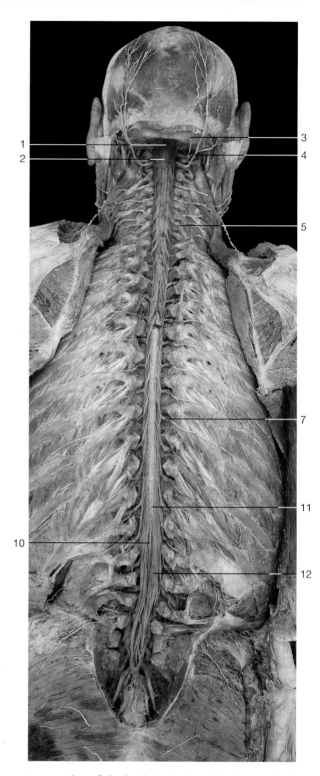

Innervation of the back. Spinal cord in the vertebral canal (opened). Longissimus dorsi and iliocostal muscles have been removed.

1	Cerebellomedullary cistern	9	Spinal arachnoid mater
2	Medulla oblongata	10	Filum terminale
3	Third cervical nerve (C$_3$)	11	Conus medullaris
4	Greater occipital nerve (C$_2$)	12	Cauda equina
5	Dorsal primary ramus	13	Lateral branches of dorsal rami of spinal nerves
6	Dorsal roots	14	Ventral ramus of spinal nerve (intercostal nerve)
7	Spinal ganglion		
8	Spinal dura mater	15	Iliocostalis muscle

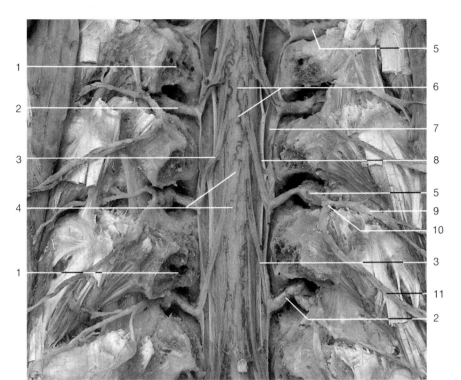

1 Arch of vertebra (divided)
2 Spinal nerve with meningeal coverings
3 Dorsal roots of thoracic spinal nerves
4 Spinal cord (thoracic portion)
5 Spinal ganglia with meningeal coverings
6 Pia mater with blood vessels
7 Dura mater (opened)
8 Denticulate ligament
9 Lateral branch of dorsal ramus
10 Dorsal ramus of spinal nerve
   (dividing into a medial and lateral branch)
11 Medial branch of dorsal ramus
   of spinal nerve
12 Spinal dura mater
13 Spinal nerves of sacral segments
14 Filum terminale

Thoracic portion of spinal cord (dorsal aspect). Vertebral canal and dura mater opened.

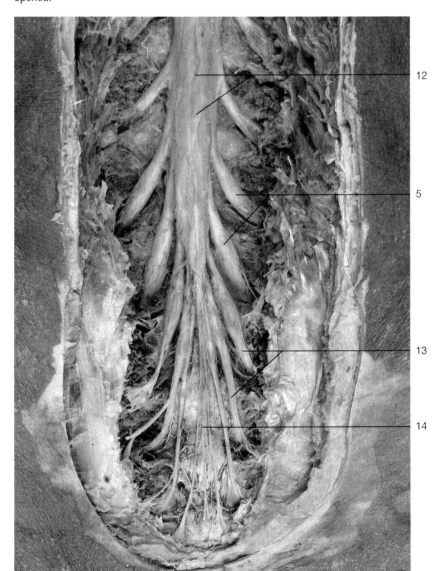

Terminal part of spinal cord with dura mater (dorsal aspect). Dorsal part of sacrum removed.

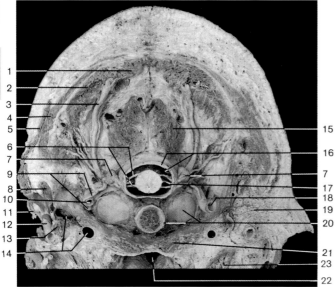

1   Trapezius muscle
2   Semispinalis capitis muscle
3   Dorsal ramus of spinal nerve
4   Sternocleidomastoid muscle
5   Platysma muscle
6   Dorsal and ventral roots of spinal nerves
7   Spinal ganglion
8   Posterior belly of digastric muscle
9   Ventral ramus of spinal nerve
10 Vertebral artery
11 Great auricular nerve
12 Superficial temporal artery
13 Styloid process
14 Internal jugular vein and internal carotid artery
15 Rectus capitis posterior major muscle
16 Dura mater and subarachnoid space
17 Denticulate ligament
18 Vertebral artery
19 Parotid gland
20 Dens of axis (divided) and inferior articular facet of atlas
21 Longus capitis muscle
22 Pharyngeal cavity
23 Medial pterygoid muscle
24 Periosteum of vertebral canal
25 Posterior spinal arteries
26 Anterior spinal artery

Meningeal coverings
27 Dura mater
28 Subdural space
29 Extradural or epidural space with venous plexus and fatty tissue
30 Arachnoid (green)
31 Subarachnoid space
32 Pia mater (pink)
33 Nucleus pulposus
34 Crus of diaphragm
35 Intervertebral disc
36 Body of first lumbar vertebra
37 Spinal cord
38 Conus medullaris
39 Cauda equina
40 Filum terminale
41 Spinous process

Horizontal section of the neck. Dissection of the second cervical spinal nerve. Posterior surface at top of figure.

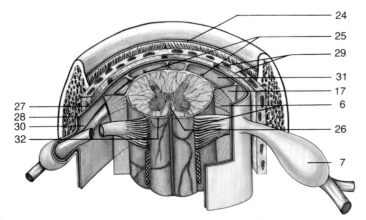

Meningeal coverings of the spinal cord (anterior aspect). (Schematic drawing.)

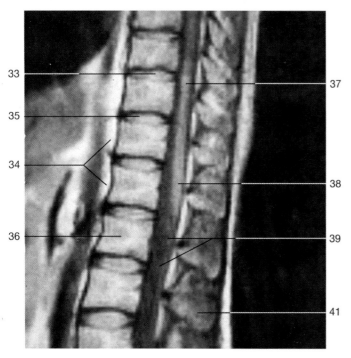

Sagittal section through the vertebral canal, T₉–L₂. (MRI scan.)

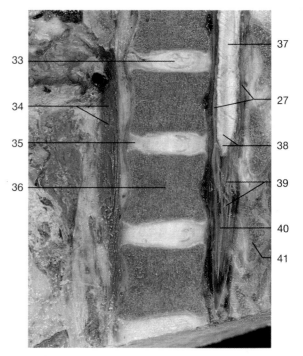

Sagittal section through the vertebral canal, T₁₂–L₂. Notice red bone marrow (unfixed).

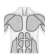

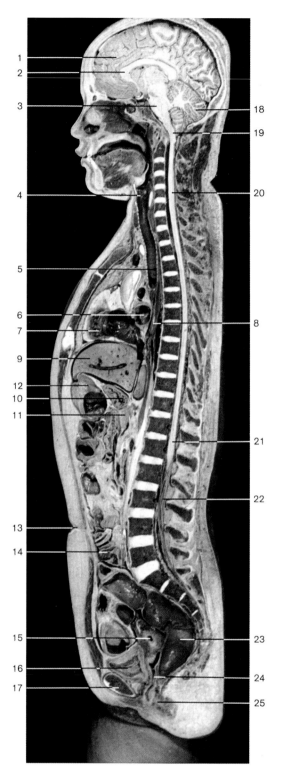

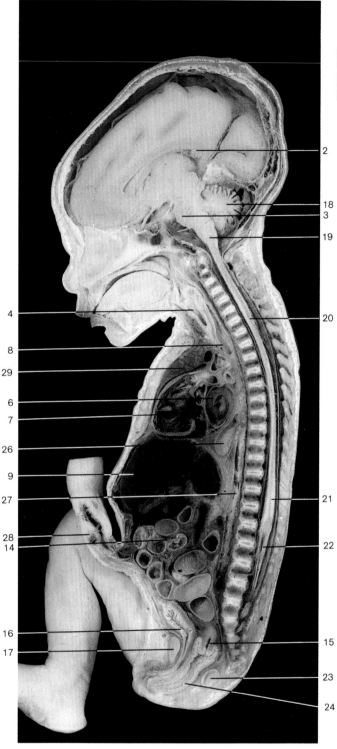

Median section of the head and trunk in the adult (female). The conus medullaris of the spinal cord is located at the level of L_1.

Median section of the head and trunk in the neonate.
Note that in the neonate the conus medullaris of the spinal cord extends far more caudally than in the adult.

1	Cerebrum	11	Pancreas
2	Corpus callosum	12	Transverse colon
3	Pons	13	Umbilicus
4	Larynx	14	Small intestine
5	Trachea	15	Uterus
6	Left atrium	16	Urinary bladder
7	Right ventricle	17	Pubic symphysis
8	Esophagus	18	Cerebellum
9	Liver	19	Medulla oblongata
10	Stomach	20	Spinal cord

21	Conus medullaris
22	Cauda equina
23	Rectum
24	Vagina
25	Anus
26	Inferior vena cava
27	Aorta
28	Umbilical cord
29	Thymus

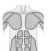

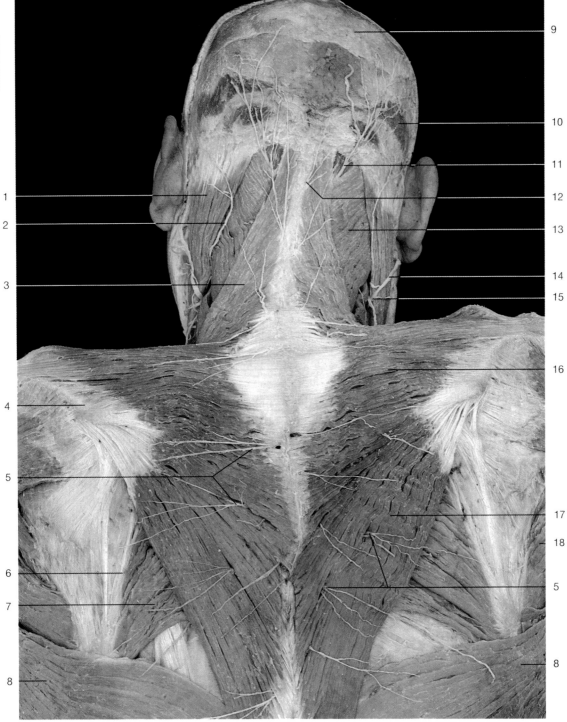

Dorsal aspect of the neck (superficial layer). Nuchal region and shoulder.

1 Sternocleidomastoid muscle
2 Lesser occipital nerve
3 Descending fibers of trapezius muscle
4 Spine of scapula
5 Medial cutaneous branches of dorsal rami of spinal nerves
6 Medial margin of scapula
7 Rhomboid major muscle
8 Latissimus dorsi muscle
9 Galea aponeurotica

10 Occipital belly of occipitofrontalis muscle
11 Greater occipital nerve
12 Third occipital nerve
13 Splenius capitis muscle
14 Great auricular nerve
15 Cutaneous nerves of cervical plexus
16 Transverse fibers of trapezius muscle
17 Ascending fibers of trapezius muscle
18 Teres major muscle

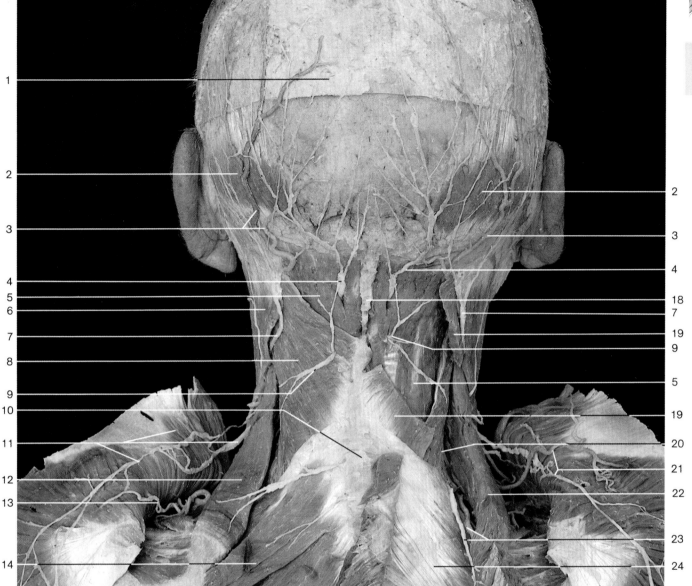

Dorsal aspect of the neck (deeper layer). The left trapezius muscle has been divided and reflected. On the right, trapezius, rhomboid, and splenius muscles have been divided. Right levator scapulae muscle has been slightly reflected.

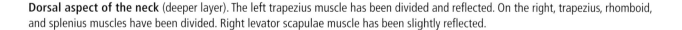

1 Galea aponeurotica	11 Left trapezius muscle and accessory nerve
2 Occipital belly of occipitofrontalis muscle	12 Levator scapulae muscle
3 Occipital artery	13 Superficial branch of transverse cervical artery
4 Greater occipital nerve (C_2)	14 Rhomboid minor muscle
5 Semispinalis capitis muscle	15 Rhomboid major muscle
6 Sternocleidomastoid muscle	16 Medial margin of scapula
7 Lesser occipital nerve	17 Medial branches of dorsal rami of spinal nerves
8 Left splenius capitis muscle	18 Ligamentum nuchae
9 Third occipital nerve (C_3)	19 Splenius capitis muscle (divided)
10 Spinous process of vertebra prominens (C_7)	

20 Splenius cervicis muscle	
21 Right accessory nerve and superficial branch of transverse cervical artery	
22 Right levator scapulae muscle	
23 Dorsal scapular nerve and deep branch of transverse cervical artery	
24 Serratus posterior superior muscle	
25 Right trapezius muscle (divided and reflected)	
26 Right rhomboid major muscle (divided and reflected)	

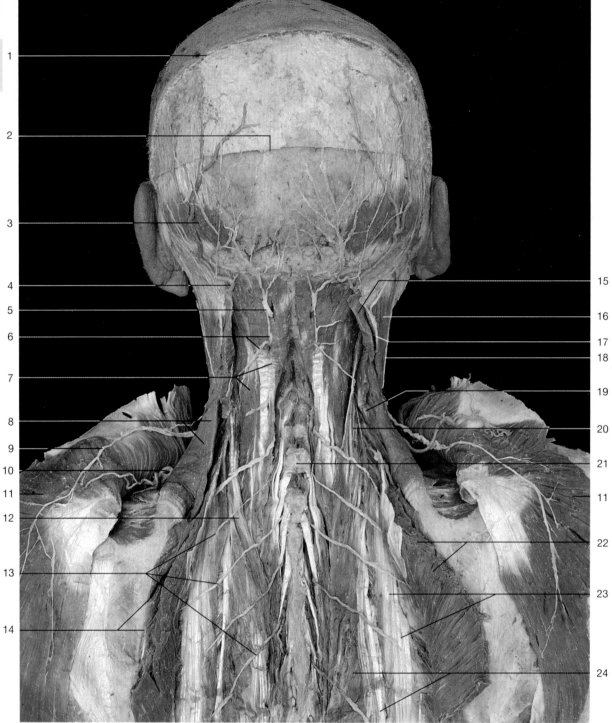

Dorsal aspect of the neck (deepest layer). Trapezius, splenius capitis, and cervicis muscles have been divided and partly removed or reflected.

1	Skin of scalp
2	Galea aponeurotica
3	Occipital belly of occipitofrontalis muscle
4	Occipital artery
5	Greater occipital nerve
6	Third occipital nerve
7	Semispinalis capitis muscle
8	Levator scapulae muscle
9	Accessory nerve (n. XI)
10	Superficial cervical artery
11	Trapezius muscle (reflected)
12	Longissimus cervicis muscle
13	Medial cutaneous branches of dorsal rami of spinal nerves
14	Medial margin of scapula
15	Splenius capitis muscle (divided)
16	Sternocleidomastoid muscle
17	Lesser occipital nerve
18	Great auricular nerve
19	Splenius cervicis muscle
20	Longissimus cervicis muscle
21	Spinous process of seventh cervical vertebra (vertebra prominens)
22	Rhomboid muscles (divided)
23	Iliocostalis thoracis muscle
24	Longissimus thoracis muscle

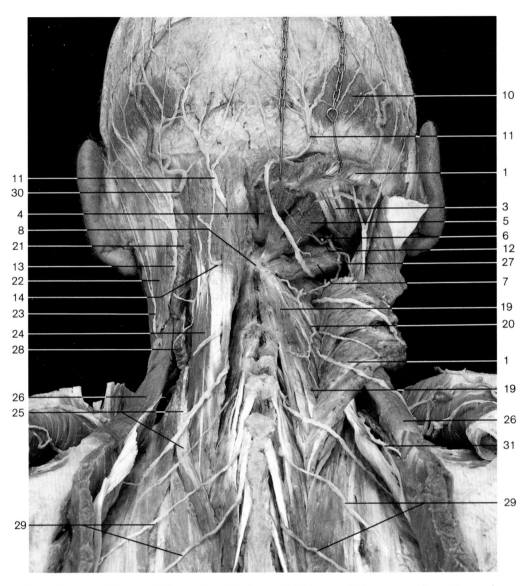

1 Semispinalis capitis muscle (divided)
2 External occipital protuberance
3 Obliquus capitis superior muscle
4 Rectus capitis posterior minor muscle
5 Rectus capitis posterior major muscle
6 Vertebral artery
7 Obliquus capitis inferior muscle
8 Spinous process of axis
9 Third cervical vertebra
10 Occipital belly of occipitofrontalis muscle
11 Greater occipital nerve
12 Suboccipital nerve (C₁)
13 Lesser occipital nerve
14 Third occipital nerve (C₃)
15 Mastoid process and splenius capitis muscle
16 Atlas
17 Axis
18 Spinous process of third cervical vertebra
19 Right semispinalis cervicis muscle
20 Deep cervical artery
21 Left splenius capitis muscle (divided)
22 Left sternocleidomastoid muscle
23 Great auricular nerve
24 Left semispinalis capitis muscle
25 Left longissimus cervicis muscle
26 Levator scapulae muscle
27 Muscular branch of vertebral artery
28 Left semispinalis cervicis muscle (divided)
29 Medial branches of dorsal rami of spinal nerves
30 Occipital artery
31 Dorsal scapular nerve

Dorsal aspect of the neck (deepest layer). **Suboccipital triangle.** Right semispinalis capitis muscle divided and reflected.

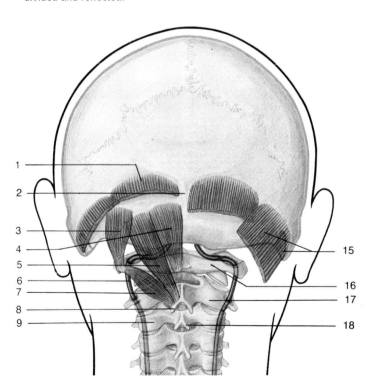

Suboccipital triangle and position of the vertebral artery (schematic drawing).

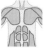

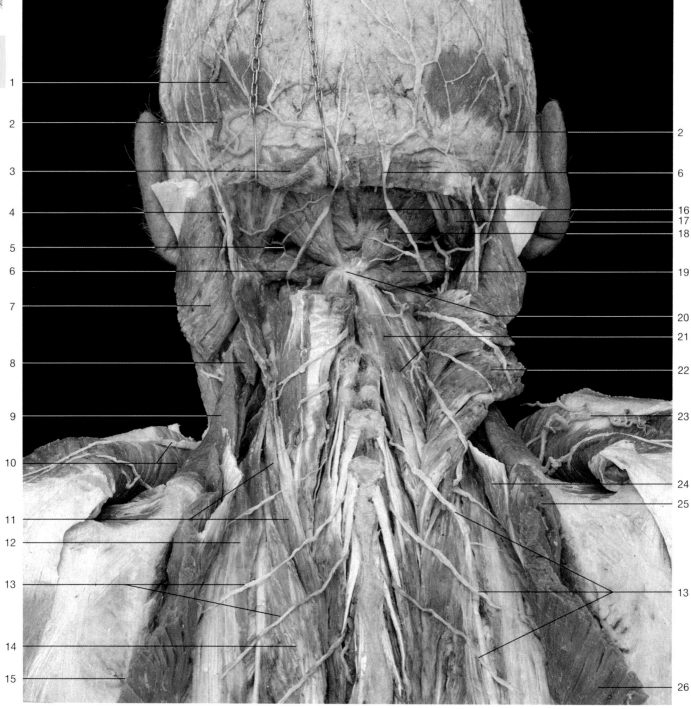

Dorsal aspect of the neck (deepest layer). Dissection of suboccipital triangle on both sides.

1   Occipital belly of occipitofrontalis muscle
2   Occipital artery
3   Insertion of semispinalis capitis muscle (divided)
4   Lesser occipital nerve (from cervical plexus)
5   Suboccipital nerve (C$_1$)
6   Greater occipital nerve (C$_2$)
7   Splenius capitis muscle (reflected)
8   Splenius cervicis muscle
9   Levator scapulae muscle
10 Accessory nerve (n. XI), trapezius muscle
11 Longissimus cervicis muscle
12 Iliocostalis cervicis muscle
13 Medial cutaneous branches of dorsal rami of spinal nerves (C$_7$, C$_8$)
14 Longissimus thoracis muscle
15 Medial margin of scapula
16 Rectus capitis posterior minor muscle
17 Obliquus capitis superior muscle
18 Rectus capitis posterior major muscle
19 Obliquus capitis inferior muscle
20 Spinous process of axis
21 Semispinalis cervicis muscle
22 Semispinalis capitis muscle (divided and reflected)
23 Transverse cervical artery (superficial branch)
24 Serratus posterior superior muscle (divided and reflected)
25 Rhomboid minor muscle (divided and reflected)
26 Rhomboid major muscle (divided and reflected)

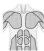

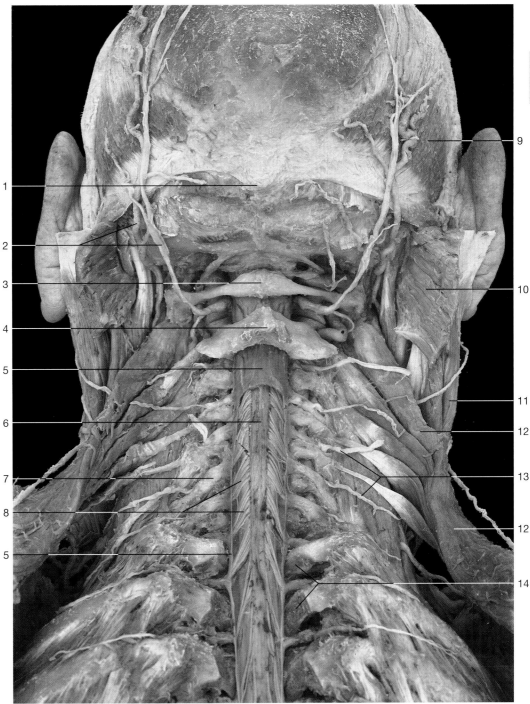

Dorsal aspect of the neck (deepest layer). The vertebral canal caudally of the atlas and axis has been opened to show the spinal cord (dura mater has been partly removed).

1 Protuberantia occipitalis externa
2 Greater occipital nerve (C₂) and occipital artery
3 Atlas (posterior arch)
4 Axis (posterior arch)
5 Dura mater
6 Spinal cord
7 Spinal ganglion

8 Posterior root filaments (fila radicularia posterior)
9 Occipital belly of occipitofrontalis muscle
10 Splenius capitis muscle (cut and reflected)
11 Sternocleidomastoid muscle
12 Levator scapulae muscle
13 Posterior branches of spinal nerves
14 Arches of cervical vertebrae (cut)

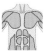

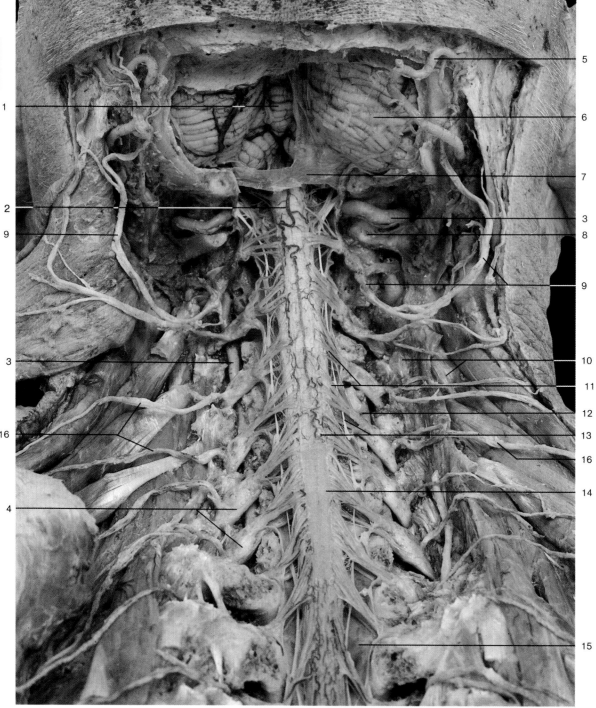

Dorsal aspect of the neck (deepest layer). Dissection of medulla oblongata and spinal cord. Cranial cavity opened.

1   Vermis of the cerebellum
2   Medulla oblongata and posterior spinal artery
3   Vertebral artery
4   Spinal ganglion
5   Occipital artery
6   Cerebellum
7   Cerebellomedullary cistern
8   Atlas

9   Greater occipital nerve (C$_2$)
10   Levator scapulae muscle and intertransverse ligament
11   Dorsal roots of spinal nerves
12   Vertebral arch
13   Denticulate ligament and arachnoid mater
14   Area where pia mater has been removed
15   Dura mater
16   Dorsal rami of spinal nerves

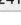

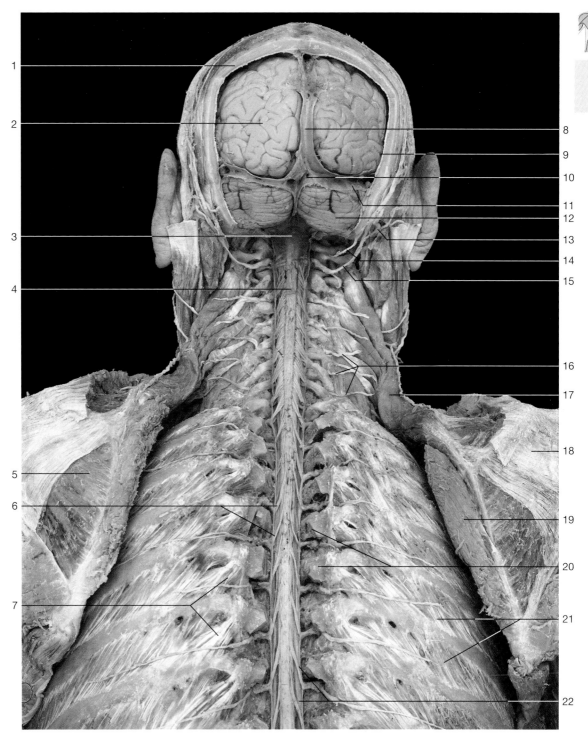

Dorsal aspect of the neck (deepest layer). Dissection of medulla oblongata and spinal cord in relation to the brain.

1	Calvaria	12	Cerebellum
2	Left hemisphere of the brain	13	Occipital artery
3	Cerebellomedullary cistern	14	Suboccipital nerve (C$_1$)
4	Spinal cord	15	Greater occipital nerve (C$_2$)
5	Scapula with infraspinous muscle	16	Posterior branches of spinal nerves
6	Root filaments (fila radicularia posterior)	17	Levator scapulae muscle
7	Levatores costarum muscles	18	Deltoid muscle
8	Falx cerebri with sinus sagittalis superior	19	Rhomboid muscles
9	Subarachnoidal space	20	Vertebral arches (cut)
10	Confluens sinuum	21	External intercostal muscle
11	Transverse sinus	22	Dura mater

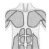

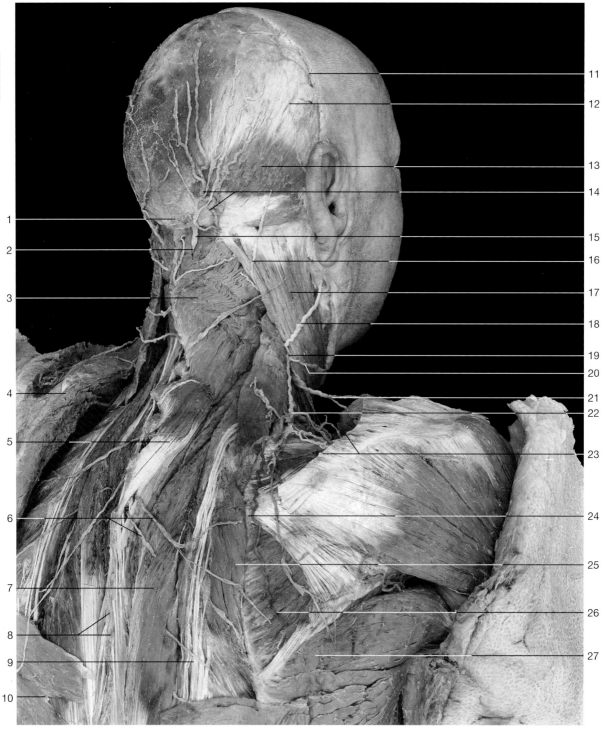

Oblique-lateral aspect of the neck and head (deeper layer). The trapezius muscle has been removed.

1   Protuberantia occipitalis externa
2   Semispinalis capitis muscle
3   Splenius capitis muscle
4   Scapula
5   Splenius cervicis muscle
6   Posterior branches of spinal nerves
7   Longissimus muscle
8   Spinous processes of thoracic vertebrae
9   Iliocostalis muscle
10 Latissimus dorsi muscle
11 Epidermis of the head (scalp)
12 Galea aponeurotica
13 Occipital belly of occipitofrontalis muscle
14 Occipital artery

15 Greater occipital nerve (C$_2$)
16 Lesser occipital nerve
17 Sternocleidomastoid muscle
18 Great auricular nerve
19 Punctum nervosum
20 Transverse cervical nerve
21 Supraclavicular nerves
22 Accessory nerve (n. XI)
23 Trapezius muscle (cut edge)
24 Medial margin of scapula
25 Rhomboid muscle
26 Infraspinous muscle
27 Teres major muscle

4 Thoracic Organs

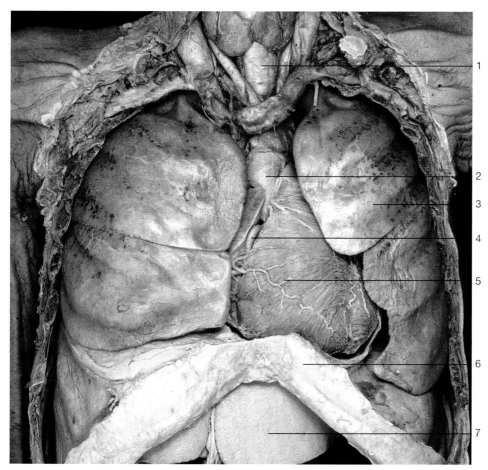

The thoracic cavity contains heart, lungs, and mediastinal organs. The thorax protects all organs but is still movable so that respiration can occur. The respiratory movements of the lung depend on the pleura covering, the thoracic wall, and the surface of the lungs.

The mediastinal organs comprise the esophagus, trachea, and the related nerves and vessels, particularly the aorta, superior vena cava, and the thoracic duct. The thoracic cavity is separated from the abdominal cavity by the diaphragm.

Thoracic organs, heart, and lungs in situ (ventral aspect). Anterior thoracic wall, parietal pleura, and pericardium have been removed.

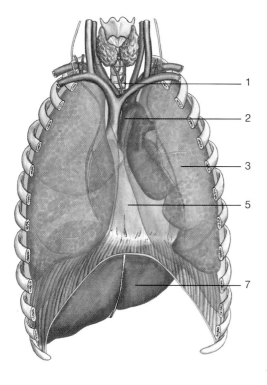

1 Trachea
2 Ascending aorta
3 Left lung
4 Right coronary artery
5 Heart (right ventricle)
6 Costal arch
7 Liver

Position of lungs and heart within the thoracic cavity (schematic drawing). The anterior part of the thorax is not depicted.

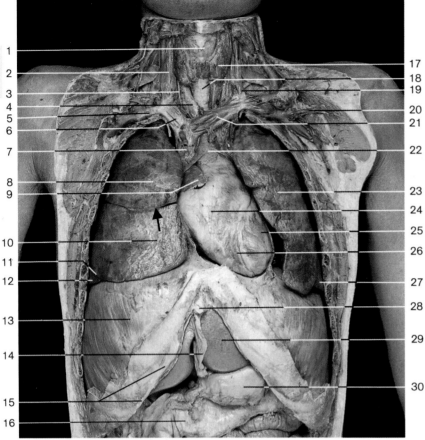

1   Cricothyroid muscle
2   Right internal jugular vein
3   Vagus nerve
4   Right common carotid artery
5   Right subclavian vein
6   Right brachiocephalic vein
7   Superior vena cava
8   Upper lobe of right lung
9   Right auricle
10 Middle lobe of right lung
11 Oblique fissure of right lung
12 Lower lobe of right lung
13 Diaphragm
14 Falciform ligament
15 Costal margin
16 Transverse colon
17 Thyroid gland
18 Trachea
19 Left internal jugular vein
20 Left cephalic vein
21 Left brachiocephalic vein
22 Pericardium (cut edge)
23 Upper lobe of left lung
24 Right ventricle
25 Left ventricle
26 Anterior interventricular sulcus
27 Lower lobe of left lung
28 Xiphoid process
29 Liver
30 Stomach
31 Pectoralis major muscle
32 Sternum
33 Left ventricle and bulb of aorta
34 Left main bronchus
35 Esophagus
36 Descending aorta
37 Spinal cord
38 Scapula
39 Right atrium
40 Right pulmonary vein
41 Right main bronchus
42 Azygos vein
43 Body of vertebra
44 Rib

Positions of thoracic organs. The anterior thoracic wall has been removed.
Arrow: horizontal fissure of right lung.

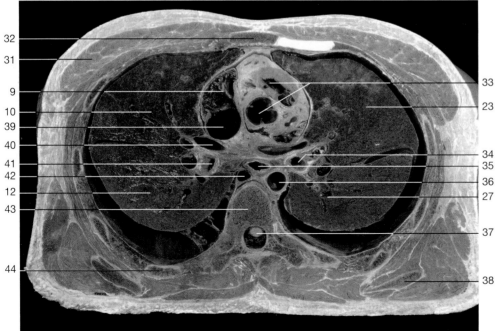

Horizontal section through the thorax at the level of the seventh thoracic vertebra (from below).

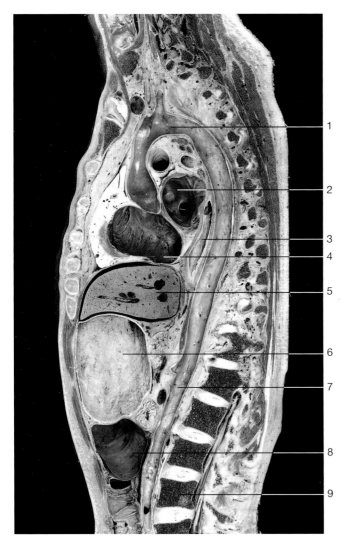

Sagittal section through the thorax, 2 cm lateral to the median plane.

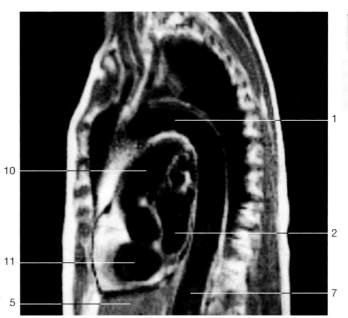

Sagittal section through the thorax (MRI scan).

1 Aortic arch
2 Left atrium of the heart
3 Esophagus
4 Right atrium of the heart
5 Liver
6 Stomach
7 Abdominal aorta
8 Transverse colon (dilated)
9 Lumbar vertebral body
10 Pulmonary trunk
11 Left ventricle of the heart
12 Trachea
13 Ascending aorta
14 Right ventricle of the heart
15 Pericardium
16 Remaining parts of thymus gland

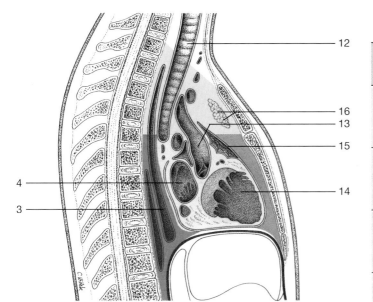

Regional anatomy of the thoracic cavity (midsagittal section).
The parts of the mediastinum are indicated by colors.

Parts of mediastinum	Content
Superior mediastinum (yellow)	Trachea, brachiocephalic vein, thymus, aortic arch, esophagus, thoracic duct
Middle portion of mediastinum (light blue)	Heart, ascending aorta, pulmonary trunk, pulmonary veins, phrenic nerves
Posterior mediastinum (red)	Esophagus with vagus nerves, descending aorta, thoracic duct, sympathetic trunks
Anterior portion of mediastinum (light red)	Smaller vessels and nerves, fat and connective tissue, thymus (only in the child)

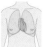

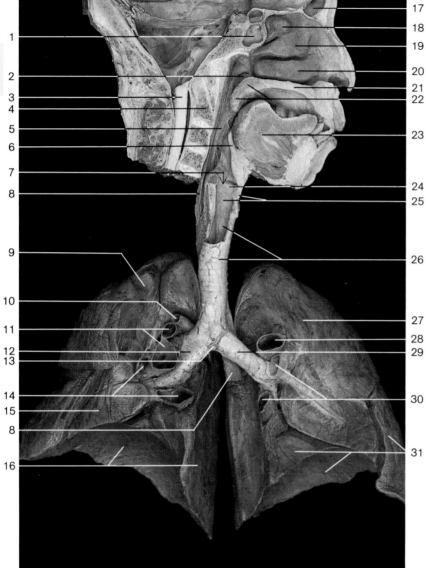

1	Sphenoid sinus
2	Pharyngeal opening of auditory tube
3	Spinal cord
4	Dens of axis
5	Oropharynx (oropharyngeal isthmus)
6	Epiglottis
7	Entrance of larynx
8	Esophagus
9	Upper lobe of right lung
10	Azygos vein
11	Branches of pulmonary artery
12	Right main bronchus
13	Bifurcation of trachea
14	Tributaries of right pulmonary veins
15	Middle lobe of right lung
16	Lower lobe of right lung
17	Frontal sinus
18	Superior nasal concha
19	Middle nasal concha
20	Inferior nasal concha
21	Hard palate
22	Soft palate with uvula
23	Tongue
24	Vocal fold
25	Larynx
26	Trachea
27	Upper lobe of left lung
28	Left pulmonary artery
29	Left main bronchus
30	Left pulmonary veins
31	Lower lobe of left lung

Respiratory system. The lungs have been fixed in expiration and turned laterally. Head bisected and turned laterally.

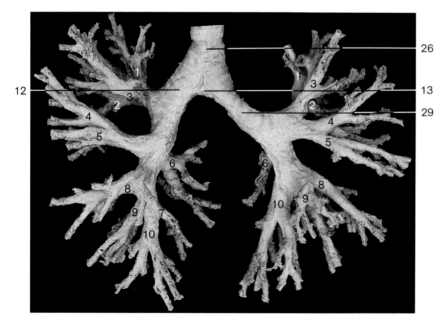

Bronchial tree (ventral aspect). The lung tissue has been removed. The bronchopulmonary segments are numbered 1–10.

▷ **To page 247:**

1	Nasal cavity
2	Pharynx
3	Larynx (thyroid cartilage)
4	Trachea
5	Upper lobe of right lung
6	Bifurcation of trachea
7	Right main bronchus
8	Horizontal fissure of right lung
9	Middle lobe of right lung
10	Oblique fissures of lungs
11	Lower lobe of right lung
12	Clavicle
13	Upper lobe of left lung
14	Left main bronchus
15	Bronchi supplying bronchopulmonary segments
16	Lower lobe of left lung
17	Costal margin
18	Hyoid bone
19	Right superior lobe bronchus
20	Right middle lobe bronchus
21	Right inferior lobe bronchus
22	Left superior lobe bronchus
23	Left inferior lobe bronchus
24	Segmental bronchi
25	Branches of pulmonary arteries
26	Branches of pulmonary veins

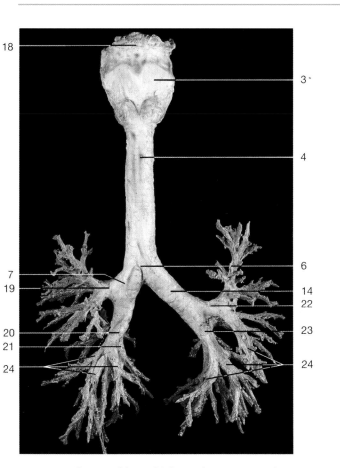

Larynx, trachea, and bronchial tree (anterior aspect).

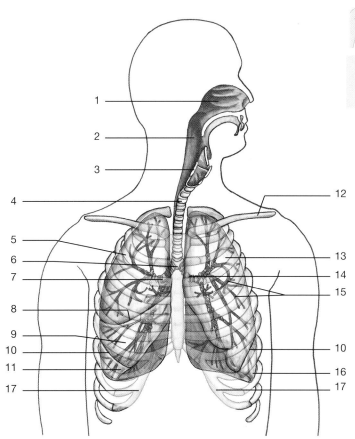

Organization and positions of respiratory organs (schematic drawing).

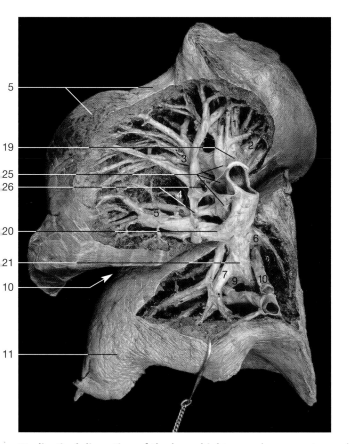

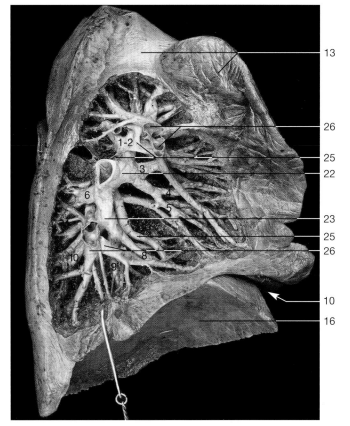

Mediastinal dissection of the bronchial tree, pulmonary veins, and pulmonary arteries of right lung (left) and left lung (right) (medial aspect). The bronchopulmonary segments are numbered 1–10.

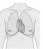

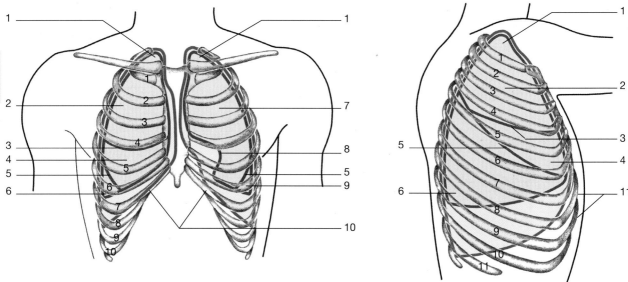

Surface projections of lungs and pleura on the thoracic wall. Left: anterior aspect; right: right-lateral aspect.
Red = margins of the lung; blue = margins of pleura. The numbers indicate ribs.

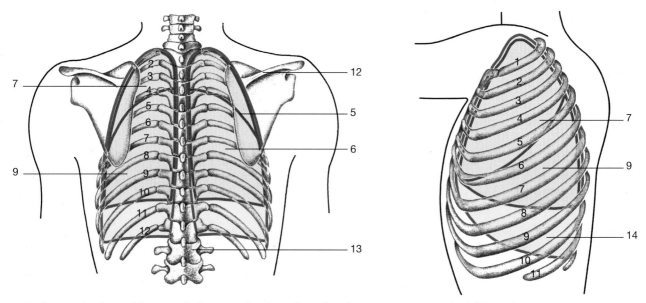

Surface projections of lungs and pleura on the thoracic wall. Left: posterior aspect; right: left-lateral aspect.
Red = margins of lung; blue = margins of pleura. The numbers indicate ribs.

1 Apex of lung	6 Lower lobe of right lung	11 Costal margin
2 Upper lobe of right lung	7 Upper lobe of left lung	12 Spine of scapula
3 Horizontal fissure of right lung	8 Cardiac notch of left lung	13 First lumbar vertebra
4 Middle lobe of right lung	9 Lower lobe of left lung	14 Space between border of lung and pleura
5 Oblique fissures of lungs	10 Infrasternal angle	(costodiaphragmatic recess)

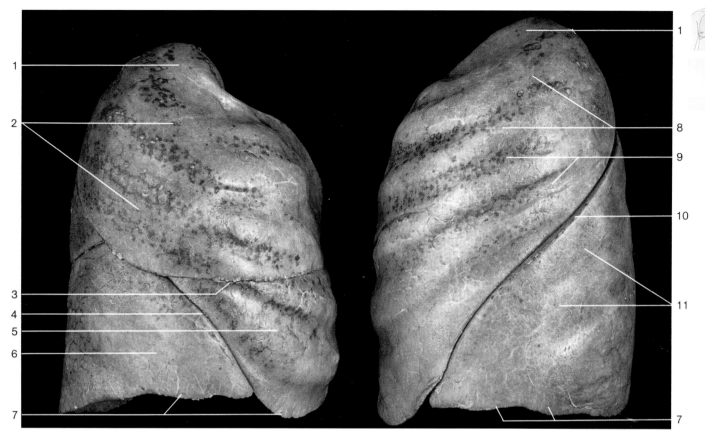

Right lung (lateral aspect).

Left lung (lateral aspect).

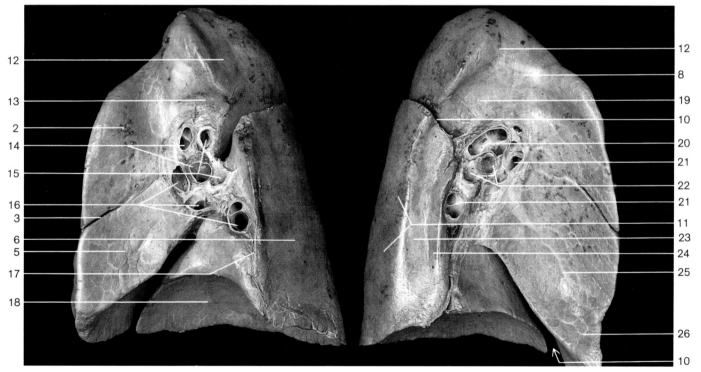

Right lung (medial aspect).

Left lung (medial aspect).

1	Apex of lung	8	Upper lobe of left lung
2	Upper lobe of right lung	9	Impressions of ribs
3	Horizontal fissure of right lung	10	Oblique fissure of left lung
4	Oblique fissure of right lung	11	Lower lobe of left lung
5	Middle lobe of right lung	12	Groove of subclavian artery
6	Lower lobe of right lung	13	Groove of azygos arch
7	Inferior border	14	Branches of right pulmonary artery
15	Bronchi	22	Left secondary bronchi
16	Right pulmonary veins	23	Groove of thoracic aorta
17	Pulmonary ligament	24	Groove of esophagus
18	Diaphragmatic surface	25	Cardiac impression
19	Groove of aortic arch	26	Lingula
20	Left pulmonary artery		
21	Branches of left pulmonary veins		

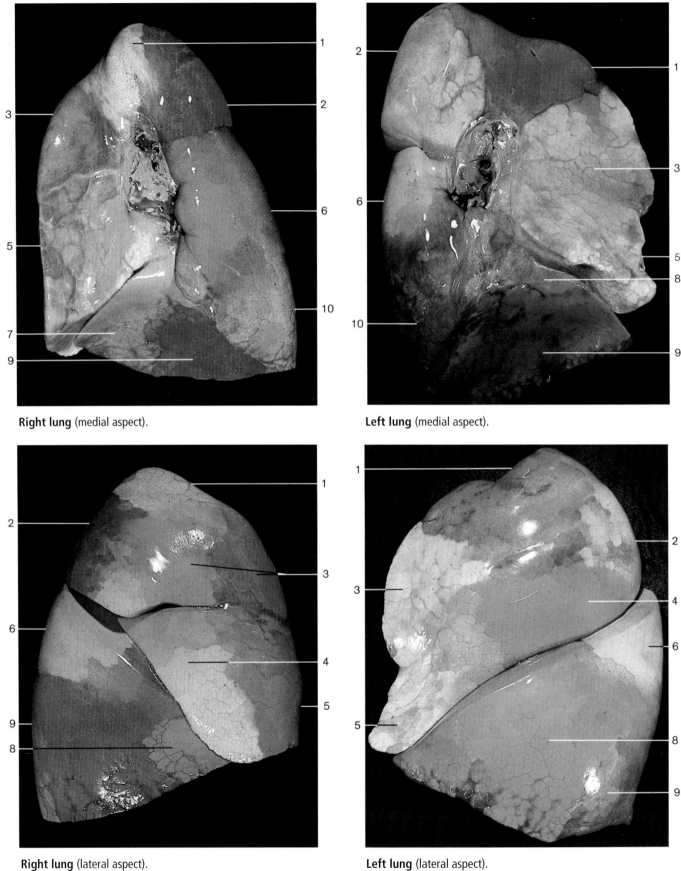

Right lung (medial aspect).

Left lung (medial aspect).

Right lung (lateral aspect).

Left lung (lateral aspect).

The bronchopulmonary segments of the lungs are differentiated by the various colors. Notice that there is no segment in the left lung that corresponds to the seventh segment of the right lung. Compare with the schematic drawing on the facing page.

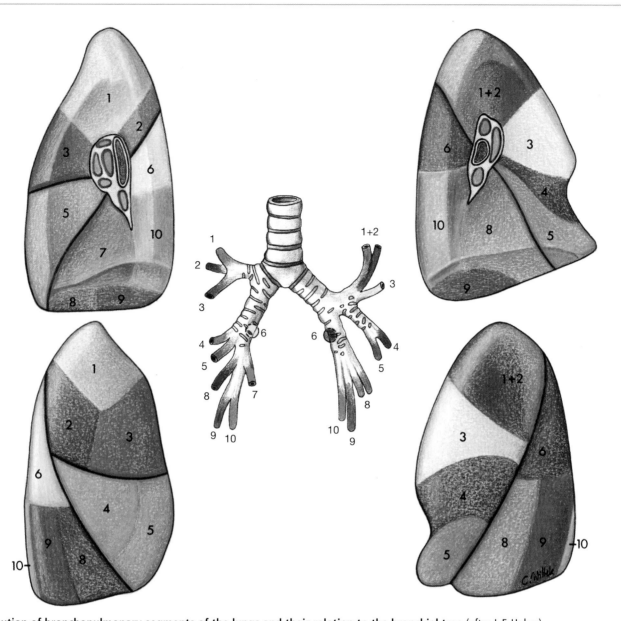

Distribution of bronchopulmonary segments of the lungs and their relation to the bronchial tree (after J. F. Huber).

The bronchopulmonary segments are morphologically and functionally separate, independent respiratory units of the lung tissue. Each segment is surrounded by connective tissue that is continuous with the visceral pleura. The segmental bronchi are centrally located in each segment and are closely accompanied by branches of the pulmonary arteries, whereas the tributaries of the pulmonary veins run **between** the segments. Thus, the veins serve two adjacent segments that drain for the most part into more than one vein. A bronchopulmonary segment is therefore not a complete vascular unit, but segmentation is the result of a specific architecture of the lung vasculature.

Right lung			Left lung			
1 Apical segment	Upper lobe bronchus		1+2 Apicoposterior segment	Superior division		Upper lobe bronchus
2 Posterior segment						
3 Anterior segment			3 Anterior segment			
4 Lateral segment	Middle lobe bronchus		4 Superior lingular segment	Inferior division		
5 Medial segment			5 Inferior lingular segment			
6 Superior (apical) segment	Lower lobe bronchus		6 Superior (apical) segment	Lower lobe bronchus		
7 Medial basal segment			7 Absent			
8 Anterior basal segment			8 Anteromedial basal segment			
9 Lateral basal segment			9 Lateral basal segment			
10 Posterior basal segment			10 Posterior basal segment			

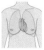

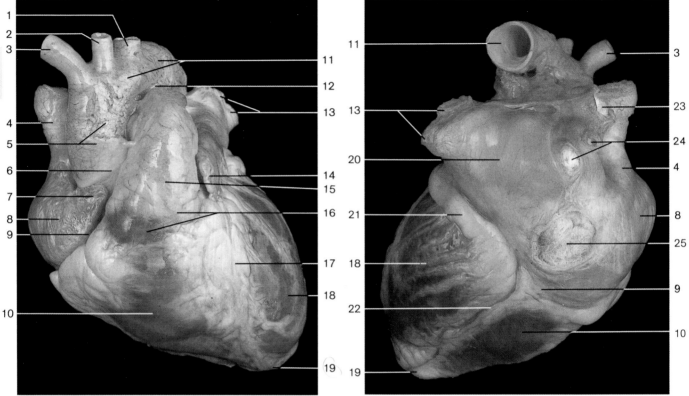

Heart of 30-year-old woman (anterior aspect).

Heart of 30-year-old woman (oblique-posterior view).

1	Left subclavian artery	9	Coronary sulcus
2	Left common carotid artery	10	Right ventricle
3	Brachiocephalic trunk	11	Aortic arch
4	Superior vena cava	12	Ligamentum arteriosum
5	Ascending aorta	13	Left pulmonary veins
6	Bulb of the aorta	14	Left auricle
7	Right auricle	15	Pulmonary trunk
8	Right atrium	16	Sinus of pulmonary trunk
		17	Anterior interventricular sulcus

18	Left ventricle
19	Apex of the heart
20	Left atrium
21	Epicardial fat overlying coronary sinus
22	Posterior interventricular sulcus
23	Right pulmonary artery
24	Right pulmonary veins
25	Inferior vena cava

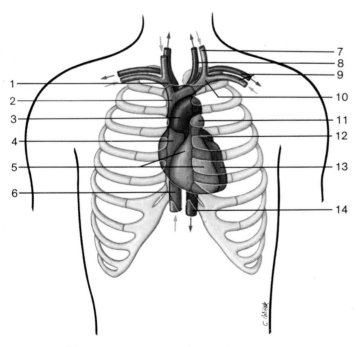

Position of heart and its vessels within the thorax (schematic drawing).

1	Right brachiocephalic vein
2	Superior vena cava
3	Ascending aorta
4	Right atrium
5	Right ventricle
6	Inferior vena cava
7	Left internal jugular vein
8	Left common carotid artery
9	Left axillary artery and vein
10	Left brachiocephalic vein
11	Pulmonary trunk
12	Left auricle
13	Left ventricle
14	Descending aorta

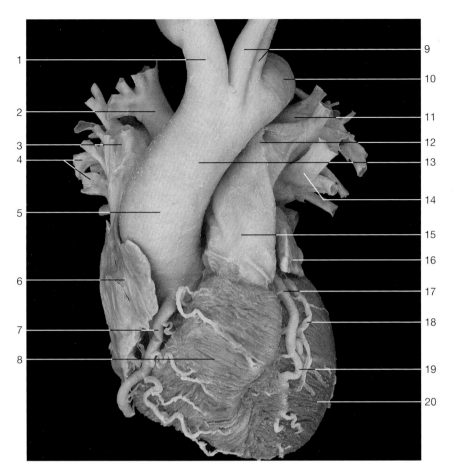

1   Brachiocephalic trunk
2   Right pulmonary artery
3   Superior vena cava
4   Right pulmonary veins
5   Ascending aorta
6   Right atrium
7   Right coronary artery
8   Right ventricle
9   Left common carotid artery and left
    subclavian artery
10 Descending aorta (thoracic part)
11 Ligamentum arteriosum (remnant of
    ductus arteriosus Botalli)
12 Left pulmonary artery
13 Aortic arch
14 Left pulmonary veins
15 Pulmonary trunk
16 Left atrium
17 Left coronary artery
18 Diagonal branch of left coronary artery
19 Interventricular branch of left coronary
    artery
20 Left ventricle
21 Right brachiocephalic vein
22 Thoracic wall
23 Liver
24 Aortic valve
25 Chordae tendineae
26 Papillary muscles
27 Stomach

Heart with related vessels. Dissection of coronary arteries (anterior aspect, systolic phase of heart action).

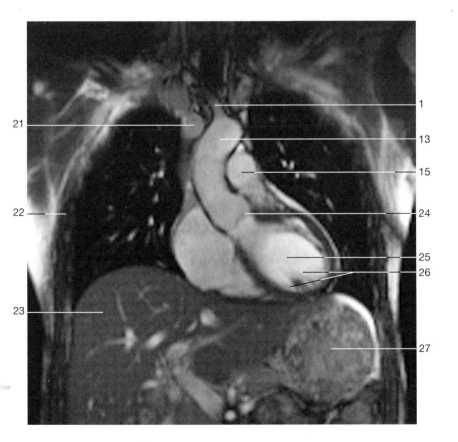

Coronal section through the thorax at the level of the ascending aorta (MRI scan, courtesy of Prof. W. Bautz and R. Janka, M. D., University of Erlangen, Germany).

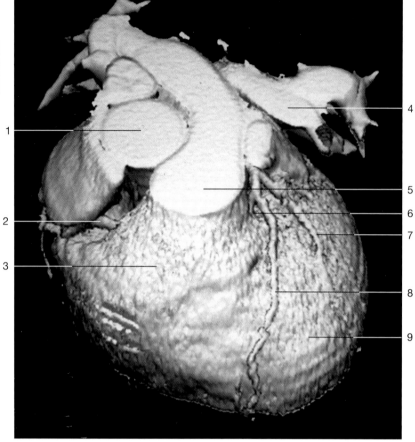

1 Ascending aorta
2 Right coronary artery
3 Right ventricle
4 Left atrium
5 Pulmonary trunk
6 Septal branch of left coronary artery
7 Diagonal branch
8 Anterior interventricular branch of left
   coronary artery
9 Left ventricle
10 Aortic root
11 Superior vena cava
12 Circumflex branch of left coronary artery
13 Sternum

Human heart (3-D reconstruction of electron beam CT scans as "Shaded Surface Display"[1]).

Electron beam tomographic image of the human heart (axial section after injection of contrast medium[1]).

[1] Courtesy of Drs. W. Moshage, S. Achenbach, and D. Ropers, Dept. of Internal Medicine II, University of Erlangen-Nürnberg, Germany.

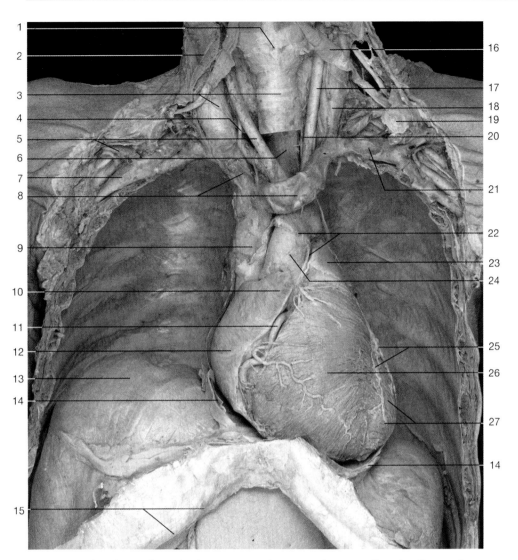

1 Larynx (thyroid cartilage)
2 Sternocleidomastoid muscle (divided)
3 Trachea (divided) and right internal jugular vein
4 Vagus nerve
5 Right common carotid artery and cephalic vein
6 Esophagus
7 Right axillary vein
8 Right and left brachiocephalic veins
9 Superior vena cava
10 Right auricle
11 Right coronary artery
12 Right atrium
13 Diaphragm
14 Pericardium (cut edges)
15 Costal margin
16 Omohyoid muscle
17 Left common carotid artery
18 Left internal jugular vein
19 Clavicle (divided)
20 Left recurrent laryngeal nerve
21 Subclavian vein
22 Pericardial reflection
23 Pulmonary trunk
24 Ascending aorta
25 Anterior interventricular sulcus and anterior interventricular branch of left coronary artery
26 Right ventricle
27 Left ventricle
28 Aortic valve
29 Tricuspid or right atrioventricular valve
30 Inferior vena cava
31 Pulmonary veins
32 Pulmonary valve
33 Left atrioventricular (bicuspid or mitral) valve

Heart and related vessels in situ (anterior aspect). Anterior thoracic wall, pericardium, and epicardium have been removed; trachea divided.

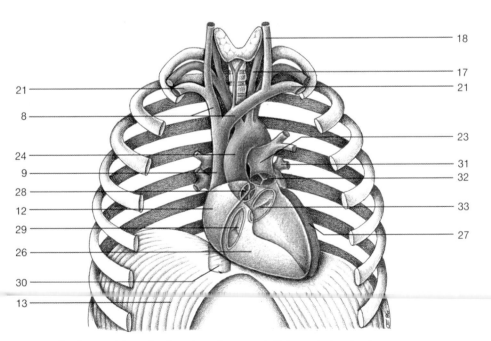

Heart in situ. Position of valves (anterior aspect). (Schematic drawing.)

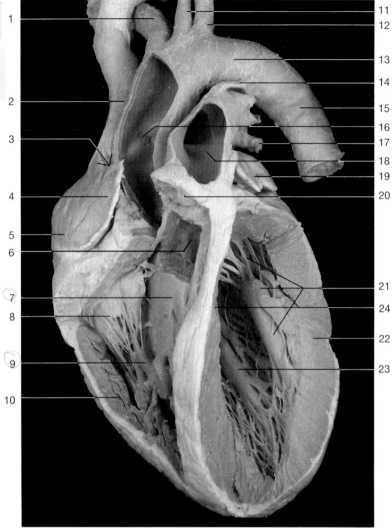

1	Brachiocephalic trunk
2	Superior vena cava
3	Sulcus terminalis
4	Right auricle
5	Right atrium
6	Aortic valve
7	Conus arteriosus (interventricular septum)
8	Right atrioventricular (tricuspid) valve
9	Anterior papillary muscle
10	Myocardium of right ventricle
11	Left common carotid artery
12	Left subclavian artery
13	Aortic arch
14	Ligamentum arteriosum (remnant of ductus arteriosus)
15	Thoracic aorta (descending aorta)
16	Ascending aorta
17	Left pulmonary vein
18	Pulmonary trunk
19	Left auricle
20	Pulmonic valve
21	Anterior papillary muscle with chordae tendineae
22	Myocardium of left ventricle
23	Posterior papillary muscle
24	Interventricular septum
25	Right and left brachiocephalic veins
26	Chordae tendineae
27	Papillary muscles of right ventricle
28	Left atrium
29	Infundibulum
30	Anterior papillary muscle of left ventricle
31	Left atrioventricular (bicuspid or mitral) valve and chordae tendineae
32	Apex of heart
33	Inferior vena cava
34	Liver
35	Aorta (pars abdominalis)

Anterior aspect of the heart. Dissection of the four valves.

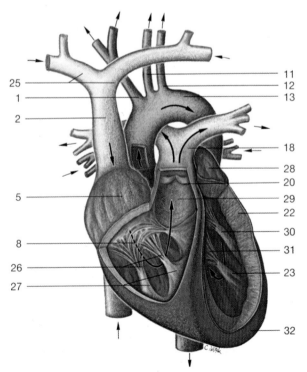

Circulation within the heart (anterior aspect).
Arrows = direction of blood flow.

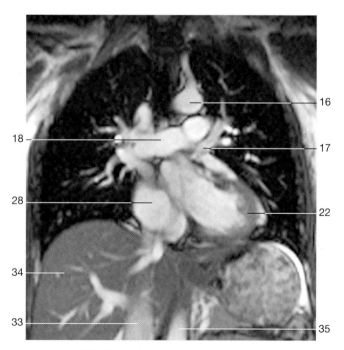

MRI scan of the heart (coronal section at the level of the left atrium; courtesy of Prof. W. Bautz and R. Janka, M. D., University of Erlangen, Germany).

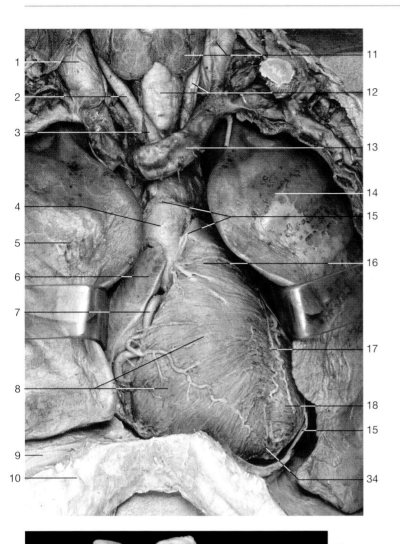

Heart in situ. Myocardium and coronary arteries (anterior aspect).

1   Internal jugular vein
2   Common carotid artery
3   Brachiocephalic trunk
4   Ascending aorta
5   Right lung
6   Right auricle
7   Right coronary artery
8   Myocardium of right ventricle
9   Diaphragm
10 Costal margin
11 Thyroid gland and internal jugular vein
12 Trachea and left common carotid artery
13 Left brachiocephalic vein
14 Left lung
15 Pericardium (cut edge)
16 Pulmonary trunk
17 Anterior interventricular artery
18 Myocardium of left ventricle
19 Muscular vortex (right ventricle)
20 Posterior interventricular sulcus
21 Anterior interventricular sulcus
22 Muscular vortex (left ventricle)
23 Aortic arch
24 Left atrium
25 Coronary sinus
26 Superior vena cava
27 Right pulmonary vein
28 Right atrium
29 Inferior vena cava
30 Coronary sulcus
31 Myocardium of left ventricle
32 Left pulmonary artery
33 Left pulmonary vein
34 Apex of heart

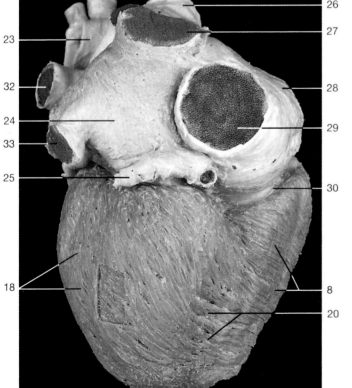

Heart (posterior aspect). The myocardium of the left ventricle has been fenestrated to show the muscle fiber bundles of the deeper layer with their more circular course.

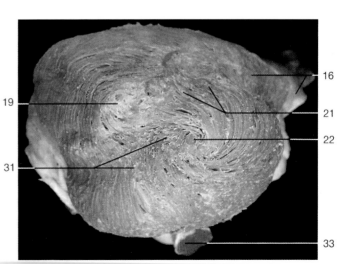

Vortex of cardiac muscle fibers (from below).

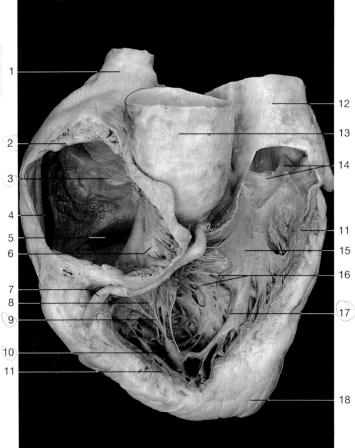

1   Superior vena cava
2   Crista terminalis
3   Fossa ovalis
4   Opening of inferior vena cava
5   Opening of coronary sinus
6   Right auricle
7   Right coronary artery and coronary sulcus
8   Anterior cusp of tricuspid valve
9   Chordae tendineae
10   Anterior papillary muscle
11   Myocardium
12   Pulmonary trunk
13   Ascending aorta
14   Pulmonic valve
15   Conus arteriosus (interventricular septum)
16   Septal papillary muscles
17   Septomarginal trabecula or moderator band
18   Apex of heart
19   Left auricle
20   Aortic valve
21   Left ventricle
22   Pulmonary veins
23   Position of fossa ovalis
24   Left atrium
25   Left atrioventricular (bicuspid or mitral) valve
26   Right atrium
27   Pericardium
28   Posterior papillary muscle
29   Right ventricle
30   Interventricular septum

Right heart (anterior aspect). Anterior wall of right atrium and ventricle removed.

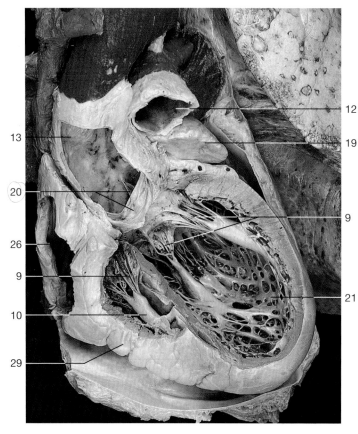

Heart, left ventricle with mitral valve, papillary muscles, and aortic valve (anterior portion of the heart removed).

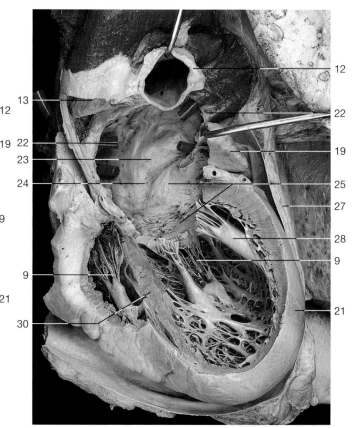

Heart, left ventricle, and atrium (opened) showing the posterior part of the mitral valve with papillary muscles.

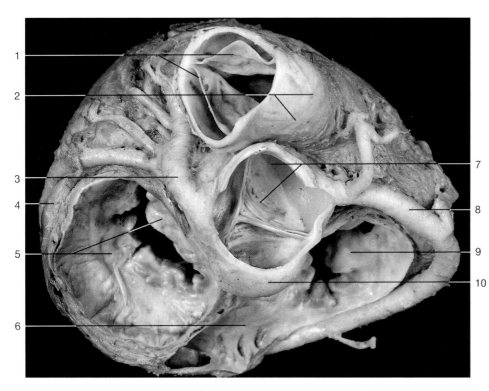

1   Pulmonic valve
2   Sinus of pulmonary trunk
3   Left coronary artery
4   Great cardiac vein
5   Left atrioventricular (mitral) valve
6   Coronary sinus
7   Aortic valve
8   Right coronary artery
9   Right atrioventricular (tricuspid) valve
10 Bulb of aorta
11 Anterior semilunar cusp of pulmonic valve
12 Left semilunar cusp of pulmonic valve
13 Right semilunar cusp of pulmonic valve
14 Left semilunar cusp of aortic valve
15 Right semilunar cusp of aortic valve
16 Posterior semilunar cusp of aortic valve
17 Right atrium
18 Anterior cusp of tricuspid valve
19 Chordae tendineae
20 Trabeculae carneae
21 Interventricular septum
22 Septal cusp of tricuspid valve
23 Anterior papillary muscle
24 Myocardium of right ventricle

Valves of heart (superior aspect). Left and right atria removed. Dissection of coronary arteries. Above: anterior wall of the heart.

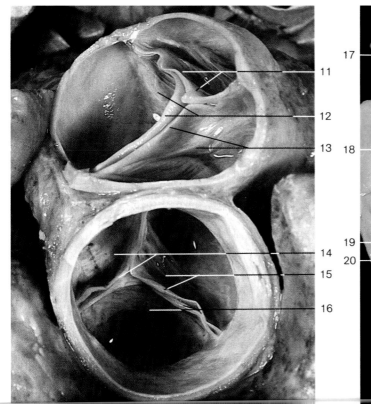

Pulmonic and aortic valves (from above). Anterior wall of the heart at the top. Both valves are closed.

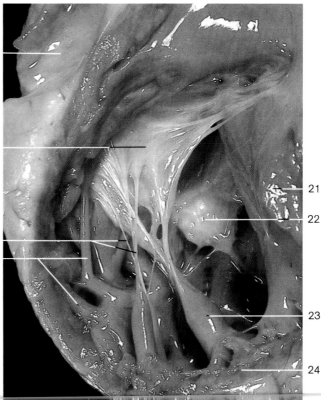

Right atrioventricular (tricuspid) valve (anterior aspect after removal of the anterior wall of the right ventricle).

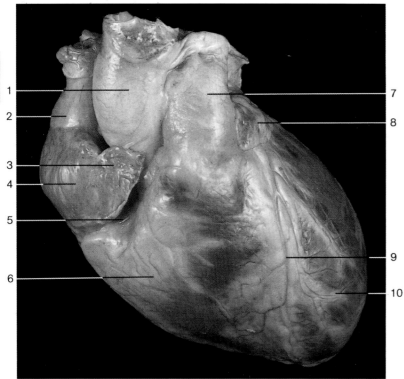

1 Ascending aorta
2 Superior vena cava
3 Right auricle
4 Right atrium
5 Coronary sulcus
6 Right ventricle
7 Pulmonary trunk
8 Left auricle
9 Anterior interventricular sulcus
10 Left ventricle
11 Right pulmonary artery
12 Sulcus terminalis with sinu-atrial node
13 Line indicating plane of position of valves
14 Myocardium of right atrium
15 Inferior vena cava
16 Valve of pulmonary trunk
17 Tricuspid valve
18 Myocardium of right ventricle

Heart, fixed in **diastole** (anterior aspect). The ventricles are relaxed, atria contracted.

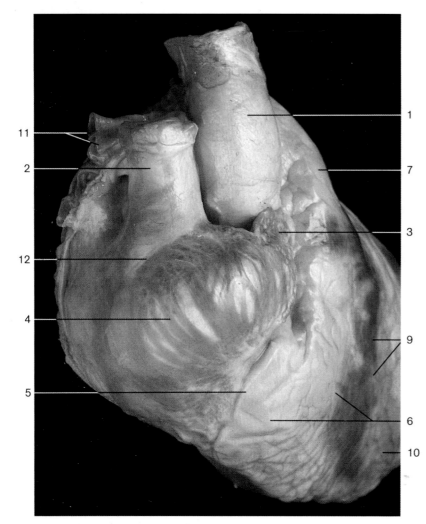

Heart, fixed in **systole** (antero-lateral aspect). The ventricles are contracted, atria dilated.

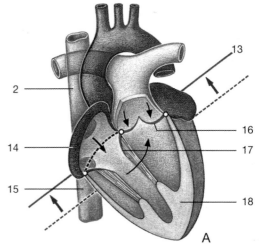

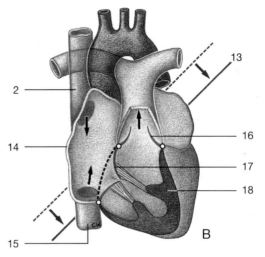

Morphological changes during heart movements.
Note the changes in position of the valves (red arrows). Contracted portions of heart are indicated in black.
A. **Diastole:** muscles of the ventricles relaxed, atrioventricular valves open, semilunar valves closed.
B. **Systole:** muscles of ventricles contracted, atrioventricular valves closed, semilunar valves open.

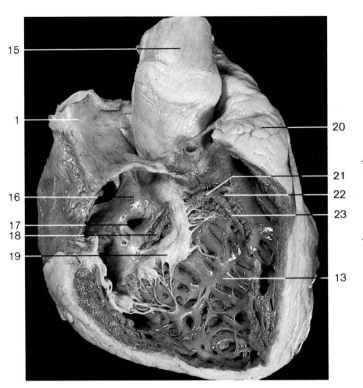

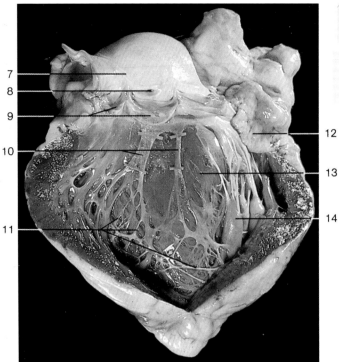

Right ventricle, dissection of **atrioventricular node, atrioventricular bundle (bundle of His),** and **right limb or bundle branch** (probes).

Left ventricle, dissection of left **limb or bundle branch of conducting system** (probes).

1 Superior vena cava	5 Muscle fiber bundles of right atrium
2 Sulcus terminalis	6 Coronary sulcus (with right coronary artery)
3 Bulb of aorta	7 Aortic sinus
4 Sinu-atrial node (arrows)	8 Entrance to left coronary artery

9 Aortic valve
10 Branches of left bundle branch
11 Purkinje fibers
12 Left auricle
13 Interventricular septum
14 Papillary muscles
15 Ascending aorta
16 Right atrium
17 Opening of coronary sinus
18 Atrioventricular node
19 Septal cusp of tricuspid valve
20 Pulmonary trunk
21 Atrioventricular bundle (bundle of His)
22 Bifurcation of atrioventricular bundle
23 Right bundle branch
24 Inferior vena cava
25 Left atrium
26 Left bundle branch
27 Papillary muscles with Purkinje fibers

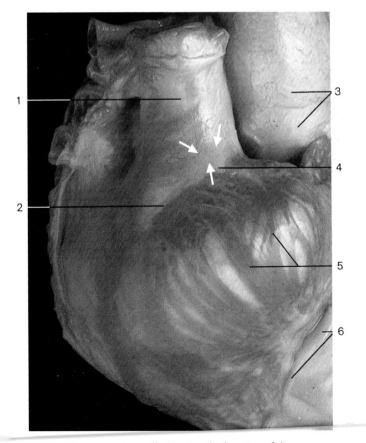

Right atrium, anterior wall, showing the location of the **sinu-atrial node** (arrows).

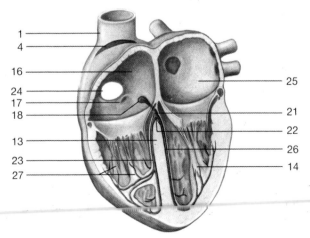

Conducting system of the heart (schematic drawing).

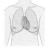

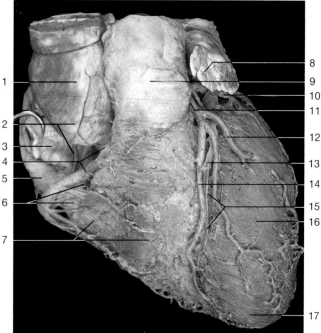

Coronary arteries (anterior aspect). The epicardium and subepicardial fatty tissue have been removed. The arteries have been injected with red resin from the aorta.

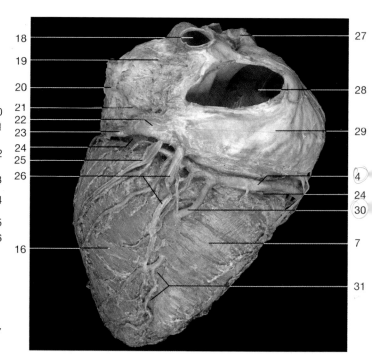

Right coronary artery and veins of the heart (dorsal aspect). The epicardium and subepicardial fatty tissue have been removed.

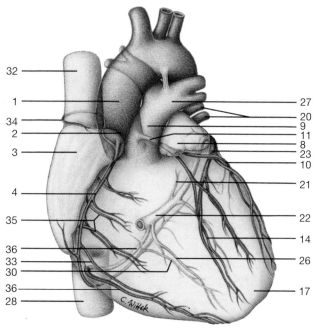

Vessels of the heart. Coronary arteries (red) and veins (blue) of the heart (anterior aspect).

1   Ascending aorta
2   Aortic bulb and (in the above specimen) sinu-atrial branch of right coronary artery
3   Right auricle
4   Right coronary artery
5   Right atrium
6   Coronary sulcus
7   Right ventricle
8   Left auricle
9   Pulmonary trunk
10 Circumflex branch of left coronary artery
11 Left coronary artery
12 Diagonal branch of left artery
13 Great cardiac vein
14 Anterior interventricular artery
15 Anterior interventricular sulcus
16 Left ventricle
17 Apex of heart
18 Right pulmonary vein
19 Left atrium
20 Left pulmonary veins
21 Oblique vein of left atrium (Marshall's vein)
22 Coronary sinus
23 Great cardiac vein
24 Coronary sulcus (posterior portion)
25 Posterior vein of left ventricle
26 Middle cardiac vein
27 Left pulmonary artery
28 Inferior vena cava
29 Right atrium
30 Posterior interventricular branch of right coronary artery
31 Posterior interventricular sulcus
32 Superior vena cava
33 Right marginal branch
34 Branch of sinu-atrial node
35 Minimal cardiac veins
36 Small cardiac vein

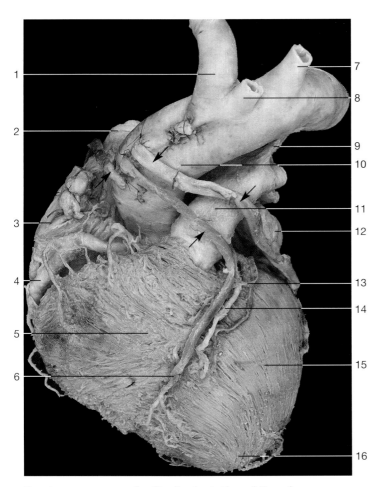

1 Brachiocephalic trunk
2 Superior vena cava
3 Right atrium
4 Right coronary artery
5 Right ventricle
6 Connection of one of the bypass vessels with the anterior interventricular artery
7 Left subclavian artery
8 Left common carotid artery
9 Ductus arteriosus (Botalli) (still open)
10 Ascending aorta with three bypass vessels implanted
11 Pulmonary trunk
12 Left atrium
13 Circumflex branch of left coronary artery
14 Anterior interventricular branch of left coronary artery
15 Left ventricle
16 Apex of heart
17 Sternum
18 Right ventricle
19 Liver
20 Spinal cord
21 Trachea
22 Aorta
23 Body of thoracic vertebrae
24 Pulmonary artery
25 Inferior vena cava
26 Hepatic vein

Heart, coronary vessels after implantation of three bypass vessels (anterior aspect). The ductus arteriosus (9) is still open.

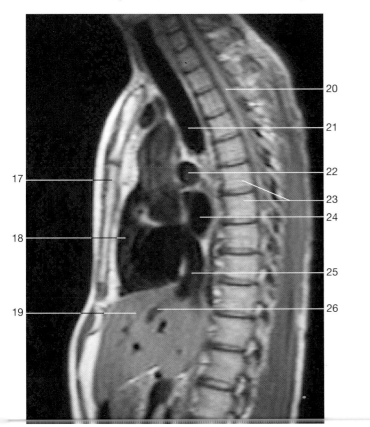

Sagittal section through the thoracic cavity (MRI scan, courtesy of Prof. W. Bautz and R. Janka, M. D., University of Erlangen, Germany).

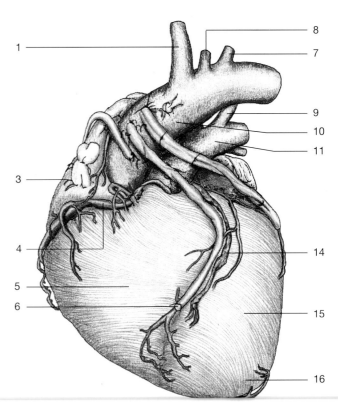

Heart, coronary vessels after implantation of three bypass vessels (yellow) (schematic drawing of the specimen above).

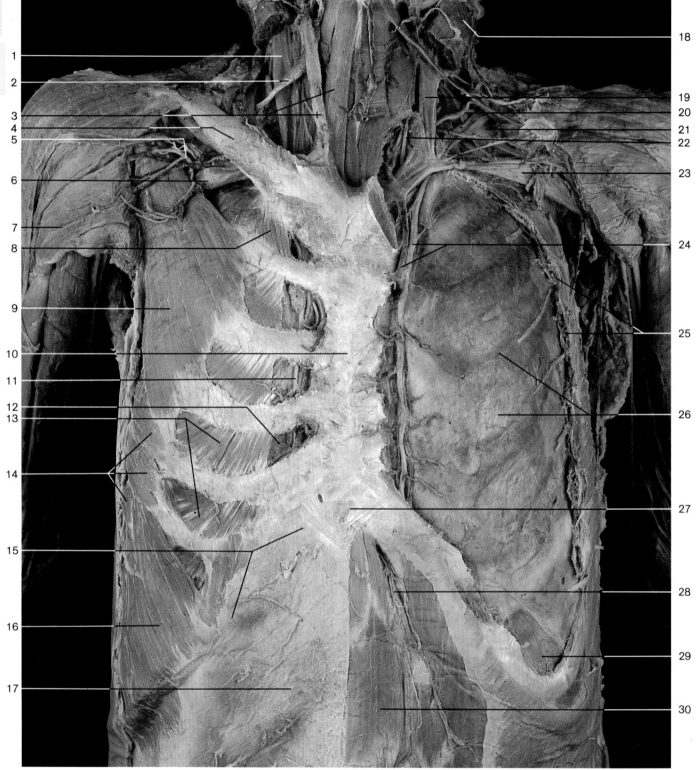

Thoracic organs (ventral aspect). The left clavicle and ribs have been partially removed, and the right intercostal spaces have been opened to show the internal thoracic vein and artery.

1	Right internal jugular vein	11	Right internal thoracic artery and vein	21	Brachial plexus
2	Omohyoid muscle	12	Fascicles of transversus thoracis muscle	22	Vagus nerve
3	Sternohyoid muscle and external jugular vein	13	Internal intercostal muscles	23	Left axillary vein
4	Clavicle	14	Serratus anterior muscle	24	Left internal thoracic artery and vein
5	Thoraco-acromial artery	15	Costal margin	25	Ribs and thoracic wall (cut)
6	Right subclavian vein	16	External abdominal oblique muscle	26	Costal pleura
7	Pectoralis major muscle	17	Anterior sheath of rectus abdominis muscle	27	Xiphoid process
8	External intercostal muscle	18	Sternocleidomastoid muscle	28	Superior epigastric artery
9	Pectoralis minor muscle	19	Left internal jugular vein	29	Diaphragm
10	Body of sternum	20	Transverse cervical artery	30	Rectus abdominis muscle

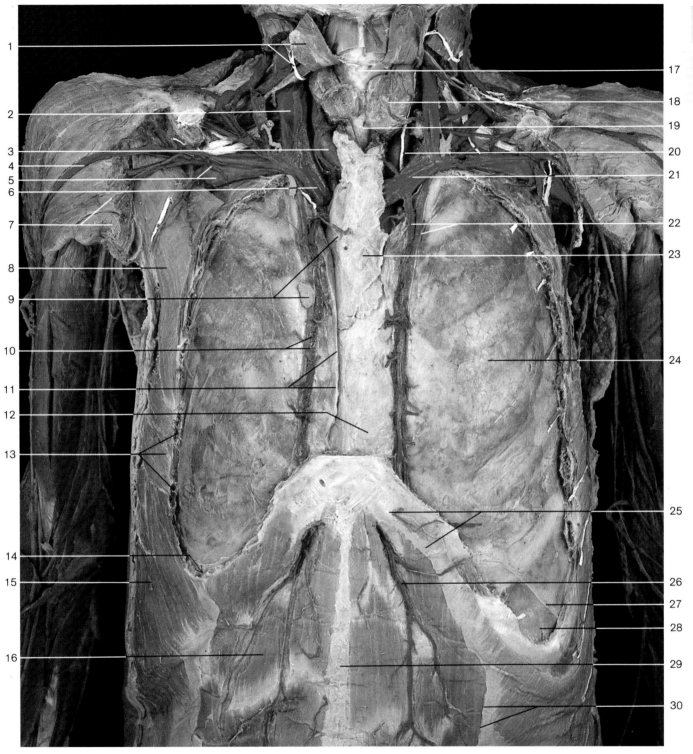

Thoracic organs, anterior mediastinum, and pleura (ventral aspect). Ribs, clavicle, and sternum have been partly removed.
Red = arteries; blue = veins; green = lymph vessels and nodes.

1	Sternothyroid muscle and its nerve (a branch of the ansa cervicalis)
2	Right internal jugular vein
3	Right common carotid artery
4	Cephalic vein
5	Right subclavian vein
6	Right brachiocephalic vein
7	Pectoralis major muscle (divided)
8	Pectoralis minor muscle (divided)
9	Parasternal lymph nodes
10	Internal thoracic artery and vein
11	Anterior margin of costal pleura
12	Pericardium
13	Fifth and sixth ribs (divided) and serratus anterior muscle
14	Costodiaphragmatic recess
15	External abdominal oblique muscle
16	Rectus abdominis muscle
17	Larynx (thyroid cartilage)
18	Thyroid gland
19	Trachea
20	Left vagus nerve
21	Left brachiocephalic vein
22	Left internal thoracic artery and vein
23	Thymus
24	Costal pleura
25	Costal margin
26	Superior epigastric artery
27	Margin of costal pleura
28	Diaphragm
29	Linea alba
30	Cut edge of anterior sheath of rectus abdominis muscle

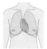

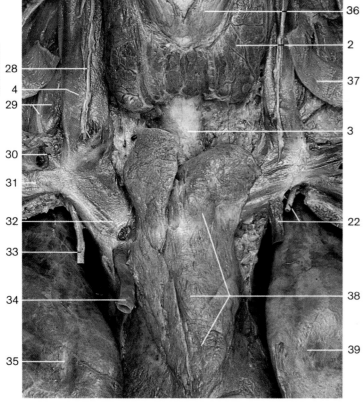

The **thymus** above the heart, showing its position and size.

1 Larynx (thyroid cartilage)
2 Thyroid gland
3 Trachea
4 Internal jugular vein
5 Brachial plexus
6 Right brachiocephalic vein and common carotid artery
7 Right phrenic nerve
8 Ascending aorta
9 Pectoralis minor muscle (divided)
10 Pulmonary trunk (covered by pericardium)
11 Costal pleura
12 Pericardium and heart
13 Serratus anterior muscle
14 Xiphoid process
15 Costal margin
16 External abdominal oblique muscle
17 Sternothyroid muscle (divided and reflected)
18 Vagus nerve
19 Left common carotid artery
20 Left sympathetic trunk
21 Left recurrent laryngeal nerve
22 Left internal thoracic artery and vein (divided)
23 Margin of costal pleura
24 Intercostal nerves and vessels
25 Superior epigastric artery
26 Rectus abdominis muscle
27 Diaphragm
28 Ansa cervicalis
29 Phrenic nerve and scalenus anterior muscle
30 External jugular vein (divided)
31 Right subclavian vein
32 Right brachiocephalic vein
33 Internal thoracic artery (divided)
34 Internal thoracic vein (divided)
35 Right lung
36 Cricothyroid muscle
37 Omohyoid muscle
38 Thymus
39 Left lung

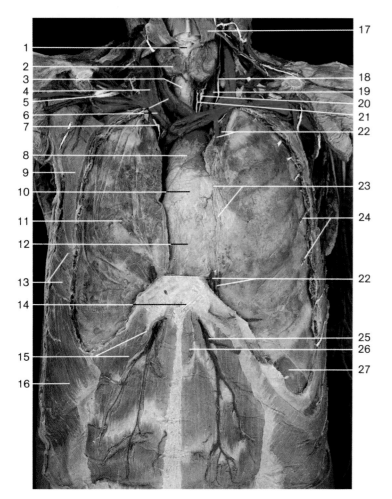

Thoracic organs (ventral aspect). The internal thoracic vessels have been removed, and the anterior margins of the pleura and lungs have been slightly reflected to display the anterior and middle mediastinum, including the heart and great vessels.

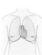

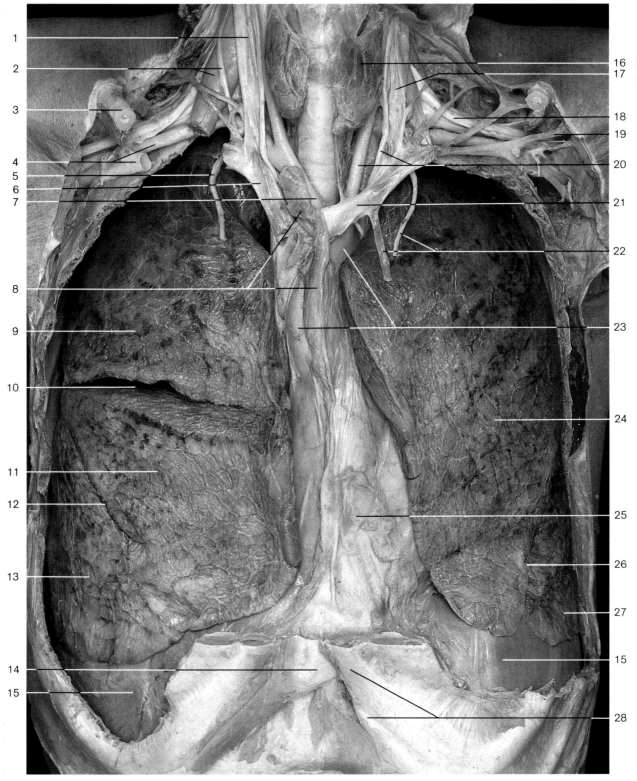

Thoracic organs (ventral aspect). The pleura has been opened and the lungs exposed. Remnants of the thymus and pericardium are seen.

1   Right internal jugular vein
2   Phrenic nerve and scalenus anterior muscle
3   Clavicle (divided)
4   Right subclavian artery and vein
5   Internal thoracic artery
6   Right brachiocephalic vein
7   Brachiocephalic trunk
8   Thymus (atrophic)
9   Upper lobe of right lung
10 Horizontal fissure of right lung (incomplete)

11 Middle lobe of right lung
12 Oblique fissure of right lung
13 Lower lobe of right lung
14 Xiphoid process
15 Diaphragm
16 Thyroid gland
17 Left internal jugular vein
18 Brachial plexus
19 Left cephalic vein

20 Left common carotid artery and
    vagus nerve
21 Left brachiocephalic vein
22 Internal thoracic artery and vein (divided)
23 Ascending aorta and aortic arch
24 Upper lobe of left lung
25 Pericardium
26 Oblique fissure of left lung
27 Lower lobe of left lung
28 Costal margin

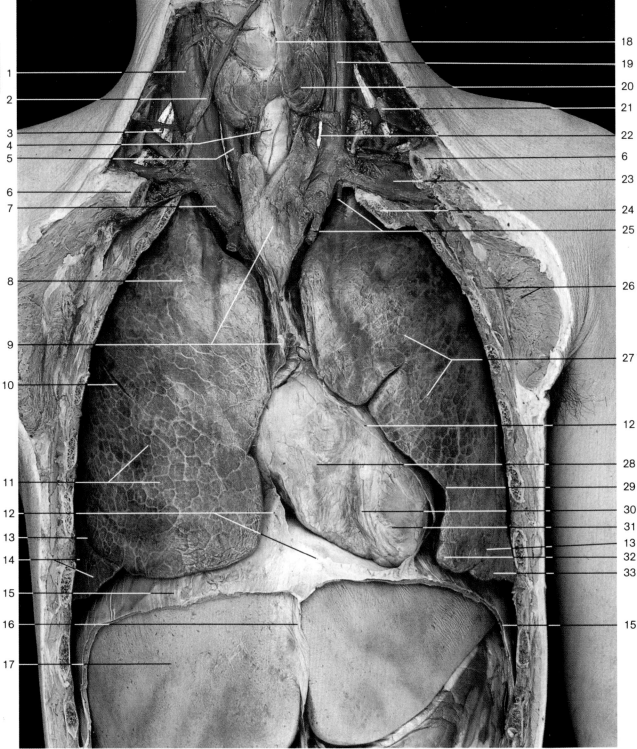

Thoracic organs (ventral aspect). The thoracic wall, costal pleura, pericardium, and diaphragm have been partly removed.

1 Internal jugular vein	13 Oblique fissure of lung	25 Internal thoracic artery and vein
2 External jugular vein (displaced medially)	14 Lower lobe of right lung	26 Pectoralis major and pectoralis minor muscles
3 Brachial plexus	15 Diaphragm	(cut edges)
4 Trachea	16 Falciform ligament	27 Upper lobe of left lung
5 Right common carotid artery	17 Liver	28 Right ventricle
6 Clavicle (divided)	18 Location of larynx	29 Cardiac notch of left lung
7 Right brachiocephalic vein	19 Left internal jugular vein	30 Interventricular sulcus of heart
8 Upper lobe of right lung	20 Thyroid gland	31 Left ventricle
9 Thymus (atrophic)	21 Omohyoid muscle (divided)	32 Lingula
10 Horizontal fissure of right lung	22 Vagus nerve	33 Lower lobe of left lung
11 Middle lobe of right lung	23 Left subclavian vein	
12 Pericardium (cut edges)	24 First rib (divided)	

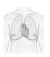

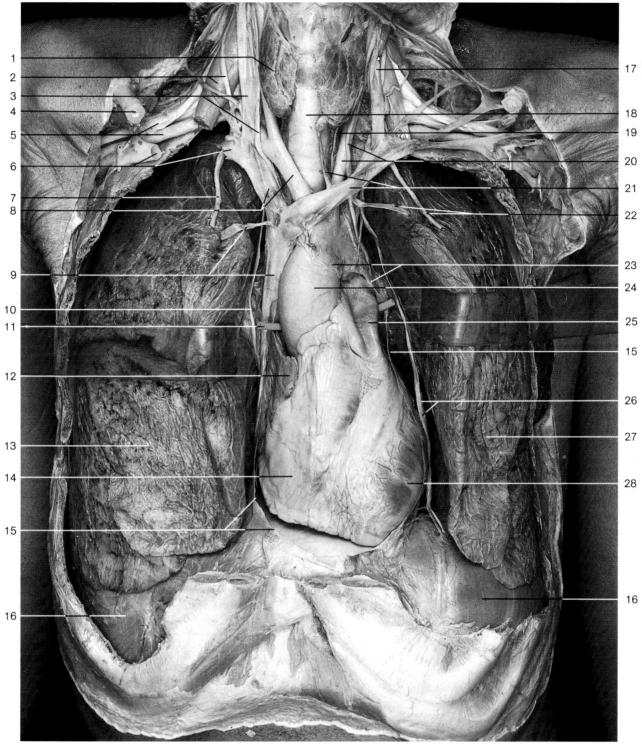

Thoracic organs (ventral aspect). Position of the heart and middle mediastinum. The anterior wall of the thorax, the costal pleura, and the pericardium have been removed and the lungs slightly reflected.

1 Thyroid gland
2 Phrenic nerve and scalenus anterior muscle
3 Vagus nerve and internal jugular vein
4 Clavicle (divided)
5 Brachial plexus and subclavian artery
6 Subclavian vein
7 Internal thoracic artery
8 Brachiocephalic trunk and right brachiocephalic vein
9 Superior vena cava and thymic vein
10 Right phrenic nerve

11 Transverse pericardial sinus (probe)
12 Right auricle
13 Middle lobe of right lung
14 Right ventricle
15 Cut edge of pericardium
16 Diaphragm
17 Internal jugular vein
18 Trachea
19 Left recurrent laryngeal nerve
20 Left common carotid artery and vagus nerve

21 Left brachiocephalic vein and inferior thyroid vein
22 Left internal thoracic artery and vein (divided)
23 Upper margin of pericardial sac
24 Ascending aorta
25 Pulmonary trunk
26 Left phrenic nerve and left peri-cardiacophrenic artery and vein
27 Upper lobe of left lung
28 Left ventricle

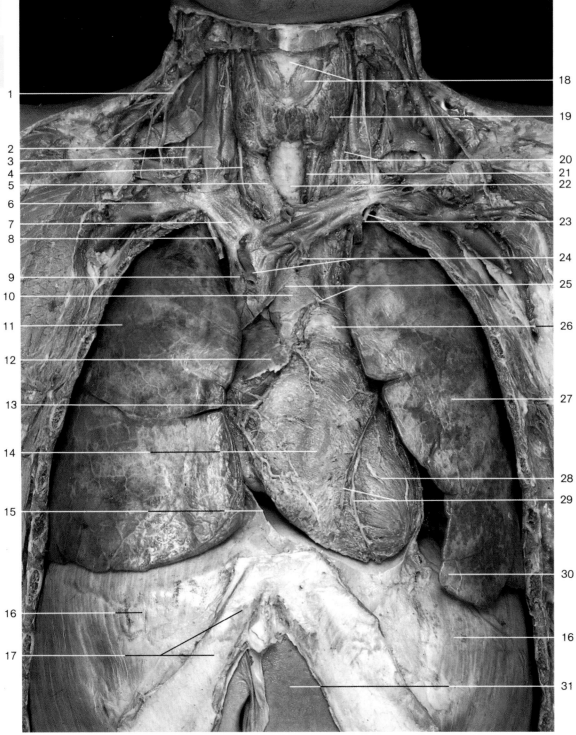

Thoracic organs (ventral aspect). Position of heart, dissection of coronary vessels in situ. The anterior wall of thorax, costal pleura, and pericardium have been removed.

1 Intermediate supraclavicular nerve
2 Internal jugular vein
3 Right phrenic nerve
4 Right vagus nerve
5 Right common carotid artery
6 Right subclavian vein
7 Right brachiocephalic vein
8 Right internal thoracic artery
9 Superior vena cava
10 Ascending aorta
11 Right lung
12 Right atrium

13 Right coronary artery and
    small cardiac vein
14 Right ventricle
15 Cut edge of pericardium
16 Diaphragm
17 Costal margin
18 Larynx (cricothyroid muscle and thyroid
    cartilage)
19 Thyroid gland
20 Left common carotid artery and
    left vagus nerve

21 Left recurrent laryngeal nerve
22 Trachea
23 Left internal thoracic artery and vein (divided)
24 Thymic veins
25 Margin of pericardial sac
26 Pulmonary trunk
27 Left lung
28 Left ventricle
29 Anterior interventricular artery and vein
30 Lingula
31 Liver

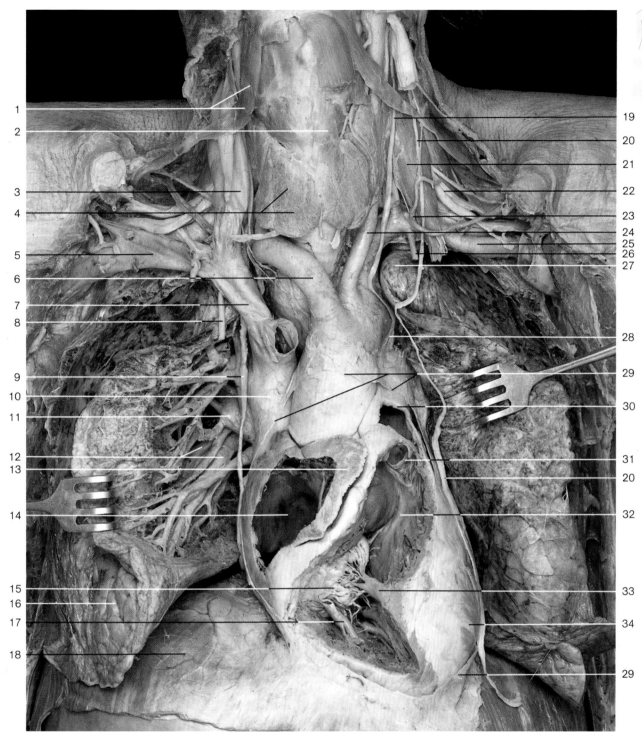

Thoracic organs (ventral aspect). Heart with valves in situ. Anterior wall of thorax, pleura, and anterior portion of pericardium have been removed. The right atrium and ventricle have been opened to show the right atrioventricular and pulmonary valves.

1	Omohyoid muscle	13	Right auricle
2	Pyramidal lobe of thyroid gland	14	Right atrium
3	Internal jugular vein	15	Right atrioventricular (tricuspid) valve
4	Thyroid gland	16	Right lung
5	Right subclavian vein	17	Posterior papillary muscle
6	Brachiocephalic trunk	18	Diaphragm
7	Right brachiocephalic vein	19	Left vagus nerve
8	Right internal thoracic artery	20	Left phrenic nerve
9	Right phrenic nerve	21	Scalenus anterior muscle
10	Superior vena cava	22	Brachial plexus
11	Pulmonary vein	23	Thyrocervical trunk
12	Branches of pulmonary artery		

24	Left common carotid artery
25	Left subclavian artery
26	Left internal thoracic artery
27	Apex of left lung
28	Left recurrent laryngeal nerve
29	Cut edge of pericardium
30	Pulmonary trunk (fenestrated)
31	Pulmonic valve
32	Supraventricular crest
33	Anterior papillary muscle
34	Left ventricle

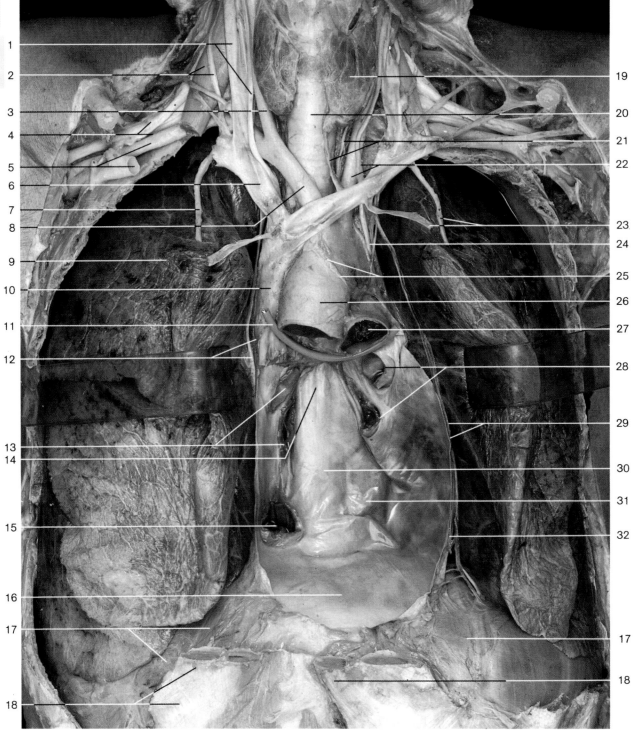

Thoracic organs (ventral aspect). Pericardium and mediastinum. Anterior wall of thorax and heart have been removed and the lungs slightly reflected. Note probe within transverse pericardial sinus.

1   Right internal jugular vein and
    right vagus nerve
2   Right phrenic nerve and scalenus anterior muscle
3   Right common carotid artery
4   Brachial plexus
5   Right subclavian artery and vein
6   Right brachiocephalic vein
7   Right internal thoracic artery (divided)
8   Brachiocephalic trunk
9   Upper lobe of right lung
10 Superior vena cava
11 Transverse pericardial sinus (probe)

12 Right phrenic nerve and right
    pericardiacophrenic artery and vein
13 Right pulmonary veins
14 Oblique sinus of pericardium
15 Inferior vena cava
16 Diaphragmatic part of pericardium
17 Diaphragm
18 Costal margin
19 Thyroid gland
20 Trachea
21 Left recurrent laryngeal nerve and
    inferior thyroid vein

22 Left common carotid artery and left vagus nerve
23 Left internal thoracic artery and vein (divided)
24 Vagus nerve at aortic arch
25 Cut edge of pericardium
26 Ascending aorta
27 Pulmonary trunk (divided)
28 Left pulmonary veins
29 Left phrenic nerve and left
    pericardiacophrenic artery and vein
30 Contour of esophagus beneath pericardium
31 Contour of aorta beneath pericardium
32 Pericardium (cut edge)

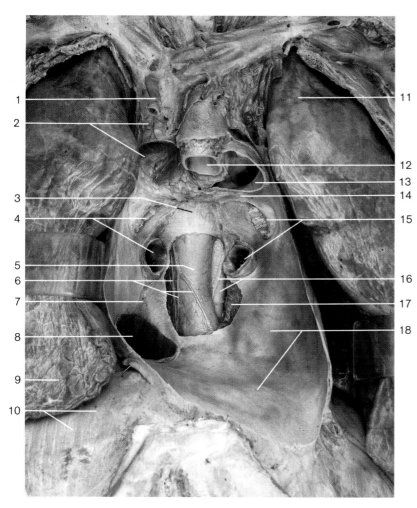

1 Internal thoracic vein
2 Superior vena cava
3 Oblique sinus of pericardium
4 Right pulmonary veins
5 Esophagus
6 Branches of right vagus nerve
7 Mesocardium
8 Inferior vena cava
9 Middle lobe of right lung
10 Diaphragm
11 Upper lobe of left lung
12 Ascending aorta
13 Pulmonary trunk
14 Transverse pericardial sinus
15 Left pulmonary veins
16 Descending aorta and left vagus nerve
17 Left lung (adjacent to pericardium)
18 Pericardium
19 Left subclavian artery
20 Vagus nerve
21 Left recurrent laryngeal nerve
22 Descending aorta
23 Pulmonary artery
24 Left atrium
25 Left ventricle
26 Coronary sinus
27 Left common carotid artery
28 Brachiocephalic trunk
29 Azygos arch
30 Right atrium
31 Right ventricle
32 Aortic arch

Pericardial sac (ventral aspect). The heart has been removed, and the posterior wall of the pericardium has been opened to show the adjacent esophagus and aorta.

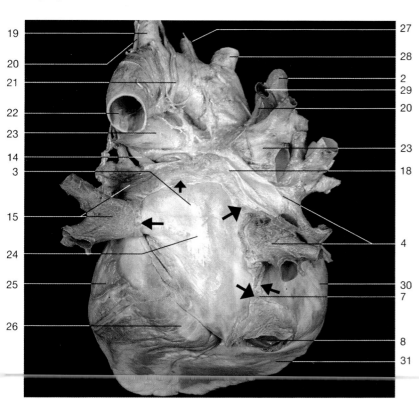

Heart with epicardium (posterior aspect). Arrows: oblique sinus.

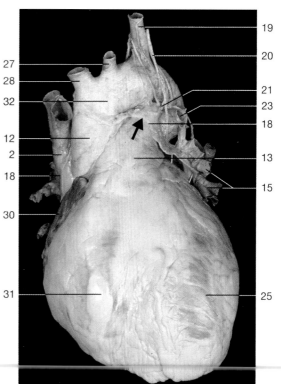

Heart with epicardium (anterior aspect).
Arrow: pericardial reflection.

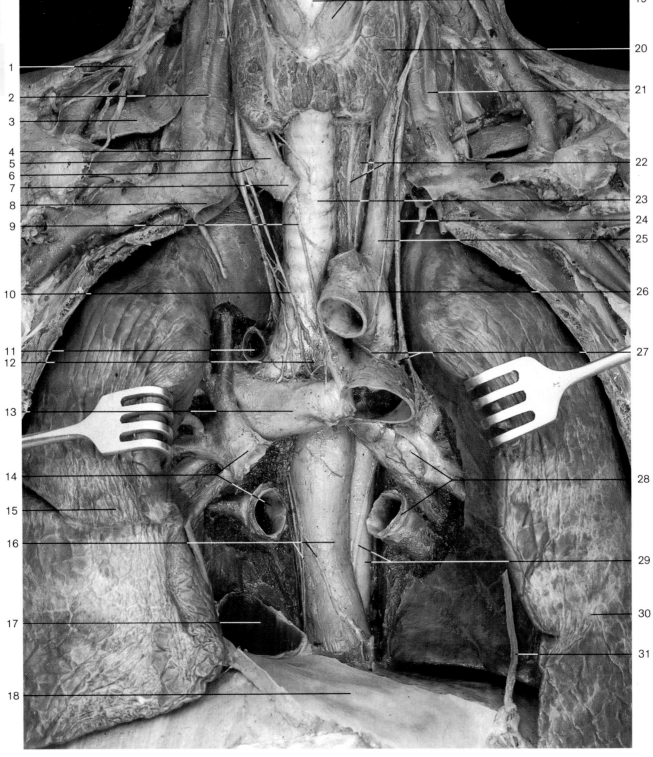

Mediastinal organs after removal of heart and pericardium (ventral aspect). Both lungs have been slightly reflected.

1	Supraclavicular nerves	11	Azygos arch (divided)
2	Internal jugular vein	12	Bifurcation of trachea
3	Omohyoid muscle	13	Right pulmonary artery
4	Right vagus nerve	14	Right pulmonary veins
5	Right common carotid artery	15	Right lung
6	Right subclavian artery	16	Esophagus and branches
7	Brachiocephalic trunk		of right vagus nerve
8	Right brachiocephalic vein	17	Inferior vena cava
9	Superior cervical cardiac branch	18	Pericardium
	of vagus nerve	19	Larynx (thyroid cartilage, cricothyroid muscle)
10	Inferior cervical cardiac branches	20	Thyroid gland
	of vagus nerve	21	Internal jugular vein

22	Esophagus and left recurrent laryngeal nerve
23	Trachea
24	Left vagus nerve
25	Left common carotid artery
26	Aortic arch
27	Left recurrent laryngeal nerve branching off from vagus nerve
28	Left pulmonary veins
29	Thoracic aorta and left vagus nerve
30	Left lung
31	Left phrenic nerve (divided)

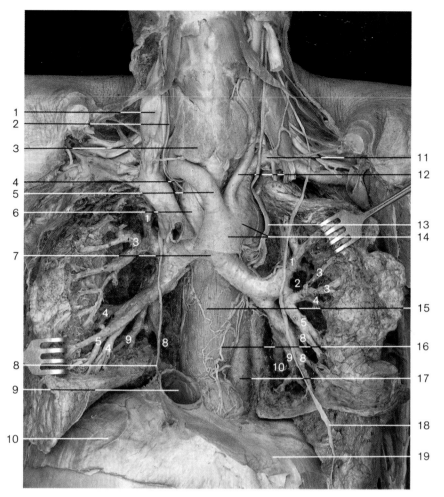

1   Internal jugular vein
2   Right vagus nerve
3   Thyroid gland
4   Right recurrent laryngeal nerve
5   Brachiocephalic trunk
6   Trachea
7   Bifurcation of trachea
8   Right phrenic nerve
9   Inferior vena cava
10 Diaphragm
11 Left subclavian artery
12 Left common carotid artery
13 Left vagus nerve
14 Aortic arch
15 Esophagus
16 Esophageal plexus
17 Thoracic aorta
18 Left phrenic nerve
19 Pericardium at the central tendon of
    diaphragm
20 Right pulmonary artery
21 Left pulmonary artery
22 Tracheal lymph nodes
23 Superior tracheobronchial lymph nodes
24 Bronchopulmonary lymph nodes

Bronchial tree in situ (ventral aspect). Heart and pericardium have been removed; the bronchi of the bronchopulmonary segments are dissected.
1–10 = numbers of segments (cf. p. 246 and 251).

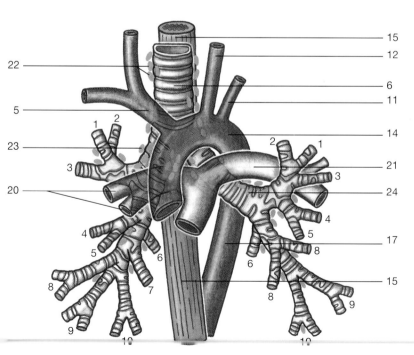

Relation of aorta, pulmonary trunk, and esophagus to trachea and bronchial tree (schematic drawing).
1–10 = numbers of segments (cf. p. 246 and 251).

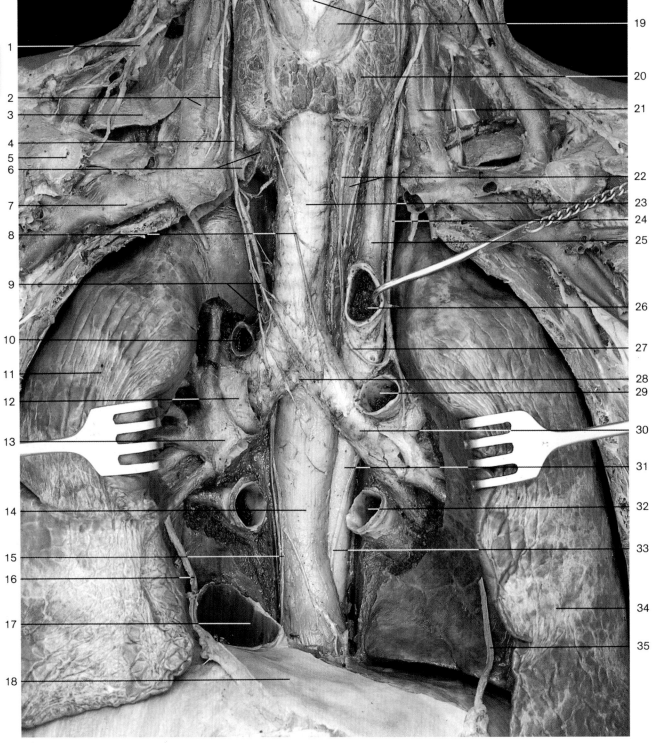

Mediastinal organs (ventral aspect). The heart with the pericardium has been removed, and the lungs and aortic arch have been slightly reflected to show the vagus nerves and their branches.

1	Supraclavicular nerves	12	Right pulmonary artery
2	Right internal jugular vein with ansa cervicalis	13	Right pulmonary veins
3	Omohyoid muscle	14	Esophagus
4	Right vagus nerve	15	Esophageal plexus
5	Clavicle	16	Right phrenic nerve (divided)
6	Right subclavian artery and recurrent laryngeal nerve	17	Inferior vena cava
7	Right subclavian vein	18	Pericardium covering the diaphragm
8	Superior cervical cardiac branch of vagus nerve	19	Larynx (thyroid cartilage and cricothyroid muscle)
9	Inferior cervical cardiac branch of vagus nerve	20	Thyroid gland
10	Azygos arch (divided)	21	Left internal jugular vein
11	Right lung	22	Esophagus and left recurrent laryngeal nerve
		23	Trachea

24	Left vagus nerve
25	Left common carotid artery
26	Aortic arch
27	Left recurrent laryngeal nerve
28	Bifurcation of trachea
29	Left pulmonary artery
30	Left primary bronchus
31	Descending aorta
32	Left pulmonary veins
33	Branch of left vagus nerve
34	Left lung
35	Left phrenic nerve (divided)

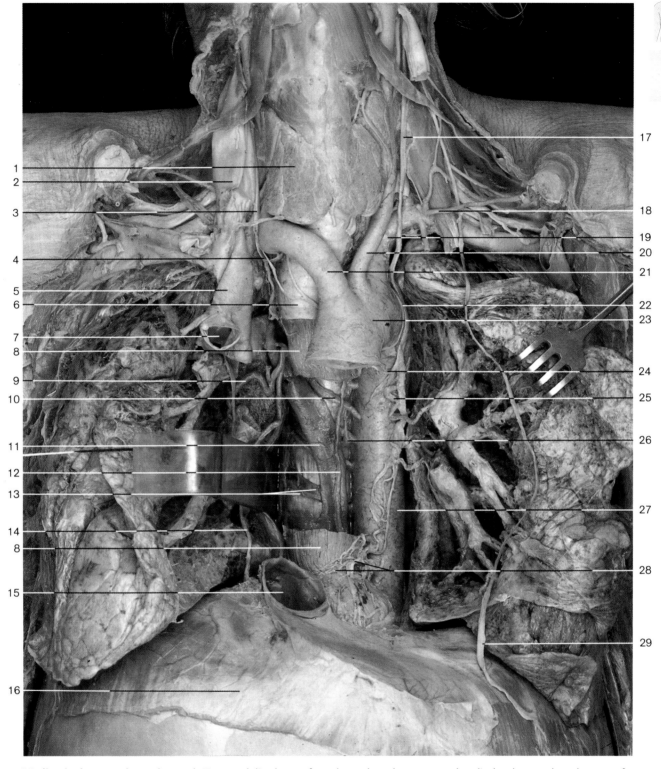

Mediastinal organs (ventral aspect). Heart and distal part of esophagus have been removed to display the vessels and nerves of the posterior mediastinum.

1	Thyroid gland	11	Azygos vein	21	Brachiocephalic trunk
2	Right internal jugular vein	12	Thoracic duct	22	Left vagus nerve
3	Right vagus nerve	13	Posterior intercostal artery and vein	23	Aortic arch
4	Point where right recurrent laryngeal nerve		(in front of the vertebral column)	24	Left recurrent laryngeal nerve
	is branching off the vagus nerve	14	Right phrenic nerve	25	Left bronchial artery
5	Right brachiocephalic vein	15	Inferior vena cava	26	Lymph node
6	Trachea	16	Diaphragm	27	Thoracic aorta
7	Left brachiocephalic vein (reflected)	17	Left vagus nerve	28	Esophageal plexus
8	Esophagus	18	Thyrocervical trunk	29	Left phrenic nerve
9	Right bronchial artery	19	Left subclavian artery		
10	Posterior intercostal artery	20	Left common carotid artery		

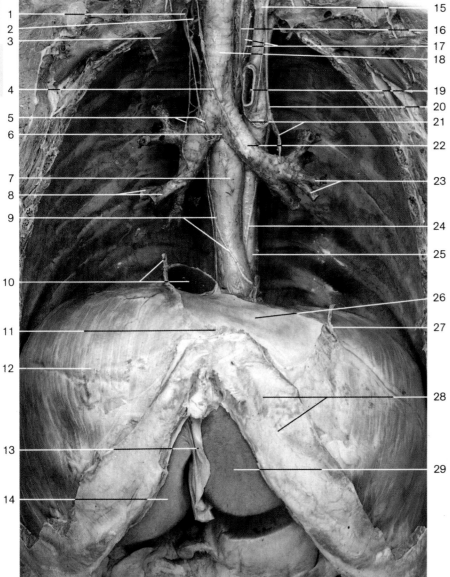

Diaphragm and organs of mediastinum (anterior aspect). Heart and lungs have been removed; the costal margin remains in place. Note the different courses of left and right vagus.

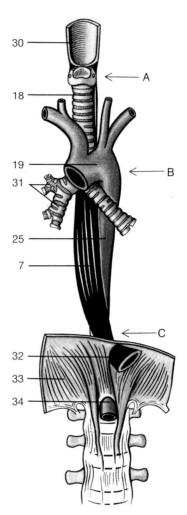

Organs of posterior mediastinum (ventral aspect, schematic drawing). Three regions in which the esophagus is narrowed are shown:
A = termed upper sphincter (at the level of the cricoid cartilage);
B = termed middle sphincter (at the level of the aortic arch);
C = termed lower sphincter (at the level of the diaphragm).

1 Right subclavian artery	11 Sternal part of diaphragm	23 Superior and inferior lingular bronchi
2 Right recurrent laryngeal nerve	12 Costal part of diaphragm	24 Esophageal plexus of left vagus nerve
3 Right brachiocephalic vein	13 Falciform ligament of liver	25 Descending aorta
4 Superior cervical cardiac nerve	14 Liver (quadrate lobe)	26 Central tendon of diaphragm covered with pericardium
5 Inferior cervical cardiac nerves and pulmonary branches	15 Left common carotid artery	27 Left phrenic nerve (divided)
6 Bifurcation of trachea	16 Left recurrent laryngeal nerve	28 Costal margin
7 Esophagus (thoracic part)	17 Esophageal branches of left vagus nerve and esophagus	29 Liver, left lobe
8 Bronchi of lateral and medial segments of middle lobe	18 Trachea	30 Pharynx
9 Esophageal plexus and branches of right vagus nerve	19 Aortic arch	31 Secondary bronchi
10 Inferior vena cava and right phrenic nerve (cut)	20 Left vagus nerve	32 Esophagus (abdominal part)
	21 Left recurrent laryngeal nerve with inferior cardiac nerve	33 Diaphragm
	22 Left primary bronchus	34 Abdominal aorta

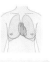

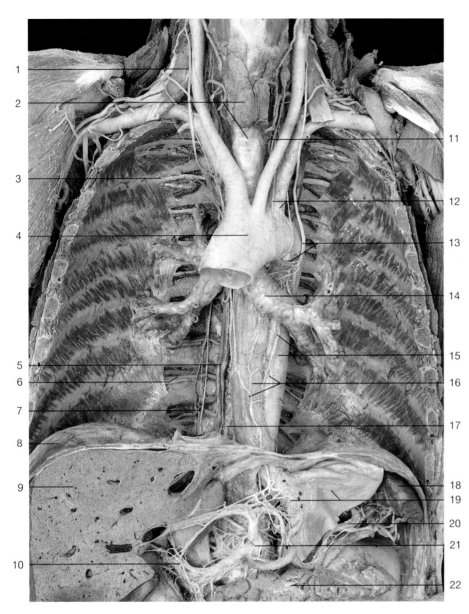

Organs of posterior mediastinum (anterior aspect).

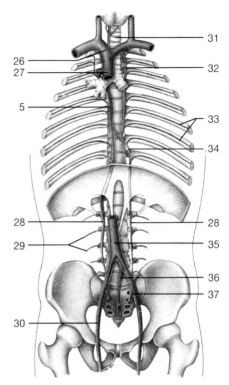

Veins of the posterior wall of thoracic and abdominal cavity (schematic drawing).

1 Right vagus nerve
2 Thyroid gland and trachea
3 Intercostal nerve
4 Aortic arch
5 Azygos vein
6 Posterior intercostal artery
7 Greater splanchnic nerve
8 Diaphragm
9 Liver
10 Proper hepatic artery and hepatic plexus
11 Left recurrent laryngeal nerve
12 Inferior cervical cardiac nerves
13 Left vagus nerve and left recurrent laryngeal nerve
14 Left primary bronchus
15 Thoracic aorta and left vagus nerve
16 Esophagus and esophageal plexus
17 Thoracic duct
18 Spleen
19 Anterior gastric plexus and stomach (divided)
20 Splenic artery and splenic plexus
21 Celiac trunk and celiac plexus
22 Pancreas
23 Ramus communicans
24 Sympathetic trunk and sympathetic ganglion
25 Posterior intercostal vein and artery and intercostal nerve
26 Right brachiocephalic vein
27 Superior vena cava
28 Ascending lumbar vein
29 Lumbar veins
30 Right external iliac vein
31 Trachea
32 Accessory hemiazygos vein
33 Posterior intercostal veins
34 Hemiazygos vein
35 Inferior vena cava
36 Median sacral vein
37 Internal iliac vein

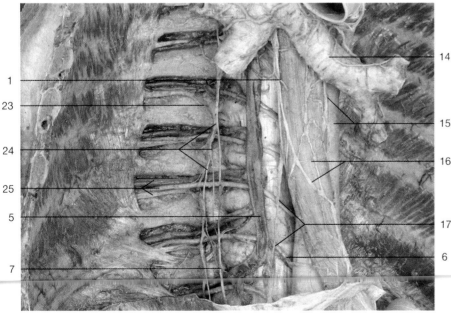

Inferior segment of posterior mediastinum (anterior aspect).

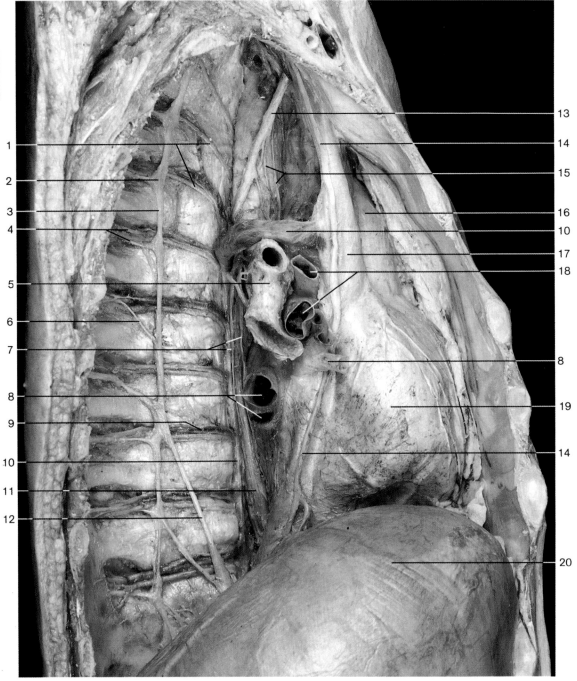

Mediastinal organs (right lateral aspect). Right lung and pleura of right half of the thorax have been removed.

1 Posterior intercostal arteries
2 Ganglion of sympathetic trunk
3 Sympathetic trunk
4 Vessels and nerves of the intercostal space (from above: posterior intercostal vein and artery and intercostal nerve)
5 Right primary bronchus
6 Ramus communicans of sympathetic trunk

7 Esophageal plexus (branches of right vagus nerve)
8 Pulmonary veins
9 Posterior intercostal vein
10 Azygos vein
11 Esophagus
12 Greater splanchnic nerve
13 Right vagus nerve

14 Right phrenic nerve
15 Inferior cervical cardiac branches of vagus nerve
16 Aortic arch
17 Superior vena cava
18 Right pulmonary artery
19 Heart with pericardium
20 Diaphragm

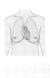

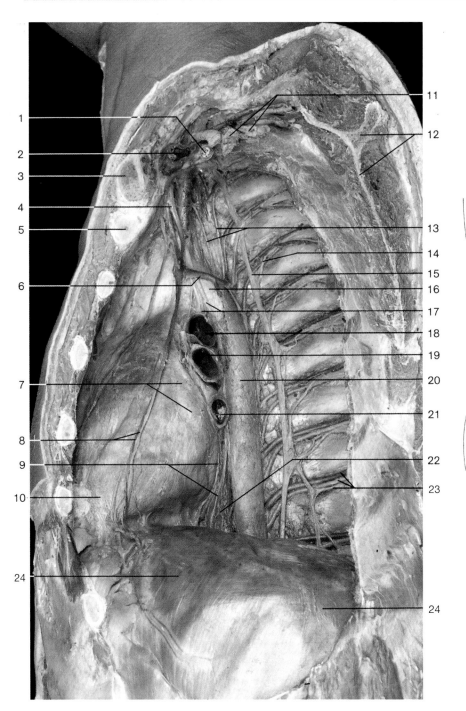

Organs of posterior and superior mediastinum (left lateral aspect).

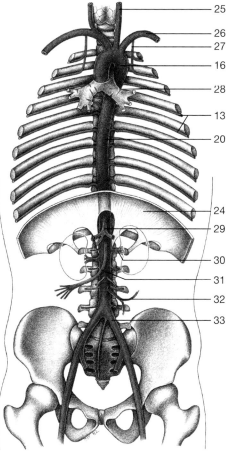

Main branches of descending aorta
(schematic drawing).

1 Subclavian artery
2 Subclavian vein
3 Clavicle (divided)
4 Left vagus nerve
5 First rib (divided)
6 Left superior intercostal vein
7 Left atrium with pericardium
8 Left phrenic nerve and pericardiacophrenic artery and vein
9 Esophageal plexus (branches derived from left vagus nerve)
10 Apex of heart with pericardium
11 Brachial plexus

12 Scapula (divided)
13 Posterior intercostal arteries
14 White ramus communicans of sympathetic trunk
15 Sympathetic trunk
16 Aortic arch
17 Left vagus nerve and left recurrent laryngeal nerve
18 Left pulmonary artery
19 Left primary bronchus
20 Thoracic aorta
21 Pulmonary vein
22 Esophagus (thoracic part)

23 Posterior intercostal artery and vein and intercostal nerve
24 Diaphragm
25 Common carotid artery
26 Subclavian artery
27 Highest intercostal artery
28 Bifurcation of trachea
29 Celiac trunk
30 Renal artery
31 Superior mesenteric artery
32 Inferior mesenteric artery
33 Common iliac artery

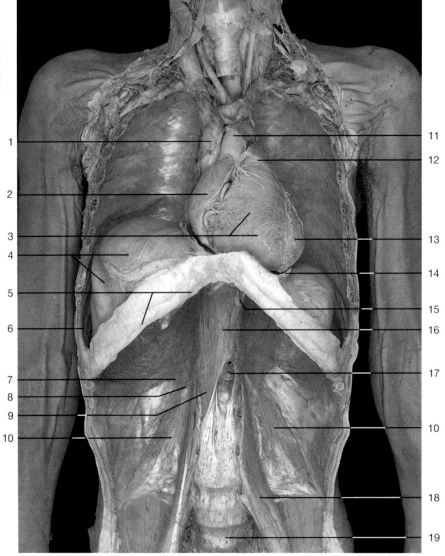

1 Superior vena cava
2 Right atrium
3 Right ventricle
4 Costal part of diaphragm
5 Costal margin
6 Position of costodiaphragmatic recess
7 Lateral arcuate ligament
8 Medial arcuate ligament
9 Right crus of lumbar part of diaphragm
10 Quadratus lumborum muscle
11 Ascending aorta
12 Pulmonary trunk
13 Left ventricle
14 Pericardium, diaphragm
15 Esophageal hiatus and abdominal
   part of esophagus (cut)
16 Lumbar part of diaphragm
17 Aortic hiatus
18 Psoas major muscle
19 Lumbar vertebra

Diaphragm in situ (anterior aspect). Anterior walls of thoracic and abdominal cavities have been removed. Natural position of the heart above the central tendon on the diaphragm is shown.

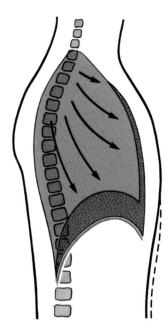

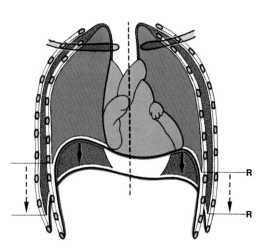

Changes in the position of the diaphragm and thoracic cage during respiration. Left: lateral aspect; right: anterior aspect. During inspiration the diaphragm moves downwards and the lower part of the thoracic cage expands forward and laterally, causing the costodiaphragmatic recess (R) to enlarge (cf. dotted arrows).

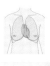

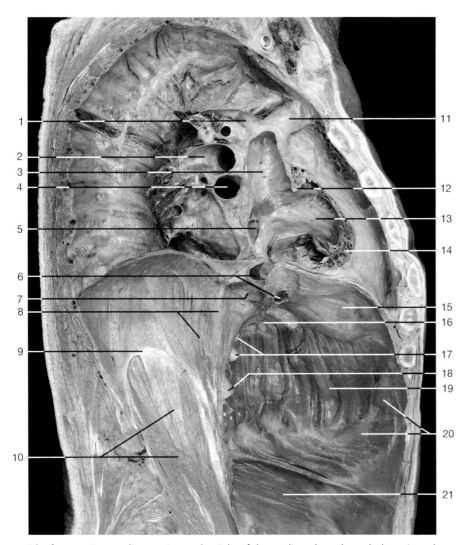

1 Azygos venous arch
2 Right pulmonary artery
3 Superior vena cava
4 Right pulmonary vein
5 Fossa ovalis
6 Hepatic veins
7 Inferior vena cava
8 Right crus of lumbar part of
   diaphragm
9 Medial arcuate ligament
10 Psoas major muscle
11 Left brachiocephalic vein
12 Terminal crista
13 Right atrium
14 Right auricle
15 Central tendon of diaphragm
16 Esophagus
17 Celiac trunk and superior
   mesenteric artery
18 Aorta
19 Costal part of diaphragm
20 Costal margin
21 Transversus abdominis muscle

Diaphragm. Paramedian section to the right of the median plane through thoracic and upper abdominal cavities. The plane passes through the superior and inferior vena cava just to the right of the vertebral bodies. Most of the heart remains in situ to the left of this plane (viewed from the right side).

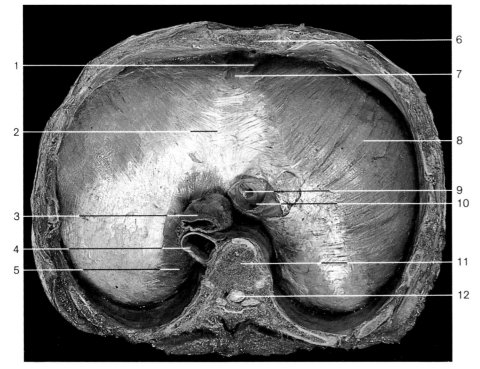

1 Sternocostal triangle
2 Central tendon (from above)
3 Esophagus
4 Aorta
5 Lumbar part of diaphragm
6 Sternum
7 Sternal part of diaphragm
8 Costal part of diaphragm
9 Entrance of hepatic veins
10 Inferior vena cava
11 Body of 9th thoracic vertebra
12 Spinal cord

Diaphragm (superior aspect). The pleura and pericardium have been removed.

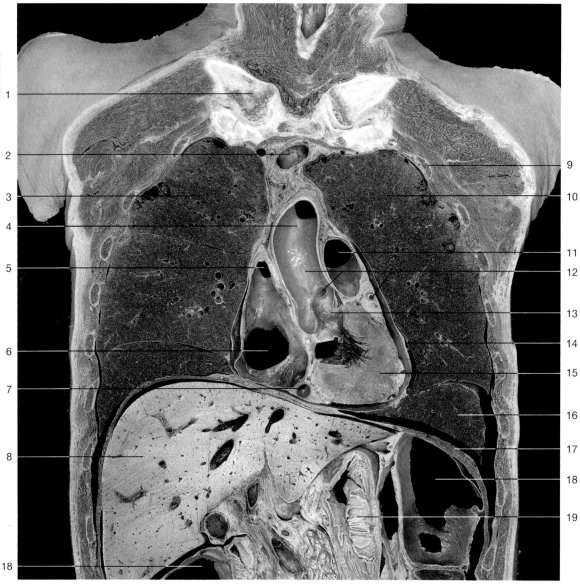

Coronal section through the thorax at the level of ascending aorta (anterior aspect).

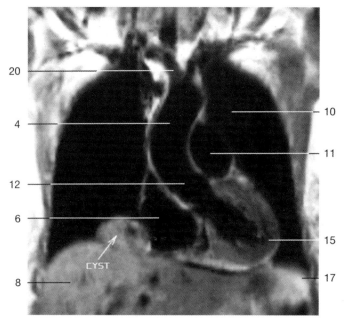

Coronal section through the thorax at the level of ascending aorta (MRI scan).

1   Clavicle
2   Left brachiocephalic vein
3   Upper lobe of right lung
4   Aortic arch
5   Superior vena cava
6   Right atrium (entrance
    of inferior vena cava)
7   Coronary sinus
8   Liver
9   Second rib
10 Upper lobe of left lung
11 Pulmonary trunk
12 Ascending aorta and left coronary
    artery
13 Aortic valve
14 Pericardium
15 Myocardium of left ventricle
16 Lower lobe of left lung
17 Diaphragm
18 Colic flexures
19 Stomach
20 Brachiocephalic trunk

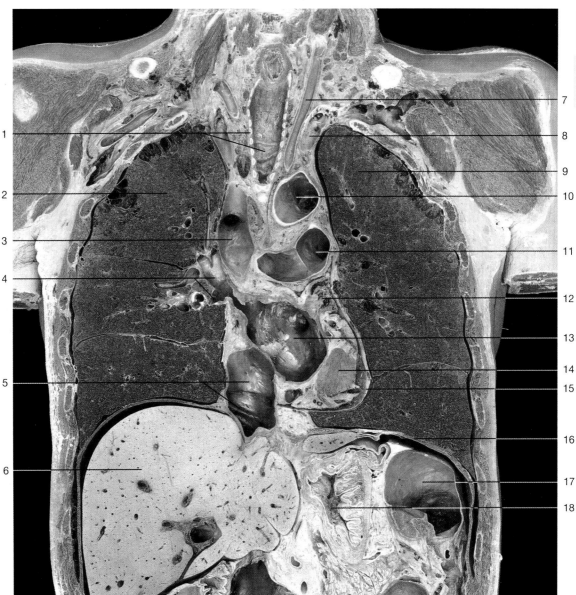

Coronal section through the thorax at the level of superior and inferior vena cava (anterior aspect).

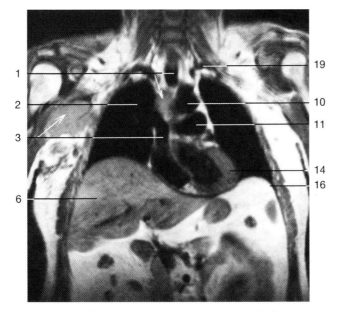

Coronal section through the thorax at the level of superior vena cava (MRI scan). Arrows = metastases of tumor.

1 Trachea
2 Upper lobe of right lung
3 Superior vena cava
4 Right pulmonary veins
5 Inferior vena cava and right atrium
6 Liver
7 Left common carotid artery
8 Left subclavian vein
9 Upper lobe of left lung
10 Aortic arch
11 Left pulmonary artery
12 Left auricle
13 Left atrium with orifices
    of pulmonary veins
14 Left ventricle (myocardium)
15 Pericardium
16 Diaphragm
17 Left colic flexure
18 Stomach
19 Left subclavian artery

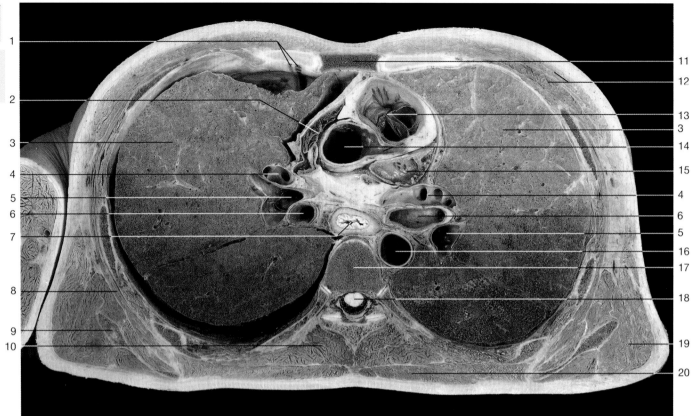

Horizontal section through the thorax at level 1 (from below).

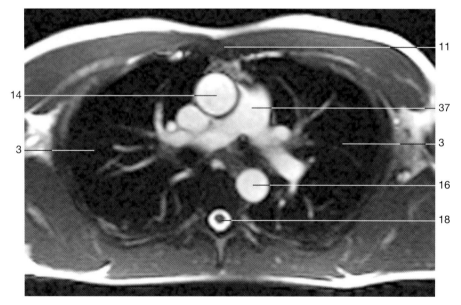

Horizontal section through the thorax at level 1 (from below). (MRI scan, courtesy of Prof. W. Bautz and R. Janka, M. D., University of Erlangen, Germany.)

1	Internal thoracic artery and vein	12	Pectoralis major and minor muscles
2	Right atrium	13	Conus arteriosus (right ventricle), pulmonic valve
3	Lung	14	Ascending aorta and left coronary artery (only in upper figure)
4	Pulmonary artery	15	Left atrium
5	Pulmonary vein	16	Descending aorta
6	Primary bronchus	17	Thoracic vertebra
7	Esophagus	18	Spinal cord
8	Serratus anterior muscle	19	Latissimus dorsi muscle
9	Scapula	20	Trapezius muscle
10	Longissimus thoracis muscle		
11	Sternum		

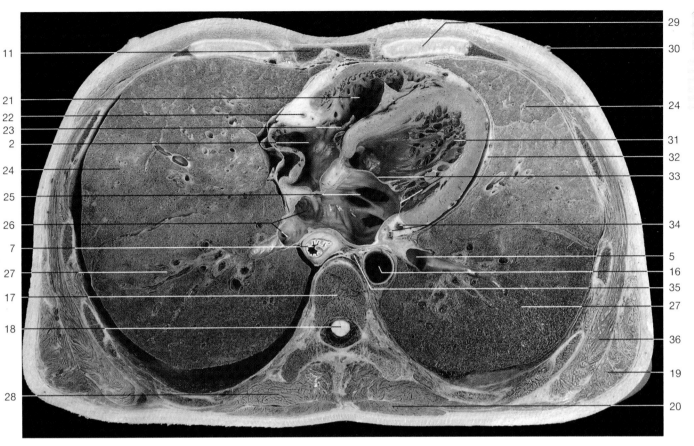

Horizontal section through the thorax at level 2 (from below).

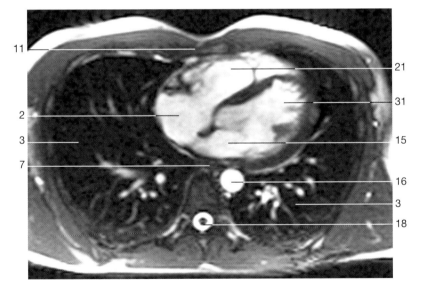

Horizontal section through the thorax at level 2 (from below). (MRI scan, courtesy of Prof. W. Bautz and R. Janka, M. D., University of Erlangen, Germany.)

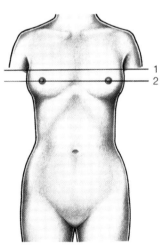

Levels of sections.

21	Right ventricle	30	Nipple
22	Right coronary artery	31	Left ventricle
23	Right atrioventricular valve	32	Pericardium
24	Lung (upper lobe)	33	Left atrioventricular valve
25	Left atrium	34	Left coronary artery and coronary sinus
26	Pulmonary veins	35	Accessory hemiazygos vein
27	Lung (lower lobe)	36	Serratus anterior muscle
28	Erector muscle of spine	37	Pulmonary trunk
29	Third costal cartilage		

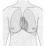

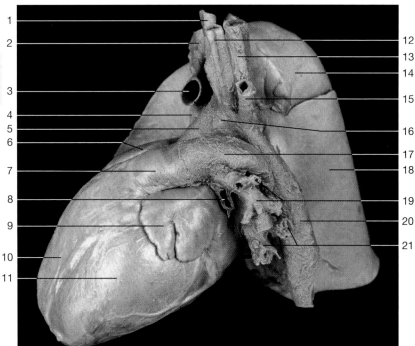

Heart and right lung of the fetus (viewed from left side). The left lung has been removed. Note the ductus arteriosus (Botalli).

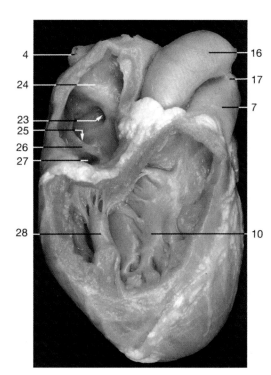

Heart of the fetus (anterior aspect). Right atrium and ventricle opened.

Shunts in the fetal circulation system		
1. Ductus venosus (of Arantius)	between umbilical vein and inferior vena cava	bypass of liver circulation
2. Foramen ovale	between right and left atrium	bypass of pulmonary circulation
3. Ductus arteriosus (Botalli)	between pulmonary trunk and aorta	

1   Right common carotid artery
2   Right brachiocephalic vein
3   Left brachiocephalic vein
4   Superior vena cava
5   Ascending aorta
6   Right auricle
7   Pulmonary trunk
8   Left primary bronchus
9   Left auricle
10 Right ventricle
11 Left ventricle
12 Left common carotid artery
13 Trachea
14 Superior lobe of right lung
15 Left subclavian artery
16 Aortic arch
17 Ductus arteriosus (Botalli)
18 Inferior lobe of right lung
19 Left pulmonary artery with branches to the left lung
20 Descending aorta
21 Left pulmonary veins
22 Inferior vena cava
23 Foramen ovale
24 Right atrium
25 Opening of inferior vena cava
26 Valve of inferior vena cava (Eustachian valve)
27 Opening of coronary sinus
28 Anterior papillary muscle of right ventricle

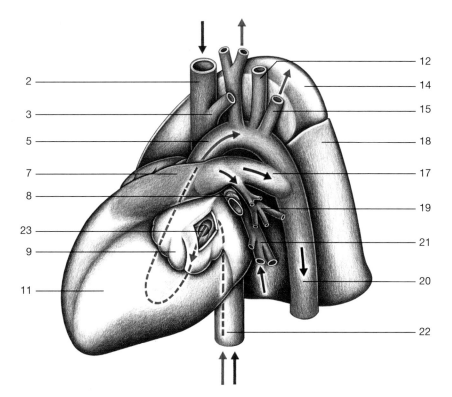

◁ **Heart of the fetus** (schematic drawing). Direction of blood flow indicated by arrows. Note the change in oxygenation of blood after ductus arteriosus entry into aorta.

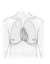

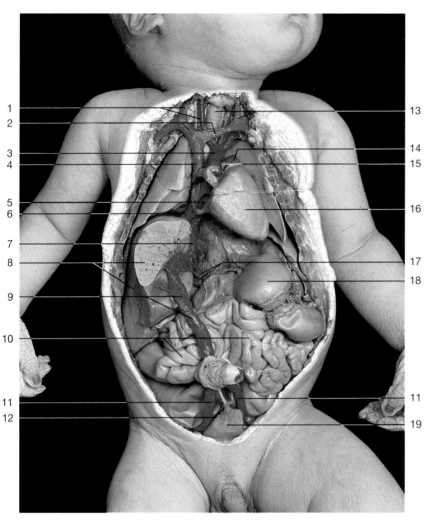

1   Internal jugular vein and right common carotid artery
2   Right and left brachiocephalic vein
3   Aortic arch
4   Superior vena cava
5   Foramen ovale
6   Inferior vena cava
7   Ductus venosus
8   Liver
9   Umbilical vein
10 Small intestine
11 Umbilical artery
12 Urachus
13 Trachea and left internal jugular vein
14 Left pulmonary artery
15 Ductus arteriosus (Botalli)
16 Right ventricle
17 Hepatic arteries (red) and portal vein (blue)
18 Stomach
19 Urinary bladder
20 Portal vein
21 Pulmonary veins
22 Descending aorta
23 Placenta

Thoracic and abdominal organs in the newborn (anterior aspect). The right atrium has been opened to show the foramen ovale. The left lobe of the liver has been removed.

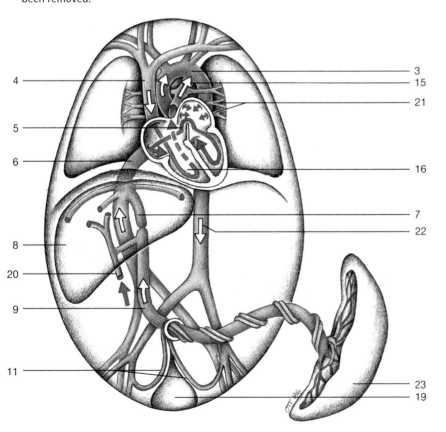

◁ **Fetal circulatory system** (schematic drawing). The oxygen gradient is indicated by color.

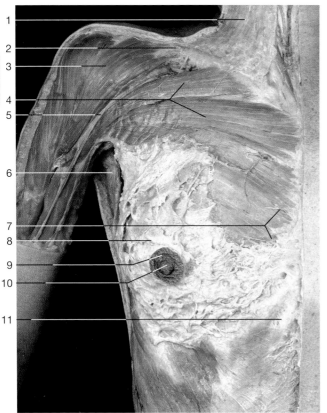

Dissection of mammary gland (anterior aspect).

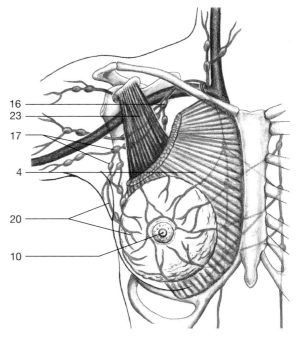

Dissection of mammary gland and axillary lymph nodes.

1	Platysma muscle	8	Breast tissue
2	Clavicle	9	Areola
3	Deltoid muscle	10	Nipple (papilla)
4	Pectoralis major muscle	11	Costal margin
5	Deltopectoral groove	12	Pectoral fascia
	and cephalic vein	13	Mammary gland
6	Latissimus dorsi muscle	14	Serratus anterior muscle
7	Medial mammarian branches		(insertion)
	of intercostal nerves	15	Lactiferous sinus

16	Apical lymph nodes
17	Axillary lymph nodes
18	Intercostobrachial nerve
19	Lateral thoracic vein
20	Lymph vessels
21	Serratus anterior muscle
22	Medial branches of intercostal
	arteries
23	Pectoralis minor muscle

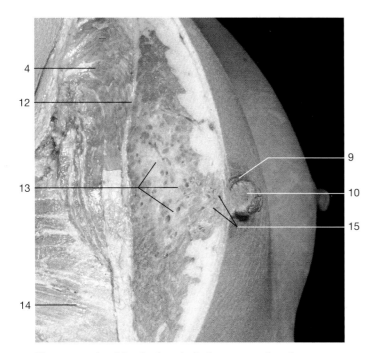

Mammary gland (sagittal section) of a pregnant female.

Lymphatics of the breast and axilla. Most lymph vessels drain into the axillary lymph nodes.

5 Abdominal Organs

The abdominal cavity located underneath the diaphragm contains the main organs of the digestive system (liver, spleen, stomach, intestine). The greater omentum partly fixed to the transverse colon covers the small intestine.

The liver, stomach, and superior part of the duodenum are connected to the lesser omentum covering the omental bursa, the entrance of which is the epiploic foramen.

The hepatoduodenal ligament contains the portal vein, the common bile duct, and the hepatic arteries. The spleen is located dorsally underneath the diaphragm.

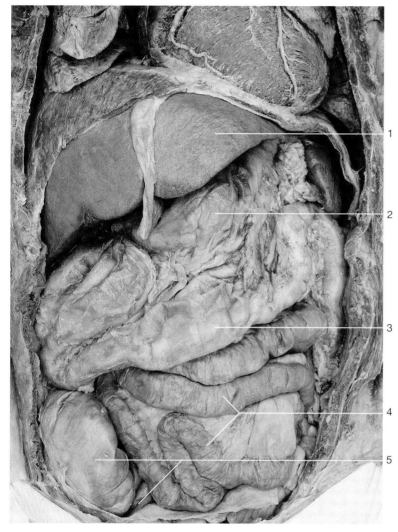

Abdominal organs in situ (anterior aspect). The greater omentum and part of the diaphragm have been removed. The heart is in contact with the diaphragm (from Lütjen-Drecoll, Rohen, Innenansichten des menschlichen Körpers, 2010).

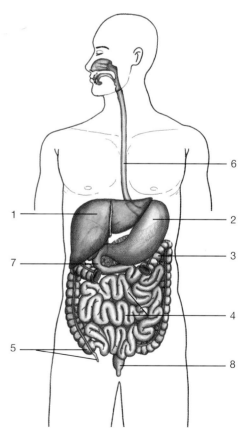

Organization of the digestive system (anterior aspect). Position of the abdominal organs.

1   Liver
2   Stomach
3   Transverse colon
4   Small intestine
5   Hindgut (cecum) with vermiform appendix
6   Esophagus
7   Duodenum
8   Rectum

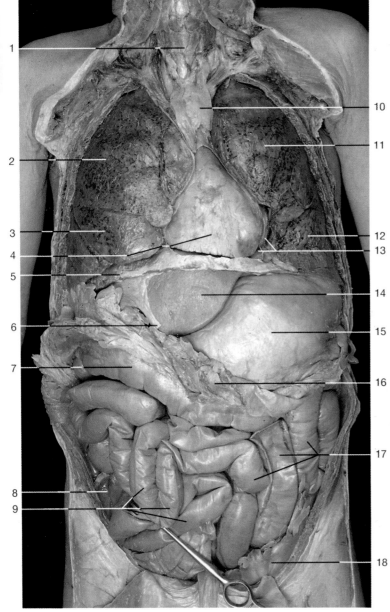

1	Thyroid gland
2	Upper lobe of right lung
3	Middle lobe of right lung
4	Heart
5	Diaphragm
6	Round ligament of liver (ligamentum teres)
7	Transverse colon
8	Cecum
9	Small intestine (ileum)
10	Thymus
11	Upper lobe of left lung
12	Lower lobe of left lung
13	Pericardium (cut edge)
14	Liver (left lobe)
15	Stomach
16	Greater omentum
17	Small intestine (jejunum)
18	Sigmoid colon
19	Rectus abdominis muscle
20	Small intestine (section)
21	Rib
22	Common bile duct, duodenum, and pancreas
23	Inferior vena cava
24	Liver
25	Body of second lumbar vertebra
26	Right kidney
27	Cauda equina and dura mater
28	Linea alba
29	Stomach and pylorus
30	Superior mesenteric artery and vein
31	Abdominal aorta
32	Left renal artery and vein
33	Left kidney
34	Psoas major muscle
35	Deep muscles of the back
36	Pancreas adjacent to lesser sac (omental bursa)
37	Falciform ligament with ligamentum teres

Abdominal organs in situ. The greater omentum has been partly removed or reflected.

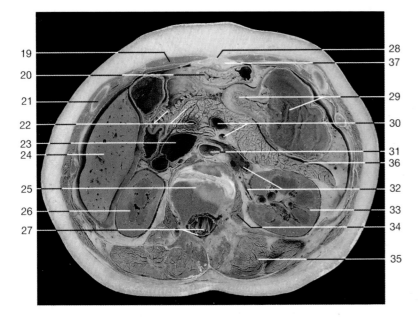

Transverse section through the abdominal cavity at the level of the second lumbar vertebra (from below).

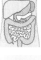

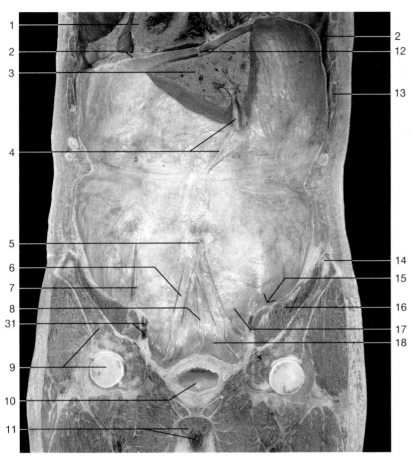

Anterior abdominal wall with pelvic cavity and thigh (frontal section, male) (internal aspect).

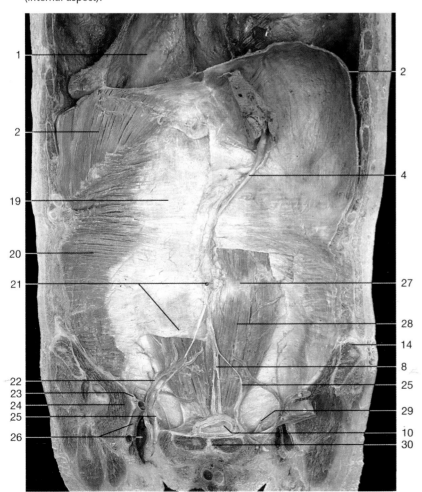

1 Left ventricle with pericardium
2 Diaphragm
3 Remnant of liver
4 Ligamentum teres
(free margin of falciform ligament)
5 Site of umbilicus
6 Medial umbilical fold
(containing the obliterated umbilical artery)
7 Lateral umbilical fold (containing inferior
epigastric artery and vein)
8 Median umbilical fold
(containing remnant of urachus)
9 Head of femur and pelvic bone
10 Urinary bladder
11 Root of penis
12 Falciform ligament of liver
13 Rib (divided)
14 Iliac crest (divided)
15 Site of deep inguinal ring and
lateral inguinal fossa
16 Iliopsoas muscle (divided)
17 Medial inguinal fossa
18 Supravesical fossa
19 Posterior layer of rectus sheath
20 Transversus abdominis muscle
21 Umbilicus and arcuate line
22 Inferior epigastric artery
23 Femoral nerve
24 Iliopsoas muscle
25 Remnant of umbilical artery
26 Femoral artery and vein
27 Tendinous intersection of rectus abdominis
muscle
28 Rectus abdominis muscle
29 Interfoveolar ligament
30 Pubic symphysis (divided)
31 External iliac artery and vein

Anterior abdominal wall (male) (internal aspect). The peritoneum and parts of the posterior layer of rectus sheath have been removed. Dissection of inferior epigastric arteries and veins.

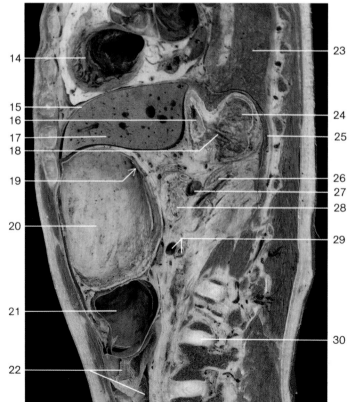

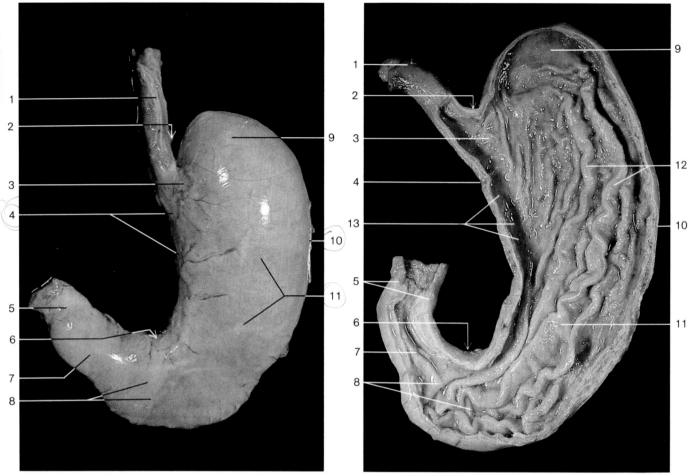

Stomach (ventral aspect).

Mucosa of posterior wall of stomach (ventral aspect).

Position of the stomach. Parasagittal section through upper part of left abdominal cavity 3.5 cm lateral to median plane.

1 Esophagus
2 Cardial notch
3 Cardial part of stomach
4 Lesser curvature of stomach
5 Pyloric sphincter
6 Angular notch (incisura angularis)
7 Pyloric canal
8 Pyloric antrum
9 Fundus of stomach
10 Greater curvature of stomach
11 Body of stomach
12 Folds of mucous membrane (gastric rugae)
13 Gastric canal
14 Right ventricle of heart
15 Diaphragm (cut edge)
16 Abdominal portion of esophagus
17 Liver
18 Cardial part of stomach (cut edge)
19 Position of pyloric canal
20 Body of stomach
21 Transverse colon
22 Small intestine
23 Lung (cut edge)
24 Fundus of stomach (section)
25 Lumbar portion of diaphragm (cut edge)
26 Suprarenal gland
27 Splenic vein
28 Pancreas
29 Superior mesenteric artery and vein
30 Intervertebral disc

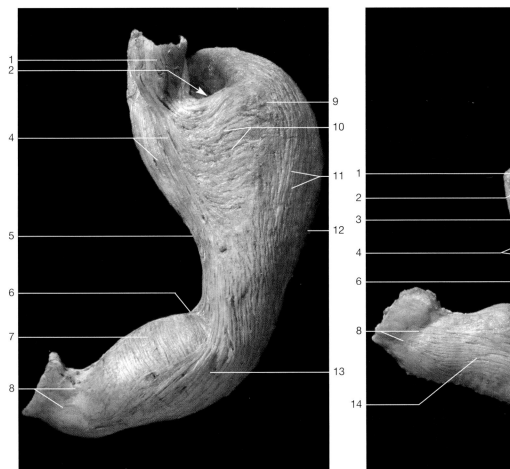

Muscular coat of stomach, outer layer (ventral aspect).

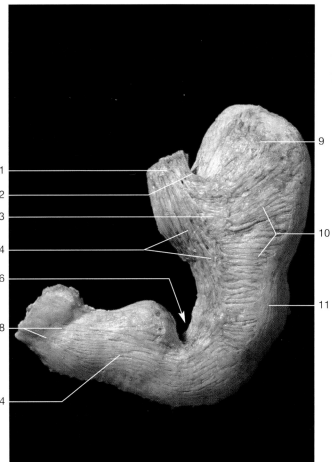

Muscular coat of stomach, middle layer (ventral aspect).

1   Esophagus (abdominal part)
2   Cardial notch
3   Cardial part of stomach
4   Longitudinal muscle layer at lesser curvature of stomach
5   Lesser curvature
6   Incisura angularis
7   Circular muscle layer of pyloric part of stomach
8   Pyloric sphincter muscle
9   Fundus of stomach
10 Circular muscle layer of fundus of stomach
11 Longitudinal muscle layer of greater curvature of stomach
12 Greater curvature of stomach
13 Longitudinal muscle layer (transition from body to pyloric part of stomach)
14 Pyloric part of stomach
15 Oblique muscle fibers

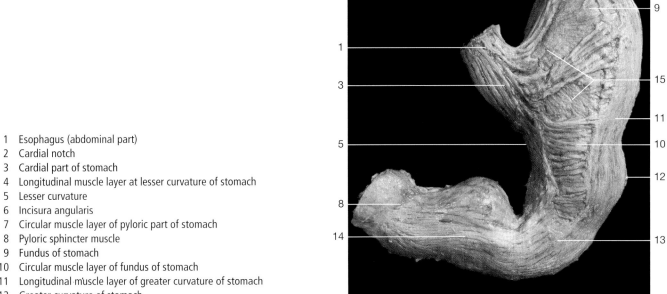

Muscular coat of stomach, inner layer (ventral aspect).

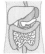

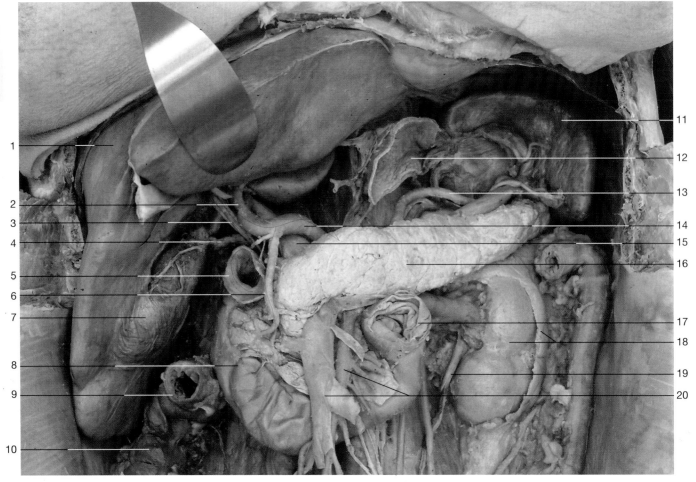

Upper abdominal organs. Pancreas, duodenum, and left kidney are shown. Stomach and transverse colon have been removed, liver elevated; superior mesenteric vein is slightly enlarged.

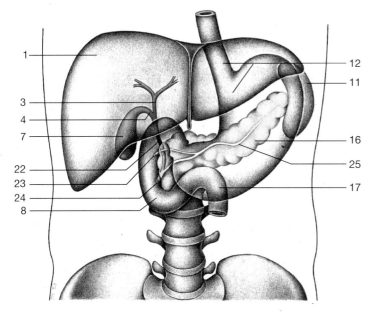

Pancreas, duodenum, and extrahepatic bile ducts (anterior aspect, schematic drawing).

1   Liver
2   Hepatic artery proper
3   Hepatic duct
4   Cystic duct
5   Pylorus
6   Gastroduodenal artery
7   Gallbladder
8   Duodenum
9   Transverse colon (cut)
10 Ascending colon
11 Spleen
12 Cardia
13 Splenic artery
14 Common hepatic artery
15 Portal vein
16 Pancreas (body)
17 Duodenojejunal flexure
18 Kidney (with capsula adiposa)
19 Ureter
20 Superior mesenteric artery and vein
21 Aorta (abdominal part)
22 Common bile duct
23 Lesser duodenal papilla
24 Greater duodenal papilla
25 Pancreatic duct

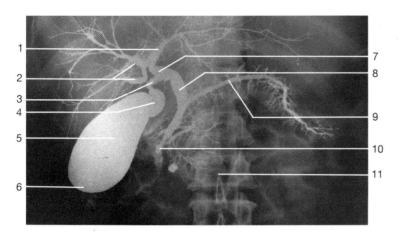

1   Left hepatic duct
2   Right hepatic duct
3   Cystic duct
4   Neck of gallbladder
5   Body of gallbladder
6   Fundus of gallbladder
7   Common hepatic duct
8   Common bile duct
9   Pancreatic duct
10 Greater duodenal papilla
11 Second lumbar vertebra
12 Folds of mucous membrane of gallbladder
13 Muscular coat of gallbladder
14 Neck of gallbladder (opened)
15 Cystic duct with spiral fold
16 Lesser duodenal papilla
17 Accessory pancreatic duct
18 Uncinate process
19 Plica circularis of duodenum (Kerckring's fold)
20 Head of pancreas
21 Body of pancreas
22 Tail of pancreas
23 Descending part of duodenum
24 Incisure of pancreas

Radiograph of biliary ducts, gallbladder, and pancreatic duct (antero-posterior view).

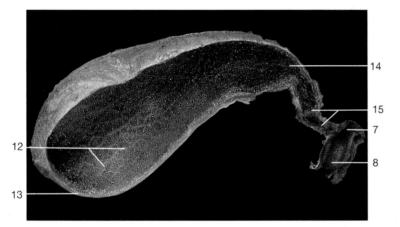

Isolated gallbladder and cystic duct (anterior aspect).
The gallbladder has been opened to display the mucous membrane.

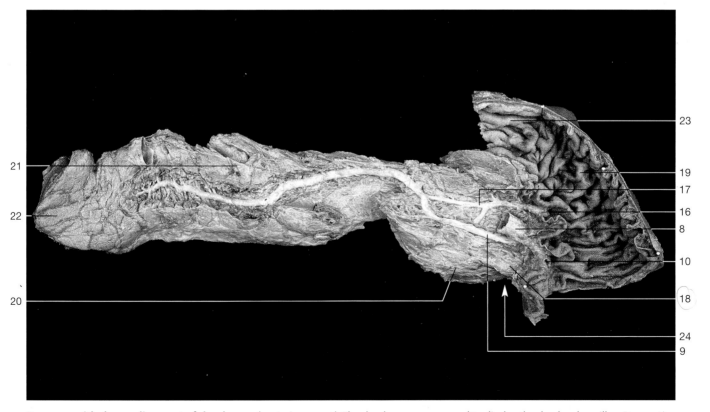

Pancreas with descending part of duodenum (posterior aspect). The duodenum was opened to display the duodenal papillae. Pancreatic duct has been dissected, the common bile duct has been divided. The sphincter of Oddi is shown.

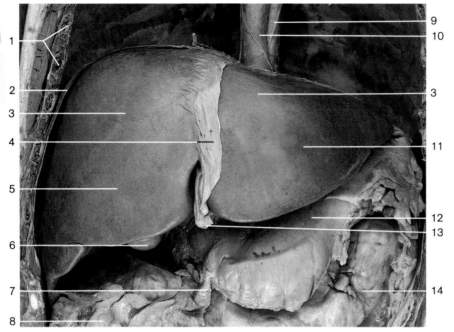

1   Ribs (cut edges)
2   Diaphragm
3   Diaphragmatic surface of liver
4   Falciform ligament of liver
5   Right lobe of liver
6   Fundus of gallbladder
7   Gastrocolic ligament
8   Greater omentum
9   Aorta
10 Esophagus
11 Left lobe of liver
12 Stomach
13 Ligamentum teres
14 Transverse colon
15 Right atrium of heart
16 Central tendon and sternal
    portion of diaphragm
17 Liver (cut edge)
18 Entrance to duodenum (pylorus)
19 Stomach
20 Duodenum
21 Transverse colon
    (divided, dilated)
22 Small intestine
23 Thoracic aorta
    (longitudinally divided)
24 Esophagus
    (longitudinally divided)
25 Esophageal hiatus of diaphragm
26 Omental bursa (lesser sac)
27 Splenic artery
28 Pancreas
29 Left renal vein
30 Intervertebral disc
31 Abdominal aorta
    (longitudinally divided)

Liver in situ (ventral aspect). Part of the diaphragm has been removed.

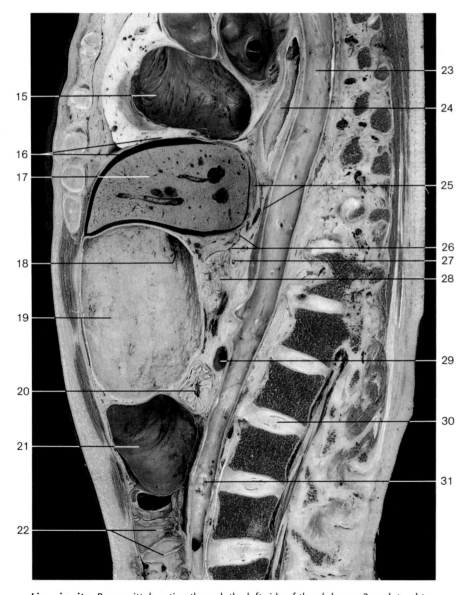

Liver in situ. Parasagittal section through the left side of the abdomen 2 cm lateral to median plane.

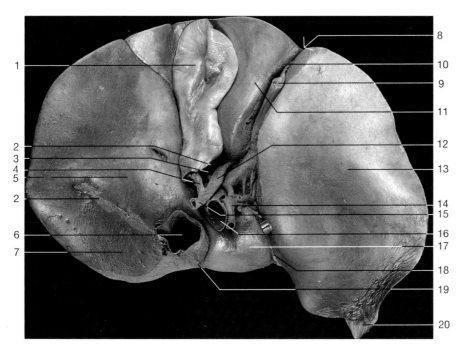

1	Fundus of gallbladder
2	Peritoneum (cut edges)
3	Cystic artery
4	Cystic duct
5	Right lobe of liver
6	Inferior vena cava
7	Bare area of liver
8	Notch for ligamentum teres and falciform ligament
9	Ligamentum teres
10	Falciform ligament of liver
11	Quadrate lobe of liver
12	Common hepatic duct
13	Left lobe of liver
14	Hepatic artery proper ⎫
15	Common bile duct ⎬ Portal triad
16	Portal vein ⎭
17	Caudate lobe of liver
18	Ligamentum venosum
19	Ligament of inferior vena cava
20	Appendix fibrosa (left triangular ligament)
21	Coronary ligament of liver
22	Hepatic veins
23	Porta hepatis

Liver (inferior aspect). Dissection of porta hepatis. Gallbladder partly collapsed. Ventral margin of liver above.

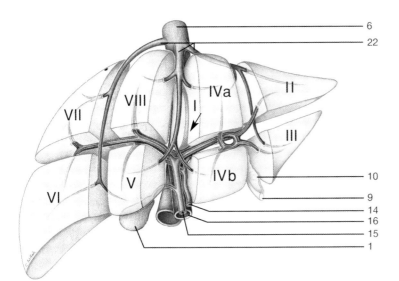

Segmentation of the liver (anterior aspect). Liver segments indicated by Roman numerals.

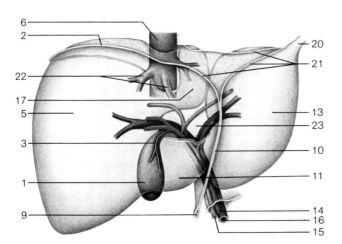

Liver (ventral aspect) (transparent drawing illustrating margins of peritoneal folds).

It should be noted that the anatomical left and right lobes of the liver do not reflect the internal distribution of the hepatic artery, portal vein, and biliary ducts. With these structures, used as criteria, the left lobe includes both the caudate and quadrate lobes, and thus the line dividing the liver into left and right functional lobes passes through the gallbladder and inferior vena cava. The three main hepatic veins drain segments of the liver that have no visible external markings.

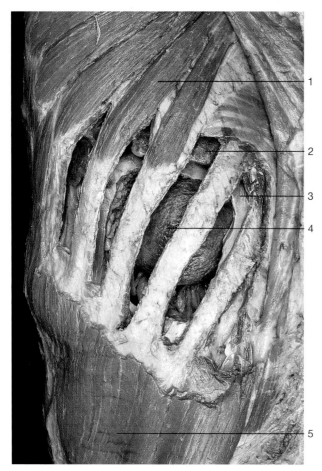

1 Serratus anterior muscle
2 Left lung
3 Diaphragm
4 Spleen
5 External abdominal oblique muscle
6 Gastrosplenic ligament
7 Splenic artery
8 Pancreas tail
9 Superior margin of spleen
10 Anterior border of spleen
11 Liver
12 Hepatic artery proper
13 Cystic duct
14 Gallbladder
15 Lesser duodenal papilla (probe)
16 Greater duodenal papilla (probe)
17 Duodenum (fenestrated)
18 Cardia
19 Pancreas and pancreatic duct
20 Kidney (with capsula adiposa, capsular fat, adipose tissue)
21 Common bile duct
22 Superior mesenteric artery and vein
23 Ureter
24 Aorta with celiac trunk
25 Suprarenal gland
26 Inferior mesenteric vein

Location of the spleen in situ (left-lateral aspect).
Intercostal spaces and diaphragm have been fenestrated.

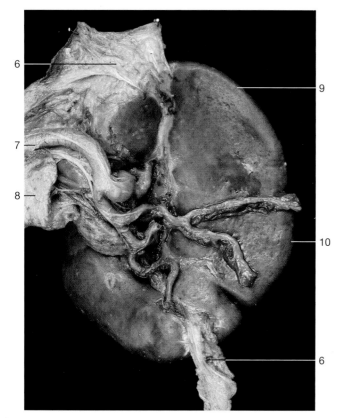

Spleen (visceral surface), hilum of spleen with vessels, nerves, and ligaments.

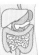

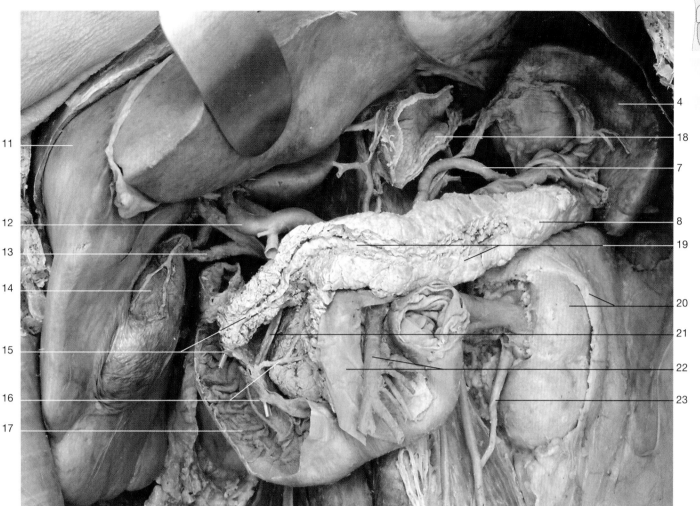

Upper abdominal organs (anterior aspect). Stomach and transverse colon have been removed, the duodenum fenestrated. The liver has been elevated to show the extrahepatic bile ducts. In this case the accessory pancreatic duct represents the main excretory duct of the pancreas.

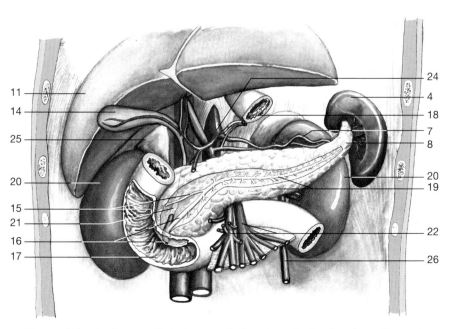

Upper abdominal organs (anterior aspect). The schematic drawing shows the most common situation of the pancreatic ducts.

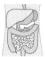

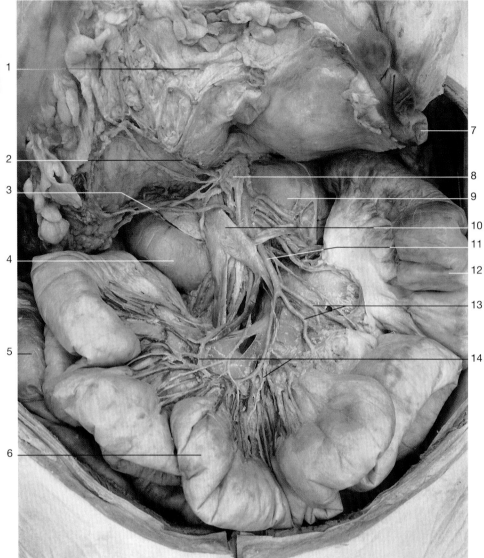

1	Greater omentum
2	Middle colic artery
3	Right colic artery
4	Duodenum
5	Ascending colon
6	Ileum
7	Transverse colon
8	Celiac ganglion
9	Duodenojejunal flexure
10	Superior mesenteric vein
11	Superior mesenteric artery
12	Jejunum
13	Jejunal arteries
14	Ileal arteries
15	Liver
16	Celiac trunk and abdominal aorta
17	Gallbladder
18	Pancreas
19	Ileocolic artery
20	Stomach
21	Spleen
22	Left colic flexure
23	Appendicular artery
24	Vermiform appendix

Vessels of abdominal organs, dissection of superior mesenteric artery and vein.
Greater omentum and transverse colon are reflected.

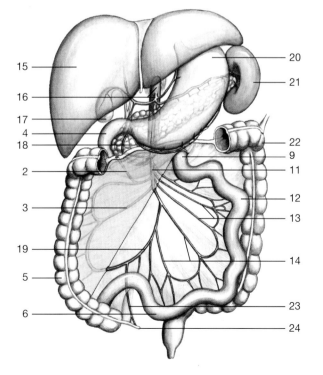

Main branches of superior mesenteric artery (schematic drawing).

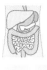

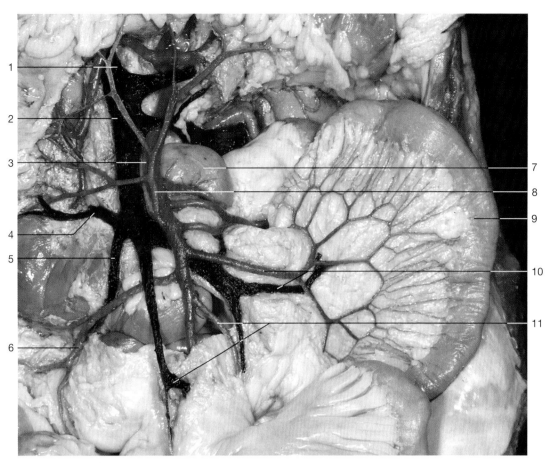

Tributaries of portal vein (blue) **and branches of superior mesenteric artery** (red) (anterior aspect).

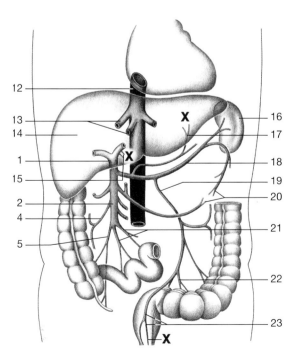

Main tributaries of portal vein (blue).
Inferior vena cava = violet; X = sites of portocaval anastomoses.

1   Portal vein
2   Superior mesenteric vein
3   Superior mesenteric artery
4   Right colic vein
5   Ileocolic vein
6   Ileocolic artery
7   Duodenojejunal flexure
8   Middle colic artery
9   Jejunum
10 Jejunal arteries and veins
11 Ileal arteries and veins
12 Inferior vena cava
13 Hepatic veins
14 Liver
15 Para-umbilical veins
     (located within the
     ligamentum teres)
16 Spleen
17 Left gastric vein with
     esophageal branches
18 Splenic vein
19 Inferior mesenteric vein
20 Gastro-omental veins
21 Ileal veins
22 Sigmoid veins
23 Superior rectal vein

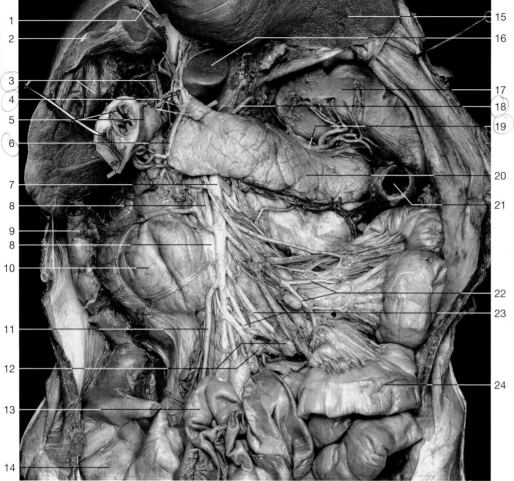

1	Ligamentum teres
2	Liver
3	Gallbladder and common bile duct
4	Hepatic artery proper and portal vein
5	Right gastric artery and pylorus
6	Gastroduodenal artery
7	Superior mesenteric artery
8	Superior mesenteric vein
9	Ascending colon
10	Duodenum
11	Ileocolic artery
12	Lymph nodes
13	Ileum
14	Cecum
15	Left lobe of liver
16	Caudate lobe of liver
17	Spleen
18	Left gastric artery
19	Splenic artery
20	Pancreas
21	Left colic flexure (cut)
22	Jejunal arteries
23	Ileal arteries
24	Jejunum
25	Middle colic artery
26	Right colic artery
27	Appendicular artery
28	Transverse mesocolon
29	Duodenojejunal flexure
30	Inferior mesenteric artery
31	Left colic artery
32	Sigmoid arteries
33	Superior rectal artery
34	Inferior vena cava
35	Abdominal aorta
36	Descending colon
37	Ileum
38	Sigmoid colon
39	Vermiform appendix
40	Cecum

Superior mesenteric artery in relation to pancreas and duodenum. Stomach and transverse colon have been removed and the liver elevated. Note the location of the spleen. A yellow probe is inserted through the omental foramen.

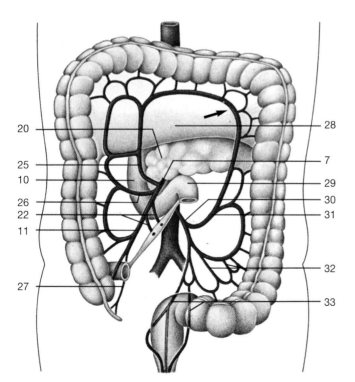

Main branches of superior and inferior mesenteric arteries (schematic drawing). Arrow = Riolan's anastomosis.

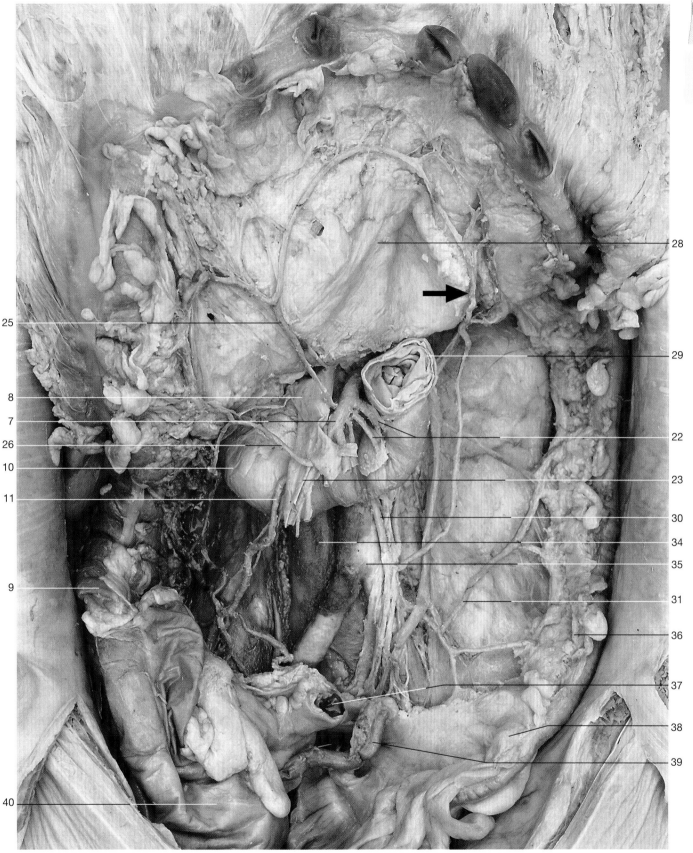

Vessels of the retroperitoneal organs. Direction of the inferior mesenteric artery and its anastomosis with the middle colic artery (arrow = Riolan's anastomosis). Greater omentum and transverse colon have been reflected, the intestine partly removed. The normally retrocecally located vermiform appendix has been replaced anteriorly. The right common iliac artery is partly obstructed by a blood thrombus.

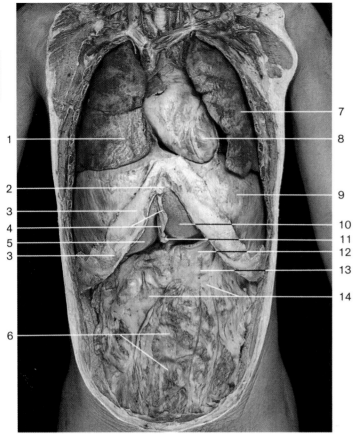

1   Middle lobe of right lung
2   Xiphoid process
3   Costal margin
4   Falciform ligament of liver
5   Quadrate lobe of liver
6   Greater omentum
7   Upper lobe of left lung
8   Heart
9   Diaphragm
10 Left lobe of liver
11 Ligamentum teres
12 Stomach
13 Gastrocolic ligament
14 Transverse colon
15 Taenia coli
16 Appendices epiploicae
17 Cecum
18 Taenia coli
19 Ileum
20 Transverse mesocolon
21 Jejunum
22 Sigmoid colon
23 Position of root of mesentery
24 Vermiform appendix
25 Duodenojejunal flexure
26 Mesentery

Abdominal organs. The anterior thoracic and abdominal walls have been removed.

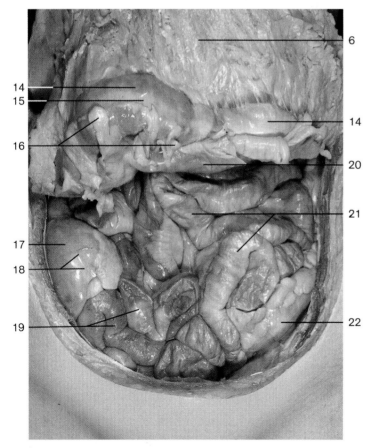

Abdominal organs (anterior aspect). The greater omentum, which is fixed to the transverse colon, has been raised.

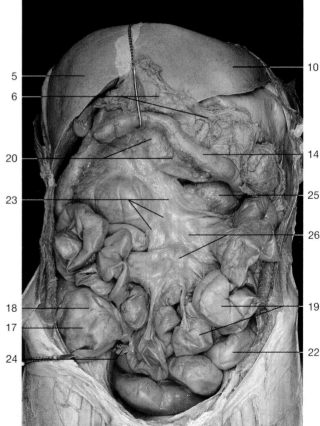

Abdominal organs (anterior aspect). The transverse colon has been reflected.

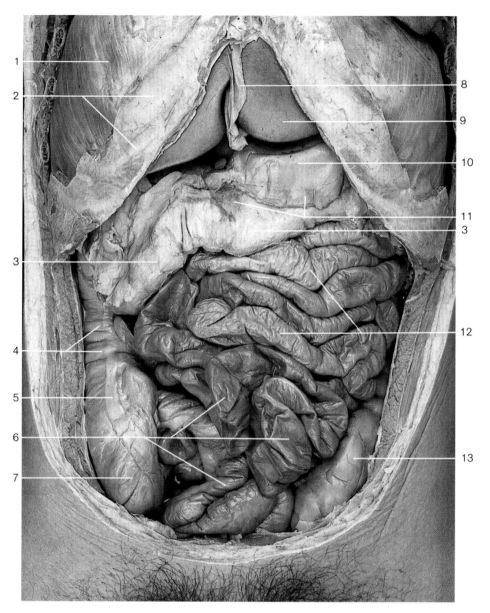

1 Diaphragm
2 Costal margin
3 Transverse colon
4 Ascending colon with haustra
5 Free taenia of cecum
6 Ileum
7 Cecum
8 Falciform ligament of liver
9 Liver
10 Stomach
11 Gastrocolic ligament
12 Jejunum
13 Sigmoid colon
14 Vermiform appendix
15 Terminal ileum
16 Meso-appendix
17 Mesentery

Abdominal organs in situ. The greater omentum has been removed.

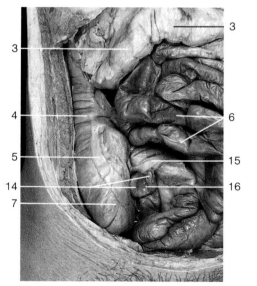

Ascending colon, cecum, and vermiform appendix (detail of the preceding figure).

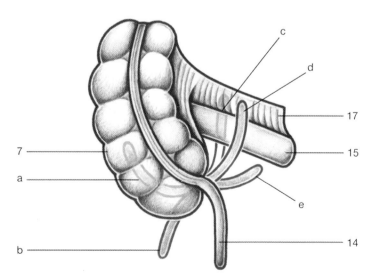

Variations in the position of the vermiform appendix.
a = retrocecal; b = paracolic; c = retro-ileal; d = pre-ileal;
e = subcecal.

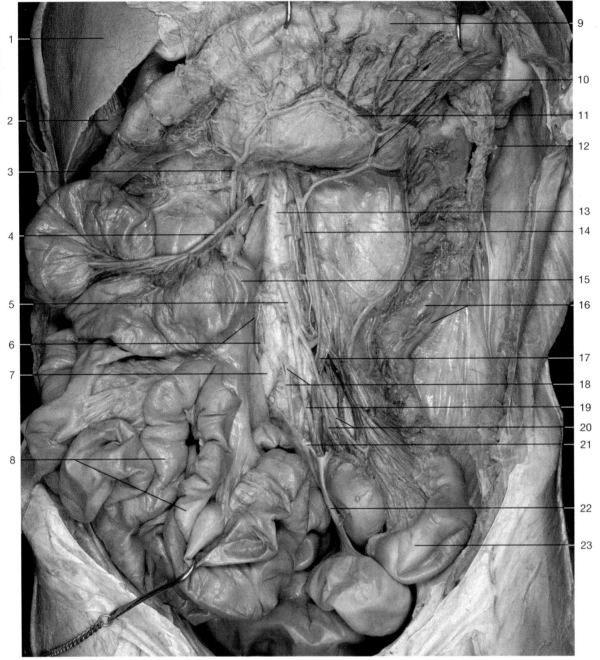

Abdominal organs. Dissection of inferior mesenteric artery and autonomic plexus. The transverse colon with mesocolon has been raised and the small intestine reflected.

1　Liver	12　Spleen
2　Gallbladder	13　Abdominal aorta
3　Middle colic artery	14　Left colic artery
4　Jejunal artery	15　Duodenojejunal flexure
5　Inferior mesenteric artery	16　Descending colon (free taenia of colon)
6　Sympathetic nerves and ganglia	17　Inferior mesenteric vein
7　Right common iliac artery	18　Superior hypogastric plexus
8　Small intestine (ileum)	19　Superior rectal artery
9　Transverse colon (reflected)	20　Sigmoid arteries
10　Transverse mesocolon	21　Peritoneum (cut edge)
11　Anastomosis between middle and left colic artery	22　Sigmoid mesocolon
	23　Sigmoid colon

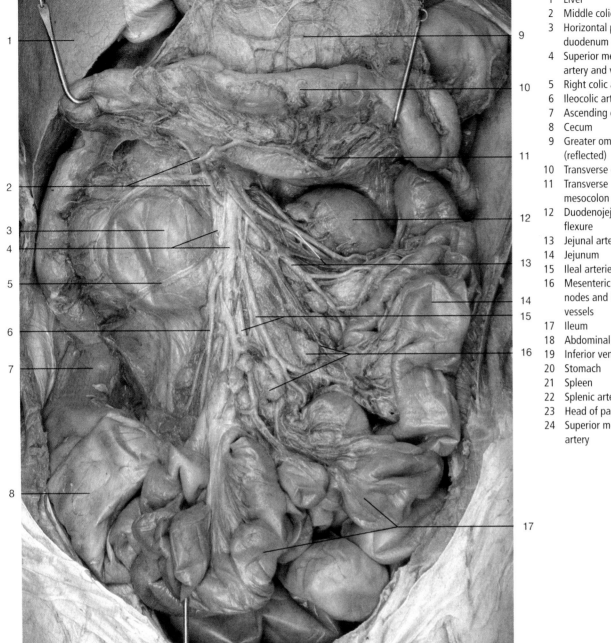

1 Liver
2 Middle colic artery
3 Horizontal part of
   duodenum (extended)
4 Superior mesenteric
   artery and vein
5 Right colic artery
6 Ileocolic artery
7 Ascending colon
8 Cecum
9 Greater omentum
   (reflected)
10 Transverse colon
11 Transverse
    mesocolon
12 Duodenojejunal
    flexure
13 Jejunal arteries
14 Jejunum
15 Ileal arteries
16 Mesenteric lymph
    nodes and lymph
    vessels
17 Ileum
18 Abdominal aorta
19 Inferior vena cava
20 Stomach
21 Spleen
22 Splenic artery
23 Head of pancreas
24 Superior mesenteric
    artery

Abdominal organs. Superior mesenteric artery. Mesenteric lymph nodes. Transverse colon reflected.

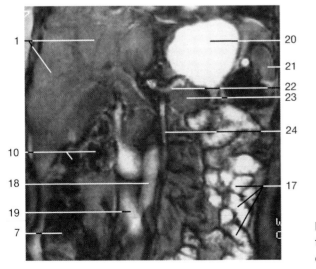

Frontal section through the abdominal cavity (MRI scan; the intestinal tract and vessels are filled with a paramagnetic substance [Gadolinium]; courtesy of Dr. W. Rödl, Erlangen, Germany).

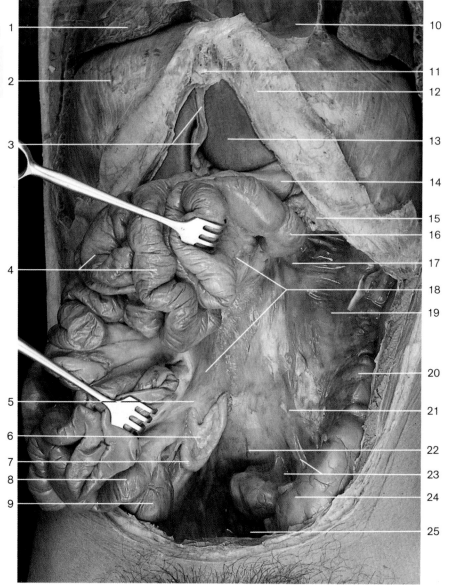

1 Lung
2 Diaphragm
3 Falciform ligament of liver
4 Jejunum
5 Ileocecal fold
6 Meso-appendix
7 Vermiform appendix
8 Ileocecal junction
9 Cecum
10 Pericardial sac
11 Xiphoid process
12 Costal margin
13 Liver
14 Stomach
15 Transverse colon
16 Duodenojejunal flexure
17 Inferior duodenal fold
18 Mesentery
19 Position of left kidney
20 Descending colon
21 Position of left common iliac artery
22 Sacral promontory
23 Sigmoid mesocolon
24 Sigmoid colon
25 Rectum
26 Beginning of jejunum
27 Peritoneum of posterior abdominal wall
28 Transverse mesocolon
29 Superior duodenal fold
30 Superior duodenal recess
31 Retroduodenal recess
32 Free taenia of ascending colon
33 Ileocecal valve
34 Frenulum of ileocecal valve
35 Orifice of vermiform appendix (probe)
36 Ileocolic artery
37 Vermiform appendix with appendicular artery
38 Ascending colon

Abdominal cavity. Mesenteries. The small intestine has been reflected laterally to demonstrate the mesentery.

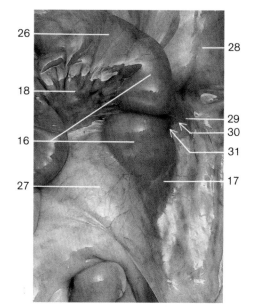

Duodenojejunal flexure
(enlargement of preceding figure).

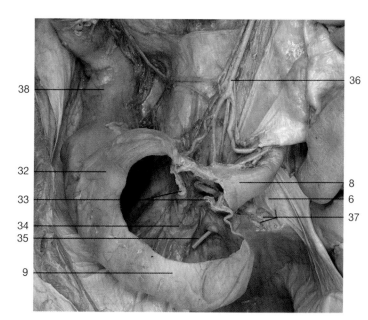

Ileocecal valve (ventral aspect). The cecum and terminal part of the ileum have been opened.

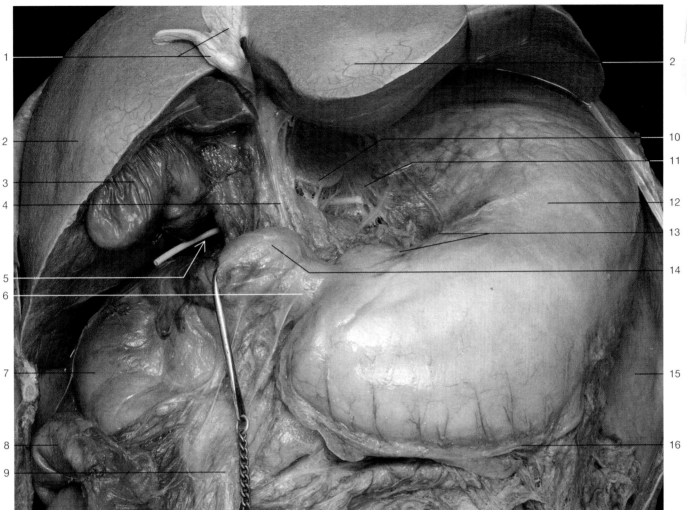

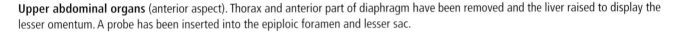

Upper abdominal organs (anterior aspect). Thorax and anterior part of diaphragm have been removed and the liver raised to display the lesser omentum. A probe has been inserted into the epiploic foramen and lesser sac.

1   Falciform ligament and ligamentum teres
2   Liver
3   Gallbladder (fundus)
4   Hepatoduodenal ligament
5   Epiploic foramen (probe)
6   Pylorus
7   Descending part of duodenum
8   Right colic flexure
9   Gastrocolic ligament
10 Caudate lobe of liver (behind lesser omentum)
11 Lesser omentum
12 Stomach
13 Lesser curvature of stomach
14 Superior part of duodenum
15 Diaphragm
16 Greater curvature of stomach with gastro-omental vessels
17 Twelfth thoracic vertebra
18 Right kidney
19 Right suprarenal gland
20 Inferior vena cava
21 Falciform ligament of liver
22 Abdominal aorta
23 Spleen
24 Lienorenal ligament
25 Gastrosplenic ligament
26 Pancreas
27 Lesser sac (omental bursa)

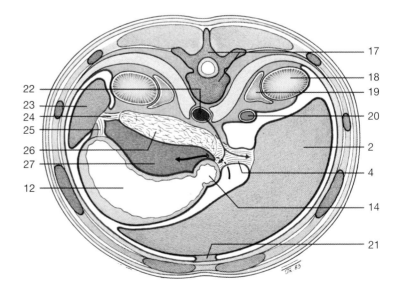

Horizontal section through the lesser sac above the level of epiploic foramen (black arrow). Viewed from above. Red arrows: routes of the arterial branches of celiac trunk to liver, stomach, duodenum, and pancreas (posterior aspect).

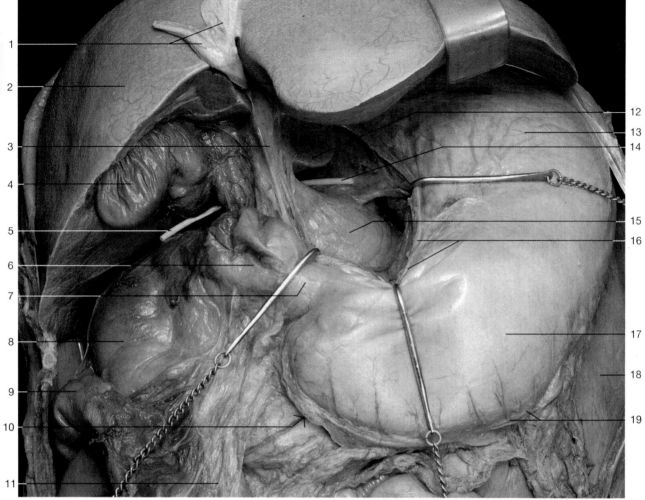

Upper abdominal organs (anterior aspect). **Lesser sac.** Lesser omentum partly removed, liver and stomach slightly reflected.

1   Falciform ligament and ligamentum teres
2   Liver
3   Hepatoduodenal ligament
4   Gallbladder
5   Probe within the epiploic foramen
6   Superior part of duodenum
7   Pylorus
8   Descending part of duodenum
9   Right colic flexure
10 Gastrocolic ligament
11 Greater omentum
12 Caudate lobe of liver
13 Fundus of stomach
14 Probe at the level of the vestibule of lesser sac
    (through epiploic foramen)
15 Head of pancreas
16 Lesser curvature of stomach
17 Body of stomach

18 Diaphragm
19 Greater curvature with gastro-omental
    vessels
20 Head of pancreas and gastropancreatic fold
21 Spleen
22 Tail of pancreas
23 Left colic flexure
24 Root of transverse mesocolon
25 Transverse mesocolon
26 Gastrocolic ligament (cut edge)
27 Transverse colon
28 Umbilicus
29 Small intestine
30 Lesser omentum
31 Lesser sac (omental bursa)
32 Duodenum
33 Mesentery
34 Sigmoid colon

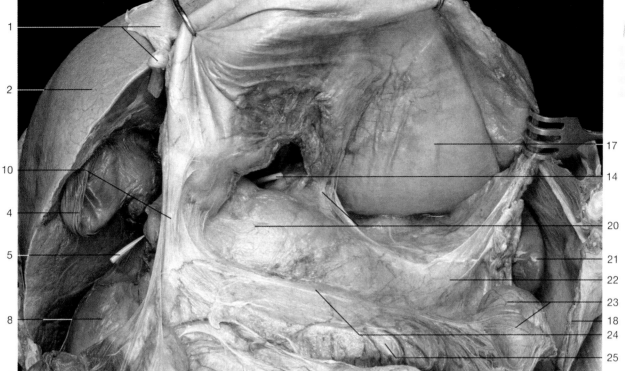

Upper abdominal organs (anterior aspect). **Lesser sac.** The gastrocolic ligament has been divided and the whole stomach raised to display the posterior wall of the lesser sac.

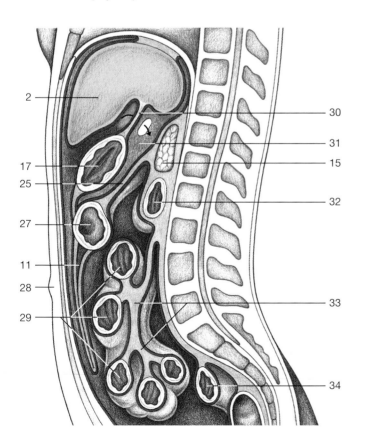

Midsagittal section through abdominal cavity, demonstrating the site of lesser sac (blue). (Schematic drawing.) The epiploic foramen, entrance to the lesser sac, is indicated by an arrow. Red = peritoneum.

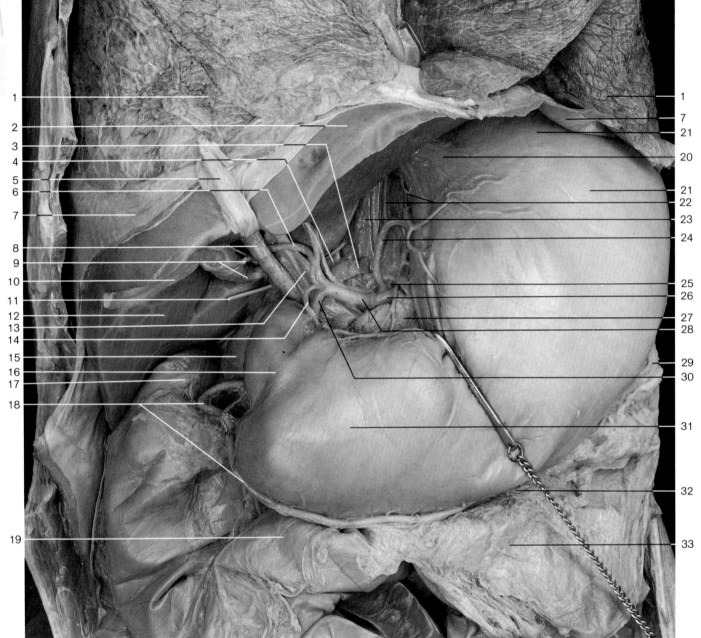

Arteries of upper abdominal organs (anterior aspect). **Dissection of celiac trunk.** The lesser omentum has been removed and the lesser curvature of the stomach reflected to display the branches of the celiac trunk. The probe is situated within the epiploic foramen.

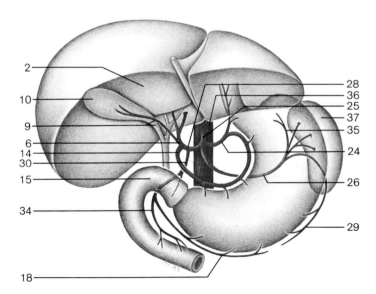

Branches of celiac trunk (schematic drawing).

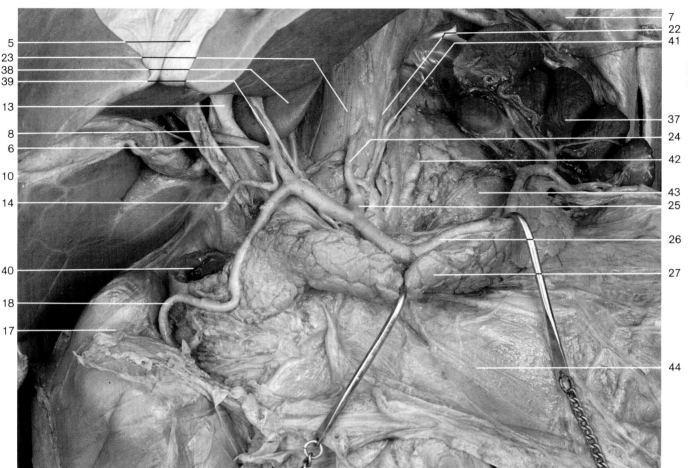

Arteries of upper abdominal organs (anterior aspect). **Branches of celiac trunk; blood supply of liver, pancreas, and spleen.**
The stomach, superior part of duodenum, and celiac ganglion have been removed to reveal the anterior aspect of the posterior wall of the lesser sac (omental bursa) and the vessels and ducts of the hepatoduodenal ligament. The pancreas has been slightly reflected anteriorly.

1	Lung	23	Lumbar part of diaphragm
2	Liver (visceral surface)	24	Left gastric artery
3	Lymph node	25	Celiac trunk
4	Inferior vena cava	26	Splenic artery
5	Ligamentum teres (reflected)	27	Pancreas
6	Right branch of hepatic artery proper	28	Common hepatic artery
7	Diaphragm	29	Left gastro-omental (gastro-epiploic) artery
8	Common hepatic duct (dilated)	30	Gastroduodenal artery
9	Cystic duct and artery	31	Pyloric part of stomach
10	Gallbladder	32	Greater curvature of stomach
11	Probe in epiploic foramen	33	Gastrocolic ligament
12	Right lobe of liver	34	Superior pancreaticoduodenal artery
13	Portal vein	35	Short gastric arteries
14	Right gastric artery	36	Aorta
15	Duodenum	37	Spleen
16	Pylorus	38	Caudate lobe of liver
17	Right colic flexure	39	Left branch of hepatic artery proper
18	Right gastro-omental (gastro-epiploic) artery	40	Descending part of duodenum (cut)
19	Transverse colon	41	Left inferior phrenic artery
20	Abdominal part of esophagus (cardiac part of stomach)	42	Suprarenal gland
21	Fundus of stomach	43	Kidney
22	Esophageal branches of left gastric artery	44	Transverse mesocolon

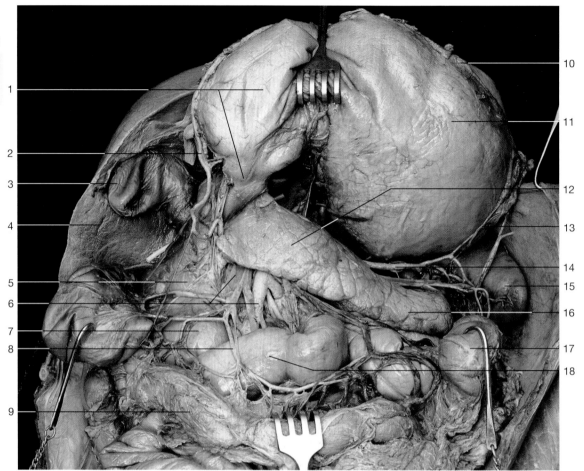

Posterior abdominal wall with pancreas and extrahepatic bile ducts in situ (anterior aspect). The gastrocolic ligament has been divided, the transverse colon and the stomach replaced to display the pancreas and superior mesenteric vessels.

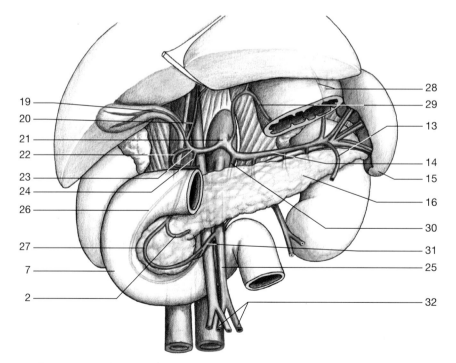

Blood supply of upper abdominal organs (branches of the celiac trunk and superior mesenteric artery). (Schematic drawing.)

1 Stomach (pyloric part) and pylorus
2 Right gastro-omental (gastro-epiploic) artery
3 Fundus of gallbladder
4 Liver (right lobe)
5 Head of pancreas
6 Superior mesenteric artery and vein
7 Duodenum
8 Middle colic artery
9 Transverse colon
10 Greater curvature of stomach
   (remnants of gastrocolic ligament)
11 Body of stomach
12 Body of pancreas
13 Left gastro-omental (gastro-epiploic) artery
14 Splenic artery
15 Spleen
16 Tail of pancreas
17 Left colic flexure
18 Jejunum
19 Cystic artery
20 Hepatic artery proper
21 Celiac trunk
22 Right gastric artery
23 Common hepatic artery
24 Gastroduodenal artery
25 Superior mesenteric artery
26 Superior posterior pancreaticoduodenal artery
27 Superior anterior pancreaticoduodenal artery
28 Short gastric arteries
29 Left gastric artery
30 Posterior pancreatic branch of splenic artery
31 Inferior pancreaticoduodenal artery
32 Jejunal arteries

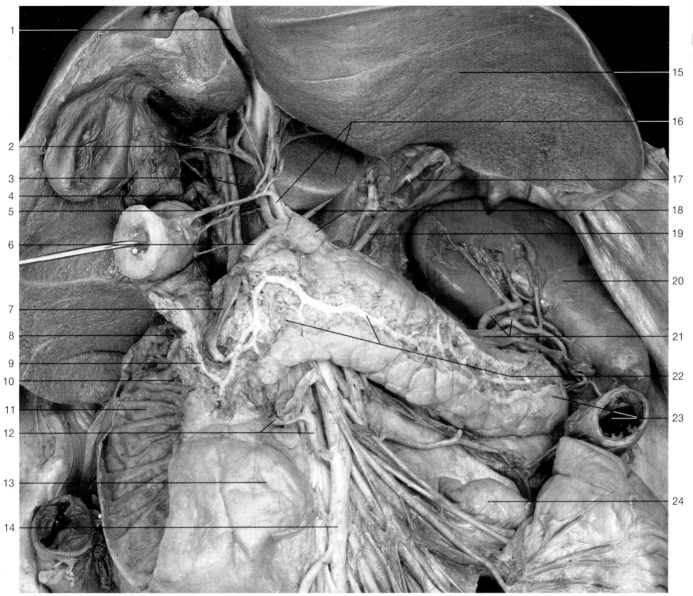

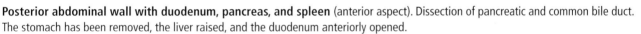

Posterior abdominal wall with duodenum, pancreas, and spleen (anterior aspect). Dissection of pancreatic and common bile duct. The stomach has been removed, the liver raised, and the duodenum anteriorly opened.

1 Ligamentum teres
2 Gallbladder and cystic artery
3 Common hepatic duct and portal vein
4 Cystic duct
5 Right gastric artery (pylorus with superior part of duodenum, cut and reflected)
6 Gastroduodenal artery
7 Common bile duct
8 Probe within the minor duodenal papilla
9 Accessory pancreatic duct
10 Probe within the major duodenal papilla
11 Descending part of duodenum (opened)
12 Middle colic artery and inferior pancreaticoduodenal artery

13 Horizontal part of duodenum (distended)
14 Superior mesenteric artery
15 Liver (left lobe)
16 Caudate lobe of liver and hepatic artery proper
17 Abdominal part of esophagus (cut)
18 Probe in epiploic foramen and lymph node
19 Left gastric artery
20 Spleen
21 Splenic vein and branches of splenic artery
22 Main pancreatic duct and head of pancreas
23 Left colic flexure and tail of pancreas
24 Duodenojejunal flexure

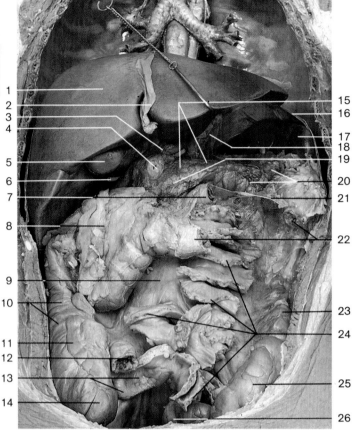

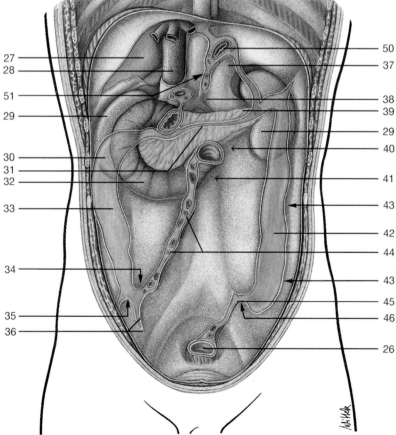

1   Liver
2   Falciform ligament
3   Hepatoduodenal ligament
4   Pylorus (divided)
5   Gallbladder
6   Probe within the epiploic foramen
7   Duodenojejunal flexure (divided)
8   Greater omentum
9   Root of mesentery
10 Ascending colon
11 Free colic taenia
12 End of ileum (divided)
13 Vermiform appendix with meso-appendix
14 Cecum
15 Pancreas and site of lesser sac
16 Diaphragm
17 Spleen
18 Cardia (part of stomach, divided)
19 Head of pancreas
20 Body and tail of pancreas
21 Transverse mesocolon
22 Transverse colon (divided)
23 Descending colon
24 Cut edge of mesentery
25 Sigmoid colon
26 Rectum
27 Attachment of bare area of liver
28 Inferior vena cava
29 Kidney
30 Attachment of right colic flexure
31 Root of transverse mesocolon
32 Junction between descending and horizontal parts of duodenum
33 Bare surface for ascending colon
34 Ileocecal recess
35 Retrocecal recess
36 Root of meso-appendix
37 Superior recess ⎫
38 Isthmus (opening) ⎬ of lesser sac
39 Splenic recess ⎭ (omental bursa)
40 Superior duodenal recess
41 Inferior duodenal recess
42 Bare surface for descending colon
43 Paracolic recesses
44 Root of mesentery
45 Root of mesosigmoid
46 Intersigmoid recess
47 Hepatic veins
48 Duodenojejunal flexure
49 Attachment of left colic flexure
50 Esophagus
51 Entrance to lesser sac through the epiploic foramen

Abdominal cavity after removal of stomach, jejunum, ileum, and part of the transverse colon. Liver has been slightly raised.

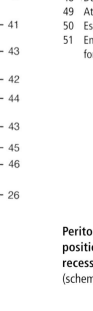

Peritoneal reflections from organs and the position of root of mesentery and peritoneal recesses on the posterior abdominal wall (schematic drawing).

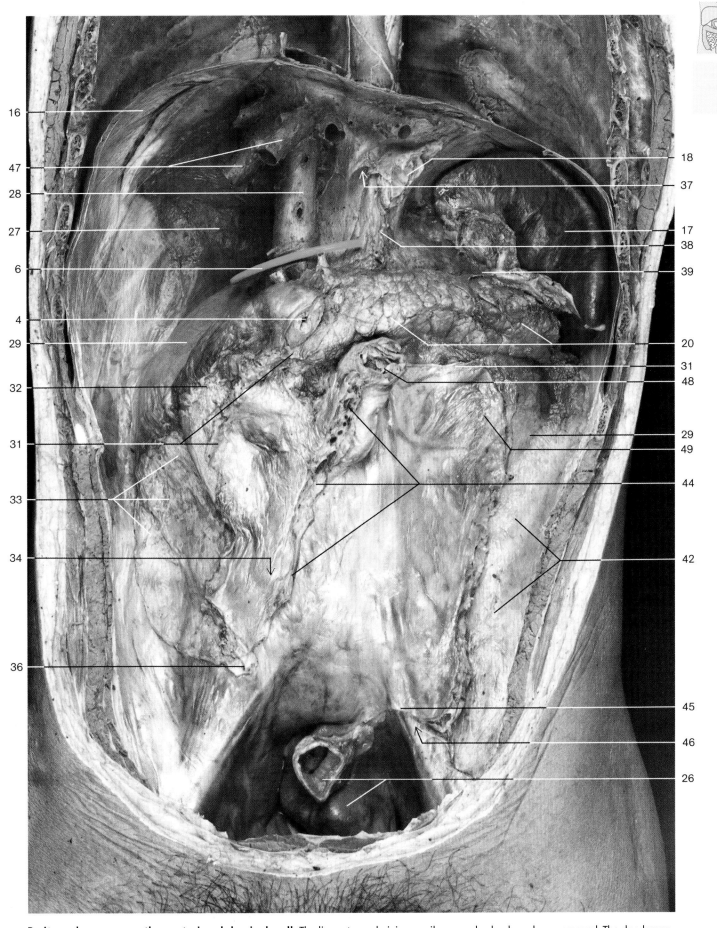

Peritoneal recesses on the posterior abdominal wall. The liver, stomach, jejunum, ileum, and colon have been removed. The duodenum, pancreas, and spleen have been left in place.

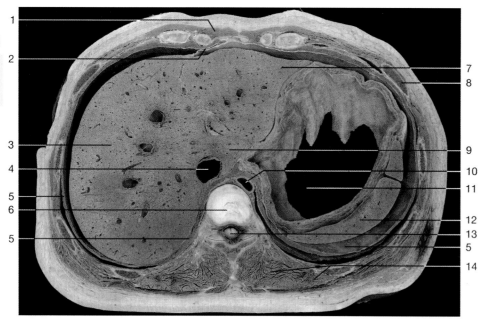

Horizontal section through the abdominal cavity at level 1 (from below).

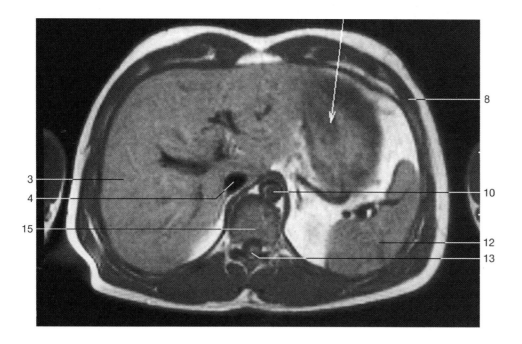

Horizontal section through the abdominal cavity (MRI scan, corresponding to level 1). Arrow: stomach.

1	Rectus abdominis muscle	20	Greater duodenal papilla
2	Falciform ligament	21	Duodenum
3	Liver (right lobe)	22	Suprarenal gland and ureter
4	Inferior vena cava	23	Kidney
5	Diaphragm	24	Round ligament of liver
6	Intervertebral disc	25	Superior mesenteric artery and vein
7	Liver (left lobe)	26	Psoas major muscle
8	Rib	27	Descending colon
9	Liver (caudate lobe)	28	Quadratus lumborum muscle
10	Abdominal (descending) aorta	29	Cauda equina
11	Stomach	30	Right renal vein
12	Spleen	31	Small intestine
13	Spinal cord	32	Iliacus muscle
14	Longissimus and iliocostalis muscles	33	Ilium
15	Body of vertebra	34	Ileocecal valve
16	Rectus abdominis muscle	35	Cecum
17	External abdominal oblique muscle	36	Common iliac artery and vein
18	Transverse colon	37	Gluteus medius muscle
19	Head of pancreas	38	Vertebral canal and dura mater

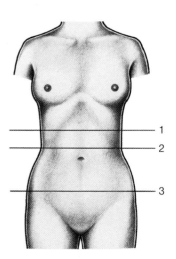

Levels of sections.

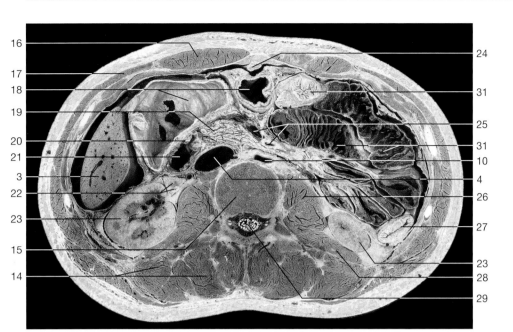

Horizontal section through the abdominal cavity at the level of greater duodenal papilla (from below).

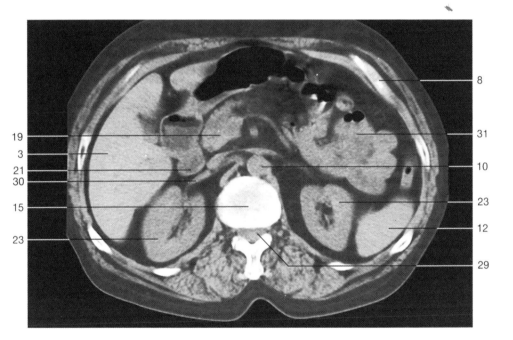

Horizontal section through the abdominal cavity (CT scan, corresponding to level 2).

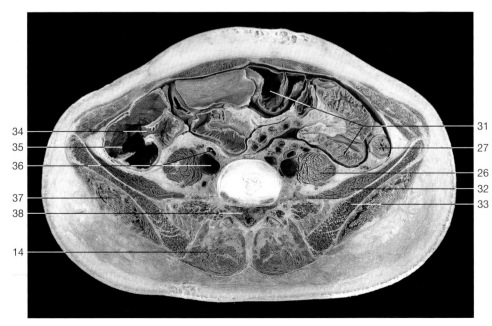

Horizontal section through the abdominal cavity at level 3 (from below).

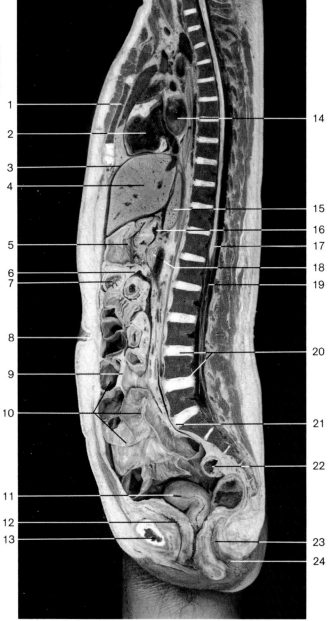

Midsagittal section through the trunk (female).

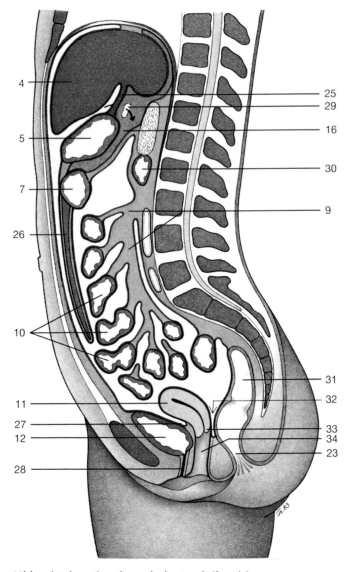

Midsagittal section through the trunk (female).
(Schematic drawing.) Blue = omental bursa; red = peritoneum.

1	Sternum	13	Pubic symphysis
2	Right ventricle of heart	14	Left atrium of heart
3	Diaphragm	15	Caudate lobe of liver
4	Liver	16	Omental bursa or lesser sac
5	Stomach	17	Conus medullaris
6	Transverse mesocolon	18	Pancreas
7	Transverse colon	19	Cauda equina
8	Umbilicus	20	Intervertebral discs
9	Mesentery		(lumbar vertebral column)
10	Small intestine	21	Sacral promontory
11	Uterus	22	Sigmoid colon
12	Urinary bladder	23	Anal canal

24	Anus
25	Lesser omentum
26	Greater omentum
27	Vesico-uterine pouch
28	Urethra
29	Epiploic (omental) foramen
30	Duodenum
31	Rectum
32	Recto-uterine pouch
33	Vaginal part of
	cervix of uterus
34	Vagina

6 Retroperitoneal Organs

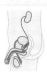

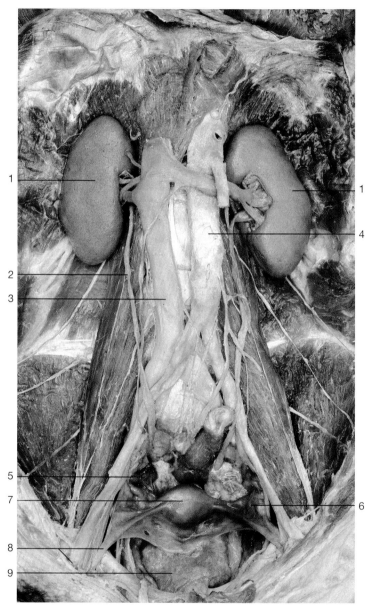

The organs of the urinary system (kidney, ureter, and, in the female, genital organs) are located together with vessels and nerves (aorta, inferior vena cava, plexus solaris, etc.) within the retroperitoneal space.

The upper part of the kidneys reaches the level of the margin of the lung. During respiration, the kidneys move slightly within their fasciae of Gerota. Parallel with the vertebral column, the ureter runs towards the urinary bladder. The great center of the autonomic nervous system, the solar plexus (celiac ganglion, etc.), is located in front of the abdominal aorta.

The genital organs of the female (uterus, uterine tube, ovary) are located within the pelvic cavity. In the male, the testis has moved out of the abdominal cavity and penetrated the inguinal canal to be finally located within the extragenital organs.

Retroperitoneal organs of the female (anterior aspect). View of the female pelvis showing uterus with uterine ligaments, ovary, and urinary bladder (from Lütjen-Drecoll, Rohen, Innenansichten des menschlichen Körpers, 2010).

1 Kidney
2 Ureter
3 Inferior vena cava
4 Abdominal aorta
5 Ovary
6 Uterine tube
7 Uterus
8 Round ligament and inguinal canal
9 Urinary bladder
10 Vagina

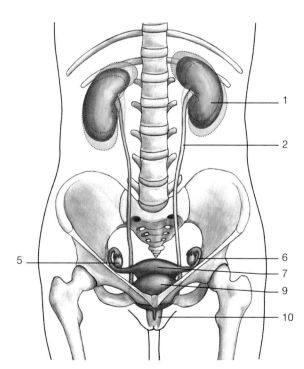

Position of kidneys, urinary and genital organs in the female (anterior aspect, schematic drawing). The excursions of the kidneys with the respiratory movements of the diaphragm are indicated.

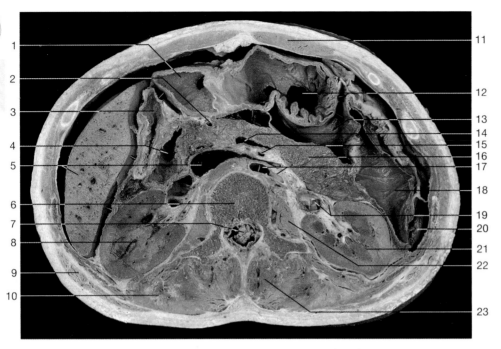

1	Pyloric antrum
2	Gastroduodenal artery
3	Descending part of duodenum
4	Vestibule of lesser sac
5	Inferior vena cava and liver
6	Body of first lumbar vertebra
7	Cauda equina
8	Right kidney
9	Latissimus dorsi muscle
10	Iliocostalis muscle
11	Rectus abdominis muscle
12	Stomach
13	Lesser sac
14	Splenic vein
15	Superior mesenteric artery
16	Pancreas
17	Aorta and left renal artery
18	Transverse colon
19	Renal artery and vein
20	Spleen
21	Left kidney
22	Psoas major muscle
23	Multifidus muscle
24	Margin of lung
25	Margin of pleura
26	Renal pelvis
27	Left ureter
28	Descending colon
29	Rectum
30	Right suprarenal gland
31	Twelfth rib
32	Ascending colon
33	Right ureter
34	Cecum
35	Vermiform appendix
36	Urinary bladder
37	Liver
38	Anterior layer of renal fascia
39	Duodenum
40	Perirenal fatty tissue
41	Posterior layer of renal fascia
42	Abdominal cavity

Horizontal section through the abdominal cavity at the level of the first lumbar vertebra (from below).

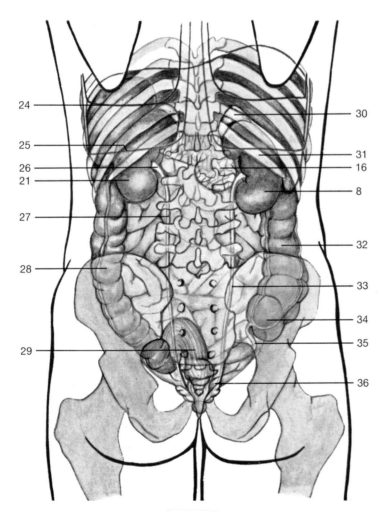

Positions of urinary organs (posterior aspect, schematic drawing). Notice that the upper part of the kidney reaches the level of the margin of pleura and lung.

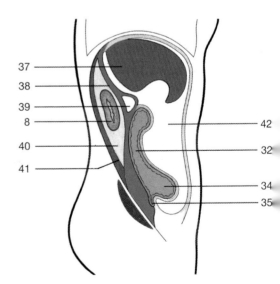

Retroperitoneal tissue, position of the right kidney (schematic drawing).
Yellow = adipose capsule of kidney.

1 Scalenus anterior, medius, and posterior muscles
2 Left subclavian artery
3 Left subclavian vein
4 Pulmonic valve
5 Arterial cone
6 Right ventricle of heart
7 Liver
8 Stomach
9 Transverse colon
10 Small intestine
11 Left lung
12 Left main bronchus
13 Branches of pulmonary vein
14 Left ventricle of heart
15 Spleen
16 Splenic artery and vein and pancreas
17 Left kidney
18 Psoas major muscle
19 Inferior vena cava
20 Renal vein
21 Body of twelfth thoracic vertebra and vertebral canal
22 Right kidney
23 Superior mesenteric artery
24 Superior mesenteric vein
25 Pancreas
26 Abdominal aorta
27 Left psoas major and quadratus lumborum muscles
28 Anterior layer of renal fascia ⎫
29 Posterior layer of renal fascia ⎬ of Gerota
30 Perirenal fatty tissue ⎭
31 Abdominal cavity
32 Descending and sigmoid colon

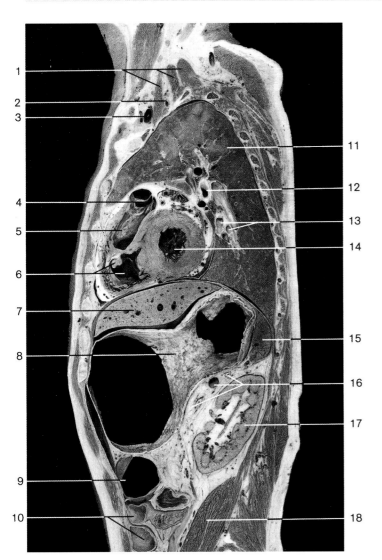

Parasagittal section through the thoracic and abdominal cavities at the level of the left kidney (5.5 cm left of median plane).

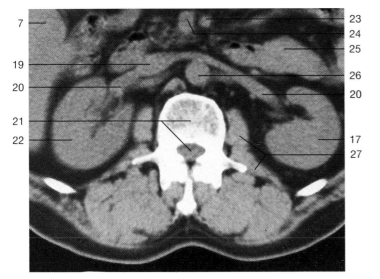

Horizontal section through the retroperitoneal region at the level of 12th thoracic vertebra (CT scan, from below).

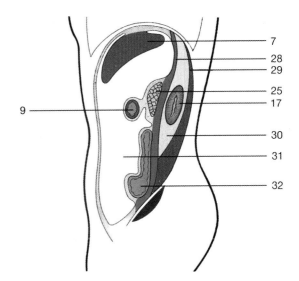

Retroperitoneal tissue, position of the left kidney (schematic drawing).

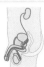

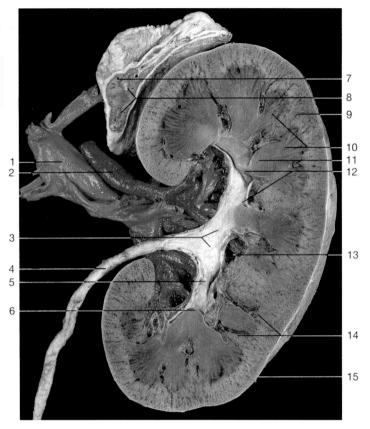

1   Renal vein
2   Renal artery
3   Renal pelvis
4   Abdominal part of ureter
5   Major renal calyx
6   Cribriform area of renal papilla
7   Cortex of suprarenal gland
8   Medulla of suprarenal gland
9   Cortex of kidney
10 Medulla of kidney
11 Renal papilla
12 Minor renal calyx
13 Renal sinus
14 Renal columns
15 Fibrous capsule of kidney

Coronal section through right kidney and suprarenal gland (posterior aspect). The renal pelvis has been opened and the fatty tissue removed to display the renal vessels.

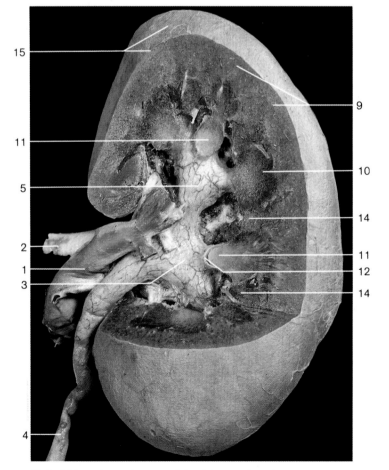

Each kidney can be divided into five segments supplied by individual interlobar arteries known as end arteries. Thus, obstruction leads to infarcts marking the trace of segment borders. The anterior kidney surface reveals four segments; the posterior, only three (Nos. 1, 4, and 5).

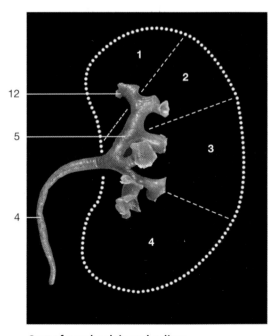

Right kidney (posterior aspect). Partial coronal section to expose internal aspect of the kidney.

Cast of renal pelvis and calices.
1–4 = Renal segments on anterior surface.

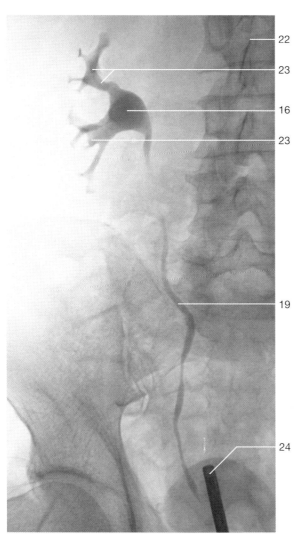

1 Hepatic vein
2 Anterior and posterior vagal trunk
3 Inferior vena cava
4 Lumbar part of diaphragm
5 Right greater and lesser splanchnic nerves
6 Celiac trunk
7 Celiac ganglion and plexus
8 Superior mesenteric artery
9 Left renal vein
10 Right sympathetic trunk and ganglion
11 Abdominal aorta
12 Left sympathetic trunk
13 Esophagus (cut),
   left greater splanchnic nerve
14 Left suprarenal gland
15 Left renal artery
16 Renal pelvis
17 Renal papilla with minor calyx
18 Left testicular vein
19 Ureter
20 Psoas major muscle
21 Quadratus lumborum muscle
22 Lumbar vertebra (L$_2$)
23 Renal calyx
24 Catheter

Renal pelvis with calices and ureter (X-ray, retrograde injection; by courtesy of Prof. Herrlinger, Fürth, Germany).

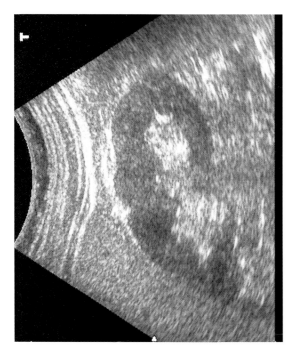

Right kidney (ultrasound image; by courtesy of Prof. Herrlinger, Fürth, Germany).

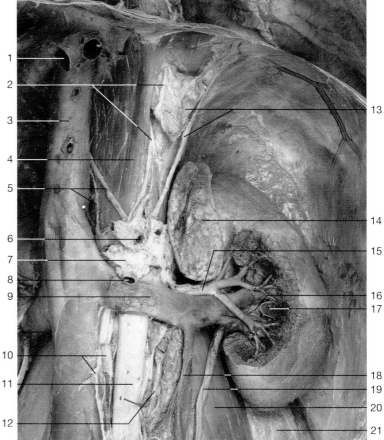

Left kidney and suprarenal gland in situ. The anterior cortical layer of the kidney has been removed to display the renal pelvis and papillae.

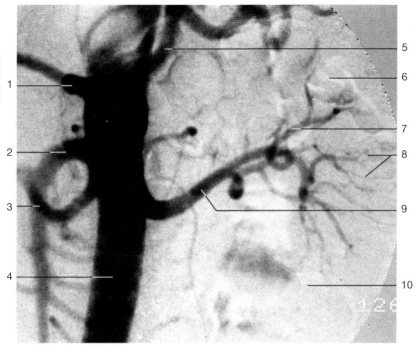

1	Celiac trunk
2	Superior mesenteric artery
3	Middle colic artery
4	Abdominal aorta (with catheter)
5	Splenic artery
6	Upper pole of kidney
7	Anterior branch of renal artery
8	Interlobular arteries
9	Left renal artery
10	Lower pole of kidney
11	Body of first lumbar vertebra
12	Posterior branch of renal artery
13	Anterior inferior segmental artery
14	Superior suprarenal artery
15	Upper capsular artery
16	Perforating artery
17	Lower capsular artery
18	Ureter
19	Right inferior phrenic artery
20	Left inferior phrenic artery
21	Middle suprarenal artery
22	Inferior suprarenal artery
23	Renal artery
24	Left testicular (or ovarian) artery
25	Inferior mesenteric artery

Abdominal aorta (subtraction angiography).

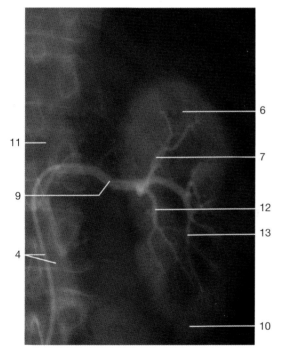

Left kidney (arteriography).

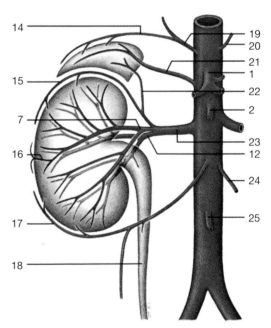

Arteries of kidney and suprarenal gland (schematic drawing).

The kidneys are perfused by app. 1.500–1.800 l of blood per day via the renal arteries. Out of more than 1.2 million renal corpuscles (glomeruli), 1% of this volume (id 150–180 l) is filtered as a cell free fluid. In the tubular system, 99% of this fluid, together with useful substances like glucose and ions, are reabsorbed. Only 1–1.5 l of urine containing waste material is excreted.

Diseases of the renal vascular system may impair the filtering process and thereby the composition of the blood.

1 Diaphragm
2 Hepatic veins
3 Inferior vena cava
4 Common hepatic artery
5 Suprarenal gland
6 Celiac trunk
7 Right renal vein
8 Kidney
9 Abdominal aorta
10 Subcostal nerve
11 Iliohypogastric nerve
12 Central tendon of
   diaphragm
13 Inferior phrenic artery
14 Cardic part of stomach
15 Spleen
16 Splenic artery
17 Superior renal artery
18 Superior mesenteric artery
19 Psoas major muscle
20 Inferior mesenteric artery
21 Ureter
22 Glomerulus
23 Afferent arteriole of
   glomerulus
24 Glomeruli
25 Radiating cortical artery
26 Subcortical or arcuate artery
27 Subcortical or arcuate vein
28 Interlobular vein
29 Interlobular artery
30 Interlobar artery and vein
31 Vessels of renal capsule
32 Efferent arteriole of glomerulus
33 Vasa recta of renal medulla
34 Spiral arteries of renal pelvis

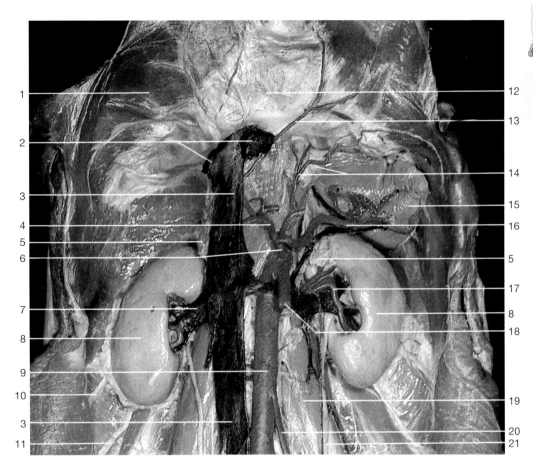

Retroperitoneal organs, kidneys, and suprarenal glands in situ (anterior aspect).
Red = arteries; blue = veins.

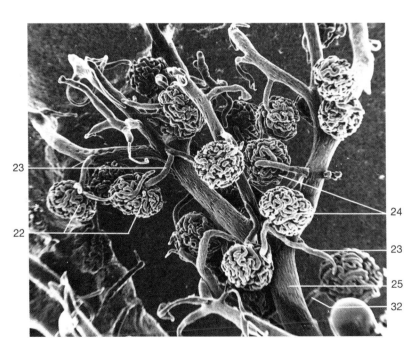

Glomeruli (210 ×). Scanning electron micrograph showing glomeruli
and associated arteries.

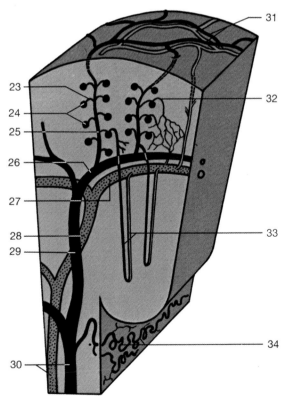

Architecture of vascular system of kidney
(schematic drawing).

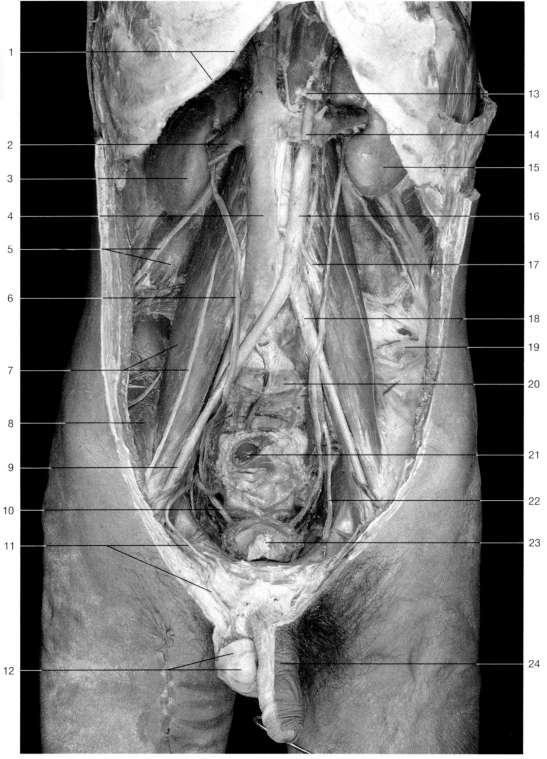

Retroperitoneal organs, urinary system in the male (anterior aspect). The peritoneum has been removed.

1	Costal arch	8	Iliacus muscle	17	Inferior mesenteric artery
2	Right renal vein	9	External iliac artery	18	Common iliac artery
3	Right kidney	10	Ureter (pelvic part)	19	Iliac crest
4	Inferior vena cava	11	Ductus deferens	20	Sacral promontory
5	Iliohypogastric nerve and quadratus lumborum muscle	12	Testis and epididymis	21	Rectum (cut)
6	Ureter (abdominal part)	13	Celiac trunk	22	Medial umbilical ligament
7	Psoas major muscle and genitofemoral nerve	14	Superior mesenteric artery	23	Urinary bladder
		15	Left kidney	24	Penis
		16	Abdominal aorta		

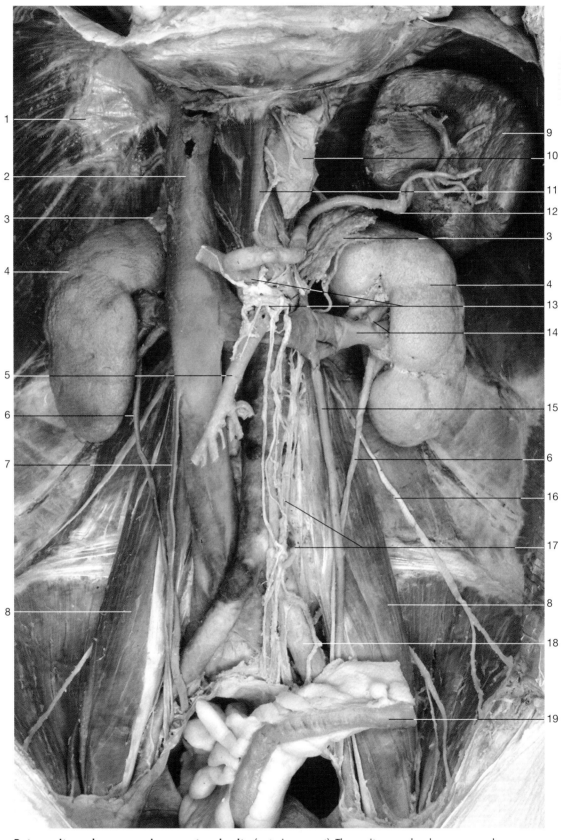

Retroperitoneal organs, urinary system in situ (anterior aspect). The peritoneum has been removed. Note the autonomic plexus and ganglia at the abdominal aorta.

1	Diaphragm	7	Right spermatic vein	11	Abdominal aorta	16	Ilio-inguinal nerve
2	Inferior vena cava	8	Psoas major	12	Splenic artery	17	Superior hypogastric
3	Suprarenal gland		muscle	13	Celiac trunk and		plexus and ganglion
4	Kidney	9	Spleen		celiac ganglion	18	Left common iliac
5	Superior mesenteric artery	10	Cardiac part of	14	Renal artery and vein		artery
6	Ureter		stomach	15	Left spermatic vein	19	Sigmoid colon

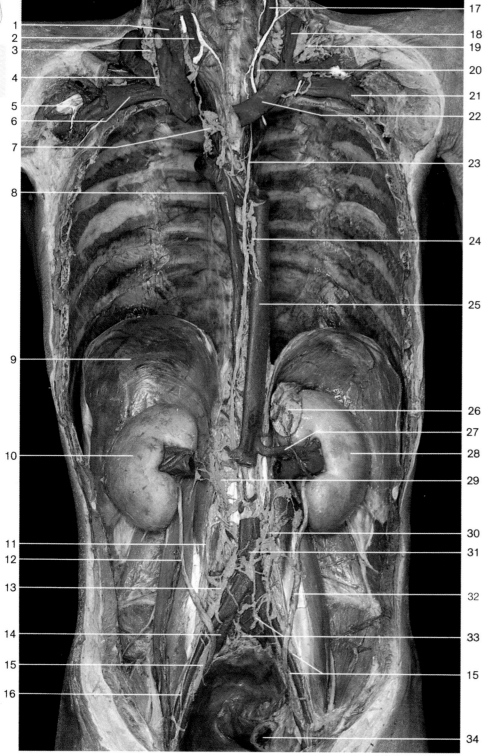

Lymph vessels and lymph nodes of the posterior wall of thoracic and abdominal cavities
(anterior aspect). Green = lymph vessels and nodes; blue = veins; red = arteries; white = nerves.

1 Internal jugular vein	9 Diaphragm	18 Internal jugular vein	27 Left renal artery
2 Right common carotid artery and right vagus nerve	10 Right kidney	19 Deep cervical lymph nodes	28 Left kidney
	11 Right lumbar trunk	20 Thoracic duct entering left jugular angle	29 Cisterna chyli
3 Jugulo-omohyoid lymph node	12 Right ureter		30 Lumbar lymph nodes
	13 Common iliac lymph nodes	21 Left subclavian vein	31 Abdominal aorta
4 Right lymphatic duct	14 Right internal iliac artery	22 Left brachiocephalic vein	32 Left ureter
5 Subclavian trunk	15 External iliac lymph nodes	23 Thoracic duct	33 Sacral lymph nodes
6 Right subclavian vein	16 Right external iliac artery	24 Mediastinal lymph nodes	34 Rectum (cut edge)
7 Bronchomediastinal trunk	17 Left common carotid artery and left vagus nerve	25 Thoracic aorta	
8 Azygos vein		26 Left suprarenal gland	

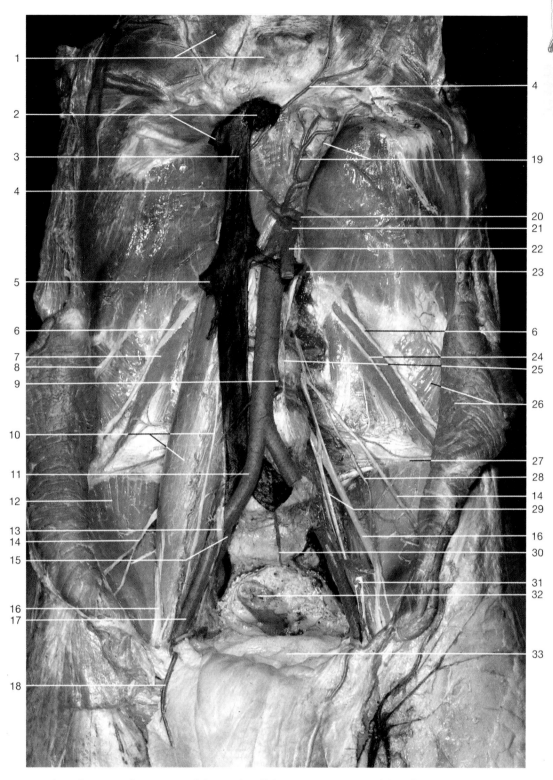

Vessels and nerves of posterior abdominal wall (anterior aspect). Part of the left psoas major muscle has been removed to display the lumbar plexus. Red = arteries; blue = veins.

1	Diaphragm	11	Common iliac artery	20	Splenic artery	31	Psoas major muscle
2	Hepatic veins	12	Iliacus muscle	21	Celiac trunk		(divided) with supplying
3	Inferior vena cava	13	Right ureter (divided)	22	Superior mesenteric artery		artery
4	Inferior phrenic artery	14	Lateral femoral cutaneous nerve	23	Left renal artery	32	Rectum (cut)
5	Right renal vein	15	Internal iliac artery	24	Ilio-inguinal nerve	33	Urinary bladder
6	Iliohypogastric nerve	16	Femoral nerve	25	Sympathetic trunk		
7	Quadratus lumborum muscle	17	External iliac artery	26	Transversus abdominis muscle		
8	Subcostal nerve	18	Inferior epigastric artery	27	Iliac crest		
9	Inferior mesenteric artery	19	Cardiac part of stomach and	28	Left genitofemoral nerve		
10	Right genitofemoral nerve		esophageal branches of left	29	Left obturator nerve		
	and psoas major muscle		gastric artery	30	Median sacral artery		

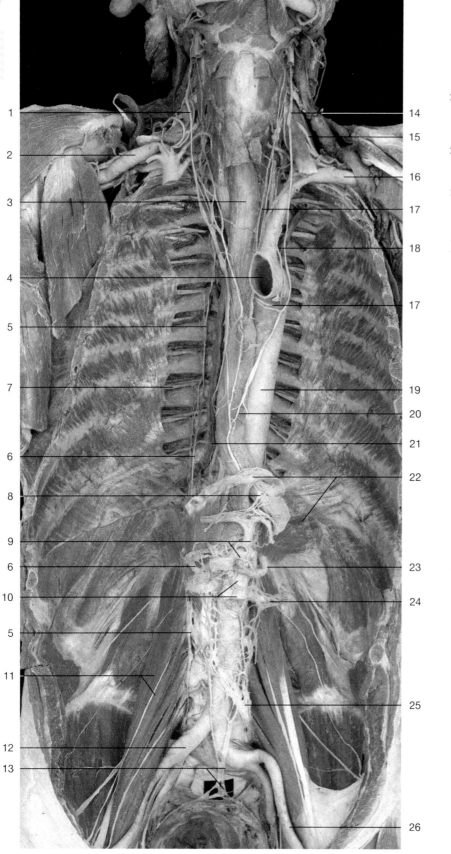

Posterior wall of thoracic and abdominal cavities with sympathetic trunk, vagus nerve, and autonomic ganglia (anterior aspect). Thoracic and abdominal organs removed, except for the esophagus and aorta.

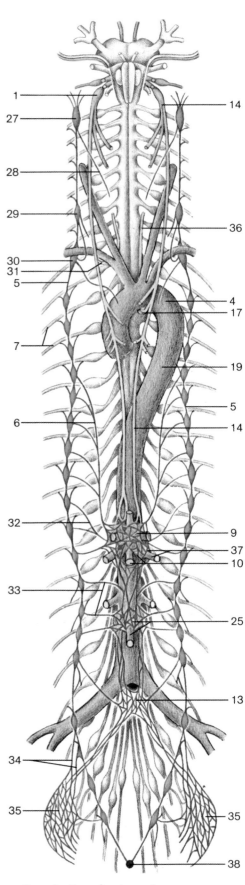

Organization of autonomic nervous system (after Mattuschka). (Schematic drawing.) Yellow = parasympathetic nerves; green = sympathetic nerves.

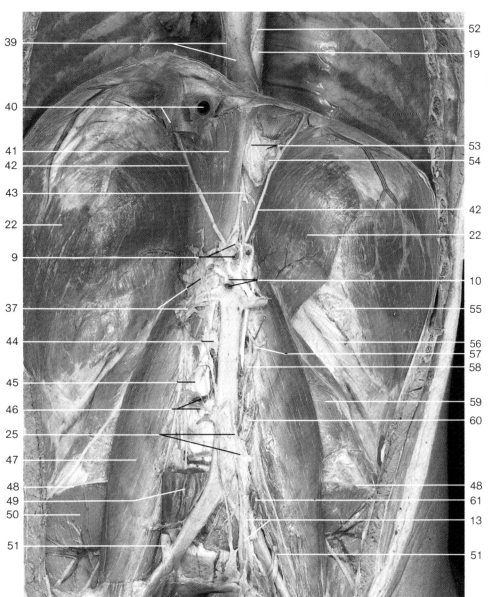

Ganglia and plexus of the autonomic nervous system within the retroperitoneal space (anterior aspect). The kidneys and the inferior vena cava with its tributaries have been removed.

1 Right vagus nerve
2 Right subclavian artery
3 Esophagus
4 Aortic arch
5 Sympathetic trunk
6 Greater splanchnic nerve
7 Intercostal nerve
8 Abdominal part of esophagus and vagal trunk
9 Celiac trunk with celiac ganglion
10 Superior mesenteric artery and ganglion
11 Psoas major muscle and genitofemoral nerve
12 Common iliac artery
13 Superior hypogastric plexus and ganglion
14 Left vagus nerve
15 Brachial plexus

16 Left subclavian artery
17 Left recurrent laryngeal nerve
18 Inferior cervical cardiac nerve
19 Thoracic aorta
20 Esophageal plexus
21 Azygos vein
22 Diaphragm
23 Splenic artery
24 Left renal artery and plexus
25 Inferior mesenteric ganglion and artery
26 Left external iliac artery
27 Superior cervical ganglion of sympathetic trunk
28 Superior cardiac branch of sympathetic trunk
29 Middle cervical ganglion of sympathetic trunk
30 Inferior cervical ganglion of sympathetic trunk

31 Right recurrent laryngeal nerve
32 Lesser splanchnic nerve
33 Lumbar splanchnic nerves
34 Sacral splanchnic nerves
35 Inferior hypogastric ganglion and plexus
36 Left recurrent laryngeal nerve
37 Aorticorenal plexus and renal artery
38 Ganglion impar
39 Esophagus with branches of vagus nerve
40 Hepatic veins
41 Right crus of diaphragm
42 Inferior phrenic artery
43 Right vagus nerve entering the celiac ganglion
44 Right lumbar lymph trunk
45 Lumbar part of right sympathetic trunk

46 Lumbar artery and vein
47 Psoas major muscle
48 Iliac crest
49 Inferior vena cava
50 Iliacus muscle
51 Ureter
52 Left vagus nerve forming the esophageal plexus
53 Left vagus nerve forming the gastric plexus
54 Esophagus continuing into the cardiac part of stomach
55 Lumbocostal triangle
56 Position of twelfth rib
57 Left lumbar lymph trunk
58 Ganglion of sympathetic trunk
59 Quadratus lumborum muscle
60 Lumbar part of left sympathetic trunk
61 Iliac lymph vessels

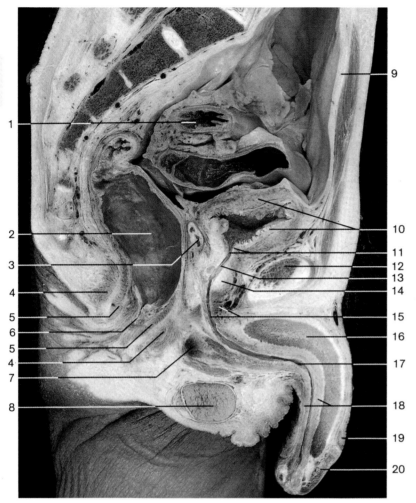

1	Sigmoid colon
2	Ampulla of rectum
3	Ampulla of ductus deferens
4	External anal sphincter muscle
5	Internal anal sphincter muscle
6	Anal canal
7	Bulb of penis
8	Testis (cut surface)
9	Median umbilical ligament
10	Urinary bladder
11	Internal urethral orifice and sphincter
12	Pubic symphysis
13	Prostatic part of urethra
14	Prostate gland
15	Membranous part of urethra and external urethral sphincter
16	Corpus cavernosum of penis
17	Spongy urethra
18	Corpus spongiosum of penis
19	Foreskin or prepuce
20	Glans penis
21	Kidney
22	Renal pelvis
23	Abdominal part of ureter
24	Pelvic part of ureter
25	Seminal vesicle
26	Ejaculatory duct
27	Bulbo-urethral or Cowper's gland
28	Ductus deferens
29	Epididymis
30	Umbilicus
31	Trigone of bladder and ureteric orifice
32	Navicular fossa of urethra
33	External urethral orifice
34	Testis

Male urogenital system, midsagittal section through the pelvis.

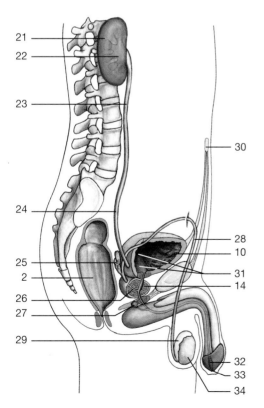

Male urogenital system (schematic drawing).

The **prostate** is located between the bladder and urogenital diaphragm. The penis includes the **urethra** and thus serves for both ejaculation and micturition. The internal (involuntary) and external (voluntary) urethral sphincters are widely separated. The **ureter,** having crossed the ductus deferens, enters the urinary bladder at its base. The peritoneum is reflected off of the posterior surface of the bladder and onto the rectum, thus forming the rectovesical pouch.

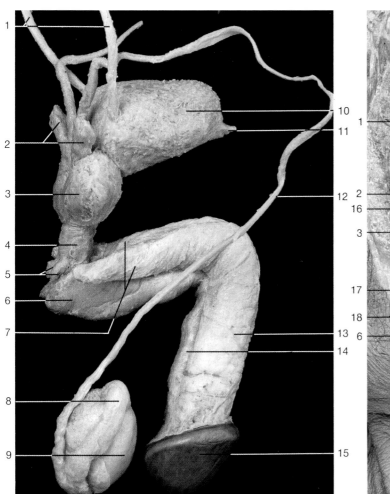

Male genital organs, isolated (right lateral aspect).

Male genital organs in situ (right lateral aspect).

Positions of male genital organs (right lateral aspect).
(Schematic drawing.)

1   Ureter
2   Seminal vesicle
3   Prostate gland
4   Urogenital diaphragm and membranous part of urethra
5   Bulbo-urethral or Cowper's gland
6   Bulb of penis
7   Left and right crus penis
8   Epididymis
9   Testis
10 Urinary bladder
11 Apex of urinary bladder
12 Ductus deferens
13 Corpus cavernosum of penis
14 Corpus spongiosum of penis
15 Glans penis
16 Ampulla of rectum
17 Levator ani muscle
18 Anal canal and external anal sphincter muscle
19 Spermatic cord (cut)
20 Sacral promontory
21 Sigmoid colon
22 Peritoneum (cut edge)
23 Rectovesical pouch
24 Ejaculatory duct
25 Lateral umbilical fold
26 Medial umbilical fold
27 Deep inguinal ring and ductus deferens
28 Pubic symphysis
29 Prostatic part of urethra
30 Spongy urethra

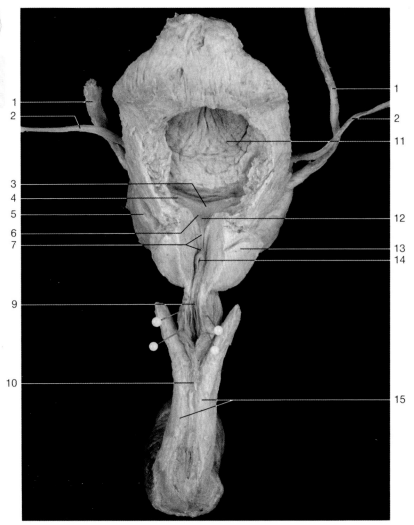

1	Ureter
2	Ductus deferens
3	Interureteric fold
4	Ureteric orifice
5	Seminal vesicle
6	Trigone of bladder
7	Prostatic urethra with seminal colliculus and urethral crest
8	Deep transverse perineal muscle
9	Membranous urethra
10	Spongy urethra
11	Mucous membrane of urinary bladder
12	Internal urethral orifice and uvula of bladder
13	Prostate
14	Prostatic utricle
15	Right and left corpus cavernosum of penis
16	Ejaculatory duct
17	Sphincter urethrae muscle
18	Median umbilical fold with remnant of urachus
19	Medial umbilical fold with remnant of umbilical artery
20	Urinary bladder
21	Rectovesical pouch
22	Rectum
23	Sacrum
24	Deep iliac circumflex artery
25	Deep inguinal ring and ductus deferens
26	External iliac artery and vein
27	Femoral nerve
28	Obturator nerve and internal iliac artery
29	Ilium and sacrum
30	Inferior epigastric artery
31	Iliopsoas muscle

Male urogenital organs, isolated (anterior aspect). Urinary bladder, prostate, and urethra have been opened. The urinary bladder is contracted.

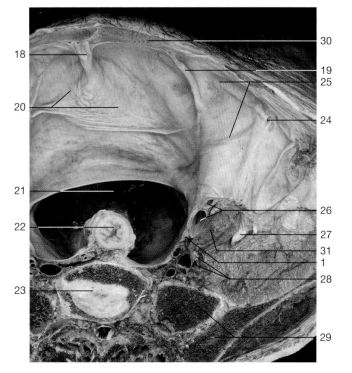

Pelvic cavity in the male (viewed from above).

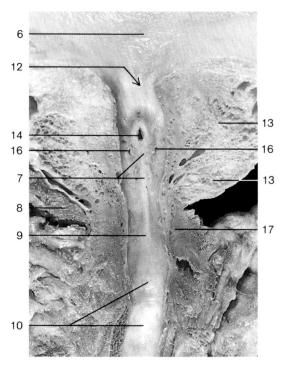

Posterior half of male urethra and prostate in continuity with neck of bladder (anterior aspect).

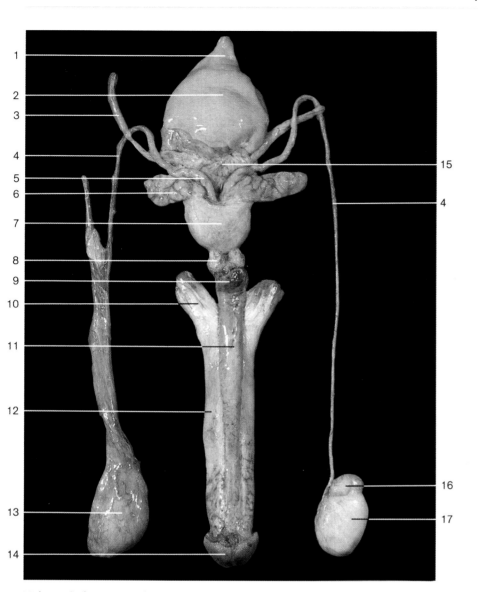

1   Apex of urinary bladder with urachus
2   Urinary bladder
3   Ureter
4   Ductus deferens
5   Ampulla of ductus deferens
6   Seminal vesicle
7   Prostate
8   Bulbo-urethral or Cowper's gland
9   Bulb of penis
10 Crus penis
11 Corpus spongiosum of penis
12 Corpus cavernosum of penis
13 Testis and epididymis with coverings
14 Glans penis
15 Fundus of bladder
16 Head of epididymis
17 Testis
18 Mucous membrane of bladder
19 Trigone of bladder
20 Ureteric orifice
21 Internal urethral orifice
22 Seminal colliculus
23 Prostate
24 Prostatic urethra
25 Membranous urethra
26 Spongy (penile) urethra
27 Skin of penis
28 Deep dorsal vein of penis (unpaired)
29 Dorsal artery of penis (paired)
30 Tunica albuginea of corpora cavernosa
31 Septum of penis
32 Deep artery of penis
33 Tunica albuginea of corpus spongiosum
34 Deep fascia of penis

Male genital organs, isolated (posterior aspect).

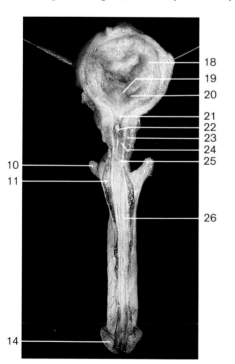

Urinary bladder, urethra, and penis
(anterior aspect, opened longitudinally).

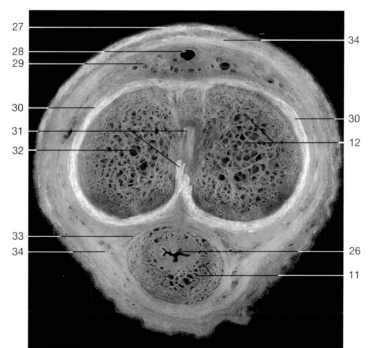

Cross section of penis (inferior aspect).

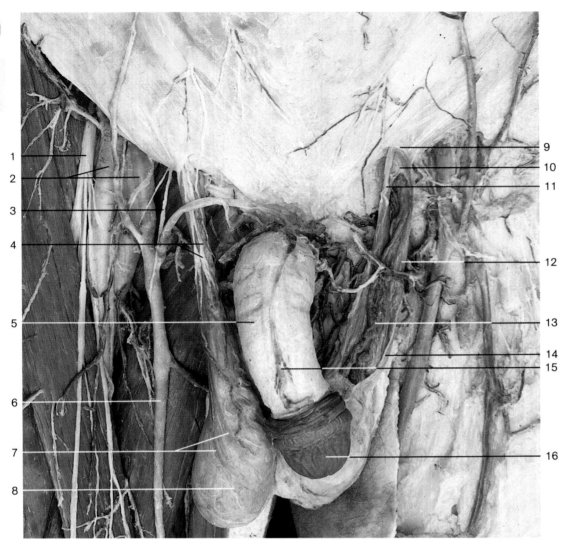

1
2
3
4
5
6
7
8

9
10
11
12
13
14
15
16

Male external genital organs with penis, testis, and spermatic cord, superficial layers (anterior aspect).

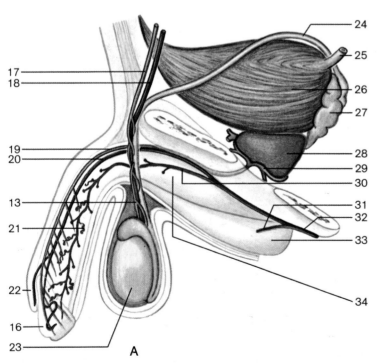

17
18
19
20
13
21
22
16
23

24
25
26
27
28
29
30
31
32
33
34

A

Vessels of male genital organs (schematic drawing).
A = lateral aspect; B = cross section of penis.

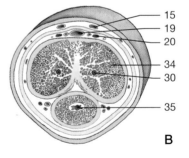

15
19
20
34
30
35

B

1 Femoral nerve
2 Femoral artery and vein
3 Femoral branch of genitofemoral nerve
4 Spermatic cord with genital branch
   of genitofemoral nerve
5 Penis with deep fascia
6 Great saphenous vein
7 Cremaster muscle
8 Testis with cremaster muscle
9 Superficial inguinal ring
10 Internal spermatic fascia (cut edge)
11 Ilio-inguinal nerve
12 Left spermatic cord
13 Pampiniform venous plexus
14 External spermatic fascia
15 Superficial dorsal vein of penis

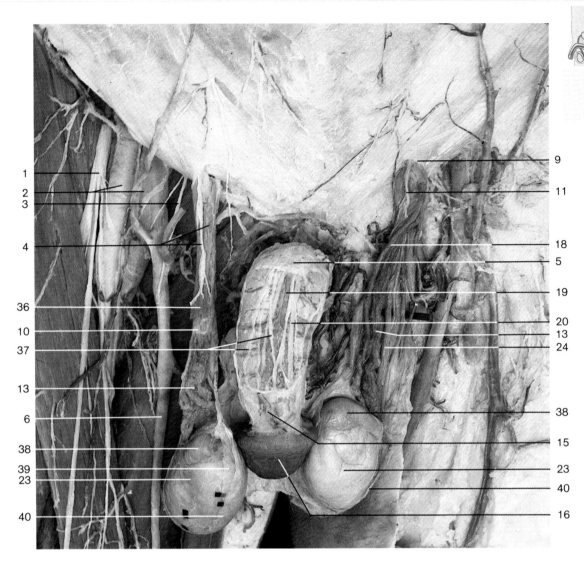

Male external genital organs with penis, testis, and spermatic cord, deeper layers (anterior aspect).
The deep fascia of the penis has been opened to display the dorsal nerves and vessels.

16 Glans penis
17 Testicular vein
18 Testicular artery
19 Deep dorsal vein of penis
20 Dorsal artery of penis
21 Helicine arteries
22 Prepuce
23 Testis with tunica albuginea
24 Ductus deferens
25 Ureter
26 Urinary bladder
27 Seminal vesicle
28 Prostate
29 Vesicoprostatic venous plexus
30 Deep artery of penis
31 Artery of bulb of penis
32 Internal pudendal artery
33 Corpus spongiosum of penis
34 Corpus cavernosum of penis
35 Urethra
36 Cremasteric fascia with cremaster muscle
37 Dorsal nerve of penis
38 Epididymis
39 Tunica vaginalis (visceral layer)
40 Tunica vaginalis (parietal layer)
41 Testis with vascular loops

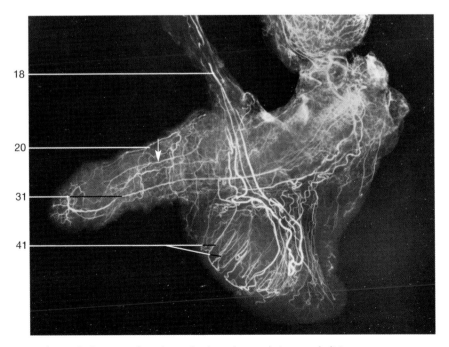

Male genital organs (arteriography, lateral aspect). Arrow = helicine artery.

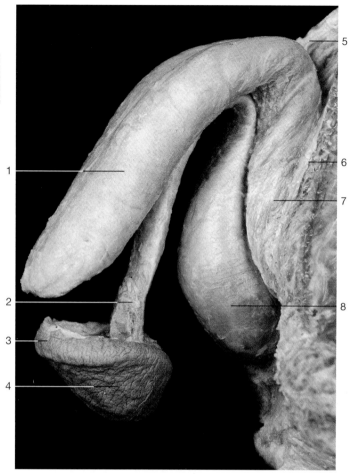

Male external genital organs (lateral aspect). The corpus spongiosum of the penis with the glans penis has been isolated and reflected.

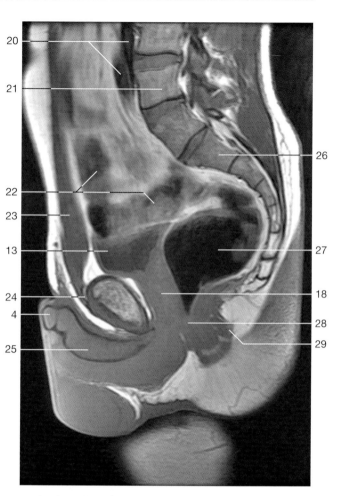

Sagittal section of the pelvic cavity with the male genital organs (MRI scan; from Heuck et al., MRT-Atlas, 2009).

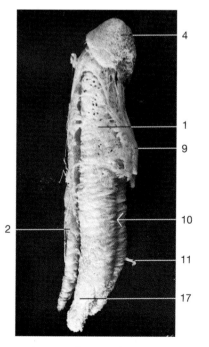

Resin cast of erected penis.

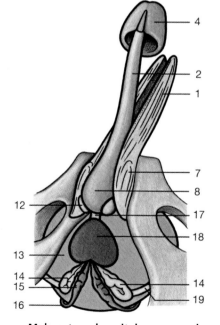

Male external genital organs and accessory glands (schematic drawing).

1 Corpus cavernosum of penis
2 Corpus spongiosum of penis
3 Corona of glans penis
4 Glans penis
5 Suspensory ligament of penis
6 Inferior pubic ramus
7 Crus penis
8 Bulb of penis
9 Deep dorsal vein of penis
10 Septum pectiniforme
11 Dorsal artery of penis
12 Bulbo-urethral or Cowper's gland
13 Urinary bladder
14 Seminal vesicle
15 Ampulla of ductus deferens
16 Ductus deferens
17 Membranous urethra
18 Prostate
19 Ureter
20 Common iliac artery and vein
21 Fifth lumbar vertebral body
22 Intestinal loops
23 Rectus abdominis muscle
24 Pubic symphysis
25 Root of penis
26 Sacral bone
27 Ampulla of rectum
28 Anal canal
29 External anal sphincter muscle

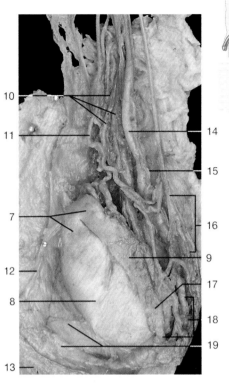

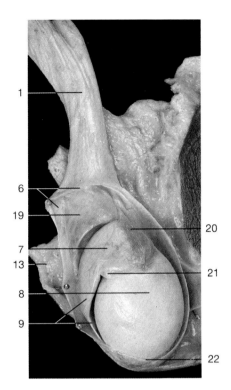

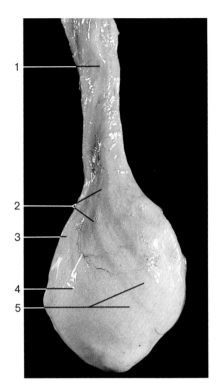

Testis and epididymis with investing layers (lateral aspect).

Testis and epididymis (lateral aspect). The tunica vaginalis has been opened.

Testis, epididymis, and spermatic cord (left side, posterolateral aspect). Dissection of spermatic cord and ductus deferens.

1	Spermatic cord covered with cremasteric fascia
2	Cremaster muscle
3	Position of epididymis
4	Internal spermatic fascia
5	Position of testis
6	Internal spermatic fascia with adjacent investing layers of testis (cut surface)
7	Head of epididymis

8	Testis with tunica vaginalis (visceral layer)
9	Body of epididymis
10	Pampiniform venous plexus (anterior veins)
11	Testicular artery
12	Tunica vaginalis (parietal layer, cut edge)
13	Skin and dartos muscle (reflected)
14	Ductus deferens

15	Artery of ductus deferens
16	Posterior veins of pampiniform plexus
17	Tail of epididymis
18	Transition of epididymal duct to ductus deferens and venous plexus
19	Parietal layer of tunica vaginalis
20	Appendix of epididymis
21	Appendix of testis
22	Gubernaculum testis

Longitudinal section through testis and epididymis. The left figure shows the testicular septa after removal of the seminiferous tubules.

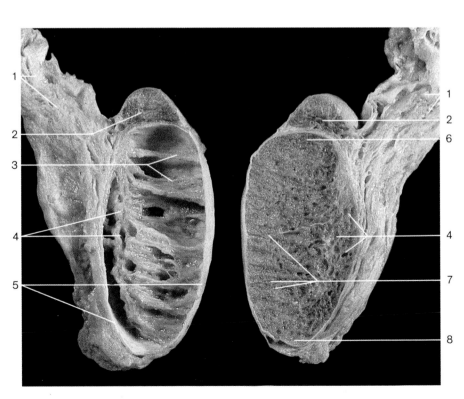

1	Spermatic cord (cut surface)
2	Head of epididymis (cut surface)
3	Septa of testis
4	Mediastinum testis
5	Tunica albuginea
6	Superior pole of testis
7	Convoluted seminiferous tubules
8	Inferior pole of testis

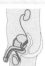

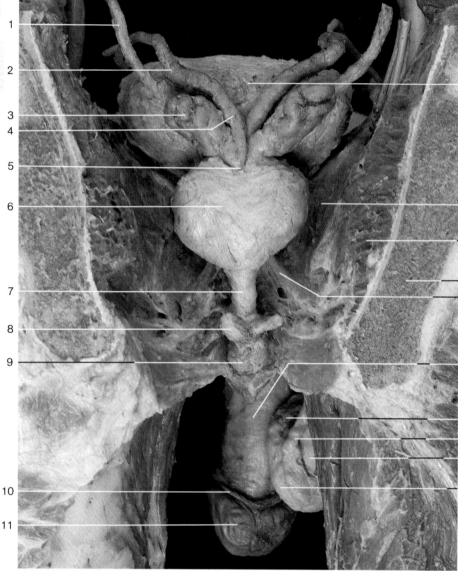

1 Ureter
2 Ductus deferens
3 Seminal vesicle
4 Ampulla of ductus deferens
5 Ejaculatory duct
   (proximal portion)
6 Prostate
7 Membranous urethra
8 Bulbo-urethral or Cowper's
   gland
9 Bulb of penis
10 Penis
11 Glans penis
12 Urinary bladder
13 Levator ani muscle
14 Obturator internus muscle
15 Pelvic bone (cut edge)
16 Puboprostatic ligament
17 Corpus spongiosum
   of penis
18 Head of epididymis
19 Beginning of ductus
   deferens
20 Testis
21 Tail of epididymis
22 Corpus cavernosum of penis
23 Spermatic cord
24 Pectineus and adductor
   muscles
25 Pubic bone
26 Prostatic part of urethra
   (seminal colliculus)
27 Rectum
28 Sciatic nerve
29 Great saphenous vein
30 Sartorius muscle
31 Femoral artery and vein
32 Rectus femoris muscle
33 Tensor fasciae latae muscle
34 Pectineus muscle
35 Iliopsoas muscle
36 Vastus lateralis muscle
37 Obturator externus muscle
38 Femur
39 Ischial tuberosity
40 Gluteus maximus muscle

Accessory glands of male genital organs in situ. Coronal section through the pelvic cavity. Posterior aspect of urinary bladder, prostate, and seminal vesicles.

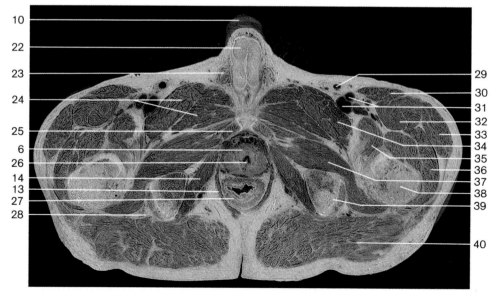

Horizontal section through pelvic cavity at the level of prostate.

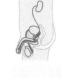

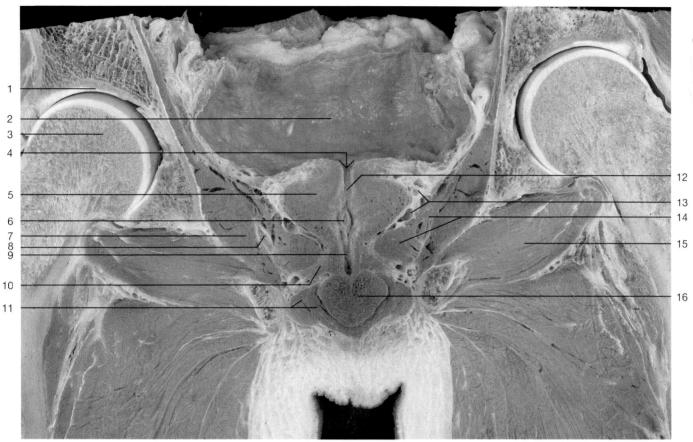

Coronal section through pelvic cavity at the level of prostate and hip joint (anterior aspect).

1	Acetabulum of hip joint	10	Deep transverse perineus muscle	19	Seminal vesicle
2	Urinary bladder	11	Crus penis and ischiocavernosus muscle	20	Internal anal sphincter muscle
3	Head of femur	12	Prostatic part of urethra	21	External anal sphincter muscle
4	Internal urethral orifice	13	Prostatic plexus	22	Anus
5	Prostate	14	Levator ani muscle	23	Psoas major muscle
6	Seminal colliculus	15	Obturator externus muscle	24	Intervertebral disc
7	Obturator internus muscle	16	Bulb of penis	25	Ilium
8	Ischiorectal fossa	17	Ampulla of rectum	26	Ligament of the head of the femur
9	Membranous urethra	18	Anal canal	27	Sacral promontory

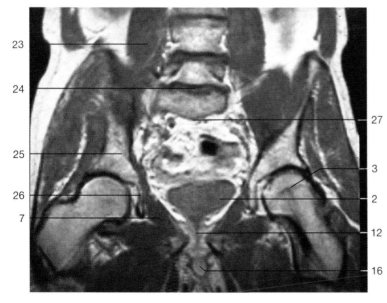

Coronal section through pelvic cavity (MRI scan).

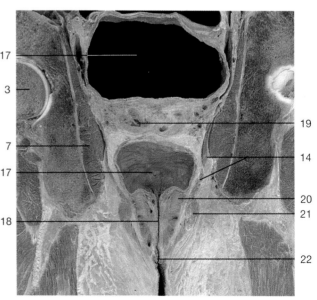

Coronal section through anal canal.

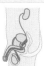

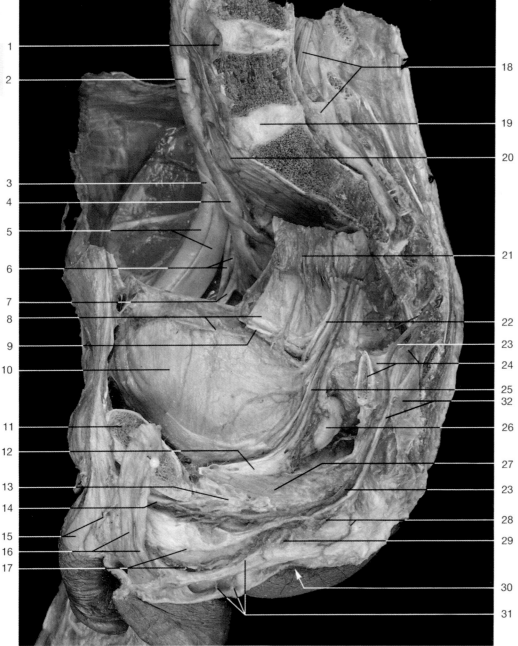

Pelvic cavity in the male (right half of parasagittal section). The arteries have been injected with red resin. The parietal layer of peritoneum has been removed. The urinary bladder is filled to a great extent.

1 Left common iliac artery	18 Cauda equina and dura mater (divided)
2 Right common iliac artery	19 Intervertebral disc between fifth
3 Right ureter	lumbar vertebra and sacrum
4 Right internal iliac artery	20 Sacral promontory
5 Right external iliac artery and vein	21 Mesosigmoid
6 Right obturator artery and nerve	22 Left ureter
7 Umbilical artery	23 Left internal pudendal artery
8 Sigmoid and superior vesical artery	24 Ischial spine (cut), sacrospinal ligament,
9 Left ductus deferens	inferior gluteal artery
10 Urinary bladder	25 Left inferior vesical artery
11 Pubic bone (cut)	26 Seminal vesicle
12 Prostate	27 Levator ani muscle
13 Vesicoprostatic venous plexus	28 Branches of inferior rectal artery
14 Deep dorsal vein of penis and	29 Perineal artery
dorsal artery of penis	30 Anus
15 Penis and superficial dorsal vein	31 Posterior scrotal branches
16 Spermatic cord and testicular artery	32 Pudendal nerve and sacrotuberal ligament
17 Bulb of penis and deep artery of penis	

1 Internal iliac artery
2 External iliac artery
3 Ureter
4 Obturator nerve
5 Umbilical artery
6 Anulus inguinalis profundus
(deep inguinal ring)
7 Urinary bladder (vesica urinaria)
8 Symphysis
9 Prostatic part of urethra
10 Sphincter muscle of urethra
11 Urethra (spongy part)
12 Cavernous body of penis
13 Glans penis
14 Sacrum
15 Promontory
16 Lateral sacral artery
17 Plexus sacralis
18 Inferior gluteal artery
19 Internal pudendal artery
20 Obturator artery
21 Inferior hypogastric plexus
22 Ductus deferens
23 Seminal vesicle (vesicula seminalis)
24 Rectum
25 Prostatic venous plexus
26 Prostate
27 Anal canal
28 Spongy part of penis
29 Pampiniform plexus
30 Testis and epididymis
31 Common iliac artery
32 Umbilical artery
33 Medial umbilical ligament
34 Branches of superior vesical artery
35 Urogenital diaphragm
36 Deep artery of penis
37 Dorsal artery of penis
38 Penis
39 Iliolumbar artery
40 Superior gluteal artery
41 Middle rectal artery
42 Levator ani muscle
43 Inferior rectal artery
44 Inferior vesical artery

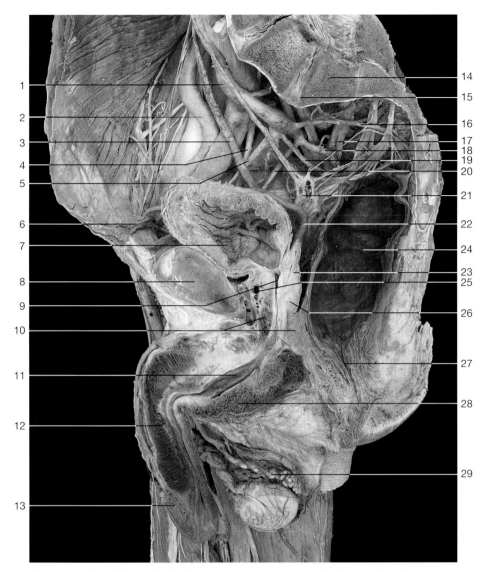

Vessels of the pelvic cavity in the male (medial aspect, midsagittal section). The gluteus maximus muscle has been removed.

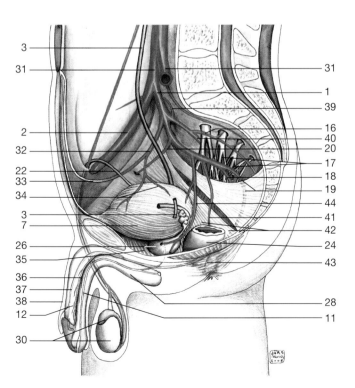

Main branches of internal iliac artery in the male (schematic drawing).

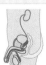

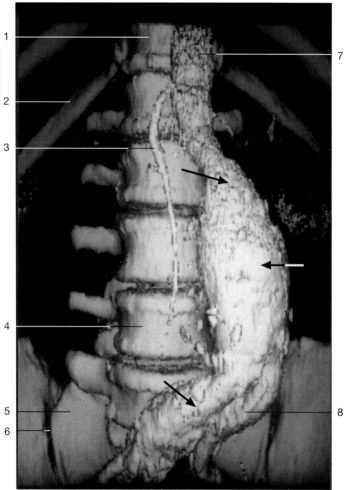

1 Twelfth thoracic vertebra (T$_{12}$)
2 Twelfth rib (rib XII)
3 Inferior mesenteric artery
4 Fourth lumbar vertebra (L$_4$)
5 Sacrum
6 Sacro-iliac articulation
7 Aorta (abdominal part)
8 Left common iliac artery (included into the aneurysm)
9 Aorta with aneurysm
10 Body of lumbar vertebra
11 Intrinsic muscles of the back
12 Thrombotic part of the aneurysm (green)
13 Inferior vena cava (compressed, blue)
14 Iliopsoas muscle
15 Vertebral canal
16 Aneurysm of the aorta (red)

Abdominal part of the aorta showing an infrarenal aneurysm with involvement of both iliac arteries (arrows) (3-D reconstruction, courtesy of Prof. H. Rupprecht and Dr. M. Rexer, Klinikum Fürth, Germany).

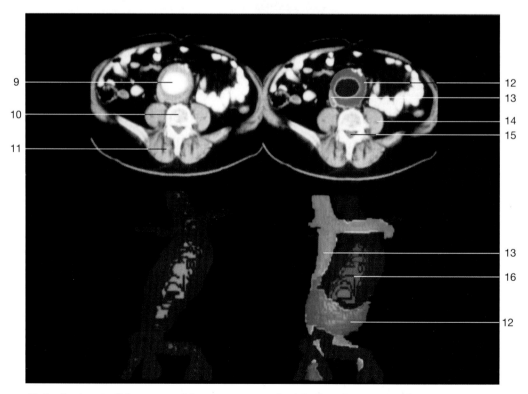

Abdominal part of the aorta with an aneurysm, after injection of contrast medium.
Above = horizontal sections through the abdominal cavity, showing different contrast medium concentrations within the aorta and the aneurysm; below = 3-D reconstruction of the aneurysm; red = aorta; green = thrombotic areas; blue = vein (vena cava inferior, partly compressed).

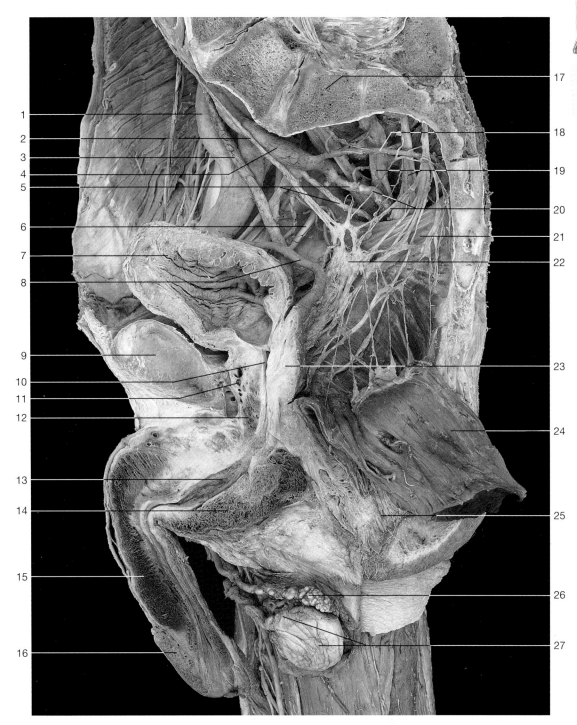

Vessels and nerves of the pelvic cavity in the male (medial aspect, midsagittal section). Rectum reflected to display the inferior hypogastric plexus.

1 External iliac artery	10 Prostatic part of urethra	20 Pelvic splanchnic nerves (nervi erigentes)
2 Right hypogastric nerve	11 Prostatic venous plexus	21 Levator ani muscle
3 Ureter	12 Sphincter urethrae muscle	22 Inferior hypogastric plexus
4 Internal iliac artery	13 Spongy part of urethra	(pelvic plexus)
5 Inferior gluteal artery and internal	14 Corpus spongiosum penis	23 Prostate
pudendal artery	15 Corpus cavernosum penis	24 Rectum (reflected)
6 Obturator artery	16 Glans penis	25 Anal canal and external anal sphincter
7 Urinary bladder	17 Sacrum	26 Pampiniform plexus continuous with
8 Ductus deferens	18 Lateral sacral artery	testicular vein
9 Symphysis pubica	19 Sacral plexus	27 Testis and epididymis

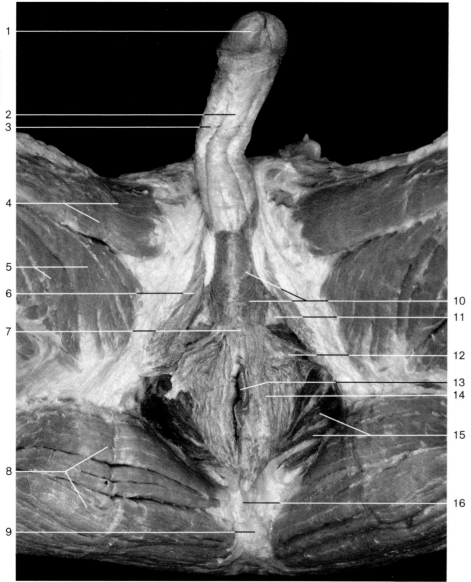

1 Glans penis
2 Corpus spongiosum of penis
3 Corpus cavernosum of penis
4 Gracilis muscle
5 Adductor muscles
6 Ischiocavernosus muscle overlying crus of penis
7 Perineal body
8 Gluteus maximus muscle
9 Coccyx
10 Bulbospongiosus muscle
11 Deep transverse perineus muscle covered by inferior fascia of urogenital diaphragm
12 Superficial transverse perineus muscle
13 Anus
14 External anal sphincter muscle
15 Levator ani muscle
16 Anococcygeal ligament
17 Obturator internus muscle
18 Urethra
19 Deep transverse perineus muscle

Muscles of urogenital and pelvic diaphragms in the male (from below).

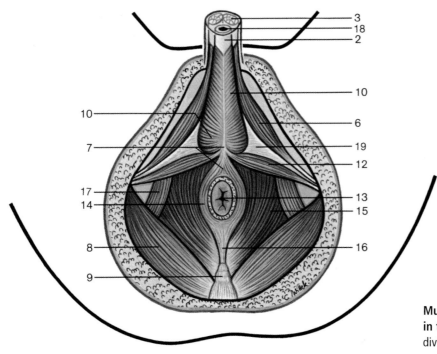

Muscles of urogenital and pelvic diaphragms in the male (from below). The penis has been divided (schematic drawing).

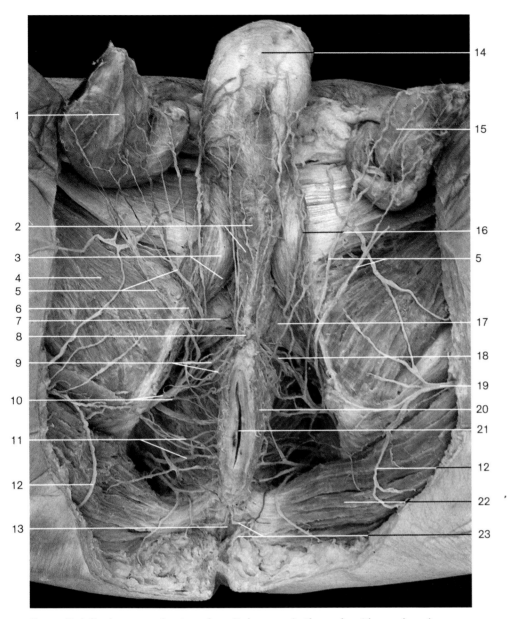

1   Right testis (reflected laterally and upward)
2   Bulbospongiosus muscle
3   Ischiocavernosus muscle
4   Adductor magnus muscle
5   Posterior scrotal nerves and superficial perineal arteries
6   Posterior scrotal artery and vein
7   Right artery of bulb of penis
8   Perineal body
9   Perineal branches of pudendal nerve
10 Pudendal nerve and internal pudendal artery
11 Inferior rectal arteries and nerves
12 Inferior cluneal nerve
13 Coccyx (location)
14 Penis
15 Left testis (reflected laterally)
16 Left posterior scrotal artery
17 Deep transverse perineal muscle
18 Left artery of bulb of penis
19 Posterior femoral cutaneous nerve
20 External anal sphincter muscle
21 Anus
22 Gluteus maximus muscle
23 Anococcygeal nerves
24 Acetabulum (femur removed)
25 Ligament of femoral head
26 Body of ischium (cut)
27 Sciatic nerve
28 Coccygeus muscle
29 Levator ani muscle
      a iliococcygeus muscle
      b pubococcygeus muscle
      c puborectalis muscle
30 Prostatic venous plexus
31 Body of pubis
32 Testis

Urogenital diaphragm and external genital organs in the male with vessels and nerves (from below). The testes have been reflected laterally.

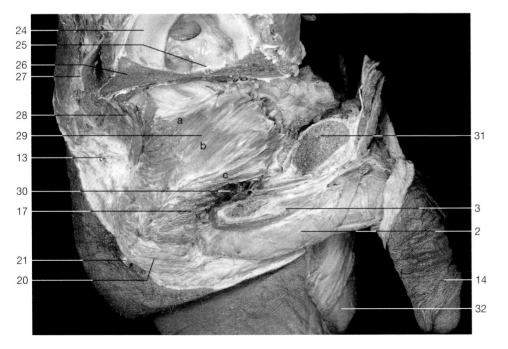

Pelvic diaphragm and external genital organs in the male. The right half of the pelvis including the obturator internus muscle and femur have been removed to display the right half of the levator ani muscle.

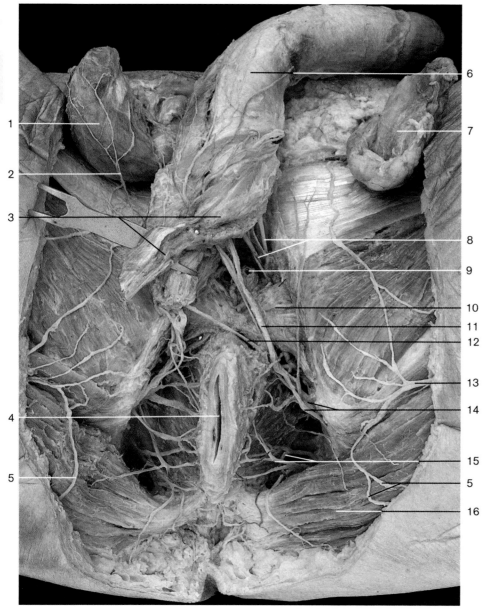

1   Right testis (reflected)
2   Posterior scrotal nerves
3   Left crus penis with ischiocavernosus muscle
4   Anus
5   Inferior cluneal nerves
6   Penis
7   Left testis (reflected)
8   Dorsal artery and nerve of penis
9   Urethra
10 Deep transverse perineus muscle
11 Perineal branch of pudendal nerve
12 Artery of bulb of penis (reflected)
13 Branch of posterior femoral cutaneous nerve
14 Internal pudendal artery and pudendal nerve
15 Inferior rectal arteries and nerves
16 Gluteus maximus muscle
17 Dorsal nerve of penis
18 Posterior femoral cutaneous nerve
19 Perineal branches of pudendal nerve
20 Inferior rectal nerves
21 Bulbospongiosus muscle (inside: dorsal artery of penis)
22 Perineal artery
23 External anal sphincter muscle
24 Inferior rectal artery and veins

Urogenital diaphragm and external genital organs in the male (from below). The left crus penis has been isolated and reflected laterally together with the bulb of the penis. The urethra has been cut.

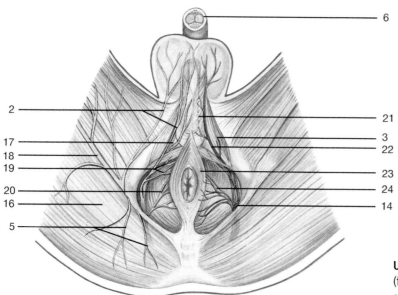

Urogenital and anal region in the male (from below). Right side: nerves; left side: arteries and veins.

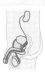

1 Right testis (reflected)
2 Corpus spongiosum of penis
3 Corpus cavernosum of penis
4 Perineal branch of posterior femoral cutaneous nerve
5 Posterior scrotal arteries and nerves
6 Deep artery of penis
7 Deep transverse perineal muscle
8 Right perineal nerves
9 Inferior rectal nerves
10 Inferior cluneal nerve
11 Anococcygeal nerves
12 Left spermatic cord
13 Left testis (cut surface)
14 Dorsal artery and nerve of penis
15 Deep dorsal vein of penis
16 Urethra (cut)
17 Artery of bulb of penis
18 Superficial transverse perineus muscle
19 Left artery of bulb of penis
20 Perineal branch of pudendal nerve
21 Anus
22 External anal sphincter muscle
23 Gluteus maximus muscle
24 Internal pudendal artery and pudendal nerve
25 Sacrotuberous ligament
26 Coccyx
27 Urogenital diaphragm (deep transverse perineus muscle)
28 Tendinous center of perineum (perineal body)
29 Levator ani muscle
30 Anococcygeal ligament
31 Obturator internus muscle
32 Dorsal artery of penis

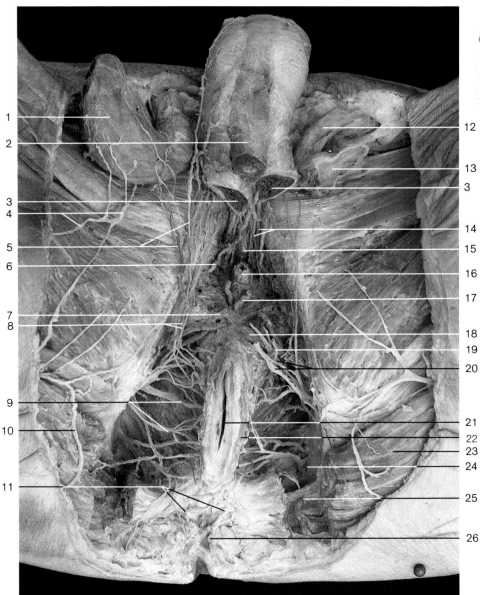

Urogenital diaphragm and external genital organs in the male (from below). The root of the penis has been cut. Dissection of the urogenital diaphragm.

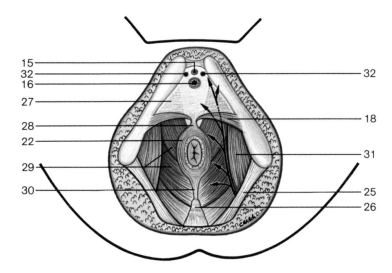

Urogenital and pelvic diaphragms in the male (from below). The penis has been removed. The arrows indicate the course of vessels and nerves (schematic drawing).

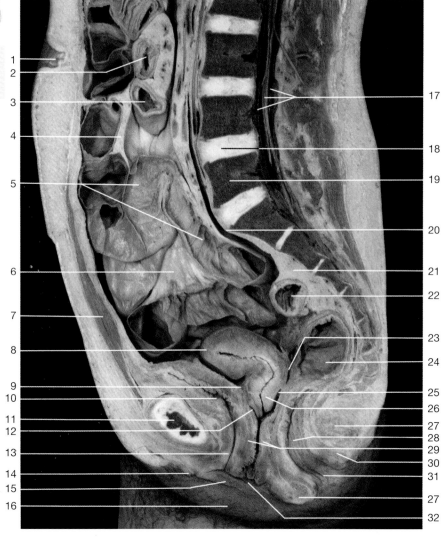

1 Umbilicus
2 Duodenum
3 Ascending part of duodenum
4 Root of mesentery
5 Small intestine
6 Mesentery
7 Rectus abdominis muscle
8 Uterus
9 Vesico-uterine pouch
10 Urinary bladder (collapsed)
11 Pubic symphysis
12 Anterior fornix of vagina
13 Urethra
14 Clitoris
15 Labium minus
16 Labium majus
17 Vertebral canal with cauda equina
18 Intervertebral disc
19 Body of fifth lumbar vertebra
20 Sacral promontory
21 Mesosigmoid
22 Sigmoid colon
23 Recto-uterine pouch
   (of Douglas)
24 Ampulla of rectum
25 Posterior fornix of vagina
26 Cervix of uterus
27 External anal sphincter muscle
28 Anal canal
29 Vagina
30 Internal anal sphincter muscle
31 Anus
32 Hymen
33 Left ureter
34 Peritoneum (cut edge)
35 Right ureter (divided)
36 Median umbilical fold
   with urachus
37 Infundibulum of uterine tube
38 Fimbriae of uterine tube
39 Ovary
40 Uterine tube (isthmus)
41 Round ligament of uterus

Female urogenital system, midsagittal section through the trunk. The urinary bladder is empty, position and shape of the uterus are normal.

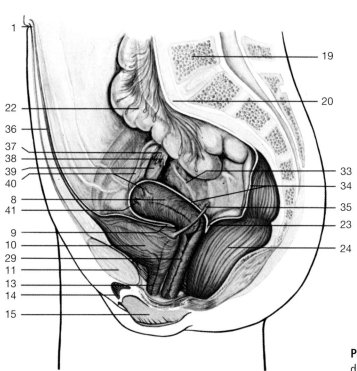

Positions of female genital organs (medial aspect, schematic drawing).

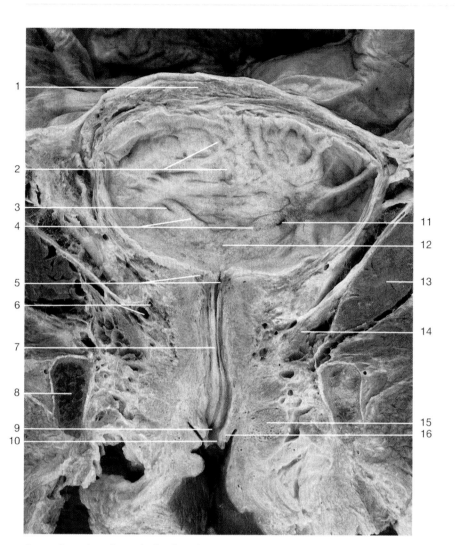

1 Muscular coat of urinary bladder
2 Folds of mucous membrane of urinary bladder
3 Right ureteric orifice
4 Interureteric fold
5 Internal urethral orifice
6 Vesico-uterine venous plexus
7 Urethra
8 Pubic bone (cut edge)
9 External urethral orifice
10 Vestibule of vagina
11 Left ureteric orifice
12 Trigone of bladder
13 Obturator internus muscle
14 Levator ani muscle
15 Bulb of the vestibule
16 Left labium minus
17 Psoas major muscle
18 Ampulla of rectum
19 Uterus
20 Urinary bladder
21 Promontory
22 Sigmoid colon
23 Uterine tube
24 Head of femur
25 Vagina

Coronal section through the female urinary bladder and urethra (anterior aspect).

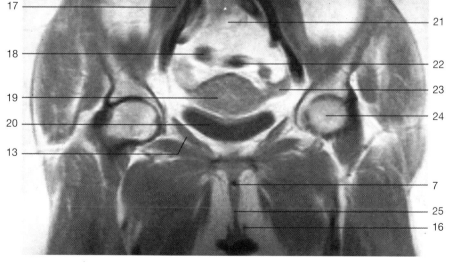

Coronal section through the pelvic cavity of the female (MRI scan).

The urogenital system of the female differs greatly from that of the male. During embryonal development, the uterus and ovary remain within the pelvic cavity where, after puberty, the ovulation takes place. Therefore, the urinary system remains functionally separated from the genital organs in the female.

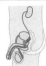

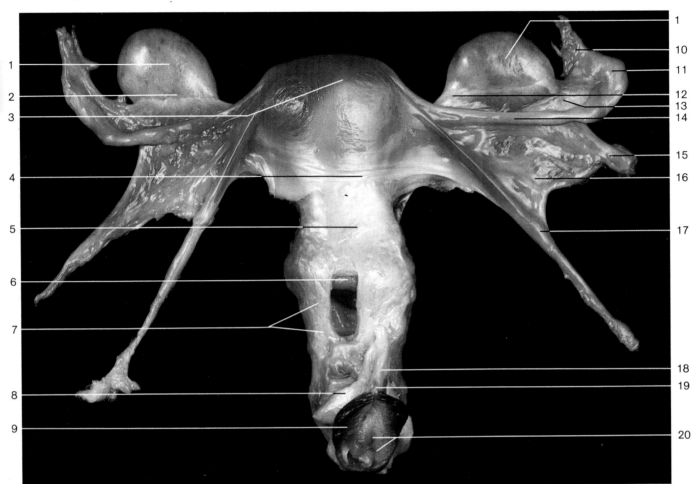

Female genital organs, isolated (anterior aspect). The anterior wall of the vagina has been opened to display the vaginal portion of the cervix.

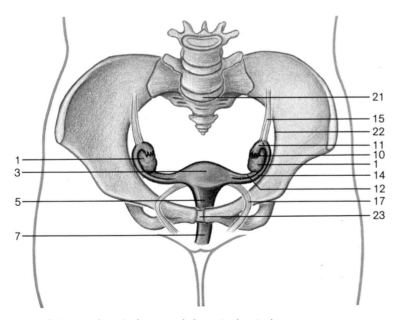

Female internal genital organs (schematic drawing).

1 Ovary
2 Mesovarium
3 Fundus of uterus
4 Vesico-uterine pouch
5 Cervix of uterus
6 Vaginal portion of cervix
7 Vagina
8 Crus of clitoris
9 Labium minus
10 Fimbriae of uterine tube
11 Infundibulum of uterine tube
12 Ligament of the ovary
13 Mesosalpinx
14 Uterine tube
15 Suspensory ligament of ovary
    (caudally displaced)
16 Broad ligament of uterus
17 Round ligament of uterus
18 Corpus cavernosum of clitoris
19 Glans of clitoris
20 Hymen, vaginal orifice
21 Promontory
22 Linea terminalis of pelvis
23 Pubic symphysis

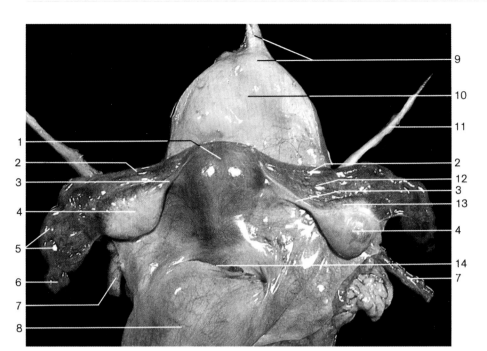

1   Fundus of uterus
2   Uterine tube
3   Ligament of the ovary
4   Ovary
5   Infundibulum of uterine tube
6   Fimbriae of uterine tube
7   Ureter
8   Rectum
9   Apex of urinary bladder and median umbilical ligament
10 Urinary bladder
11 Round ligament of uterus
12 Mesosalpinx
13 Mesovarium
14 Recto-uterine pouch (of Douglas)
15 Suspensory ligament of ovary
16 Scarring of ovary (following ovulation)
17 Abdominal opening of uterine tube
18 Body of uterus
19 Cervical canal
20 Vaginal portion of cervix of uterus (congestion)
21 Vagina
22 Mucous membrane of uterus
23 Anterior fornix of vagina

Female genital organs, isolated (supero-posterior aspect).

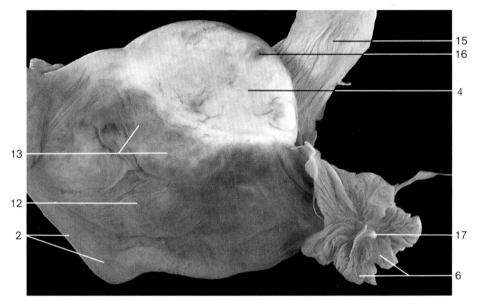

Right ovary and uterine tube, isolated (supero-posterior aspect). The fimbriae of the uterine tube have been reflected to show the abdominal ostium.

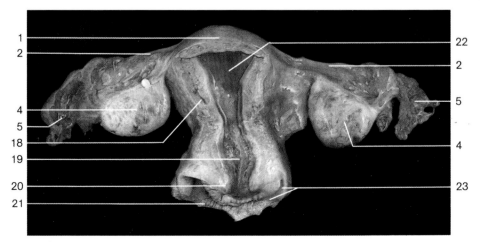

Uterus and related organs (posterior aspect). The posterior wall of the uterus has been opened.

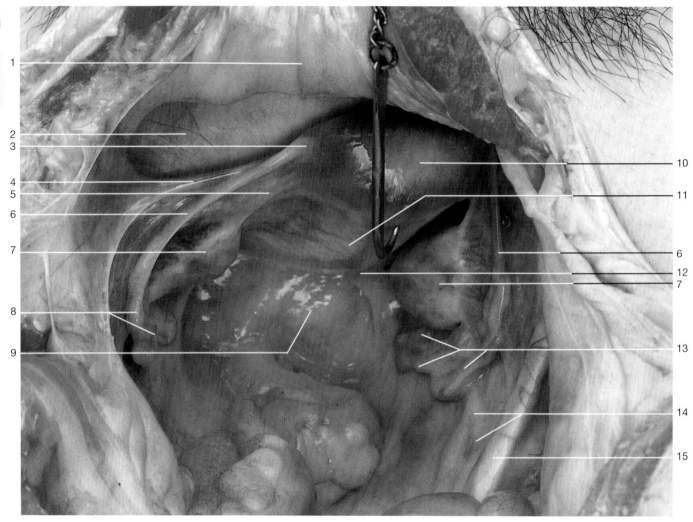

Female internal genital organs. Pelvic cavity (seen from above). The uterus has been reflected to the right.

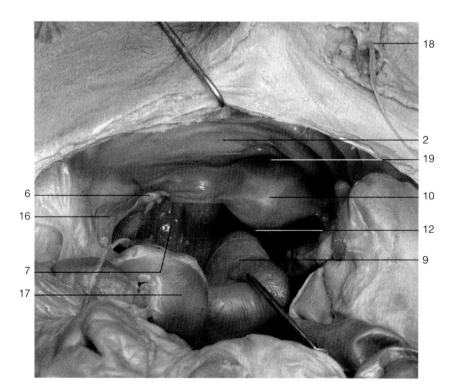

Female internal genital organs. Pelvic cavity (seen from above).

1   Median umbilical fold with urachus
2   Urinary bladder
3   Insertion of uterine tube
    at fundus of uterus
4   Round ligament of uterus
5   Ligament of ovary
6   Uterine tube (isthmus)
7   Ovary
8   Ampulla of uterine tube
9   Rectum
10 Uterus
11 Vagina
12 Recto-uterine pouch
    (of Douglas)
13 Fimbriae of uterine tube
14 Suspensory ligament of ovary
15 Right common iliac artery
    (covered by peritoneum)
16 Mesosalpinx
17 Sigmoid colon
18 Saphenous opening
19 Vesico-uterine pouch

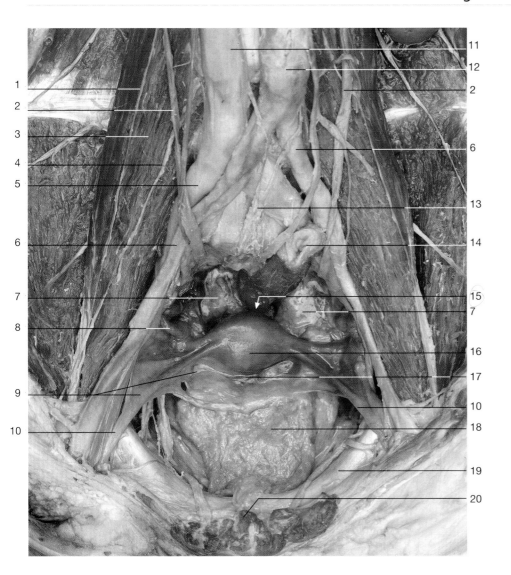

1 Ilio-inguinal nerve
2 Ureter
3 Psoas major muscle
4 Genitofemoral nerve
5 Common iliac vein
6 Common iliac artery
7 Ovary
8 Uterine tube
9 Peritoneum
10 Round ligament of uterus
11 Inferior vena cava
12 Abdominal aorta
13 Superior hypogastric plexus
14 Rectum
15 Recto-uterine pouch
   (of Douglas)
16 Uterus
17 Vesico-uterine pouch
18 Urinary bladder
19 Iliac crest
20 Pubic symphysis
21 Placenta
22 Amnion and chorion
23 Adnexa of uterus
   (uterine tube and ovaries)
24 Myometrium
25 Internal orifice of uterus
26 Cervix of uterus
27 Umbilical cord

**View of the female pelvis
showing uterus and related
organs** (superior aspect).

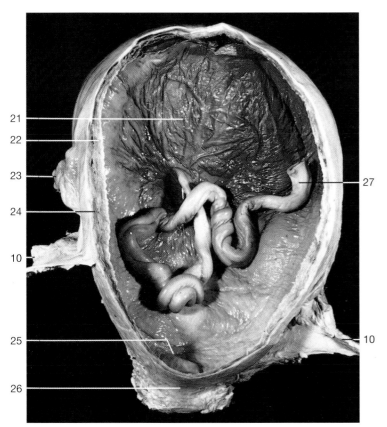

Fullterm uterus with placenta (anterior aspect).
The anterior wall of the uterus has been removed to
show the location of the placenta.

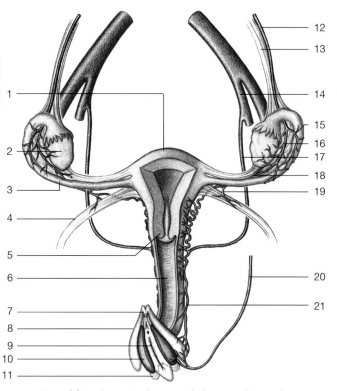

Arteries of female genital organs (schematic drawing).

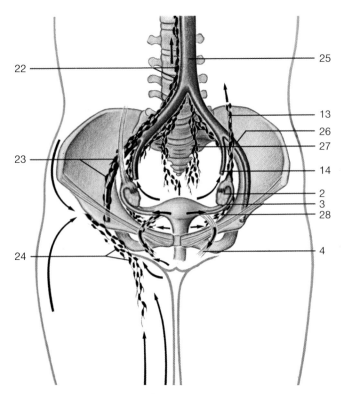

Main drainage routes of lymph vessels of uterus and its adnexa (indicated by arrows). (Schematic drawing.) Red = arteries; black = lymph vessels and nodes.

1 Uterus	10 Bulb of vestibule
2 Ovary	11 Greater vestibular gland
3 Uterine tube	12 Ovarian artery
4 Round ligament of uterus	13 Suspensory ligament of ovary
5 Vaginal portion of cervix of uterus	14 Internal iliac artery
6 Vagina	15 Tubal branch of ovarian artery
7 Clitoris	16 Ovarian branch of ovarian artery
8 Corpus cavernosum of clitoris	17 Uterine artery
9 Vaginal orifice	18 Ovarian branch of uterine artery

19 Artery of round ligament	28 Internal iliac lymph nodes
20 Internal pudendal artery	29 Superior gluteal artery
21 Vaginal artery	30 Obturator artery
22 Lumbar lymph nodes	31 Inferior gluteal artery
23 External iliac lymph nodes	32 Middle sacral artery
24 Inguinal lymph nodes	33 Femoral artery
25 Abdominal aorta	34 Vessels of labium majus
26 External iliac artery	35 Femur
27 Sacral lymph nodes	

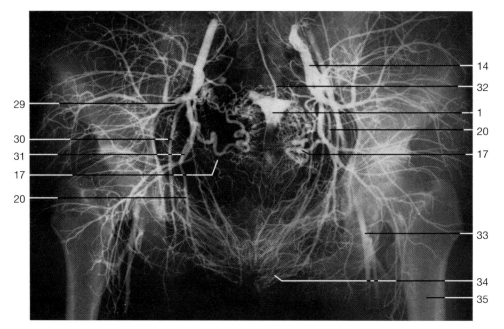

Pelvic vessels in the female (arteriography, antero-posterior view).

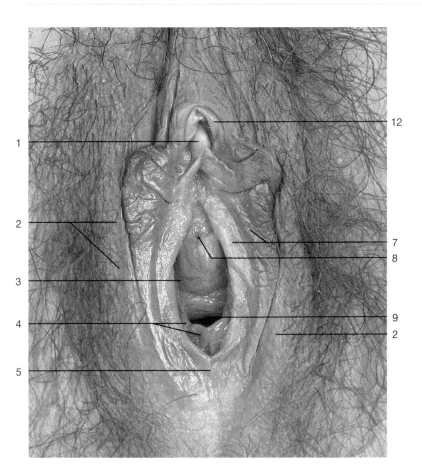

1 Glans of clitoris
2 Labium majus
3 Vestibule of vagina
4 Hymen
5 Posterior labial commissure
6 Body of clitoris
7 Labium minus
8 External orifice of urethra
9 Vaginal orifice
10 Ureter
11 Adnexa of uterus
12 Prepuce of clitoris
13 Crus of clitoris
14 Greater vestibular glands
15 Anus and internal anal sphincter muscle
16 Median umbilical ligament containing urachus
17 Urinary bladder
18 Infundibulum of uterine tube
19 Ovary
20 Ampulla of uterine tube
21 Suspensory ligament of the ovary
22 Bulbospongiosus muscle and bulb of vestibule
23 Central tendon of perineum (perineal body)
24 External anal sphincter muscle

Female external genital organs (anterior aspect). Labia reflected.

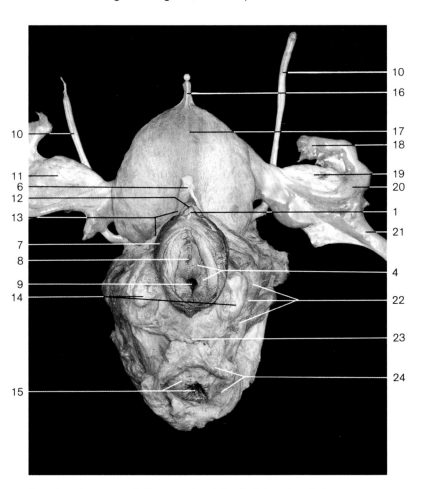

Female external genital organs in relation to internal genital organs and urinary system, isolated (anterior aspect).

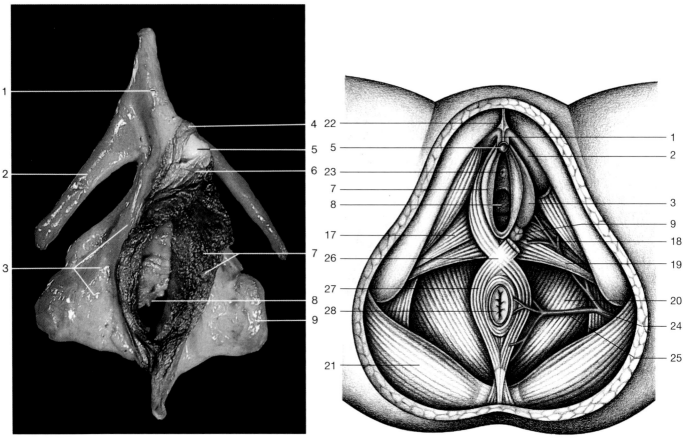

Cavernous tissue of female external genital organs, isolated (anterior aspect).

Urogenital and pelvic diaphragms (anterior aspect, schematic drawing). Blue = cavernous tissue of clitoris and bulb of vestibule.

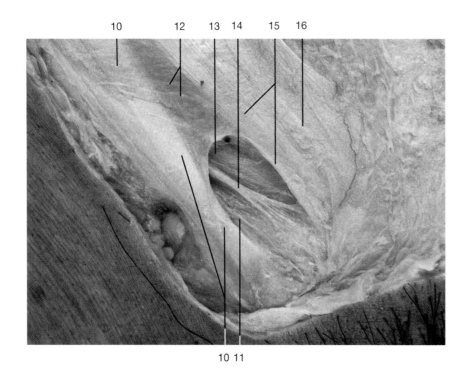

Inguinal canal and round ligament of uterus in situ (right side, ventral aspect).

1　Body of clitoris
2　Crus of clitoris
3　Bulb of vestibule
4　Prepuce of clitoris
5　Glans of clitoris
6　Frenulum of clitoris
7　Labium minus
8　Vaginal orifice
9　Greater vestibular gland
10　Lateral crus of superficial inguinal ring
11　Ilio-inguinal nerve
12　Intercrural fibers
13　Superficial inguinal ring
14　Round ligament of uterus
15　Medial crus of superficial inguinal ring
16　Aponeurosis of external abdominal oblique muscle
17　Deep transverse perineal muscle with fascia
18　Deep artery of clitoris
19　Superficial transverse perineus muscle
20　Levator ani muscle
21　Gluteus maximus muscle
22　Suspensory ligament of clitoris
23　External orifice of urethra
24　Internal pudendal artery
25　Inferior rectal artery
26　Perineal body
27　External anal sphincter muscle
28　Anus

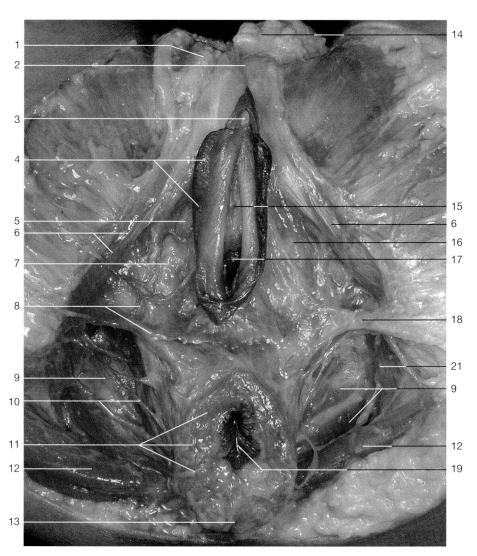

Urogenital diaphragm and external genital organs in the female, superficial layer (from below).

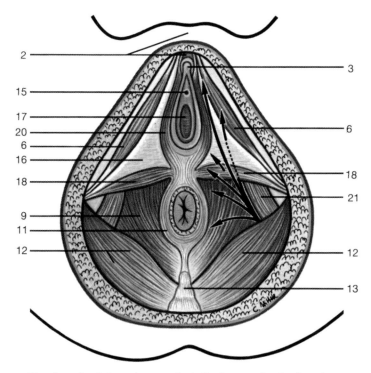

Muscles of pelvic and urogenital diaphragms in the female (from below, schematic drawing).

1   Fatty tissue encasing round ligament
2   Position of pubic symphysis
3   Clitoris
4   Labium minus
5   Bulb of vestibule
6   Ischiocavernosus muscle
7   Greater vestibular gland
8   Perineal branches of pudendal nerve
9   Levator ani muscle
10   Inferior rectal nerves
11   External anal sphincter muscle
12   Gluteus maximus muscle
13   Coccyx
14   Fatty tissue of mons pubis
15   External orifice of urethra
16   Urogenital diaphragm with fascia of deep transverse perineus muscle
17   Vaginal orifice
18   Superficial transverse perineal muscle
19   Anus
20   Bulbospongiosus muscle
21   Obturator internus muscle

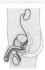

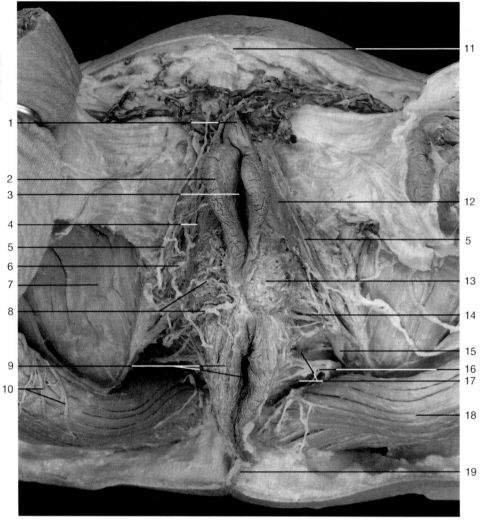

Urogenital diaphragm and external genital organs in the female, superficial layer (from below). On the right side the bulb of vestibule has been removed.

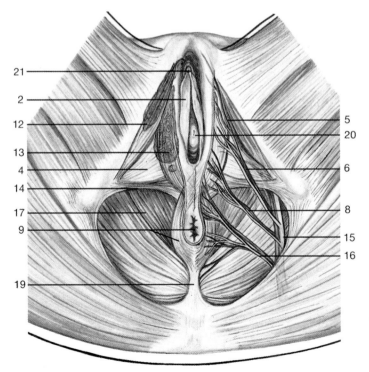

External female genital organs. Position of arteries and nerves; bulb of vestibule in blue (schematic drawing).

1 Prepuce of clitoris
2 Labium minus
3 Vaginal orifice
4 Deep transverse perineus muscle
5 Dorsal nerve of clitoris
6 Posterior labial nerves
7 Great adductor muscle
8 Perineal branches of pudendal nerve
9 Anus and external anal sphincter muscle
10 Inferior cluneal nerves
11 Mons pubis
12 Crus of clitoris with ischiocavernosus muscle
13 Bulb of vestibule
14 Superficial transverse perineus muscle
15 Pudendal nerve and internal pudendal artery
16 Inferior rectal nerves
17 Levator ani muscle
18 Gluteus maximus muscle
19 Anococcygeal ligament
20 External urethral orifice
21 Glans of clitoris

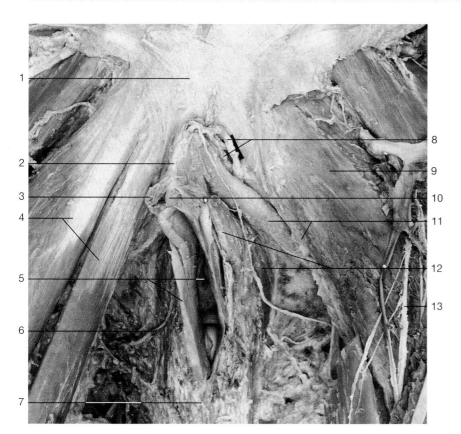

1   Position of pubic symphysis
2   Body of clitoris
3   Prepuce of clitoris
4   Adductor longus and gracilis muscles
5   External orifice of vagina and
     labium minus
6   Posterior labial nerve
7   Perineal body
8   Deep artery of clitoris and
     dorsal nerve of clitoris
9   Adductor brevis muscle
10 Glans of clitoris
11 Crus of clitoris and
     ischiocavernosus muscle
12 Bulb of vestibule and
     bulbospongiosus muscle
13 Anterior branch of obturator nerve
14 Labium minus
15 Vaginal orifice
16 Posterior labial nerves
17 Branches of pudendal nerve
18 External sphincter of anus
19 Anus
20 Bulb of vestibule (divided)
21 Dorsal artery of clitoris
22 Superficial transverse perineus muscle
23 Perineal branch of posterior femoral
     cutaneous nerve
24 Levator ani muscle
25 Pudendal nerve and
     internal pudendal artery
26 Inferior rectal nerves
27 Gluteus maximus muscle
28 Anococcygeal ligament

External genital organs in the female (inferior aspect). The clitoris has been dissected and slightly reflected to the right. The prepuce of clitoris has been divided to display the glans.

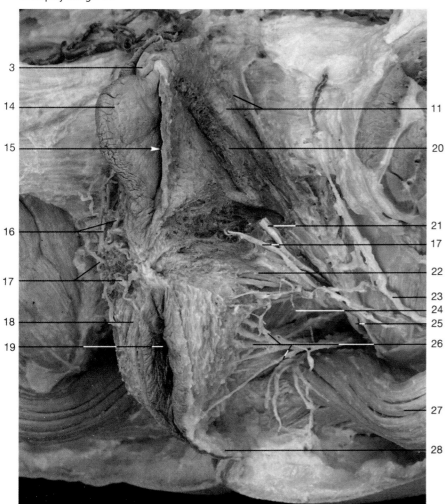

Urogenital diaphragm and external genital organs in the female (latero-inferior aspect). The bulb of vestibule has partly been removed; the left labium minus was cut away.

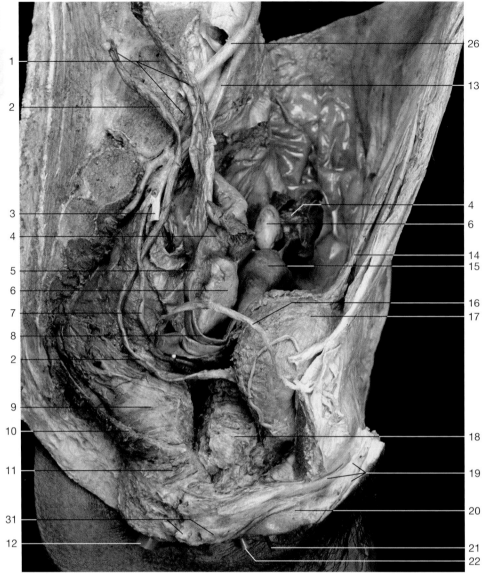

1	Body of fifth lumbar vertebra, suspensory ligament of ovary, and sacral promontory
2	Ureter
3	Medial umbilical ligament (remnant of umbilical artery) (cut)
4	Infundibulum of uterine tube
5	Ampulla of uterine tube
6	Ovary
7	Uterine artery
8	Uterine tube
9	Rectum
10	Levator ani muscle (pelvic diaphragm – cut edge)
11	External anal sphincter muscle
12	Anus (probe)
13	Internal iliac artery
14	Remnant of urachus (median umbilical ligament)
15	Uterus
16	Round ligament of uterus
17	Urinary bladder
18	Vagina
19	Clitoris
20	Labium minus
21	External orifice of urethra (red probe)
22	Vaginal orifice (green probe)
23	Lateral umbilical ligament
24	Inferior epigastric artery
25	Obturator artery, vein, and nerve
26	External iliac artery
27	Recto-uterine pouch (of Douglas)
28	Recto-uterine fold
29	Vesico-uterine pouch
30	Suspensory ligament of ovary
31	Greater vestibular gland and bulb of the vestibule

Pelvic cavity in the female, internal genital organs in situ (lateral aspect). Right half of the pelvis and sacrum have been removed.

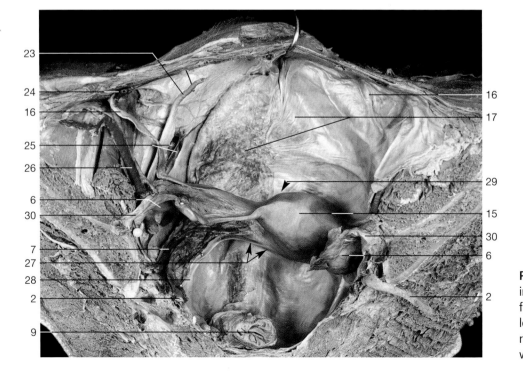

Pelvic cavity in the female, internal genital organs in situ (seen from above). The peritoneum at the left half of pelvic cavity has been removed to display uterine tube, vessels, and nerves.

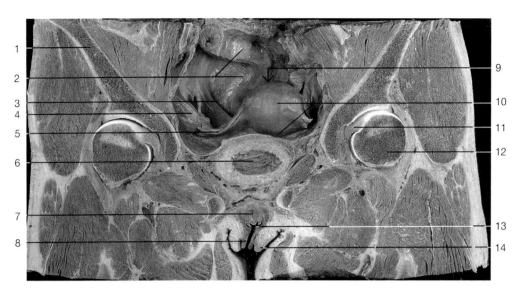

1   Ilium
2   Rectum
3   Recto-uterine fold
4   Ovary
5   Uterine tube
6   Urinary bladder
7   Urethra
8   Labium minus
9   Recto-uterine pouch of Douglas
10   Uterus (uterovesical pouch)
11   Ligament of the head of the femur
12   Head of femur
13   Vestibule of vagina
14   Labium majus
15   Anal cleft
16   Coccyx
17   Rectum
18   Myometrium of uterus
19   Uterine cavity
20   Obturator internus muscle
21   Iliopsoas muscle
22   Sartorius muscle
23   Sciatic nerve and gluteus maximus muscle
24   Uterine venous plexus
25   Broad ligament
26   Small intestine
27   Femoral artery and vein
28   Femoral nerve
29   Pyramidalis muscle
30   Rectum (anal canal)
31   Vagina
32   Urethral sphincter muscle (base of urinary bladder)
33   Pubic symphysis
34   Levator ani muscle
35   Obturator externus muscle
36   Mons pubis
37   Pectineus muscle

Coronal section through the pelvic cavity of the female (cf. MRI scan on p. 355).

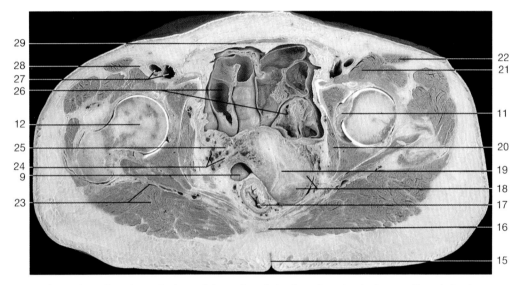

Horizontal section through the pelvic cavity of the female at level of uterus (from below). The uterus is retroverted to the left.

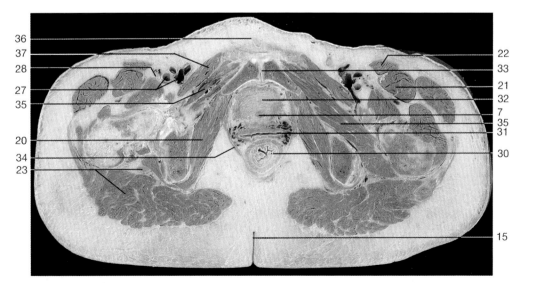

Horizontal section through the pelvic cavity of the female at level of the urethral sphincter and vagina (from below).

7 Upper Limb

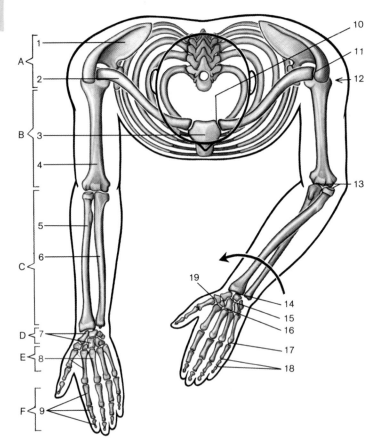

A = Shoulder girdle
B = Arm
C = Forearm
D = Wrist
E = Palm of hand
F = Finger

Bones
1 Scapula
2 Clavicle
3 Sternum
4 Humerus
5 Radius
6 Ulna
7 Carpal bones
8 Metacarpal bones
9 Phalanges

Joints
10 Sternoclavicular joint
11 Acromioclavicular joint
12 Shoulder joint
13 Elbow joint
14 Wrist joint
15 Midcarpal joint
16 Carpometacarpal joint
17 Metacarpophalangeal joint
18 Interphalangeal joints of the hand
19 Carpometacarpal joint of thumb

Organization of shoulder girdle and upper limb (superior aspect). The two positions of the forearm essential to manual skills in the human, supination (right arm) and pronation (left arm), are shown.

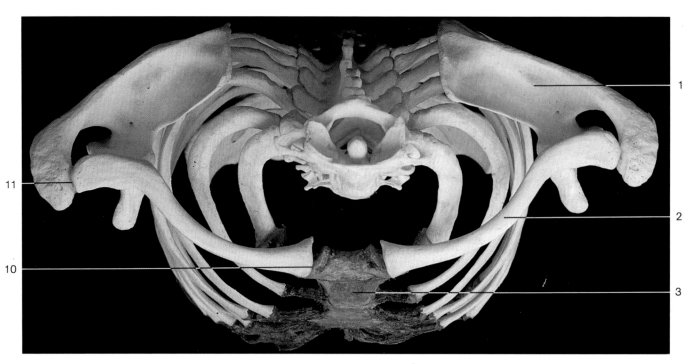

Bones of shoulder girdle articulated with the thorax (superior aspect).

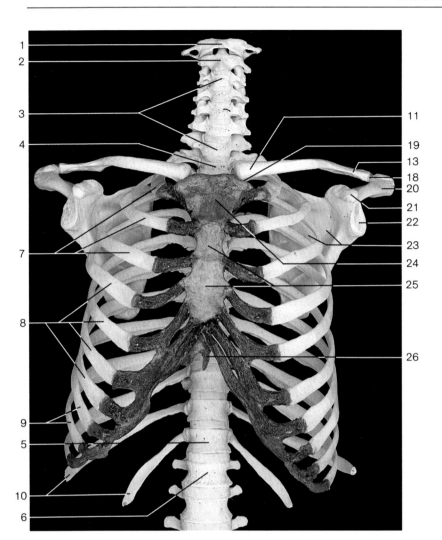

Skeleton of shoulder girdle and thorax (anterior aspect).
The cartilaginous parts of the ribs appear dark brown.

Vertebral column
1 Atlas
2 Axis
3 Third–seventh cervical vertebrae
4 First thoracic vertebra
5 Twelfth thoracic vertebra
6 First lumbar vertebra

Ribs
7 First–third ribs   } True ribs
8 Fourth–seventh ribs   }
9 Eighth–tenth ribs   } False ribs
10 Eleventh and twelfth ribs }
   (floating ribs)

Clavicle
11 Sternal end
12 Articular facet for sternum
13 Acromial end
14 Articular facet for acromion
15 Impression for costoclavicular ligament
16 Conoid tubercle
17 Trapezoid line
18 Site of acromioclavicular joint
19 Site of sternoclavicular joint

Scapula
20 Acromion
21 Coracoid process
22 Glenoid cavity
23 Costal surface

Sternum
24 Manubrium
25 Body
26 Xiphoid process

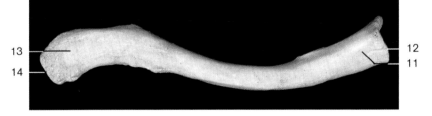

Right clavicle (superior aspect).

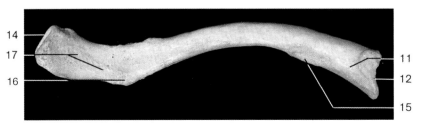

Right clavicle (inferior aspect).

Because of the human body's upright posture, the upper limb has developed a high degree of mobility. The shoulder girdle is to a great extent movable in the thorax and is connected with the trunk only by the sternoclavicular joint. A further characteristic of the forearm is the capacity for rotation (i.e., pronation and supination).

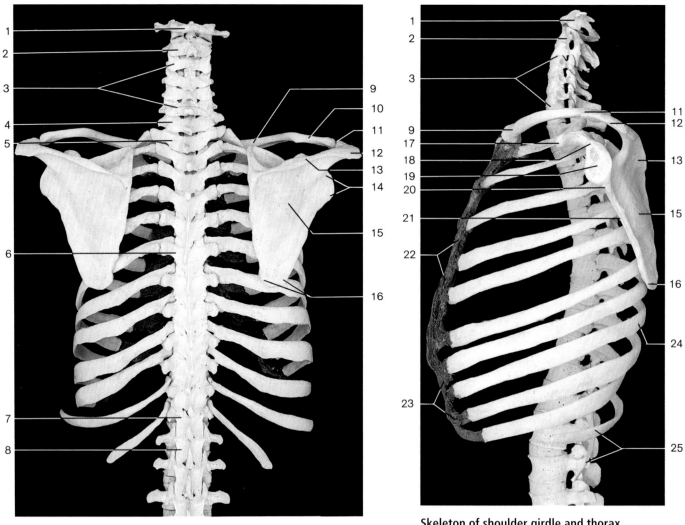

Skeleton of shoulder girdle and thorax (posterior aspect).

Skeleton of shoulder girdle and thorax (lateral aspect).

Vertebral column
1 Atlas
2 Axis
3 Third–sixth cervical vertebrae
4 Seventh vertebra (vertebra prominens)
5 First thoracic vertebra
6 Sixth thoracic vertebra
7 Twelfth thoracic vertebra
8 First lumbar vertebra

Clavicle
9 Sternal end
10 Acromial end
11 Site of acromioclavicular joint

Scapula
12 Acromion
13 Spine of scapula
14 Lateral angle
15 Posterior surface
16 Inferior angle
17 Coracoid process
18 Supraglenoid tubercle
19 Glenoid cavity
20 Infraglenoid tubercle
21 Lateral margin

Thorax
22 Body of sternum
23 Costal arch
24 Angle of ribs
25 Floating ribs

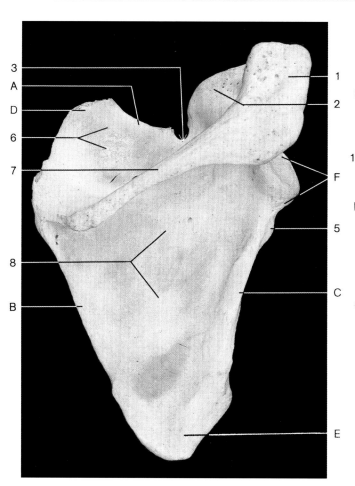

3
A
D
6
7
8
B

1
2
F
5
C
E

Right scapula (posterior aspect).

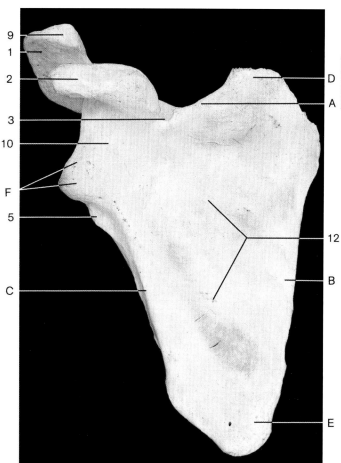

9
1
2
3
10
F
5
C

D
A
12
B
E

Right scapula (anterior aspect, costal surface).

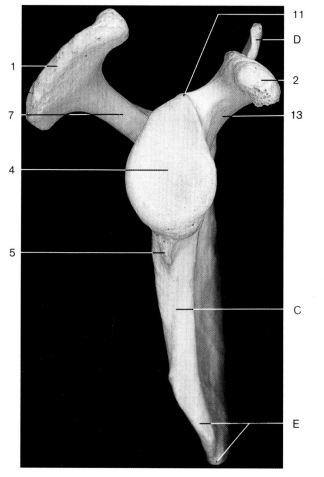

11
D
2
13

1
7
4
5

C
E

Right scapula (lateral aspect).

Scapula

A = superior border
B = medial border
C = lateral border
D = superior angle
E = inferior angle
F = lateral angle

1 Acromion
2 Coracoid process
3 Scapular notch
4 Glenoid cavity
5 Infraglenoid tubercle
6 Supraspinous fossa
7 Spine
8 Infraspinous fossa
9 Articular facet for acromion
10 Neck
11 Supraglenoid tubercle
12 Costal (anterior) surface
13 Base of coracoid process

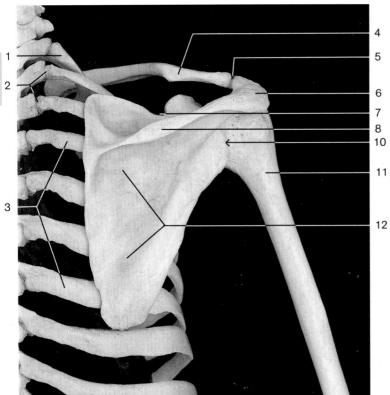

1 First rib
2 Position of costotransverse joints
3 Fourth–seventh ribs
4 Clavicle
5 Position of acromioclavicular joint
6 Acromion
7 Scapular notch
8 Spine of scapula
9 Head of humerus
10 Glenoid cavity
11 Surgical neck of humerus
12 Posterior surface of scapula
13 Coracoid process
14 Infraglenoid tubercle
15 Greater tubercle of humerus
16 Anatomical neck of humerus

Bones of shoulder joint (posterior aspect).

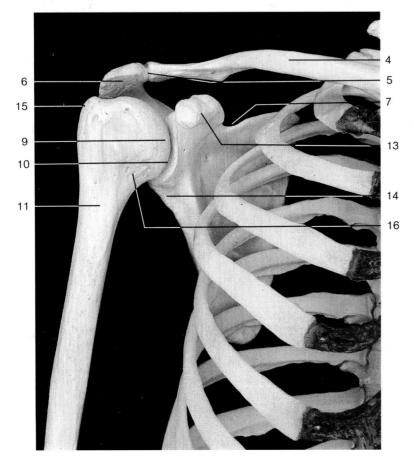

Bones of shoulder joint (anterior aspect).

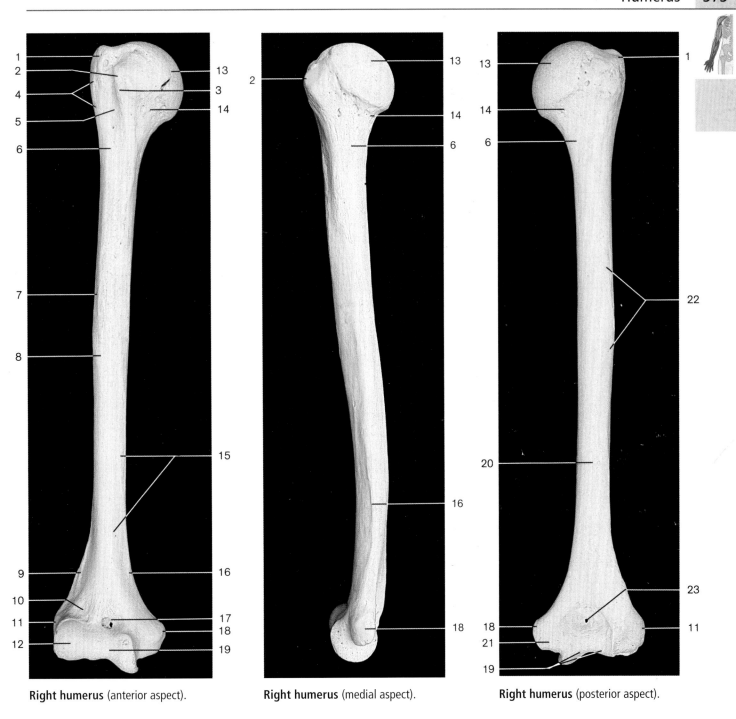

Right humerus (anterior aspect).   **Right humerus** (medial aspect).   **Right humerus** (posterior aspect).

Humerus

1	Greater tubercle	7	Deltoid tuberosity	13	Head	19	Trochlea
2	Lesser tubercle	8	Anterolateral surface	14	Anatomical neck	20	Posterior surface
3	Crest of lesser tubercle	9	Lateral supracondylar ridge	15	Anteromedial surface	21	Groove for ulnar nerve
4	Crest of greater tubercle	10	Radial fossa	16	Medial supracondylar ridge	22	Groove for radial nerve
5	Intertubercular sulcus /groove	11	Lateral epicondyle	17	Coronoid fossa	23	Olecranon fossa
6	Surgical neck	12	Capitulum	18	Medial epicondyle		

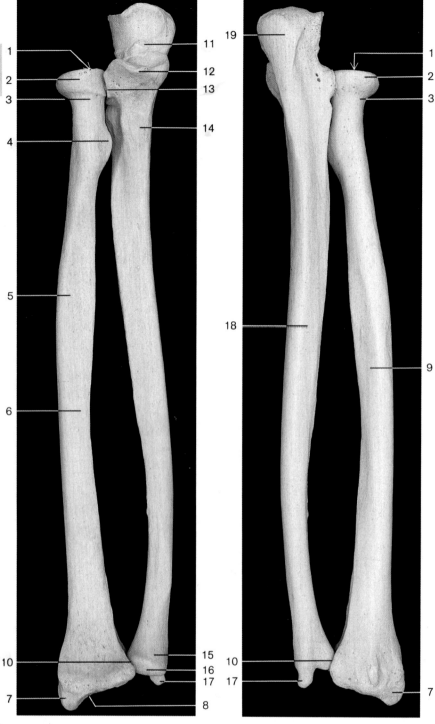

Radius
1 Head
2 Articular circumference
3 Neck
4 Radial tuberosity
5 Shaft
6 Anterior surface
7 Styloid process
8 Articular surface
9 Posterior surface
10 Ulnar notch

Ulna
11 Trochlear notch
12 Coronoid process
13 Radial notch
14 Ulnar tuberosity
15 Head
16 Articular circumference
17 Styloid process
18 Posterior surface
19 Olecranon

Bones of right forearm, radius, and ulna (anterior aspect).

Bones of right forearm, radius, and ulna (posterior aspect).

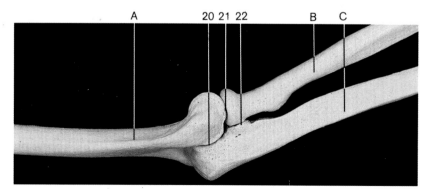

Bones of right elbow joint (lateral aspect).

Articulations at the right elbow
20 Site of humero-ulnar joint
21 Site of humeroradial joint
22 Site of proximal radio-ulnar joint

A = humerus
B = radius
C = ulna

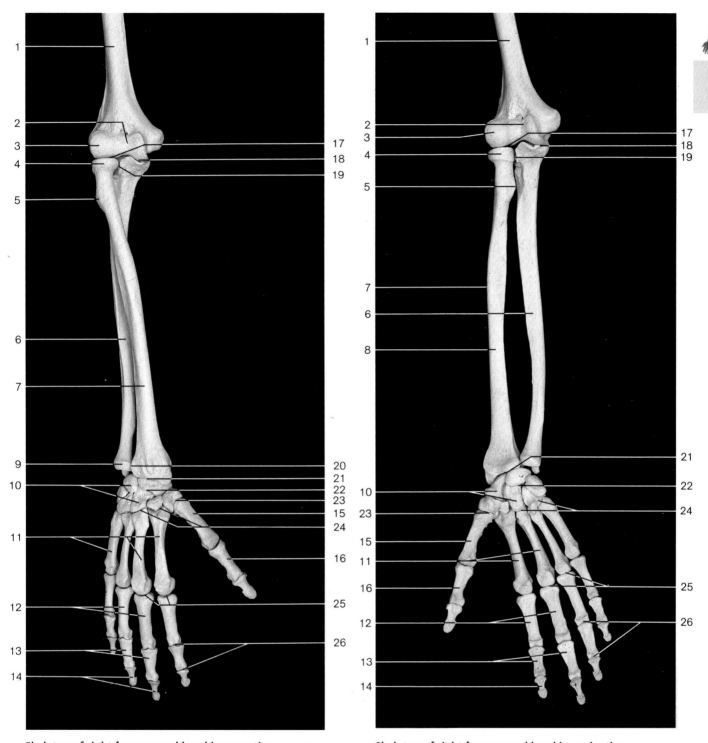

Skeleton of right forearm and hand in pronation.

Skeleton of right forearm and hand in supination.

1	Humerus	9	Articular circumference of ulna	**Sites of joints**	
2	Trochlea of humerus	10	Carpal bones	17	Humeroradial joint
3	Capitulum of humerus	11	Metacarpal bones	18	Humero-ulnar joint
4	Articular circumference of radius	12	Proximal phalanges	19	Proximal radio-ulnar joint
5	Radial tuberosity	13	Middle phalanges	20	Distal radio-ulnar joint
6	Anterior surface of ulna	14	Distal phalanges	21	Wrist joint
7	Posterior surface of radius	15	Metacarpal bone of thumb	22	Midcarpal joint
8	Anterior surface of radius	16	Proximal phalanx of thumb	23	Carpometacarpal joint of thumb
				24	Carpometacarpal joints
				25	Metacarpophalangeal joints
				26	Interphalangeal joints of the hand

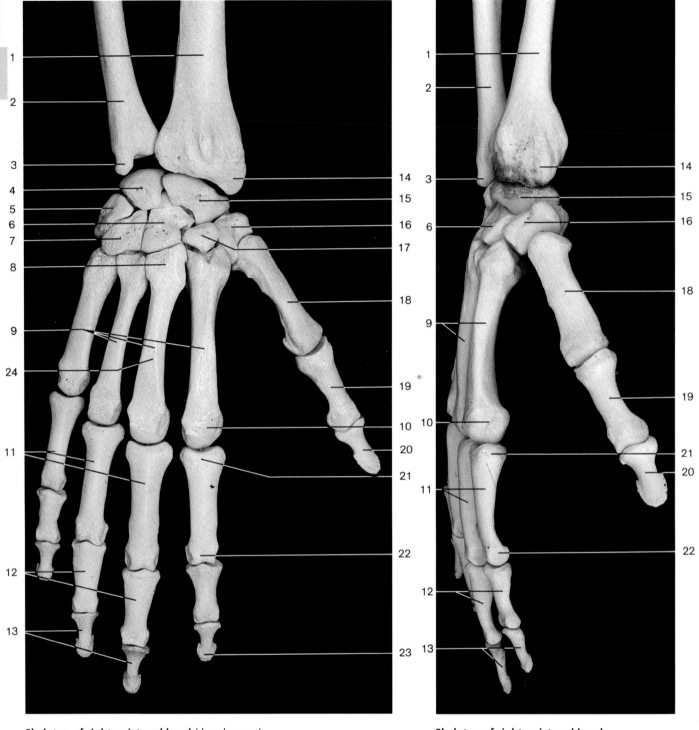

Skeleton of right wrist and hand (dorsal aspect).

Skeleton of right wrist and hand
(medial aspect).

1	Radius	8	Base of third metacarpal bone	15	Scaphoid bone
2	Ulna	9	Metacarpal bones	16	Trapezium bone
3	Styloid process of ulna	10	Head of metacarpal bone	17	Trapezoid bone
4	Lunate bone	11	Proximal phalanges of hand	18	Metacarpal bone of thumb
5	Triquetral bone	12	Middle phalanges of hand	19	Proximal phalanx of thumb
6	Capitate bone	13	Distal phalanges of hand	20	Distal phalanx of thumb
7	Hamate bone	14	Styloid process of radius	21	Base of second proximal phalanx

Carpal bones (4, 5, 6, 7)

Carpal bones (15, 16, 17)

22 Head of second
    proximal phalanx
23 Tuberosity of distal
    phalanx
24 Body of
    third metacarpal
    bone

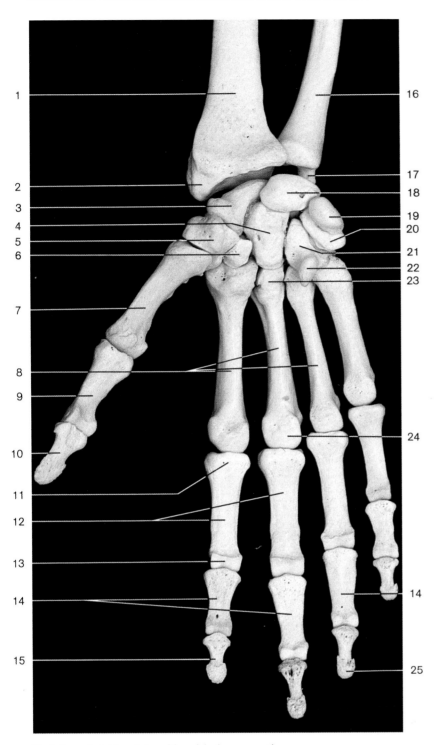

1   Radius
2   Styloid process of radius
3   Scaphoid bone ⎫
4   Capitate bone ⎪
5   Trapezium   ⎬ Carpal bones
6   Trapezoid bone ⎭
7   First metacarpal bone
8   Second to fourth metacarpal bones
9   Proximal phalanx of thumb
10 Distal phalanx of thumb
11 Base of second proximal phalanx
12 Proximal phalanges
13 Head of second proximal phalanx
14 Middle phalanges
15 Distal phalanx
16 Ulna
17 Styloid process of ulna
18 Lunate bone   ⎫
19 Pisiform bone   ⎪
20 Triquetral bone ⎬ Carpal bones
21 Hamate bone   ⎭
22 Hamulus or hook
    of hamate bone
23 Base of third metacarpal bone
24 Head of metacarpal bone
25 Tuberosity of distal phalanx

Skeleton of right wrist and hand (palmar aspect).

The human hand is one of the most admirable structures of the human body. The carpometacarpal joint of the thumb, a saddle joint, enjoys wide mobility so that the thumb can come into contact with all other fingers, thus enabling the hand to become an instrument for grasping and psychologic expression. During evolution, these newly developed functions appeared after the erect posture of the human body was achieved. An inevitable prerequisite for the development of human cultures is not only the differentiation of the brain but also the development of an organ capable of realizing its ideas: the human hand.

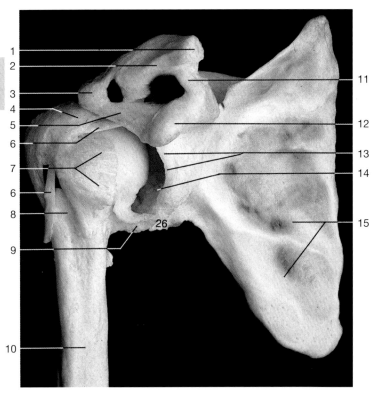

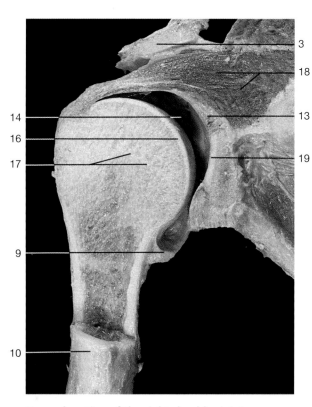

Right shoulder joint. The anterior part of the articular capsule has been removed and the head of the humerus has been slightly rotated outward to show the cavity of the joint.

Coronal section of the right shoulder joint (anterior aspect).

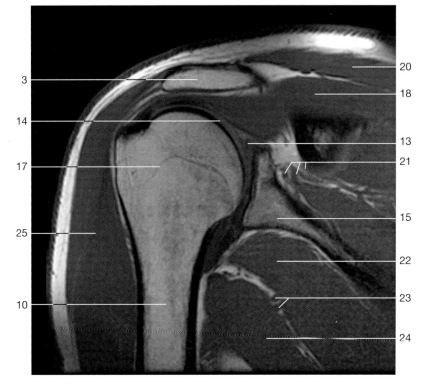

Coronal section of the right shoulder joint (MRI scan; from Heuck et al., MRT-Atlas, 2009).

1   Acromial end of clavicle
2   Acromioclavicular joint
3   Acromion
4   Tendon of supraspinatus muscle
     (attached to the articular capsule)
5   Coraco-acromial ligament
6   Tendon of long head of biceps brachii muscle
7   Tendon of subscapularis muscle
     (attached to the articular capsule)
8   Intertubercular sulcus
9   Articular capsule of shoulder joint
10 Humerus
11 Trapezoid ligament
12 Coracoid process
13 Glenoid labrum
14 Shoulder joint (joint cavity)
15 Scapula
16 Head of humerus
17 Epiphysial line
18 Supraspinatus muscle
19 Glenoid cavity
20 Trapezius muscle
21 Suprascapular artery, vein, and nerve
22 Teres major muscle
23 Circumflexa scapular artery and vein
24 Latissimus dorsi muscle
25 Deltoid muscle
26 Tendon of long head of triceps brachii muscle

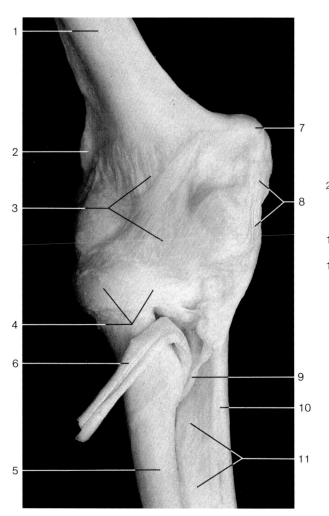

Ligaments of the elbow joint (anterior aspect).

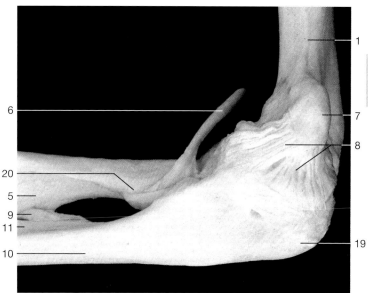

Elbow joint with collateral ligaments (medial aspect).

1	Humerus	11	Interosseous membrane
2	Lateral epicondyle of humerus	12	Radial fossa
3	Articular capsule	13	Capitulum of humerus
4	Anular ligament of proximal radio-ulnar joint	14	Head of radius
5	Radius	15	Radial collateral ligament
6	Tendon of biceps brachii muscle	16	Coronoid fossa
7	Medial epicondyle of humerus	17	Trochlea of humerus
8	Ulnar collateral ligament	18	Coronoid process of ulna
9	Oblique chord	19	Olecranon
10	Ulna	20	Radial tuberosity

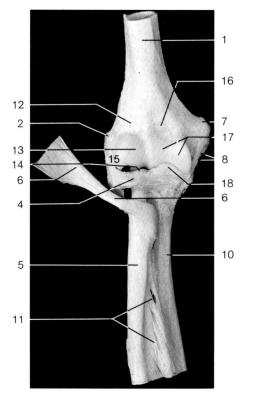

Elbow joint with ligaments (anterior aspect). Articular capsule has been removed to show the anular ligament.

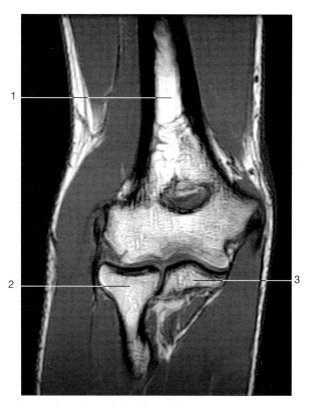

Coronal section of the elbow joint
(MRI scan, courtesy of Prof. Dr. A. Heuck, Munich).

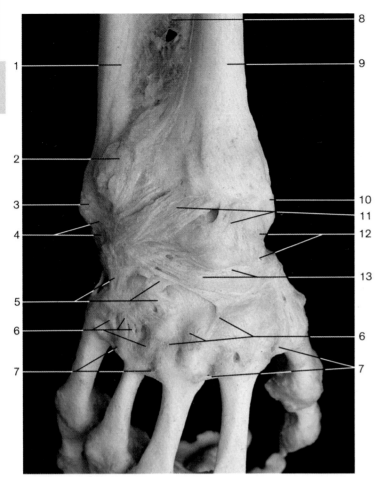

1   Ulna
2   Exostosis (pathological)
3   Head of ulna
4   Ulnar carpal collateral ligament
5   Deep intercarpal ligaments
6   Dorsal carpometacarpal ligaments
7   Dorsal metacarpal ligaments
8   Interosseous membrane
9   Radius
10   Styloid process of radius
11   Dorsal radiocarpal ligament
12   Radial collateral ligament
13   Articular capsule and dorsal intercarpal ligaments
14   Palmar radiocarpal ligament
15   Tendon of flexor carpi radialis muscle (cut)
16   Radiating carpal ligament
17   Palmar carpometacarpal ligaments
18   First metacarpal bone
19   Palmar ulnocarpal ligament
20   Tendon of flexor carpi ulnaris muscle (cut)
21   Pisohamate ligament
22   Pisometacarpal ligament
23   Palmar metacarpal ligaments
24   Fifth metacarpal bone
25   Articular disc (ulnocarpal)
26   Lunate bone
27   Triquetral bone
28   Hamate bone
29   Scaphoid bone (navicular)
30   Capitate bone
31   Trapezoid bone
32   Second and third metacarpal bones
33   Dorsal interosseus muscles

Ligaments of hand and wrist (dorsal aspect).

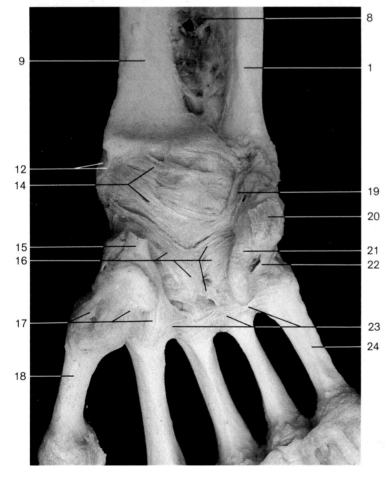

Ligaments of hand and wrist (palmar aspect).

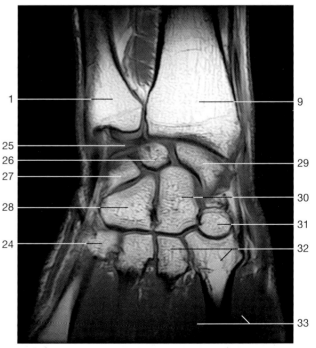

Coronal section of the hand and wrist (MRI scan; from Heuck et al., MRT-Atlas, 2009). Note the location of the wrist joint.

1 Radius
2 Styloid process of radius
3 Palmar radiocarpal ligament
4 Tendon of flexor carpi radialis muscle (cut)
5 Radiating carpal ligament
6 Articular capsule of carpometacarpal joint of thumb
7 Articular capsule of metacarpophalangeal joint of thumb
8 Palmar ligaments and articular capsule of metacarpophalangeal joints
9 Palmar ligaments and articular capsule of interphalangeal joints
10 Articular capsule
11 Interosseous membrane
12 Ulna
13 Distal radio-ulnar joint
14 Styloid process of ulna
15 Palmar ulnocarpal ligament
16 Pisiform bone with tendon of flexor carpi ulnaris muscle
17 Pisometacarpal ligament
18 Pisohamate ligament
19 Metacarpal bone
20 Deep transverse metacarpal ligament
21 Tendons of extensor muscles and articular capsule
22 Collateral ligament of interphalangeal joint
23 Collateral ligaments of metacarpophalangeal joints
24 Second metacarpal bone

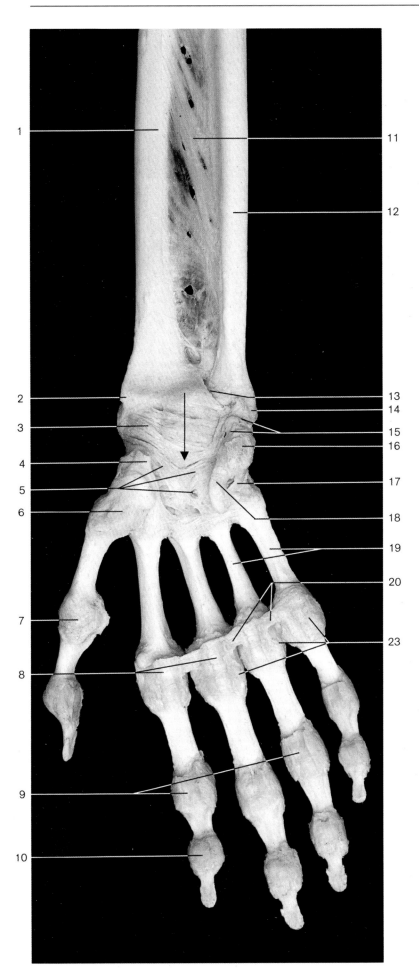

Ligaments of right forearm, hand, and fingers (palmar aspect).
The arrow indicates the location of the carpal tunnel.

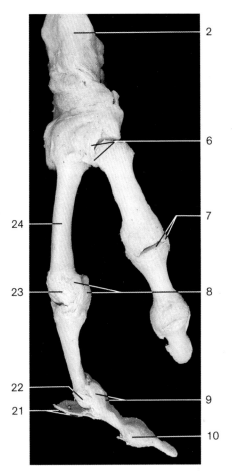

Ligaments of fingers
(lateral aspect).

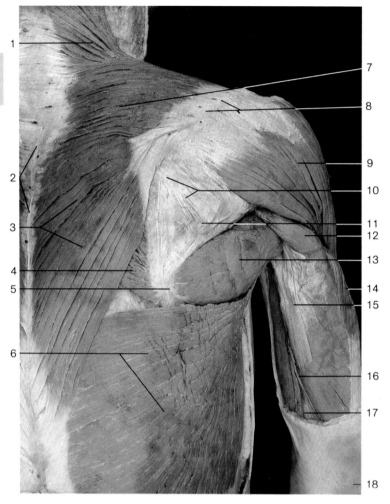

1 Descending fibers of trapezius muscle
2 Spinous processes of thoracic vertebrae
3 Ascending fibers of trapezius muscle
4 Rhomboid major muscle
5 Inferior angle of scapula
6 Latissimus dorsi muscle
7 Transverse fibers of trapezius muscle
8 Spine of scapula
9 Posterior fibers of deltoid muscle
10 Infraspinatus muscle and infraspinous fascia
11 Teres minor muscle and fascia
12 Long head of triceps brachii muscle
13 Teres major muscle
14 Lateral head of triceps brachii muscle
15 Medial head of triceps brachii muscle
16 Medial intermuscular septum
17 Ulnar nerve
18 Olecranon

Muscles of shoulder and arm, superficial layer (right side, dorsal aspect).

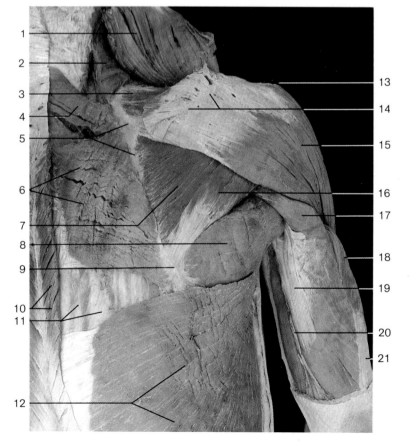

1 Trapezius muscle (reflected)
2 Levator scapulae muscle
3 Supraspinatus muscle
4 Rhomboid minor muscle
5 Medial border of scapula
6 Rhomboid major muscle
7 Infraspinatus muscle
8 Teres major muscle
9 Inferior angle of scapula
10 Cut edge of trapezius muscle
11 Intrinsic muscles of back with fascia
12 Latissimus dorsi muscle
13 Acromion
14 Spine of scapula
15 Deltoid muscle
16 Teres minor muscle
17 Long head of triceps brachii muscle
18 Lateral head of triceps brachii muscle
19 Medial head of triceps brachii muscle
20 Medial intermuscular septum
21 Tendon of triceps brachii muscle

Muscles of shoulder and arm, deeper layer (right side, dorsal aspect). The trapezius muscle has been cut near its origin at the vertebral column and reflected upward.

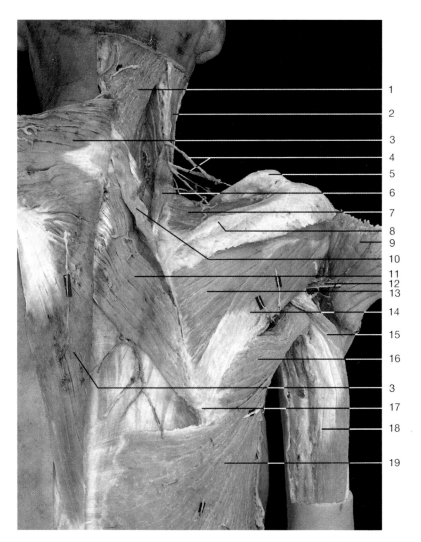

1   Splenius capitis muscle
2   Sternocleidomastoid muscle
3   Trapezius muscle (reflected)
4   Lateral supraclavicular nerves
5   Clavicle
6   Levator scapulae muscle
7   Supraspinatus muscle
8   Spine of scapula
9   Deltoid muscle (reflected)
10 Rhomboid minor muscle
11 Rhomboid major muscle
12 Axillary nerve and posterior
    circumflex humeral artery
13 Infraspinatus muscle
14 Teres minor muscle
15 Long head of triceps brachii muscle
16 Teres major muscle
17 Inferior angle of scapula
18 Triceps brachii muscle
19 Latissimus dorsi muscle

Muscles of shoulder and arm, deeper layer (right side, dorsal aspect).
The trapezius and deltoid muscles have been divided and reflected.

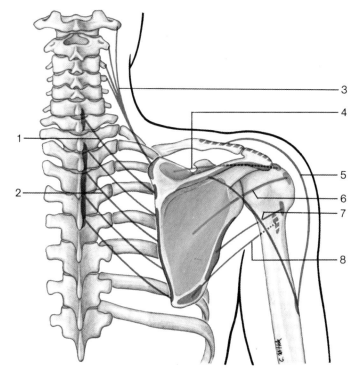

Shoulder muscles, schematic diagram illustrating the course of
the main muscles of the dorsal aspect of the shoulder.

1   Rhomboid minor muscle (red)
2   Rhomboid major muscle (red)
3   Levator scapulae muscle (red)
4   Supraspinatus muscle (blue)
5   Deltoid muscle (red)
6   Infraspinatus muscle (blue)
7   Teres minor muscle (red)
8   Teres major muscle (red)

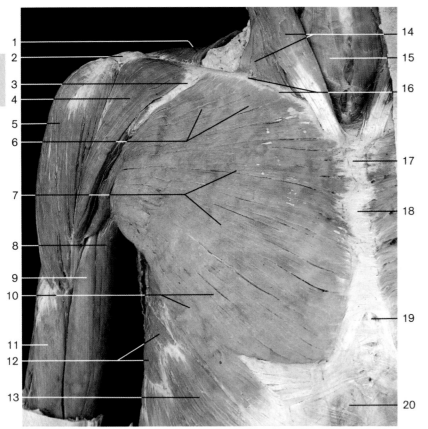

1   Trapezius muscle
2   Acromion
3   Deltopectoral triangle
4   Clavicular part of deltoid muscle
    (anterior fibers)
5   Acromial part of deltoid muscle
    (central fibers)
6   Clavicular part of pectoralis major muscle
7   Sternocostal part of pectoralis major muscle
8   Short head of biceps brachii muscle
9   Long head of biceps brachii muscle
10 Abdominal part of pectoralis major muscle
11 Brachialis muscle
12 Serratus anterior muscle
13 External abdominal oblique muscle
14 Sternocleidomastoid muscle
15 Infrahyoid muscles
16 Clavicle
17 Manubrium sterni
18 Body of sternum
19 Xiphoid process
20 Anterior layer of sheath of rectus
    abdominis muscle

Shoulder, arm, and pectoral muscles, superficial layer (ventral aspect).

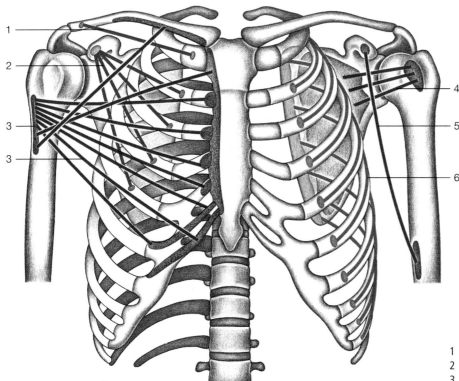

Arrangement of pectoral and shoulder muscles (ventral aspect).
(Schematic drawing.)

1   Subclavius muscle (blue)
2   Pectoralis minor muscle (blue)
3   Pectoralis major muscle (red)
4   Subscapularis muscle (red)
5   Coracobrachialis muscle (red)
6   Serratus anterior muscle (green)

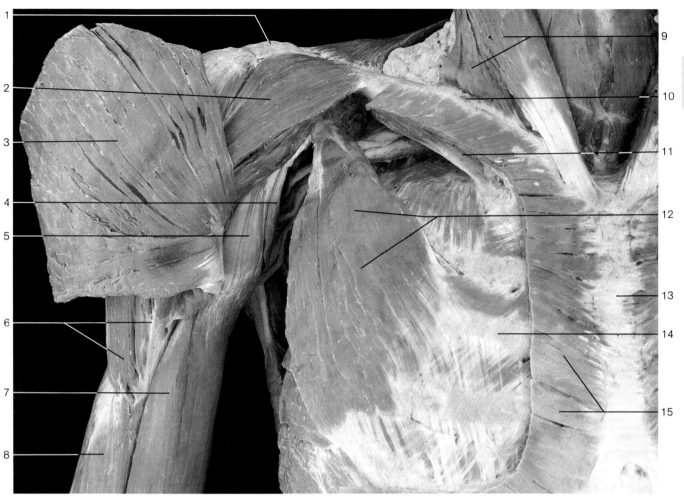

Shoulder, arm, and pectoral muscles, deep layer (ventral aspect).

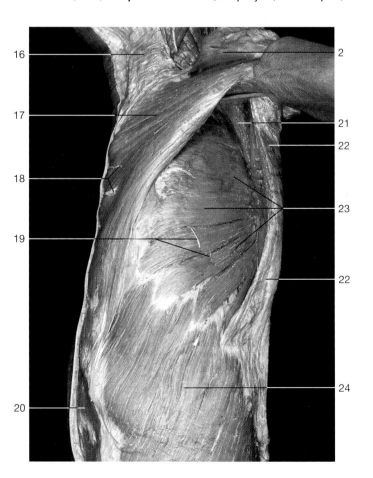

1 Acromion
2 Clavicular part of deltoid muscle
3 Pectoralis major muscle (reflected)
4 Coracobrachialis muscle
5 Short head of biceps brachii muscle
6 Deltoid muscle (insertion on humerus)
7 Long head of biceps brachii muscle
8 Brachialis muscle
9 Sternocleidomastoid muscle
10 Clavicle
11 Subclavius muscle
12 Pectoralis minor muscle
13 Sternum
14 Third rib
15 Pectoralis major muscle
16 Platysma muscle
17 Pectoralis major muscle forming the anterior axillary fold
18 Anterior cutaneous branches of intercostal nerves
19 Lateral cutaneous branches of intercostal nerves
20 Rectus abdominis muscle
21 Subscapularis muscle
22 Latissimus dorsi muscle forming the posterior axillary fold
23 Serratus anterior muscle forming the medial wall of the axilla
24 External abdominal oblique muscle

Axillary fossa and serratus anterior muscle
(left side, lateral aspect).

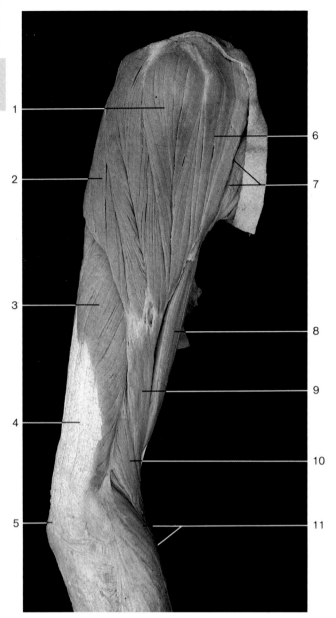

Muscles of the right arm (lateral aspect).

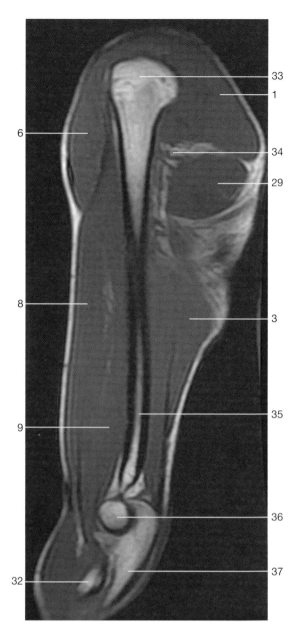

Sagittal section of the right arm (MRI scan; from Heuck et al., MRT-Atlas, 2009).

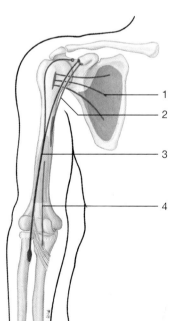

Position and course of flexors of arm (schematic drawing).

1 Subscapularis muscle (red)
2 Coracobrachialis muscle (blue)
3 Biceps brachii muscle (red)
4 Brachialis muscle (blue)

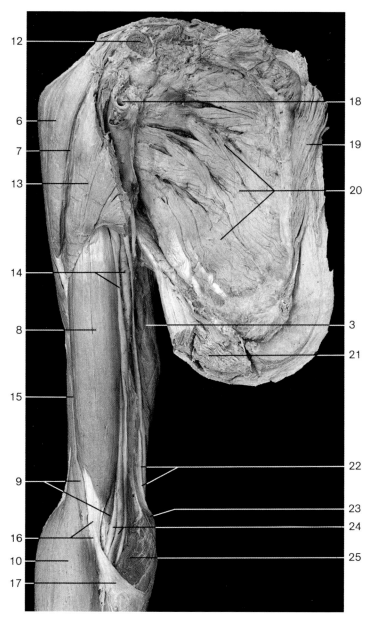

Muscles of the right arm (ventral aspect). The arm with the scapula and attached muscles has been removed from the trunk.

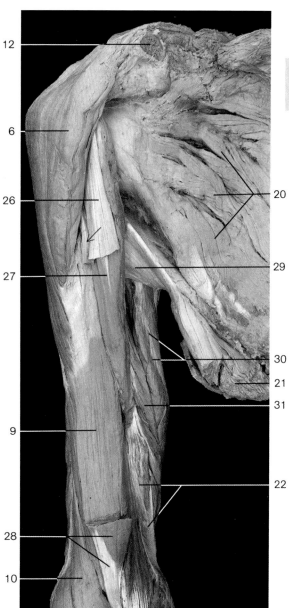

Muscles of the right arm (ventral aspect). Part of the biceps brachii muscle has been removed. Arrow: tendon of long head of biceps brachii muscle.

1   Acromial part of deltoid muscle (central fibers)
2   Scapular part of deltoid muscle (posterior fibers)
3   Triceps brachii muscle
4   Tendon of triceps brachii muscle
5   Olecranon
6   Clavicular part of deltoid muscle (anterior fibers)
7   Deltopectoral groove
8   Biceps brachii muscle
9   Brachialis muscle
10 Brachioradialis muscle
11 Extensor carpi radialis longus muscle
12 Clavicle (divided)
13 Pectoralis major muscle
14 Medial intermuscular septum with vessels and nerves
15 Lateral intermuscular septum
16 Tendon of biceps brachii muscle
17 Bicipital aponeurosis
18 Axillary artery
19 Rhomboid major muscle

20 Subscapularis muscle
21 Latissimus dorsi muscle (divided)
22 Medial intermuscular septum
23 Medial epicondyle of humerus
24 Brachial artery and median nerve
25 Pronator teres muscle
26 Tendon of short head of biceps brachii muscle
27 Coracobrachialis muscle
28 Distal part of biceps brachii muscle
29 Teres major muscle
30 Long head of triceps brachii muscle
31 Medial head of triceps brachii muscle
32 Radius
33 Head of humerus
34 Axillary nerve
35 Humerus
36 Trochlea
37 Ulna

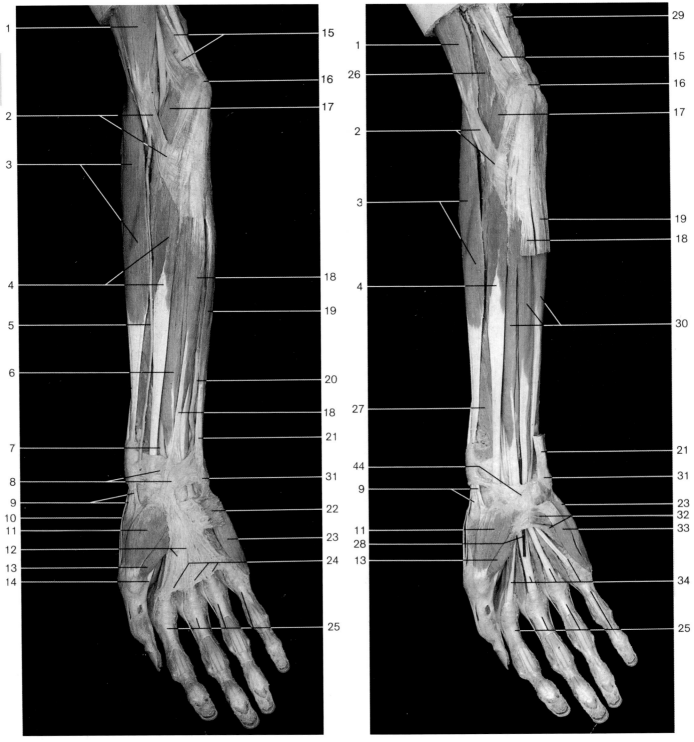

Flexor muscles of forearm and hand, superficial layer (ventral aspect).

Flexor muscles of forearm and hand, superficial layer (ventral aspect). The palmaris longus and flexor carpi ulnaris muscles have been removed.

1	Biceps brachii muscle
2	Bicipital aponeurosis
3	Brachioradialis muscle
4	Flexor carpi radialis muscle
5	Radial artery
6	Flexor digitorum superficialis muscle
7	Median nerve
8	Antebrachial fascia and tendon of palmaris longus muscle
9	Tendon of abductor pollicis longus muscle
10	Tendon of extensor pollicis brevis muscle
11	Abductor pollicis brevis muscle

12	Palmar aponeurosis
13	Superficial head of flexor pollicis brevis muscle
14	Tendon of flexor pollicis longus muscle
15	Medial intermuscular septum
16	Medial epicondyle of humerus
17	Humeral head of pronator teres muscle
18	Palmaris longus muscle
19	Flexor carpi ulnaris muscle
20	Ulnar artery
21	Tendon of flexor carpi ulnaris muscle
22	Palmaris brevis muscle

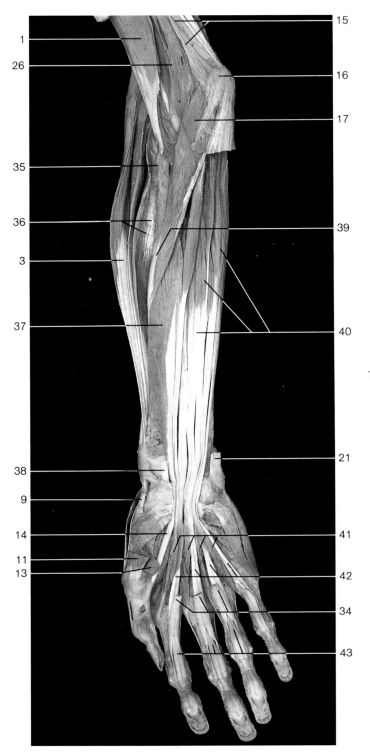

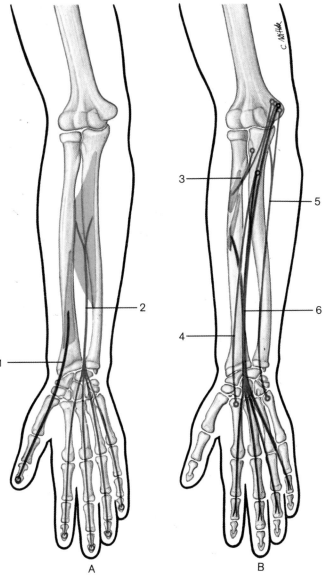

Position of flexors of fingers and hand (schematic drawing).

A   Deep layer

1   Flexor pollicis
    longus muscle (blue)
2   Flexor digitorum
    profundus muscle (red)

B   Superficial layer

3   Pronator teres muscle (red)
4   Flexor carpi radialis
    muscle (red)
5   Flexor carpi ulnaris
    muscle (red)
6   Flexor digitorum superficialis
    muscle (blue)

Flexor muscles of forearm and hand, middle layer (ventral aspect).
The palmaris longus, flexor carpi radialis, and ulnaris muscles have
been removed. The flexor retinaculum has been divided.

23   Abductor digiti minimi muscle
24   Transverse fasciculi of palmar aponeurosis
25   Digital fibrous sheaths of tendons of flexor digitorum muscle
26   Brachialis muscle
27   Flexor pollicis longus muscle
28   Carpal tunnel (canalis carpi, probe)
29   Triceps brachii muscle
30   Flexor digitorum superficialis muscle
31   Pisiform bone
32   Opponens digiti minimi muscle
33   Flexor digiti minimi brevis muscle
34   Tendons of flexor digitorum superficialis muscle

35   Supinator muscle
36   Extensor carpi radialis brevis muscle
37   Flexor pollicis longus muscle
38   Tendon of flexor carpi radialis muscle
39   Pronator teres muscle (insertion of radius)
40   Flexor digitorum profundus muscle
41   Lumbrical muscles
42   Tendons of flexor digitorum profundus muscle
43   Tendons of flexor digitorum profundus muscle having passed
     through the divided tendons of the flexor digitorum superficialis
     muscle
44   Flexor retinaculum

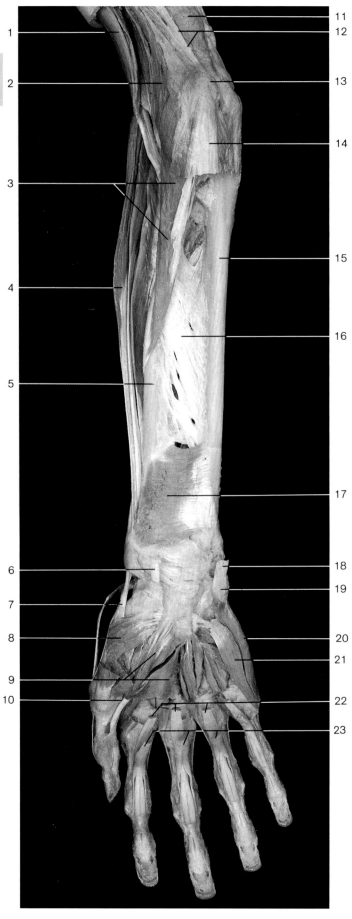

1. Biceps brachii muscle
2. Brachialis muscle
3. Pronator teres muscle
4. Brachioradialis muscle
5. Radius
6. Tendon of flexor carpi radialis muscle
7. Tendon of abductor pollicis longus muscle
8. Opponens pollicis muscle
9. Adductor pollicis muscle
10. Tendon of flexor pollicis longus muscle
11. Triceps brachii muscle
12. Medial intermuscular septum
13. Medial epicondyle of humerus
14. Common flexor mass (divided)
15. Ulna
16. Interosseous membrane
17. Pronator quadratus muscle
18. Tendon of flexor carpi ulnaris muscle
19. Pisiform bone
20. Abductor digiti minimi muscle
21. Flexor digiti minimi brevis muscle
22. Tendons of flexor digitorum profundus muscle
23. Tendons of flexor digitorum superficialis muscle
24. Flexor retinaculum
25. Hypothenar muscles
26. Thenar muscles
27. Common synovial sheath of flexor tendons
28. Synovial sheath of tendon of flexor pollicis longus muscle
29. Digital synovial sheaths of flexor tendons

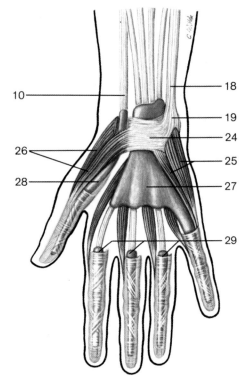

Flexor muscles of forearm and hand, deep layer (ventral aspect). All flexors have been removed to display the pronator quadratus and pronator teres muscles together with the interosseous membrane. Forearm in supination.

Synovial sheaths of flexor tendons (palmar aspect of right hand, semischematic drawing).

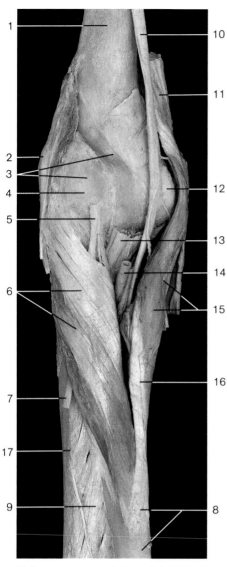

1 Humerus
2 Lateral epicondyle of humerus
3 Articular capsule
4 Position of capitulum of humerus
5 Deep branch of radial nerve
6 Supinator muscle
7 Entrance of deep branch of radial nerve to extensor muscles
8 Radius and insertion of pronator teres muscle
9 Interosseous membrane
10 Median nerve
11 Triceps brachii muscle
12 Trochlea of humerus
13 Tendon of biceps brachii muscle
14 Brachial artery
15 Pronator teres muscle
16 Tendon of pronator teres muscle
17 Ulna
18 Pronator quadratus muscle
19 Tendon of flexor carpi radialis muscle
20 Thenar muscles
21 Synovial sheath of tendon of flexor pollicis longus muscle
22 Fibrous sheath of flexor tendons
23 Digital synovial sheath of flexor tendons
24 Flexor digitorum superficialis muscle
25 Tendon of flexor carpi ulnaris muscle
26 Common synovial sheath of flexor tendons
27 Position of pisiform bone
28 Flexor retinaculum
29 Hypothenar muscles

Right supinator and elbow joint
(ventral aspect). Forearm in pronation.

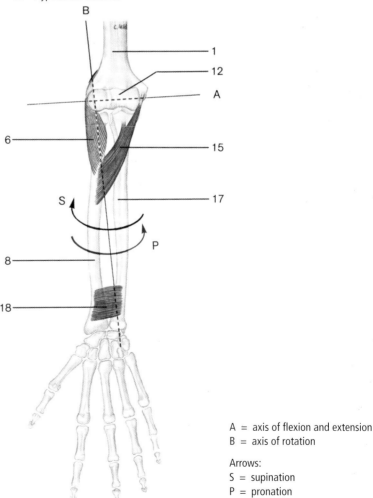

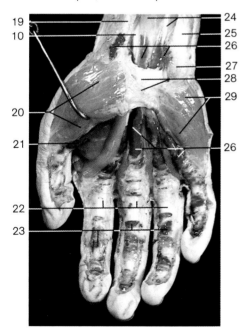

Synovial sheaths of flexor tendons
(palmar aspect of right hand). Blue PVA
solution has been injected into the sheaths.

A = axis of flexion and extension
B = axis of rotation

Arrows:
S = supination
P = pronation

Diagram illustrating the two axes of the elbow joint.

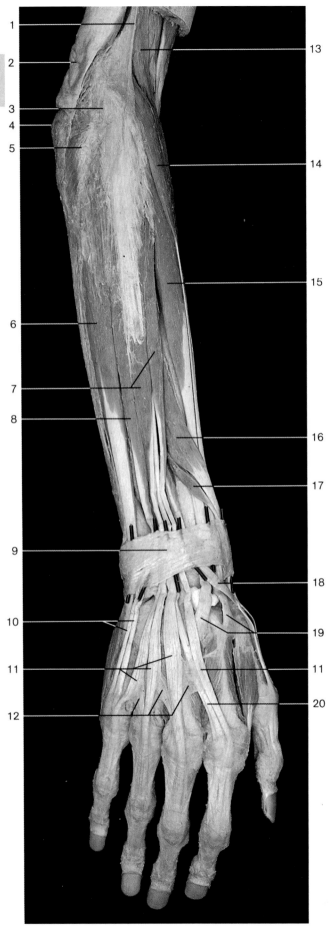

1   Lateral intermuscular septum
2   Tendon of triceps brachii muscle
3   Lateral epicondyle of humerus
4   Olecranon
5   Anconeus muscle
6   Extensor carpi ulnaris muscle
7   Extensor digitorum muscle
8   Extensor digiti minimi muscle
9   Extensor retinaculum
10 Tendons of extensor digiti minimi muscle
11 Tendons of extensor digitorum muscle
12 Intertendinous connections
13 Brachioradialis muscle
14 Extensor carpi radialis longus muscle
15 Extensor carpi radialis brevis muscle
16 Abductor pollicis longus muscle
17 Extensor pollicis brevis muscle
18 Tendon of extensor pollicis longus muscle
19 Tendons of both extensor carpi radialis longus
    and extensor carpi radialis brevis muscles
20 Tendon of extensor indicis muscle
21 First tunnel: Abductor pollicis longus muscle,
                     extensor pollicis brevis muscle
22 Second tunnel: Extensor carpi radialis longus and brevis muscles
23 Third tunnel: Extensor pollicis longus muscle
24 Fourth tunnel: Extensor digitorum muscle,
                     extensor indicis muscle
25 Fifth tunnel: Extensor digiti minimi muscle
26 Sixth tunnel: Extensor carpi ulnaris muscle

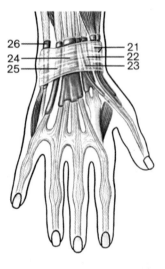

Synovial sheaths of extensor tendons on the back of the right wrist (indicated in blue). Notice the six tunnels for the passage of the extensor tendons beneath the extensor retinaculum (schematic drawing).

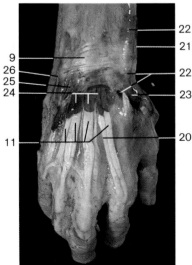

Extensor muscles of forearm and hand, superficial layer (dorsal aspect). Tunnels for extensor tendons indicated by probes.

Synovial sheaths of extensor tendons. The sheaths have been injected with blue gelatin.

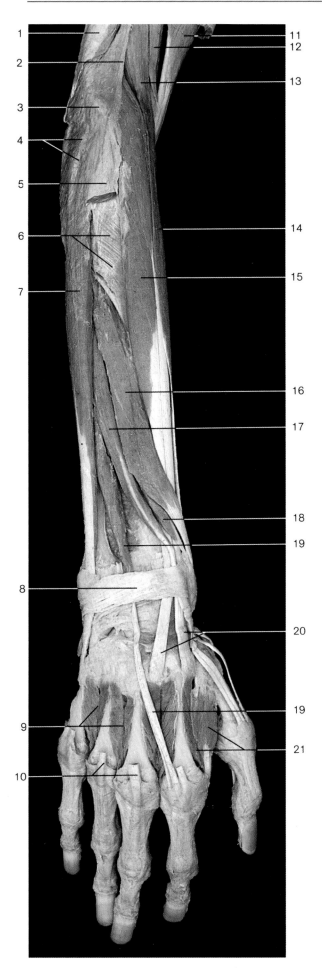

1 Triceps brachii muscle
2 Lateral intermuscular septum
3 Lateral epicondyle of humerus
4 Anconeus muscle
5 Extensor digitorum and extensor digiti minimi muscles (cut)
6 Supinator muscle
7 Extensor carpi ulnaris muscle
8 Extensor retinaculum
9 Third and fourth dorsal interosseous muscles
10 Tendons of extensor digitorum muscle (cut)
11 Biceps brachii muscle
12 Brachialis muscle
13 Brachioradialis muscle
14 Extensor carpi radialis longus muscle
15 Extensor carpi radialis brevis muscle
16 Abductor pollicis longus muscle
17 Extensor pollicis longus muscle
18 Extensor pollicis brevis muscle
19 Extensor indicis muscle
20 Tendons of the extensor carpi radialis longus and extensor carpi radialis brevis muscles
21 First dorsal interosseous muscle

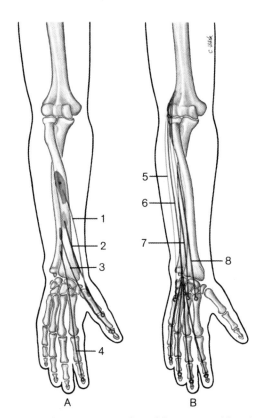

Position of extensor muscles of forearm and hand (schematic drawing).

A Extensors of thumb

1 Abductor pollicis longus muscle (red)
2 Extensor pollicis brevis muscle (blue)
3 Extensor pollicis longus muscle (red)
4 Extensor indicis muscle (blue)

B Extensors of fingers and hand

5 Extensor carpi ulnaris muscle (blue)
6 Extensor digitorum muscle (red)
7 Extensor carpi radialis brevis muscle (blue)
8 Extensor carpi radialis longus muscle (blue)

Extensor muscles of forearm and hand, deep layer (dorsal aspect).

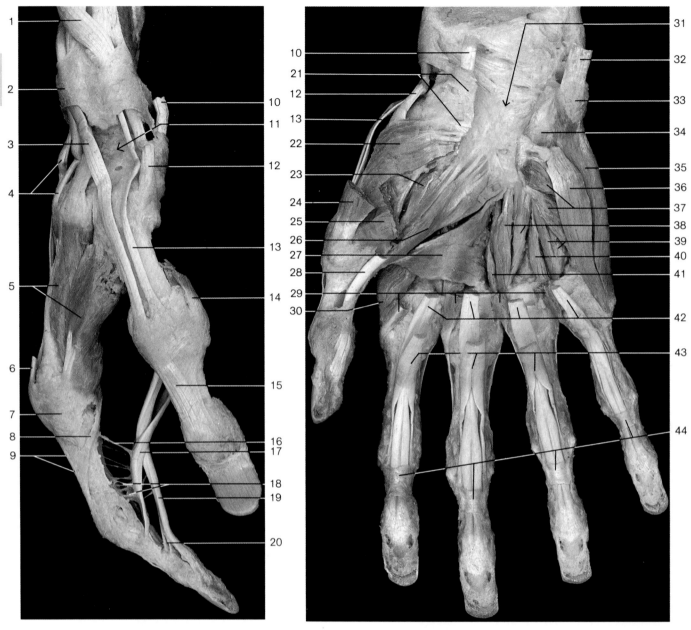

Muscles of thumb and index finger (medial aspect). The tendons of the extensor muscles of the thumb and the insertion of the flexor tendons of the index finger are displayed.

Muscles of right hand (palmar aspect). The tendons of the flexor muscles and parts of the thumb muscles have been removed. The carpal tunnel has been opened.

1	Tendons of extensor pollicis brevis and abductor pollicis longus muscle
2	Extensor retinaculum
3	Tendon of extensor pollicis longus muscle
4	Tendons of extensor carpi radialis longus and brevis muscles
5	First dorsal interosseous muscle
6	Tendon of extensor digitorum muscle for index finger
7	Location of metacarpophalangeal joint
8	Tendon of lumbrical muscle
9	Extensor expansion of index finger
10	Tendon of flexor carpi radialis muscle (cut)
11	Anatomical snuffbox
12	Tendon of abductor pollicis longus muscle
13	Tendon of extensor pollicis brevis muscle
14	Tendon of abductor pollicis brevis muscle

15	Extensor expansion of extensor of thumb
16	Vinculum longum
17	Tendons of flexor digitorum superficialis muscle dividing to allow passage of deep tendons
18	Vincula of flexor tendons
19	Tendon of flexor digitorum profundus muscle
20	Vinculum breve
21	Radial carpal eminence (cut edge of flexor retinaculum)
22	Opponens pollicis muscle
23	Deep head of flexor pollicis brevis muscle
24	Abductor pollicis brevis muscle (cut)
25	Superficial head of flexor pollicis brevis muscle (cut)
26	Oblique head of adductor pollicis muscle
27	Transverse head of adductor pollicis muscle
28	Tendon of flexor pollicis longus muscle (cut)

29	Lumbrical muscles (cut)
30	First dorsal interosseous muscle
31	Position of carpal tunnel
32	Tendon of flexor carpi ulnaris muscle
33	Location of pisiform bone
34	Hook of hamate bone
35	Abductor digiti minimi muscle
36	Flexor digiti minimi brevis muscle
37	Opponens digiti minimi muscle
38	Second palmar interosseous muscle
39	Third palmar interosseous muscle
40	Fourth dorsal interosseous muscle
41	Third dorsal interosseous muscle
42	Tendon of flexor digitorum profundus muscle (cut)
43	Tendons of flexor digitorum superficialis muscle (cut)
44	Fibrous flexor sheaths

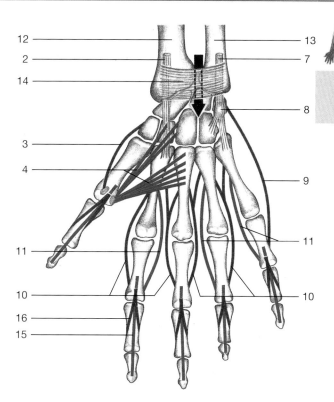

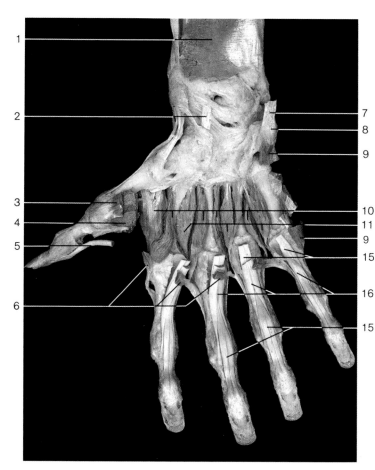

Muscles of right hand, deep layer (palmar aspect). The thenar and hypothenar muscles have been removed to display the interosseous muscles.

Actions of interosseous muscles in abduction and adduction of fingers (palmar aspect, schematic drawing).
Arrow: carpal tunnel.
Red = abduction (dorsal interosseous, abductor digiti minimi, and abductor pollicis brevis muscles)
Blue = adduction (palmar interosseous muscles, adductor pollicis muscle)

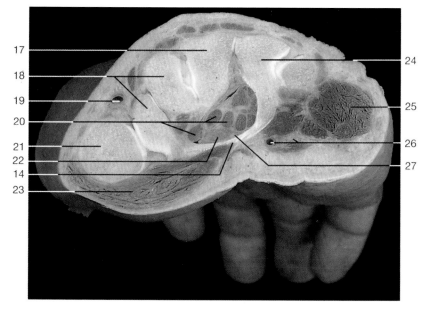

Transverse section through the right hand, showing the carpal tunnel (canalis carpi).

1   Pronator quadratus muscle
2   Tendon of flexor carpi radialis muscle
3   Abductor pollicis brevis muscle (divided)
4   Adductor pollicis muscle (divided)
5   Tendon of flexor pollicis longus muscle
6   Lumbrical muscles (cut)
7   Tendon of flexor carpi ulnaris muscle
8   Pisiform bone
9   Abductor digiti minimi muscle (divided)
10 Dorsal interosseous muscles
11 Palmar interosseous muscles
12 Radius
13 Ulna
14 Flexor retinaculum
15 Tendons of flexor digitorum profundus muscle
16 Tendons of flexor digitorum superficialis muscle
17 Capitate bone
18 Trapezium bone and trapezoid bone
19 Radial artery
20 Tendon of flexor muscles
21 First metacarpal bone
22 Median nerve
23 Thenar muscles
24 Hamate bone
25 Hypothenar muscles
26 Ulnar artery and nerve
27 Carpal tunnel (canalis carpi)

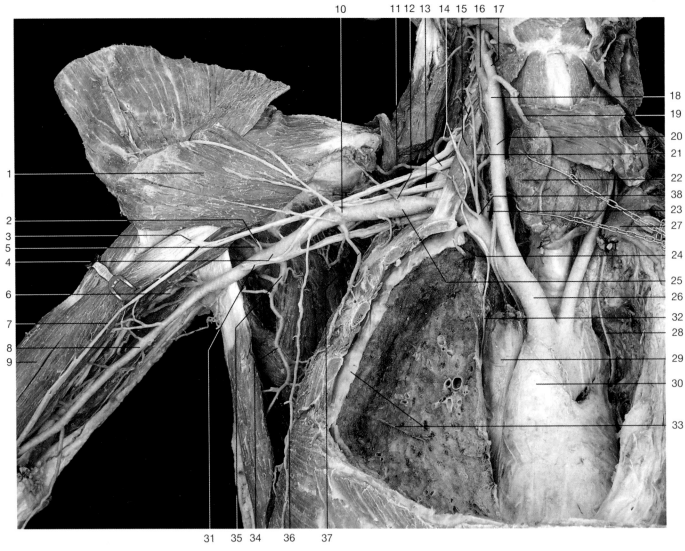

Main branches of right subclavian and axillary arteries (anterior aspect). Pectoralis muscles have been reflected, clavicle and anterior wall of thorax removed, and right lung divided. Left lung with pleura and thyroid gland have been reflected laterally to display aortic arch and common carotid artery with their branches.

1	Pectoralis minor muscle (reflected)	22	Thyroid gland	43	Radial collateral artery
2	Anterior circumflex humeral artery	23	Inferior thyroid artery	44	Radial recurrent artery
3	Musculocutaneous nerve (divided)	24	Internal thoracic artery	45	Radial artery
4	Axillary artery	25	Right subclavian artery	46	Anterior and posterior interosseous
5	Posterior circumflex humeral artery	26	Brachiocephalic trunk		arteries
6	Profunda brachii artery	27	Left brachiocephalic vein (divided)	47	Princeps pollicis artery
7	Median nerve (var.)	28	Left vagus nerve	48	Deep palmar arch
8	Brachial artery	29	Superior vena cava (divided)	49	Common palmar digital arteries
9	Biceps brachii muscle	30	Ascending aorta	50	Ulnar recurrent artery
10	Thoraco-acromial artery	31	Median nerve (divided)	51	Recurrent interosseous artery
11	Suprascapular artery	32	Phrenic nerve	52	Common interosseous artery
12	Descending scapular artery	33	Right lung (divided) and pulmonary pleura	53	Ulnar artery
13	Brachial plexus (middle trunk)	34	Thoracodorsal artery	54	Superficial palmar arch
14	Transverse cervical artery	35	Subscapular artery	55	Median nerve and brachial artery
15	Scalenus anterior muscle and phrenic nerve	36	Lateral mammary branches (variant)	56	Biceps brachii muscle
16	Right internal carotid artery	37	Lateral thoracic artery	57	Ulnar nerve
17	Right external carotid artery	38	Thyrocervical trunk	58	Flexor pollicis longus muscle
18	Carotid sinus	39	Superior thoracic artery	59	Palmar digital arteries
19	Superior thyroid artery	40	Superior ulnar collateral artery	60	Anterior interosseous artery
20	Right common carotid artery	41	Inferior ulnar collateral artery	61	Flexor carpi ulnaris muscle
21	Ascending cervical artery	42	Middle collateral artery	62	Superficial palmar branch of radial artery

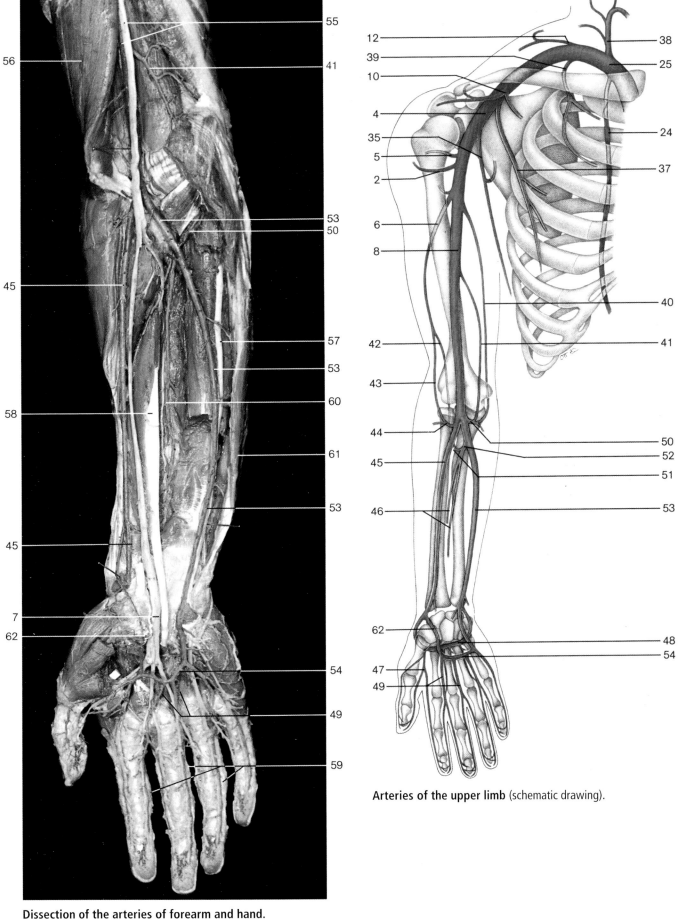

Dissection of the arteries of forearm and hand.
The superficial flexor muscles have been removed, the carpal
tunnel opened, and the flexor retinaculum cut. The arteries have
been filled with colored resin.

Arteries of the upper limb (schematic drawing).

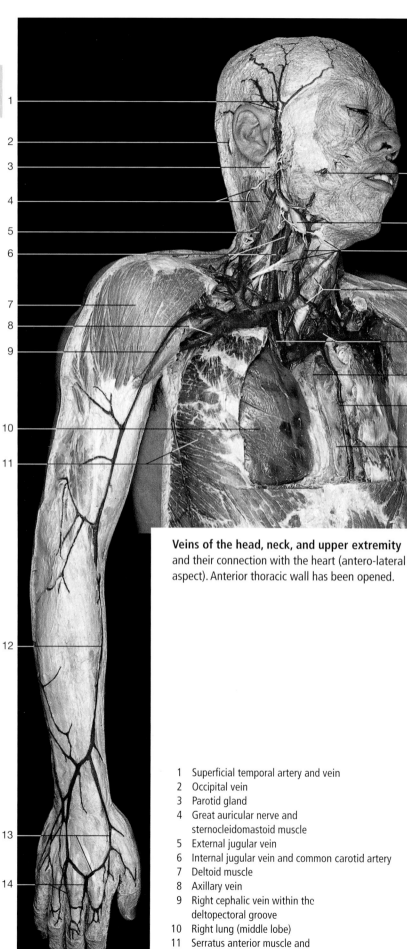

Veins of the head, neck, and upper extremity and their connection with the heart (antero-lateral aspect). Anterior thoracic wall has been opened.

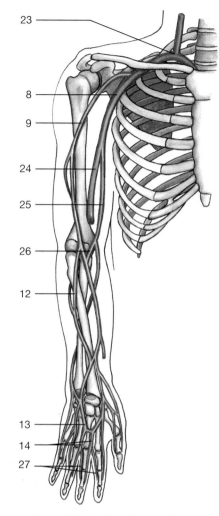

Superficial veins of upper limb (schematic drawing).

1	Superficial temporal artery and vein
2	Occipital vein
3	Parotid gland
4	Great auricular nerve and sternocleidomastoid muscle
5	External jugular vein
6	Internal jugular vein and common carotid artery
7	Deltoid muscle
8	Axillary vein
9	Right cephalic vein within the deltopectoral groove
10	Right lung (middle lobe)
11	Serratus anterior muscle and lateral thoracic vein
12	Cephalic vein on forearm
13	Venous network on dorsum of hand
14	Dorsal metacarpal veins
15	Facial artery and vein
16	Submandibular gland
17	Anterior jugular vein, hyoid bone, and omohyoid muscle
18	Jugular venous arch and thyroid gland
19	Right and left brachiocephalic veins
20	Retrosternal body (remnant of thymus gland)
21	Internal thoracic artery and vein
22	Heart with pericardium
23	Right venous angle
24	Brachial vein
25	Basilic vein
26	Median cubital vein
27	Digital veins

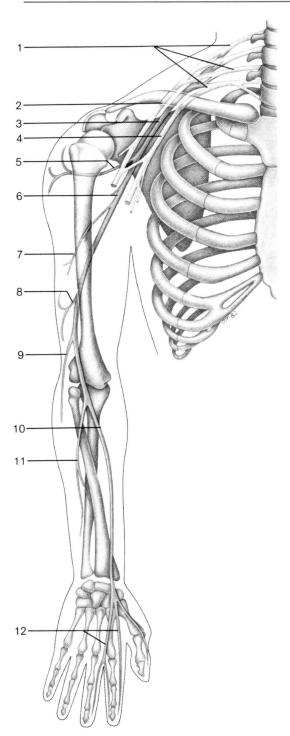

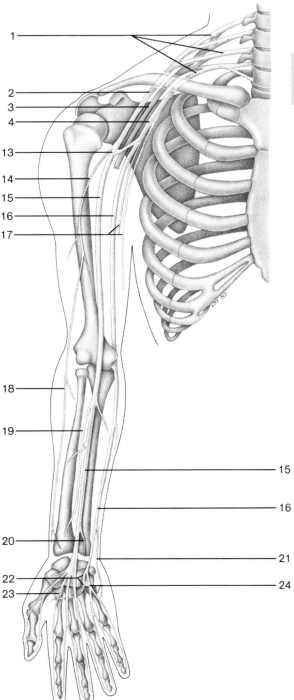

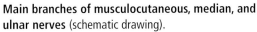

Main branches of radial nerve (schematic drawing). Posterior divisions of trunks and posterior cord and its branches are indicated in green.

Main branches of musculocutaneous, median, and ulnar nerves (schematic drawing). Anterior divisions of the trunks and all the components arising from them are indicated in yellow.

1 Brachial plexus
2 Lateral cord of brachial plexus
3 Posterior cord of brachial plexus
4 Medial cord of brachial plexus
5 Axillary nerve
6 Radial nerve
7 Posterior cutaneous nerve of arm
8 Lower lateral cutaneous nerve of arm
9 Posterior cutaneous nerve of forearm
10 Superficial branch of radial nerve
11 Deep branch of radial nerve
12 Dorsal digital nerves

13 Roots of median nerve
14 Musculocutaneous nerve
15 Median nerve
16 Ulnar nerve
17 Medial cutaneous nerves of arm and forearm
18 Lateral cutaneous nerve of forearm
19 Anterior interosseous nerve
20 Palmar branch of median nerve
21 Dorsal branch of ulnar nerve
22 Deep branch of ulnar nerve
23 Common palmar digital nerves of median nerve
24 Superficial branch of ulnar nerve

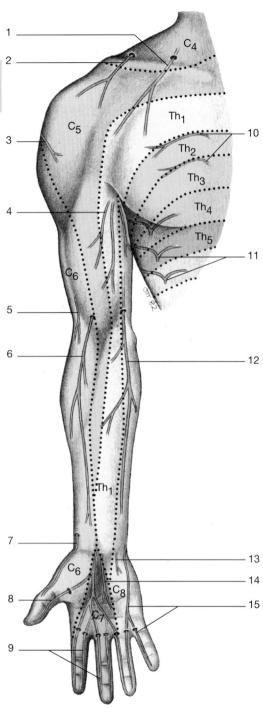

Cutaneous nerves of the right upper limb (ventral aspect, schematic drawing).

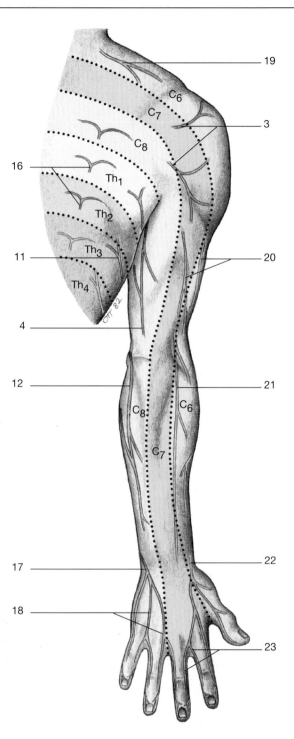

Cutaneous nerves of the right upper limb (dorsal aspect, schematic drawing).

1	Medial supraclavicular nerve	13	Palmar cutaneous branch of ulnar nerve
2	Intermediate supraclavicular nerve	14	Palmar branch of median nerve
3	Upper lateral cutaneous nerve of arm	15	Palmar digital branches of ulnar nerve
4	Terminal branches of intercostobrachial nerves	16	Cutaneous branches of dorsal rami of spinal nerves
5	Lower lateral cutaneous nerve of arm	17	Dorsal branch of ulnar nerve
6	Lateral cutaneous nerve of forearm	18	Dorsal digital nerves
7	Terminal branch of superficial branch of radial nerve	19	Posterior supraclavicular nerve
8	Palmar digital nerve of thumb (branch of median nerve)	20	Posterior cutaneous nerve of arm
9	Palmar digital branches of median nerve	21	Posterior cutaneous nerve of forearm
10	Anterior cutaneous branches of intercostal nerves	22	Superficial branch
11	Lateral cutaneous branches of intercostal nerves	23	Dorsal digital branches
12	Medial cutaneous nerve of forearm		

20–23 from radial nerve

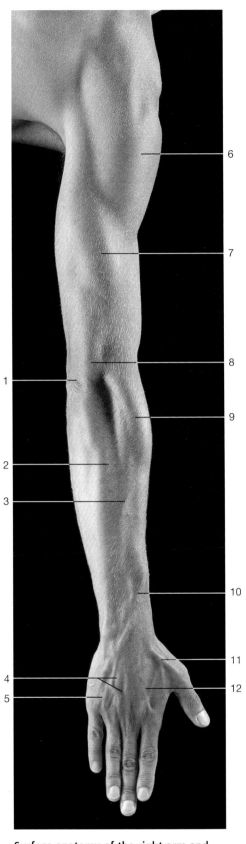

Surface anatomy of the right arm and hand (posterior aspect).

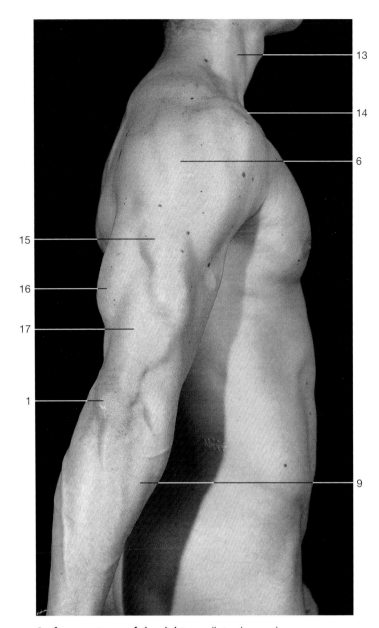

Surface anatomy of the right arm (lateral aspect).
Triceps brachii muscle is strongly contracted.

1	Olecranon	11	Tendon of abductor pollicis longus muscle
2	Extensor muscles of forearm	12	Tendon of extensor indicis muscle
3	Accessory cephalic vein	13	Sternocleidomastoid muscle
4	Tendons of extensor digitorum muscle	14	Clavicle
5	Dorsal venous network of hand	15	Lateral head of triceps brachii muscle
6	Deltoid muscle	16	Medial head of triceps brachii muscle
7	Triceps brachii muscle	17	Tendon of triceps brachii muscle
8	Lateral epicondyle of humerus		
9	Brachioradialis muscle		
10	Cephalic vein		

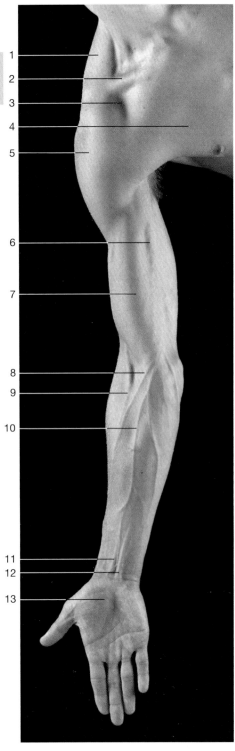

Surface anatomy of the right arm and hand (anterior aspect).

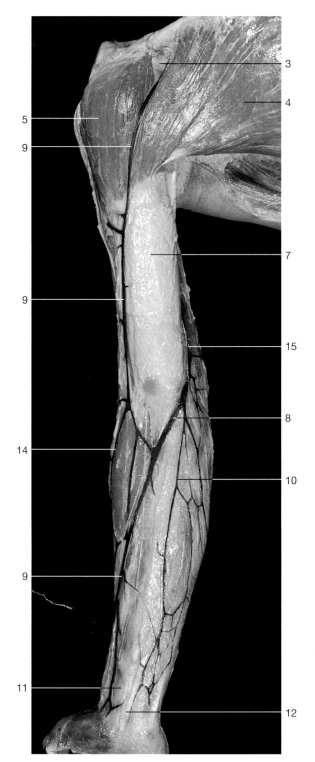

Superficial veins of the right arm, injected with blue gelatine (anterior aspect).

1   Trapezius muscle
2   Clavicle
3   Deltopectoral triangle
4   Pectoralis major muscle
5   Deltoid muscle
6   Brachial vein
7   Biceps brachii muscle

8   Median cubital vein
9   Cephalic vein
10 Median vein of forearm
11 Tendon of flexor carpi radialis
12 Tendon of palmaris longus muscle
13 Location of adductor pollicis muscle
14 Accessory cephalic vein
15 Basilic vein

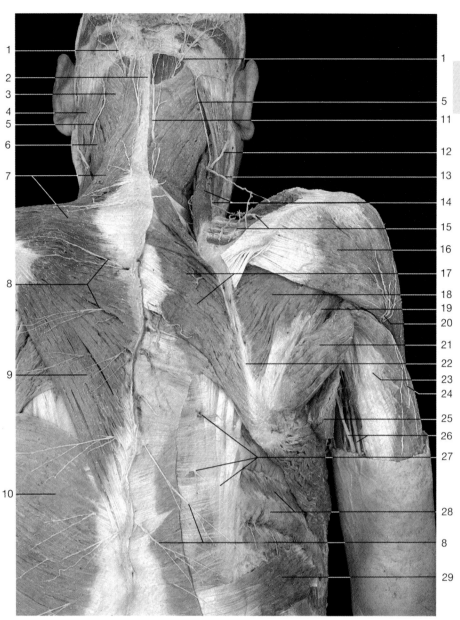

Posterior regions of neck and shoulder (dorsal aspect). Left side: superficial layer. Right side: trapezius and latissimus dorsi muscles have been removed. Dissection of dorsal branches of spinal nerves.

1 Greater occipital nerve	16 Deltoid muscle
2 Ligamentum nuchae	17 Rhomboid major muscle
3 Splenius capitis muscle	18 Infraspinatus muscle
4 Sternocleidomastoid muscle	19 Teres minor muscle
5 Lesser occipital nerve	20 Upper lateral cutaneous nerve of arm (branch of axillary nerve)
6 Splenius cervicis muscle	21 Teres major muscle
7 Descending and transverse fibers of trapezius muscle	22 Medial margin of scapula
8 Medial cutaneous branches of dorsal rami of spinal nerves	23 Long head of triceps muscle
9 Ascending fibers of trapezius muscle	24 Posterior cutaneous nerve of arm (branch of radial nerve)
10 Latissimus dorsi muscle	25 Latissimus dorsi muscle (divided)
11 Cutaneous branch of third occipital nerve	26 Ulnar nerve and brachial artery
12 Great auricular nerve	27 Lateral cutaneous branches of dorsal rami of spinal nerves and iliocostalis thoracis muscle
13 Accessory nerve (n. XI)	28 External intercostal muscle and seventh rib
14 Posterior supraclavicular nerve and levator scapulae muscle	29 Serratus posterior inferior muscle
15 Branches of suprascapular artery	

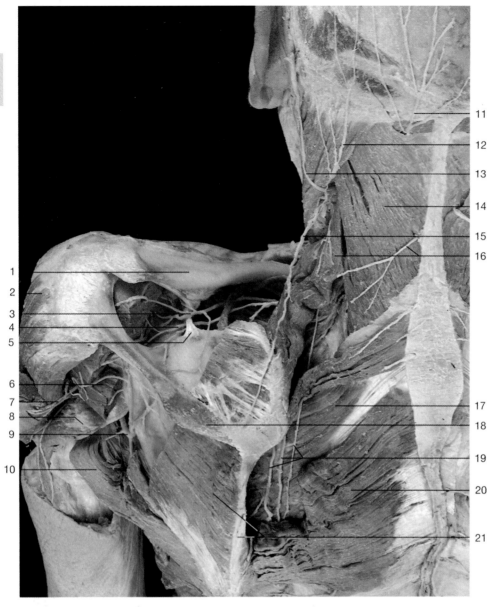

1	Clavicle
2	Deltoid muscle
3	Suprascapular artery
4	Suprascapular nerve
5	Superior transverse scapular ligament
6	Teres minor muscle
7	Axillary nerve and posterior circumflex humeral artery
8	Long head of triceps muscle
9	Circumflex scapular artery
10	Teres major muscle
11	Greater occipital nerve
12	Lesser occipital nerve
13	Great auricular nerve
14	Splenius capitis muscle
15	Accessory nerve (n. XI)
16	Third occipital nerve and levator scapulae muscle
17	Serratus posterior superior muscle
18	Spine of scapula
19	Descending scapular artery and dorsal scapular nerve
20	Rhomboid major muscle
21	Infraspinatus muscle and medial margin of scapula
22	Radial nerve and profunda brachii artery
23	Thoracodorsal artery
24	Thyrocervical trunk
25	Roots of brachial plexus

Posterior region of shoulder, deepest layer. Rhomboid and scapular muscles fenestrated; posterior part of deltoid muscle reflected.

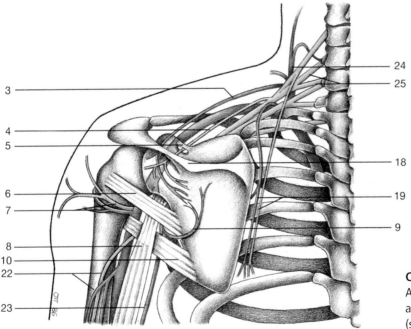

Collateral circulation of shoulder.
Anastomosis of suprascapular
and circumflex scapular arteries
(schematic drawing).

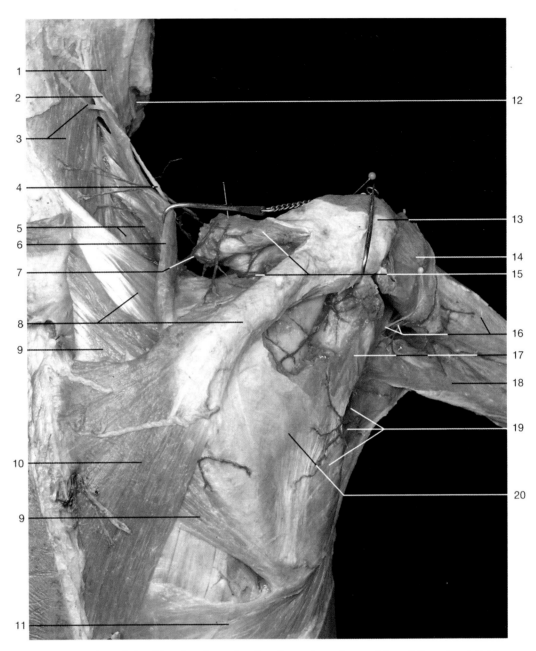

Posterior region of shoulder, deep layer. Arteries of scapular region are injected. Trapezius, deltoid, and infraspinatus muscles are partially removed or reflected.

1   Sternocleidomastoid muscle
2   Lesser occipital nerve
3   Splenius capitis muscle and
    third occipital nerve
4   Accessory nerve (n. XI)
5   Splenius cervicis muscle and transverse
    cervical artery (deep branch)
6   Levator of scapula muscle
7   Transverse cervical artery (superficial
    branch)
8   Spine of scapula and serratus posterior
    superior muscle
9   Rhomboid major muscle

10 Trapezius muscle
11 Latissimus dorsi muscle
12 Facial artery
13 Acromion
14 Deltoid muscle
15 Suprascapular artery and supraspinatus muscle
    (reflected)
16 Axillary nerve, posterior circumflex humeral
    artery, and lateral head of triceps brachii muscle
17 Teres minor muscle
18 Long head of triceps brachii muscle
19 Circumflex scapular artery and teres major
20 Infraspinatus muscle

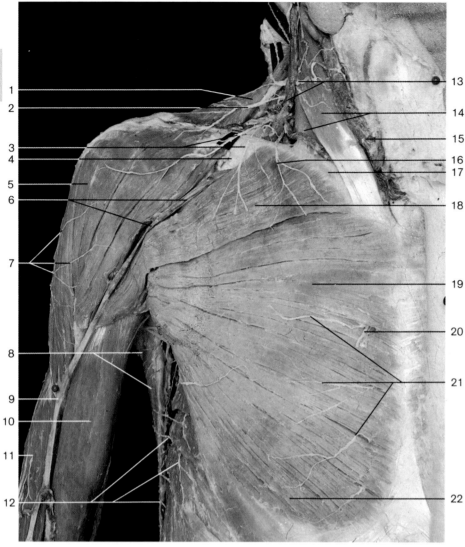

1   Trapezius muscle
2   Posterior supraclavicular nerve
3   Middle supraclavicular nerve
4   Deltopectoral triangle
5   Deltoid muscle
6   Cephalic vein within the deltopectoral groove
7   Upper lateral cutaneous nerve of arm (branch of axillary nerve)
8   Latissimus dorsi muscle
9   Cephalic vein
10 Biceps brachii muscle
11 Triceps brachii muscle
12 Lateral cutaneous branches of intercostal nerves
13 Transverse cervical nerve and external jugular vein
14 Sternocleidomastoid muscle
15 Anterior jugular vein
16 Anterior supraclavicular nerve
17 Clavicle
18 Clavicular part of pectoralis major muscle
19 Sternocostal part of pectoralis major muscle
20 Perforating branch of internal thoracic artery
21 Anterior cutaneous branches of intercostal nerves
22 Abdominal part of pectoralis major muscle
23 Sternocleidomastoid muscle, cervical branch of facial nerve, and anterior jugular vein
24 External jugular vein and transverse cervical nerve (inferior branch)
25 Sternoclavicular joint (opened) with articular disc
26 Pectoralis major muscle
27 Omohyoid muscle and external jugular vein
28 Jugular venous arch and sternohyoid muscle
29 Sternoclavicular joint (not opened)

Right shoulder and thoracic wall, superficial layer (anterior aspect). Dissection of the cutaneous nerves and veins.

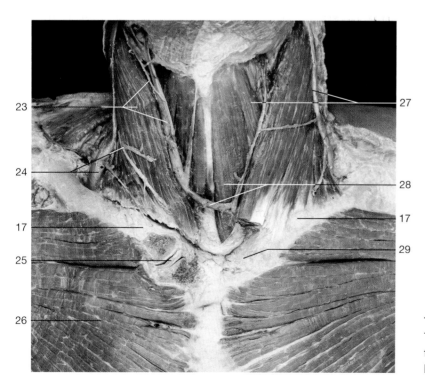

Thoracic wall with neck region (anterior aspect). The sternoclavicular joint is depicted. On the right side the joint has been opened by a coronal section. Note the articular disc.

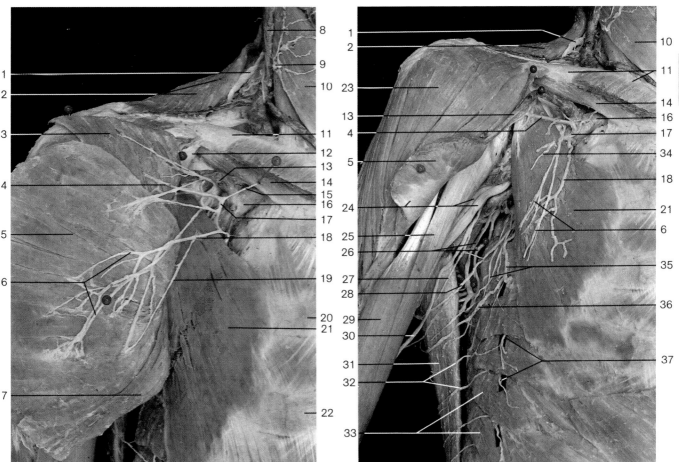

Right deltopectoral triangle, infraclavicular region
(anterior aspect). The pectoralis major muscle has been cut and
reflected.

Right shoulder and thoracic wall with axillary region, deep
layer (anterior aspect). The pectoralis major muscle has been cut
and partly removed.

1   Accessory nerve
2   Trapezius muscle
3   Pectoralis major muscle (clavicular part)
4   Acromial branch of thoraco-acromial artery
5   Pectoralis major muscle
6   Lateral pectoral nerves
7   Abdominal part of pectoralis major muscle
8   External jugular vein
9   Cutaneous branches of cervical plexus
10 Sternocleidomastoid muscle
11 Clavicle
12 Clavipectoral fascia
13 Cephalic vein
14 Subclavius muscle
15 Clavicular branch of thoraco-acromial artery
16 Subclavian vein
17 Thoraco-acromial artery
18 Pectoral branch of thoraco-acromial artery
19 Medial pectoral nerve
20 Second rib

21 Pectoralis minor muscle
22 Third rib
23 Deltoid muscle
24 Pectoralis major muscle (reflected), brachial artery, and
    median nerve
25 Short head of biceps brachii muscle
26 Thoracodorsal artery and nerve
27 Medial cutaneous nerve of arm
28 Intercostobrachial nerve (T$_2$)
29 Long head of biceps brachii muscle
30 Medial cutaneous nerve of forearm
31 Latissimus dorsi muscle
32 Lateral cutaneous branches of intercostal nerves
    (posterior branches)
33 Serratus anterior muscle
34 Medial pectoral nerve
35 Long thoracic nerve and lateral thoracic artery
36 Intercostobrachial nerve (T$_3$)
37 Lateral cutaneous branches of intercostal nerves
    (anterior branches)

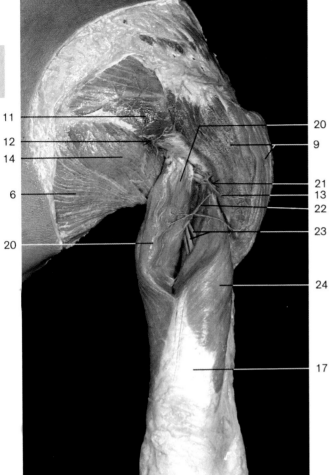

Shoulder and arm (dorsal aspect). Dissection of the quadrangular and triangular spaces of the axillary region.

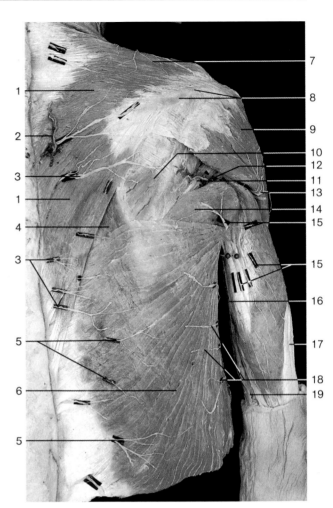

Posterior region of shoulder and arm, superficial layer. Note the segmental arrangement of the cutaneous nerves of the back.

1 Trapezius muscle
2 Dorsal branches of posterior intercostal artery and vein (medial cutaneous branches)
3 Medial branches of dorsal rami of spinal nerves
4 Rhomboid major muscle
5 Lateral branches of dorsal rami of spinal nerves
6 Latissimus dorsi muscle
7 Posterior supraclavicular nerves
8 Spine of scapula
9 Deltoid muscle
10 Infraspinatus muscle
11 Teres minor muscle
12 Triangular space with circumflex scapular artery and vein
13 Upper lateral cutaneous nerve of arm with artery
14 Teres major muscle
15 Terminal branches of intercostobrachial nerve
16 Medial cutaneous nerve of arm
17 Tendon of triceps brachii muscle
18 Lateral cutaneous branches of intercostal nerves
19 Medial cutaneous nerve of forearm
20 Long head of triceps brachii muscle
21 Quadrangular space with axillary nerve and posterior humeral circumflex artery
22 Anastomosis between profunda brachii artery and posterior humeral circumflex artery
23 Course of radial nerve and profunda brachii artery
24 Lateral head of triceps brachii muscle
25 Medial collateral artery
26 Radial collateral artery
27 Radial nerve

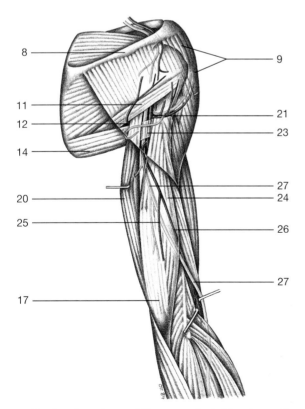

Regional anatomy of the upper limb (dorsal aspect). Localization of vessels and nerves.

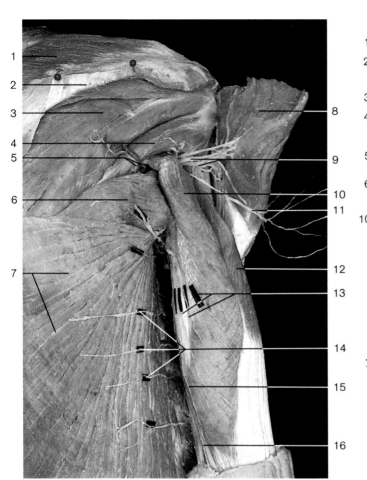

Scapular region, arm and shoulder, deep layer (dorsal aspect). Part of deltoid muscle has been cut and reflected to display the quadrangular and triangular spaces of the axillary region.

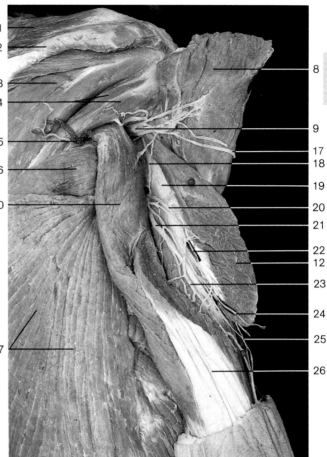

Scapular region, arm and shoulder, deep layer (dorsal aspect). The lateral head of the triceps brachii muscle has been cut to display the radial nerve and accompanying vessels.

1	Trapezius muscle
2	Spine of scapula
3	Infraspinatus muscle
4	Teres minor muscle
5	Triangular space containing circumflex scapular artery and vein
6	Teres major muscle
7	Latissimus dorsi muscle
8	Deltoid muscle (cut and reflected)
9	Quadrangular space containing axillary nerve and posterior circumflex humeral artery and vein
10	Long head of triceps brachii muscle
11	Cutaneous branch of axillary nerve
12	Lateral head of triceps brachii muscle
13	Terminal branches of intercostobrachial nerve

14	Lateral cutaneous branches of intercostal nerves
15	Medial cutaneous nerve of arm
16	Medial cutaneous nerve of forearm
17	Upper lateral cutaneous nerve of arm
18	Anastomosis between profunda brachii artery and posterior humeral circumflex artery
19	Humerus
20	Profunda brachii artery
21	Radial nerve
22	Radial collateral artery
23	Middle collateral artery
24	Lower lateral cutaneous nerve of arm
25	Posterior cutaneous nerve of forearm
26	Tendon of triceps brachii muscle

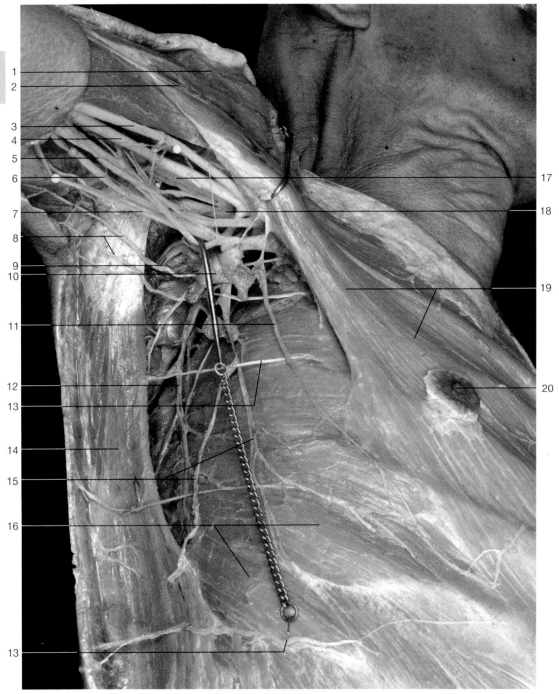

Right axillary region (inferior aspect). **Dissection of superficial axillary nodes and lymphatic vessels.**
The pectoralis major muscle has been slightly elevated.

1	Deltoid muscle	11	Lateral thoracic artery
2	Cephalic vein	12	Thoracodorsal artery
3	Median nerve	13	Lateral cutaneous branch of intercostal nerve
4	Brachial artery	14	Latissimus dorsi muscle
5	Medial cutaneous nerves of arm and forearm	15	Thoraco-epigastric vein
6	Ulnar nerve	16	Serratus anterior muscle
7	Basilic vein	17	Musculocutaneous nerve
8	Intercostobrachial nerves	18	Radial nerve
9	Circumflex scapular artery	19	Pectoralis major muscle
10	Superficial axillary nodes	20	Nipple

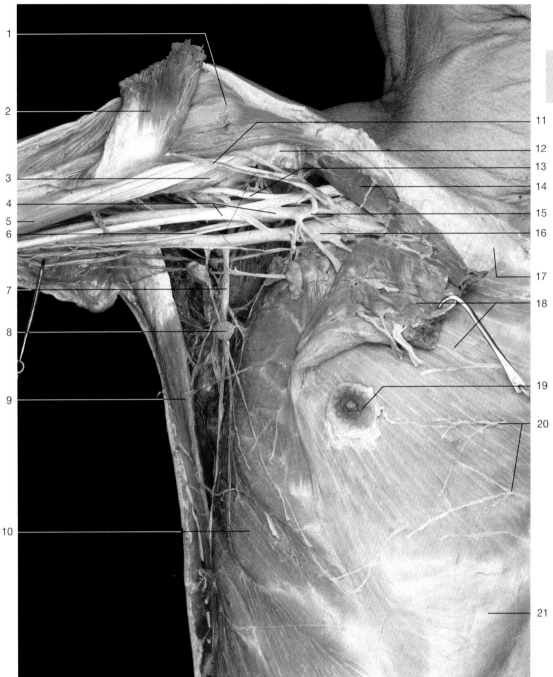

Right axillary region (anterior aspect). **Dissection of deep axillary nodes.** Pectoralis major and minor muscles divided and reflected. Shoulder girdle and arm elevated and reflected.

1   Deltoid muscle
2   Insertion of pectoralis major muscle
3   Coracobrachialis muscle
4   Roots of median nerve, axillary artery
5   Short head of biceps brachii muscle
6   Ulnar nerve and medial cutaneous nerve of forearm
7   Thoraco-epigastric vein
8   Deep axillary node
9   Latissimus dorsi muscle
10 Serratus anterior muscle

11 Cephalic vein
12 Insertion of pectoralis minor muscle (coracoid process)
13 Musculocutaneous nerve
14 Subclavius muscle
15 Thoraco-acromial artery
16 Axillary vein
17 Clavicle
18 Pectoralis major and minor muscles (reflected)
19 Nipple
20 Anterior cutaneous branches of intercostal nerves
21 Anterior layer of rectus sheath

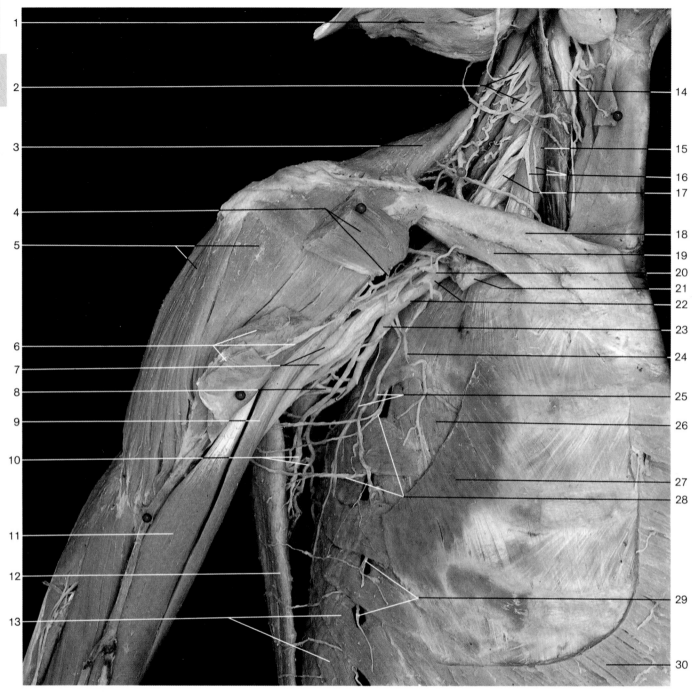

Right axillary region (anterior aspect). The pectoralis major and minor muscles have been cut and reflected to display the vessels and nerves of the axilla.

1 Sternocleidomastoid muscle (cut and reflected)
2 Cervical plexus
3 Trapezius muscle
4 Pectoralis minor muscle and medial pectoral nerve
5 Deltoid muscle
6 Pectoralis major muscle and lateral pectoral nerve
7 Median nerve and brachial artery
8 Circumflex scapular artery
9 Short head of biceps brachii muscle
10 Thoracodorsal artery and nerve
11 Long head of biceps brachii muscle
12 Latissimus dorsi muscle
13 Serratus anterior muscle
14 Internal jugular vein
15 Scalenus anterior muscle

16 Phrenic nerve and ascending cervical artery
17 Brachial plexus (at the levels of the trunks)
18 Clavicle
19 Subclavius muscle
20 Thoraco-acromial artery
21 Subclavian vein (cut)
22 Axillary artery
23 Subscapular artery
24 Superior thoracic artery
25 Lateral thoracic artery and long thoracic nerve
26 External intercostal muscle
27 Insertion of pectoralis minor muscle
28 Intercostobrachial nerves
29 Lateral cutaneous branches of intercostal nerves
30 Insertion of pectoralis major muscle

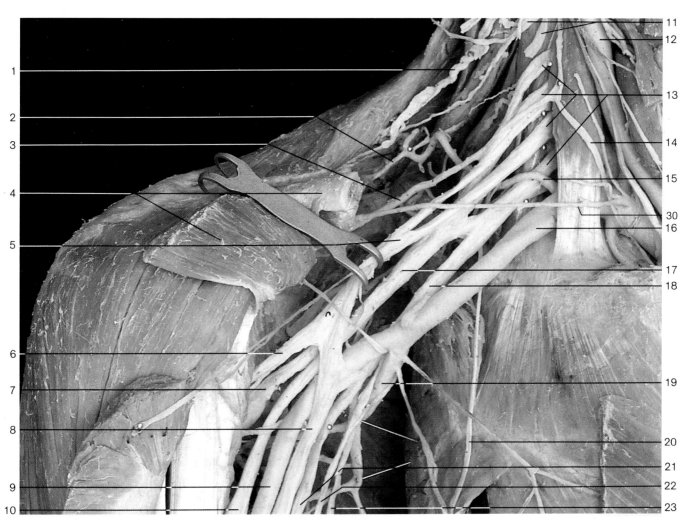

Brachial plexus (anterior aspect). Clavicle and the two pectoralis muscles have been partly removed.

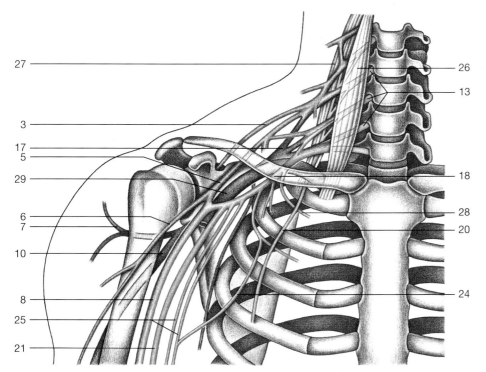

Main branches of brachial plexus. Posterior cord in purple, lateral cord in orange, and medial cord in green (schematic drawing).

1   Accessory nerve
2   Dorsal scapular artery
3   Suprascapular nerve
4   Clavicle and pectoralis minor muscle
5   Lateral cord of brachial plexus
6   Musculocutaneous nerve
7   Axillary nerve
8   Median nerve
9   Brachial artery
10 Radial nerve
11 Cervical plexus
12 Common carotid artery
13 Roots of brachial plexus (C_5–T_1)
14 Phrenic nerve
15 Transverse cervical artery
16 Subclavian artery
17 Posterior cord of brachial plexus
18 Medial cord of brachial plexus
19 Subscapular artery
20 Long thoracic nerve
21 Ulnar nerve
22 Medial cutaneous nerve of forearm
23 Thoracodorsal nerve
24 Intercostobrachial nerve
25 Medial cutaneous nerves of arm and forearm
26 Scalenus anterior muscle
27 Scalenus medius muscle
28 Intercostal nerve (T_1)
29 Axillary artery
30 Suprascapular artery

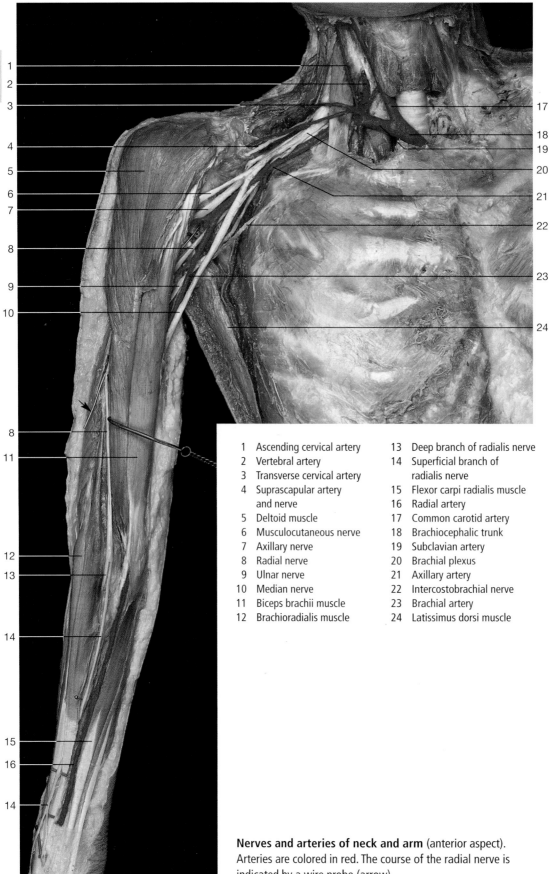

1 Ascending cervical artery	13 Deep branch of radialis nerve
2 Vertebral artery	14 Superficial branch of
3 Transverse cervical artery	radialis nerve
4 Suprascapular artery	15 Flexor carpi radialis muscle
and nerve	16 Radial artery
5 Deltoid muscle	17 Common carotid artery
6 Musculocutaneous nerve	18 Brachiocephalic trunk
7 Axillary nerve	19 Subclavian artery
8 Radial nerve	20 Brachial plexus
9 Ulnar nerve	21 Axillary artery
10 Median nerve	22 Intercostobrachial nerve
11 Biceps brachii muscle	23 Brachial artery
12 Brachioradialis muscle	24 Latissimus dorsi muscle

Nerves and arteries of neck and arm (anterior aspect).
Arteries are colored in red. The course of the radial nerve is
indicated by a wire probe (arrow).

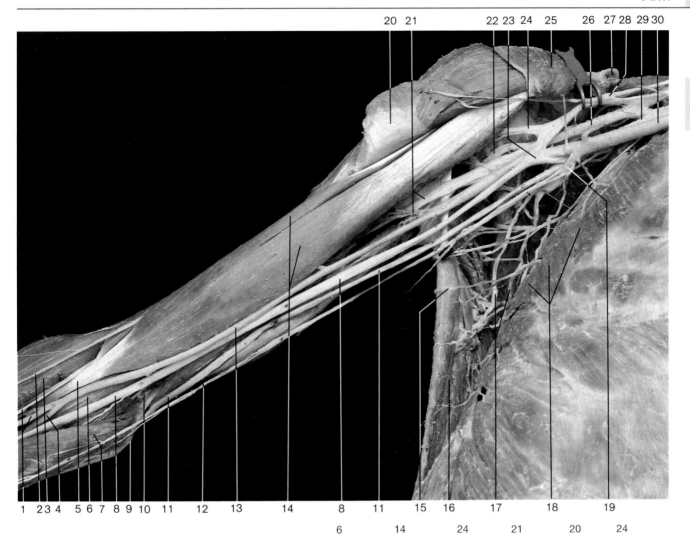

Right arm. Dissection of vessels and nerves (medial aspect). Shoulder girdle has been reflected slightly.

Right arm. Dissection of vessels and nerves, deeper layer. Biceps muscle has been reflected.

1 Radial artery and superficial branch of radial nerve	8 Median nerve	17 Thoracodorsal nerve and artery	24 Musculocutaneous nerve
2 Lateral cutaneous nerve of forearm	9 Medial epicondyle of humerus	18 Serratus anterior muscle	25 Pectoralis minor muscle (reflected) and medial pectoral nerve
3 Brachioradialis muscle	10 Inferior ulnar collateral artery	19 Subscapular artery	26 Posterior cord of brachial plexus
4 Ulnar artery	11 Ulnar nerve	20 Pectoralis major muscle (reflected) and lateral pectoral nerve	27 Clavicle (cut)
5 Tendon of biceps brachii muscle	12 Medial cutaneous nerve of forearm	21 Radial nerve and profunda brachii artery	28 Lateral cord of brachial plexus
6 Brachialis muscle	13 Brachial artery	22 Axillary nerve	29 Medial cord of brachial plexus
7 Pronator teres muscle	14 Biceps brachii muscle	23 Roots of the median nerve with axillary artery	30 Subclavian artery
	15 Intercostobrachial nerve (T$_3$)		31 Brachial vein
	16 Latissimus dorsi muscle		

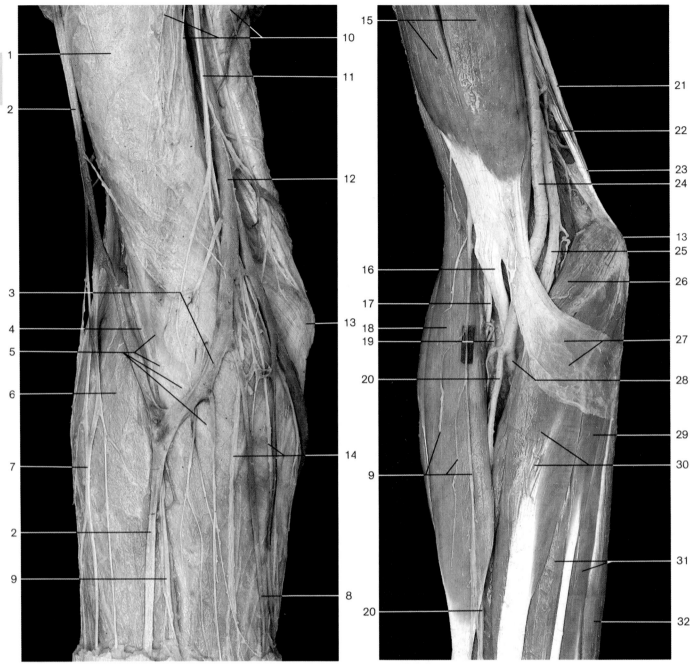

Cubital region (anterior aspect). Dissection of cutaneous nerves and veins.

Cubital region, superficial layer (anterior aspect). The fasciae of the muscles have been removed.

1   Biceps brachii muscle with fascia
2   Cephalic vein
3   Median cubital vein
4   Lateral cutaneous nerve of forearm
5   Tendon and aponeurosis of biceps brachii muscle
    (covered by the antebrachial fascia)
6   Brachioradialis muscle with fascia
7   Accessory cephalic vein
8   Median vein of forearm
9   Branches of lateral cutaneous nerve of forearm
10 Terminal branches of medial cutaneous nerve of arm
11 Medial cutaneous nerve of forearm
12 Basilic vein
13 Medial epicondyle of humerus
14 Terminal branches of medial cutaneous nerve
    of forearm
15 Biceps brachii muscle

16 Tendon of biceps brachii muscle
17 Radial nerve
18 Brachioradialis muscle
19 Radial recurrent artery
20 Radial artery
21 Ulnar nerve
22 Superior ulnar collateral artery
23 Medial intermuscular septum
24 Brachial artery
25 Median nerve
26 Pronator teres muscle
27 Bicipital aponeurosis
28 Ulnar artery
29 Palmaris longus muscle
30 Flexor carpi radialis muscle
31 Flexor digitorum superficialis muscle
32 Flexor carpi ulnaris muscle

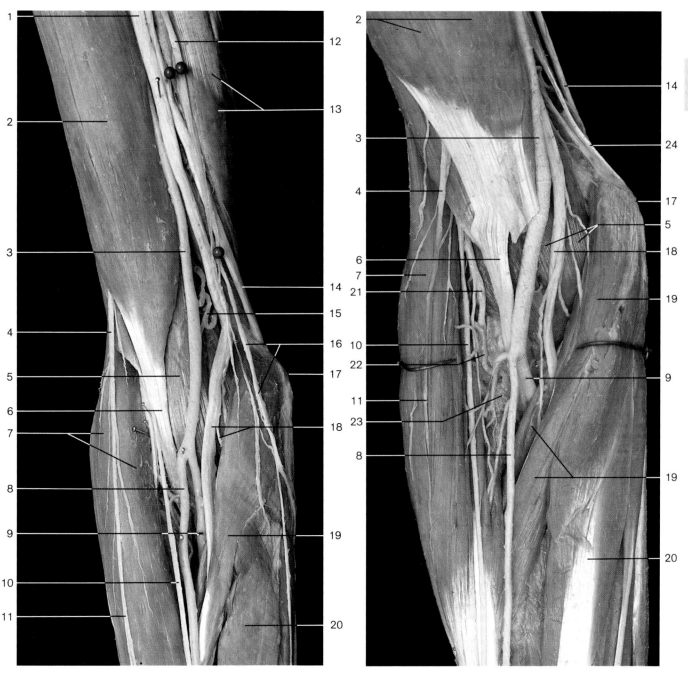

Cubital region, middle layer (anterior aspect). The bicipital aponeurosis has been removed.

Cubital region, middle layer (anterior aspect). The pronator teres and brachioradialis muscles have been slightly reflected.

1 Median nerve
2 Biceps brachii muscle
3 Brachial artery
4 Lateral cutaneous nerve of forearm
   (terminal branch of musculocutaneous nerve)
5 Brachialis muscle
6 Tendon of biceps brachii muscle
7 Brachioradialis muscle
8 Radial artery
9 Ulnar artery
10 Superficial branch of radial nerve
11 Lateral cutaneous nerve of forearm
12 Medial cutaneous nerve of forearm

13 Triceps brachii muscle
14 Ulnar nerve
15 Inferior ulnar collateral artery
16 Anterior branch of medial cutaneous nerve of forearm
17 Medial epicondyle of humerus
18 Median nerve with branches to pronator teres muscle
19 Pronator teres muscle
20 Flexor carpi radialis muscle
21 Deep branch of radial nerve
22 Radial recurrent artery
23 Supinator muscle
24 Medial intermuscular septum of arm

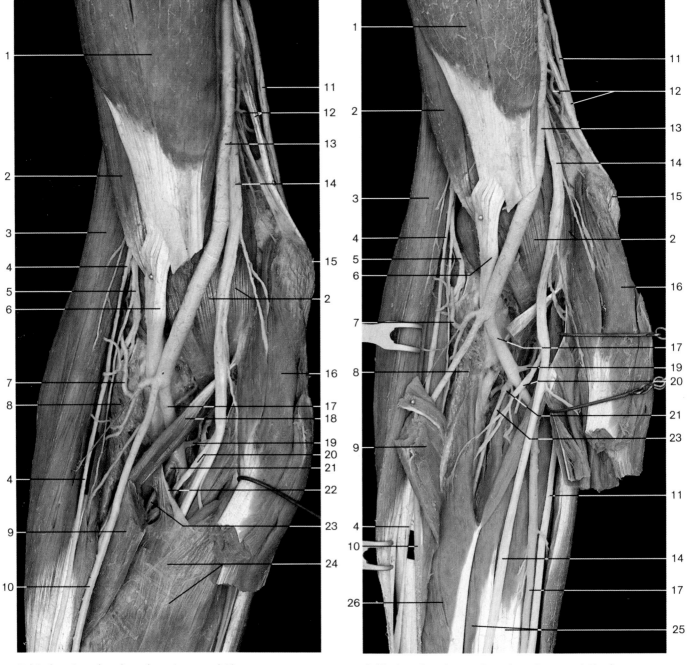

Cubital region, deep layer (anterior aspect). The pronator teres and flexor carpi ulnaris muscles have been cut and reflected.

Cubital region, deepest layer (anterior aspect). The flexor digitorum superficialis muscle and the ulnar head of the pronator teres muscle have been cut and reflected.

1	Biceps brachii muscle
2	Brachialis muscle
3	Brachioradialis muscle
4	Superficial branch of radial nerve
5	Deep branch of radial nerve
6	Tendon of biceps brachii muscle
7	Radial recurrent artery
8	Supinator muscle
9	Insertion of pronator teres muscle
10	Radial artery
11	Ulnar nerve
12	Medial intermuscular septum of arm and superior ulnar collateral artery
13	Brachial artery

14	Median nerve
15	Medial epicondyle of humerus
16	Humeral head of pronator teres muscle
17	Ulnar artery
18	Ulnar head of pronator teres muscle
19	Ulnar recurrent artery
20	Anterior interosseous nerve
21	Common interosseous artery
22	Tendinous arch of flexor digitorum superficialis muscle
23	Anterior interosseous artery
24	Flexor digitorum superficialis muscle
25	Flexor digitorum profundus muscle
26	Flexor pollicis longus muscle

1 Radial artery
2 Basilic vein
3 Pronator teres muscle
4 Flexor carpi radialis muscle
5 Ulnar artery
6 Palmaris longus muscle
7 Median nerve
8 Tendon of biceps brachii muscle
9 Flexor digitorum superficialis muscle
10 Ulnar nerve
11 Tendon of brachialis muscle
12 Flexor carpi ulnaris muscle
13 Flexor digitorum profundus muscle
14 Ulna
15 Median cubital vein
16 Cephalic antebrachii vein
17 Radial vein
18 Brachioradialis muscle
19 Superficial branch of radial nerve,
    radial artery and vein
20 Extensor carpi radialis longus muscle
21 Extensor carpi radialis brevis muscle
22 Supinator muscle
23 Deep branch of radial nerve
24 Radius
25 Extensor digitorum muscle
26 Extensor carpi ulnaris muscle
27 Anconeus muscle

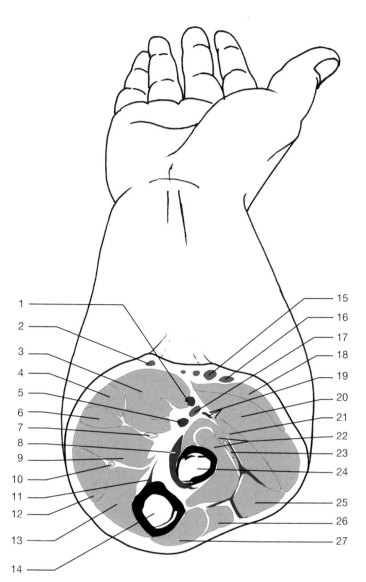

Muscles, nerves, and blood vessels of the forearm (axial section distally of the elbow joint, cf. MRI scan).

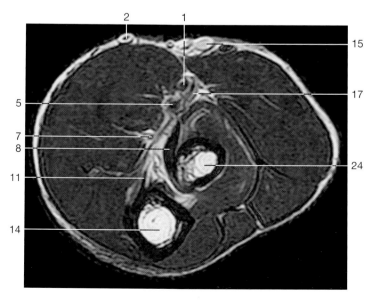

Axial section of the forearm (distally of the elbow joint, MRI scan; from Heuck et al., MRT-Atlas, 2009). For details see schematic drawing above.

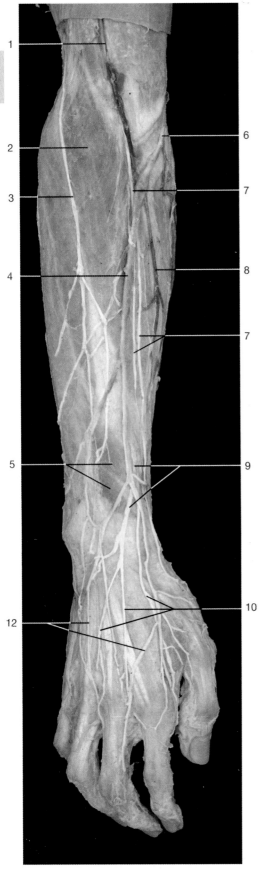

Superficial veins and cutaneous nerves of forearm and hand (posterior aspect).

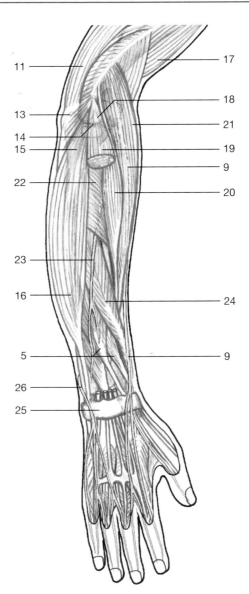

Course of the nerves to forearm and hand (posterior aspect).
Yellow = radial and ulnar nerves.

1 Cephalic vein
2 Brachioradialis muscle covered by its fascia
3 Posterior cutaneous nerve of forearm (branch of radialis nerve)
4 Cephalic vein of forearm
5 Extensor pollicis longus and brevis muscles covered by their fascia
6 Median cubital vein
7 Lateral cutaneous nerves of forearm (branch of musculocutaneous nerve)
8 Intermedian vein of forearm
9 Superficial branch of radial nerve
10 Dorsal digital branches of radial nerve

11 Triceps brachii muscle
12 Dorsal venous network of hand
13 Olecranon
14 Humeroradial joint
15 Ulna
16 Extensor carpi ulnaris muscle
17 Biceps brachii muscle
18 Trochlea of humerus
19 Extensor digitorum muscle
20 Extensor carpi radialis muscle
21 Brachioradialis muscle
22 Supinator muscle
23 Deep branch of radial nerve
24 Abductor pollicis longus muscle
25 Extensor retinaculum
26 Ulnar nerve

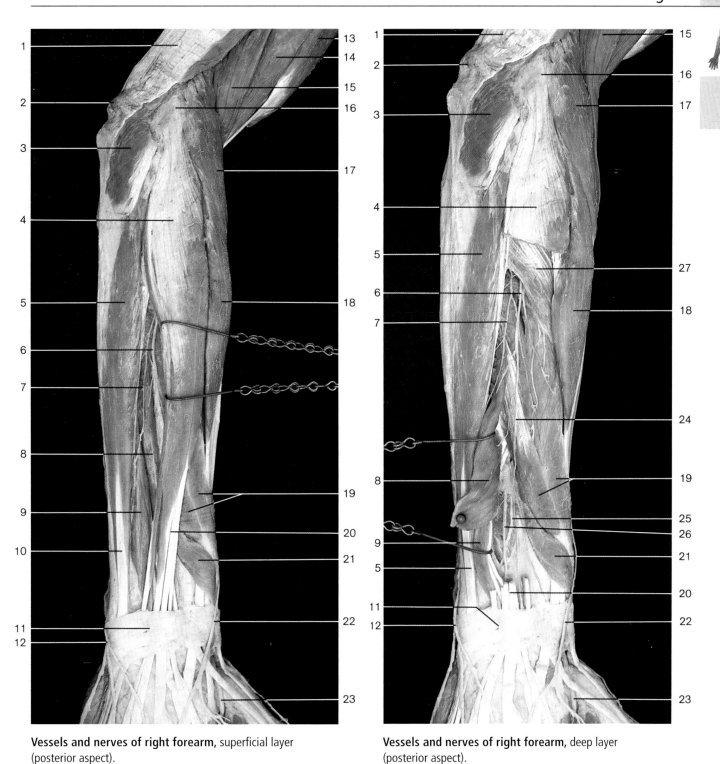

Vessels and nerves of right forearm, superficial layer (posterior aspect).

Vessels and nerves of right forearm, deep layer (posterior aspect).

1 Tendon of triceps brachii muscle	11 Extensor retinaculum	21 Extensor pollicis brevis muscle
2 Olecranon	12 Dorsal branch of ulnar nerve	22 Superficial branch of radial nerve
3 Anconeus muscle	13 Biceps brachii muscle	23 Radial artery
4 Extensor digitorum muscle	14 Brachialis muscle	24 Posterior interosseous nerve
5 Extensor carpi ulnaris muscle	15 Brachioradialis muscle	25 Posterior interosseous branch of
6 Deep branch of radial nerve	16 Lateral epicondyle of humerus	radial nerve
7 Posterior interosseous artery	17 Extensor carpi radialis longus muscle	26 Posterior branch of anterior
8 Extensor pollicis longus muscle	18 Extensor carpi radialis brevis muscle	interosseous artery
9 Extensor indicis muscle	19 Abductor pollicis longus muscle	27 Supinator muscle
10 Tendon of extensor carpi ulnaris muscle	20 Tendons of extensor digitorum muscle	

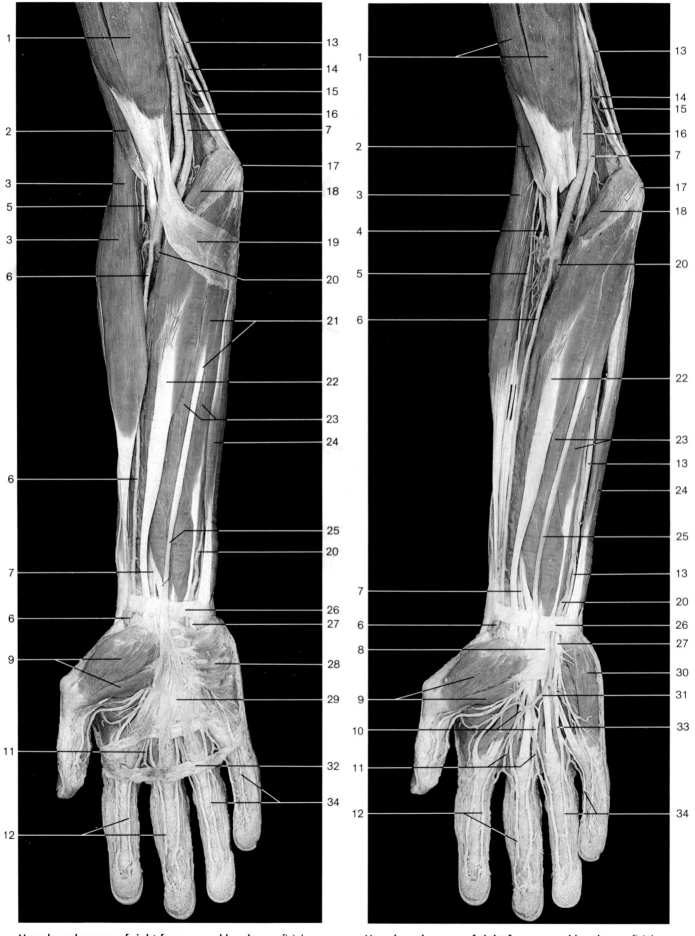

Vessels and nerves of right forearm and hand, superficial layer (palmar aspect).

Vessels and nerves of right forearm and hand, superficial layer (palmar aspect). The palmar aponeurosis of the hand and the bicipital aponeurosis have been removed.

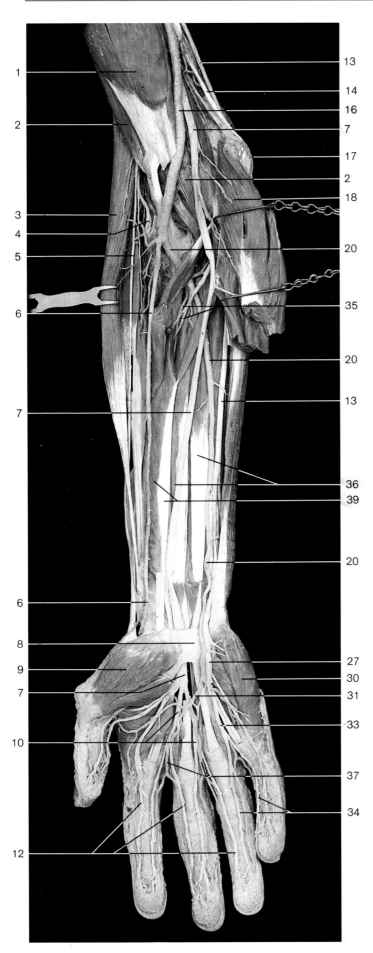

1   Biceps brachii muscle
2   Brachialis muscle
3   Brachioradialis muscle
4   Deep branch of radial nerve
5   Superficial branch of radial nerve
6   Radial artery
7   Median nerve
8   Flexor retinaculum
9   Thenar muscles
10 Common palmar digital branches of median nerve
11 Common palmar digital arteries
12 Proper palmar digital nerves (median nerve)
13 Ulnar nerve
14 Medial intermuscular septum of arm
15 Superior ulnar collateral artery
16 Brachial artery
17 Medial epicondyle of humerus
18 Pronator teres muscle
19 Bicipital aponeurosis
20 Ulnar artery
21 Palmaris longus muscle
22 Flexor carpi radialis muscle
23 Flexor digitorum superficialis muscle
24 Flexor carpi ulnaris muscle
25 Tendon of palmaris longus muscle
26 Remnant of antebrachial fascia
27 Superficial branch of ulnar nerve
28 Palmaris brevis muscle
29 Palmar aponeurosis
30 Hypothenar muscles
31 Superficial palmar arch
32 Superficial transverse metacarpal ligament
33 Common palmar digital branch of ulnar nerve
34 Proper palmar digital branches of ulnar nerve
35 Anterior interosseous artery and nerve
36 Flexor digitorum profundus muscle
37 Common palmar digital arteries
38 Palmar branch of median nerve
39 Flexor pollicis longus muscle
40 Palmar branch of ulnar nerve

Vessels and nerves of forearm and hand, deep layer (palmar aspect). The superficial layer of the flexor muscles has been removed.

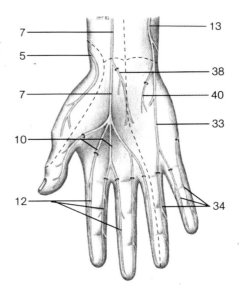

Innervation pattern of palmar surfaces of hand.
3½ digits by median nerve, 1½ digits by ulnar nerve.

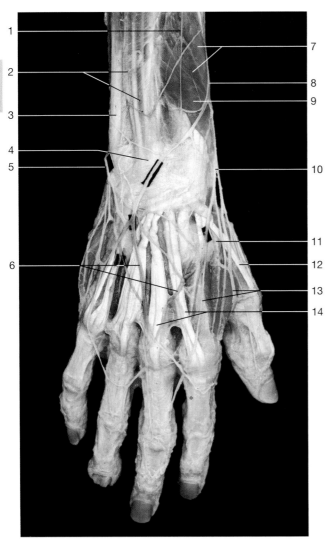

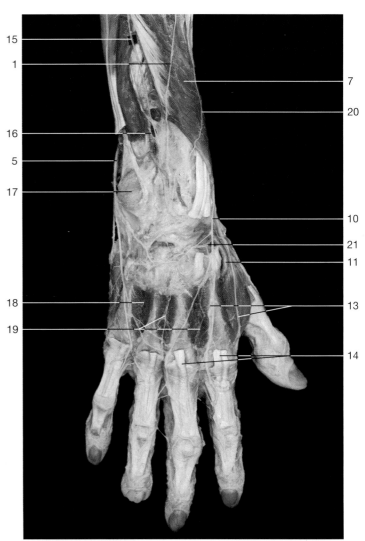

Posterior region of hand (superficial layer). Cutaneous nerves and veins are depicted.

Posterior region of hand (deeper layer). Extensor digitorum muscle has been partly removed.

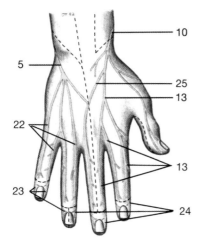

Innervation pattern of posterior surfaces of hand.
2½ digits by radial nerve, 2½ digits by ulnar nerve. Note that the terminal branches to the dorsal surfaces of the distal phalanges are derived from the palmar digital nerves. The cutaneous distribution varies; often 3½ digits are innervated by the radial and 1½ digits by the ulnar nerve.

1 Posterior cutaneous nerve of forearm (branch of radial nerve)
2 Extensor digitorum muscle
3 Tendon of extensor carpi ulnaris muscle
4 Extensor retinaculum
5 Ulnar nerve
6 Dorsal venous network of hand
7 Abductor pollicis longus muscle
8 Cephalic vein
9 Extensor pollicis brevis muscle
10 Radial nerve, superficial branch
11 Radial artery
12 Tendon of extensor pollicis longus muscle
13 Dorsal digital branches of radial nerve
14 Tendons of extensor digitorum muscle with intertendinous connections
15 Posterior interosseus nerve (branch of the deep radial nerve)
16 Posterior interosseous artery
17 Styloid process of ulna
18 Dorsal interosseus muscle IV
19 Dorsal carpal branch of radial artery
20 Lateral cutaneous nerve of forearm (branch of musculocutaneous nerve)
21 Dorsal metacarpal artery
22 Proper dorsal digital branches of ulnar nerve
23 Regions supplied by palmar digital nerves (ulnar nerve)
24 Regions supplied by palmar digital nerves (median nerve)
25 Communicating branch with ulnar nerve

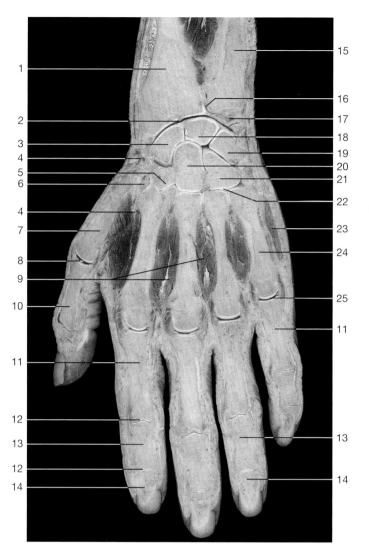

Coronal section through the left hand (posterior aspect).

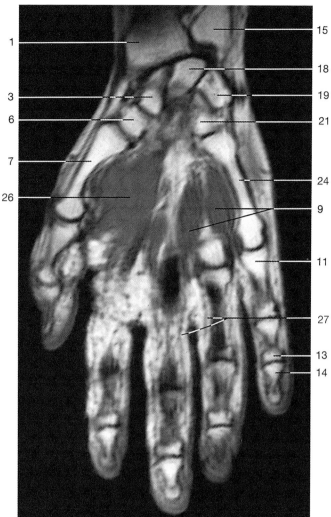

Coronal section through the left hand (posterior aspect)
(MRI scan, courtesy of Prof. Heuck, Munich).

Axial section through the left hand (MRI scan;
from Heuck et al., MRT-Atlas, 2009).

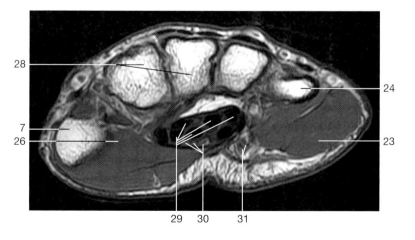

1	Radius	
2	Wrist joint	
3	Scaphoid (navicular) bone	
4	Radial artery	
5	Trapezoid bone	
6	Trapezium bone	
7	First metacarpal bone	
8	Metacarpophalangeal joint of thumb	
9	Interosseous muscles	
10	Proximal phalanx of thumb	
11	Proximal phalanx of fingers	
12	Interphalangeal joints	
13	Middle phalanx	
14	Distal phalanx	
15	Ulna	
16	Distal radio-ulnar joint	
17	Articular disc	
18	Lunate bone	
19	Triquetral bone	
20	Capitate bone	
21	Hamate bone	
22	Carpometacarpal joints	
23	Abductor digiti minimi muscle	
24	Fifth metacarpal bone	
25	Metacarpophalangeal joint	
26	Adductor pollicis muscle	
27	Proper palmar digital arteries	
28	Second and third metacarpal bones	
29	Tendons of flexor digitorum superficialis and profundus muscles	
30	Median nerve	
31	Ulnar artery and vein	

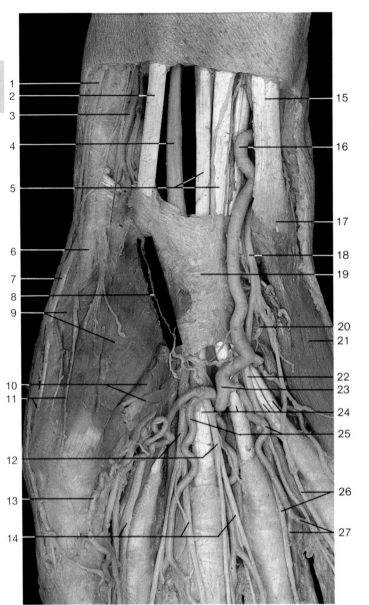

1
2
3
4
5
6
7
8
9
10
11
12
13
14

15
16
17
18
19
20
21
22
23
24
25
26
27

1
4
3

32
19
8

31
12

14

34
16

43
18

30
23
25

27

35

Arteries and nerves of the right hand
(palmar aspect, schematic drawing).

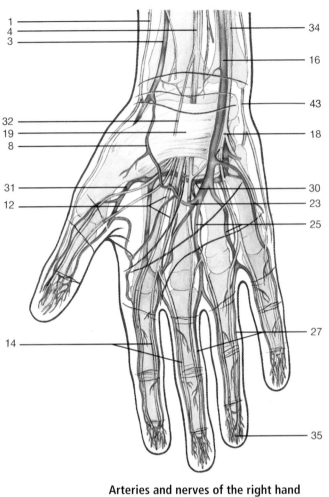

◁

Right hand, superficial layer (palmar aspect).
Dissection of the superficial palmar arch.

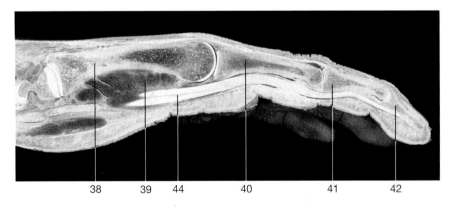

38   39   44   40   41   42

Longitudinal section through the hand
at the level of the third finger.

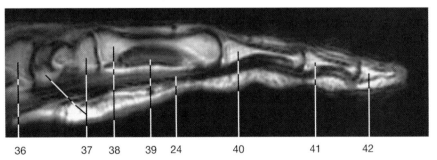

36   37   38   39   24   40   41   42

Longitudinal section through the hand
at the level of the third finger (MRI scan,
courtesy of Prof. Heuck, Munich).

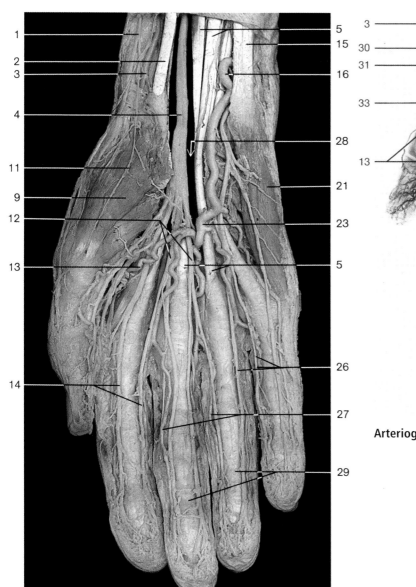

Right hand, middle layer (palmar aspect). The flexor retinaculum has been removed.

Arteriogram of the right hand (palmar aspect).

1   Superficial branch of radial nerve
2   Tendon of flexor carpi radialis muscle
3   Radial artery
4   Median nerve
5   Tendon of flexor digitorum superficialis muscle
6   Tendon of abductor pollicis longus muscle
7   Tendon of extensor pollicis brevis muscle
8   Superficial palmar branch of radial artery
9   Abductor pollicis brevis muscle
10 Superficial head of flexor pollicis brevis muscle
11 Terminal branches of superficial branch of radial nerve
12 Common palmar digital nerves (median nerve)
13 Proper palmar digital arteries of thumb
14 Proper palmar digital nerves (median nerve)
15 Tendon of flexor carpi ulnaris muscle
16 Ulnar artery
17 Position of pisiform bone
18 Superficial branch of ulnar nerve
19 Flexor retinaculum
20 Deep branch of ulnar nerve
21 Abductor digiti minimi muscle
22 Common palmar digital nerves (ulnar nerve)

23 Superficial palmar arch
24 Tendons of flexor digitorum muscles
25 Common palmar digital arteries
26 Palmar digital nerves (ulnar nerve)
27 Proper palmar digital arteries
28 Carpal tunnel
29 Fibrous sheaths for the tendons of flexor digitorum muscles
30 Deep palmar arch
31 Princeps pollicis artery
32 Palmar branch of median nerve
33 Common digital palmar artery
34 Ulnar nerve
35 Capillary network of finger
36 Radius
37 Carpal bones
38 Metacarpal bone
39 Interosseous muscles
40 Proximal phalanx
41 Middle phalanx
42 Distal phalanx
43 Dorsal branch of ulnar nerve
44 Tendons of flexor digitorum profundus (upper) and superficialis (lower) muscles

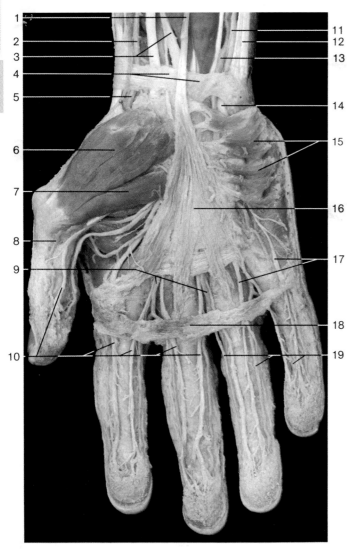

Right hand, superficial layer (palmar aspect). Dissection of vessels and nerves.

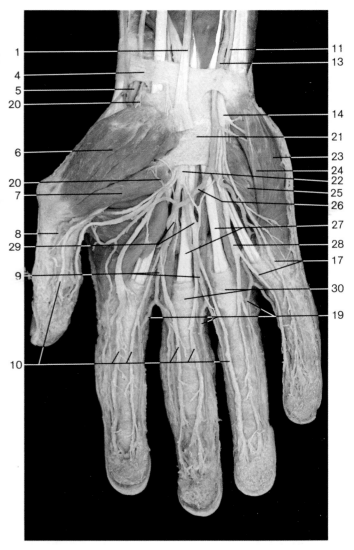

Right hand, superficial layer (palmar aspect). Dissection of vessels and nerves. The palmar aponeurosis has been removed to display the superficial palmar arch.

1	Tendon of palmaris longus muscle
2	Radial artery
3	Tendon of flexor carpi radialis muscle and median nerve
4	Distal part of antebrachial fascia
5	Radial artery passing into the anatomical snuffbox
6	Abductor pollicis brevis muscle
7	Superficial head of flexor pollicis brevis muscle
8	Palmar digital artery of thumb
9	Common palmar digital arteries
10	Proper palmar digital nerves (median nerve)
11	Ulnar nerve
12	Tendon of flexor carpi ulnaris muscle
13	Ulnar artery
14	Superficial branch of ulnar nerve
15	Palmaris brevis muscle
16	Palmar aponeurosis

17	Palmar digital nerves (ulnar nerve)
18	Superficial transverse metacarpal ligament
19	Proper palmar digital arteries
20	Superficial palmar branch of radial artery (contributing to the superficial palmar arch)
21	Flexor retinaculum
22	Median nerve
23	Abductor digiti minimi muscle
24	Flexor digiti minimi brevis muscle
25	Opponens digiti minimi muscle
26	Superficial palmar arch
27	Tendons of flexor digitorum superficialis muscle
28	Common palmar digital branch of ulnar nerve
29	Common palmar digital branch of median nerve
30	Fibrous sheath of flexor tendons

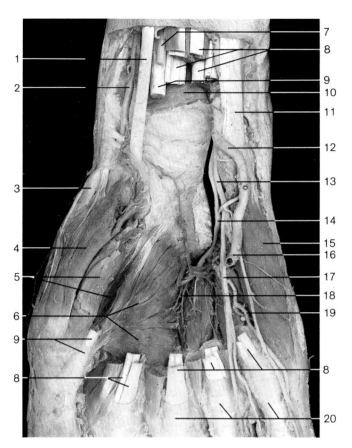

Right hand, deep layer (palmar aspect). The carpal tunnel has been opened, the tendons of the flexor muscles have been removed, and the superficial palmar arch has been cut.

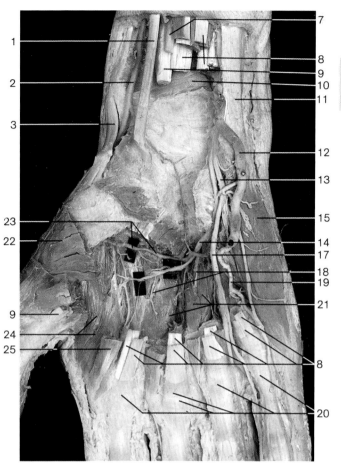

Right hand, deep layer (palmar aspect). Dissection of the deep palmar arch.

1	Tendon of flexor carpi radialis muscle
2	Radial artery
3	Tendon of abductor pollicis longus muscle
4	Abductor pollicis brevis muscle
5	Superficial and deep heads of flexor pollicis brevis muscle
6	Oblique and transverse heads of adductor pollicis muscle
7	Median nerve
8	Tendons of flexor digitorum superficialis and profundus muscles
9	Tendon of flexor pollicis longus muscle
10	Pronator quadratus muscle
11	Tendon of flexor carpi ulnaris muscle

12	Ulnar artery
13	Superficial branch of ulnar nerve
14	Deep branch of ulnar nerve
15	Abductor digiti minimi muscle
16	Superficial palmar arch (cut end)
17	Common palmar digital nerves (ulnar nerve)
18	Palmar metacarpal arteries of deep palmar arch
19	Palmar digital artery of the fifth finger
20	Fibrous sheaths of tendons of flexor muscles
21	Palmar interosseous muscles
22	Opponens pollicis muscle (cut)
23	Deep palmar arch
24	First dorsal interosseous muscle
25	First lumbrical muscle

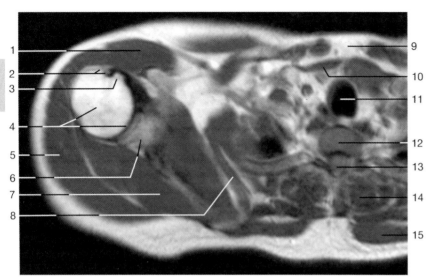

Horizontal section through the right shoulder joint (section 1; MRI scan; inferior aspect).

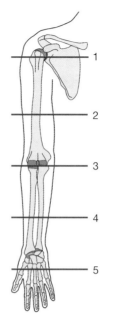

Upper limb, location of sections 1–5
(MRI scans, p. 430: courtesy of Prof. Heuck, Munich, Germany; MRI scans, p. 431: courtesy of Prof. Bautz and R. Janka, M. D., University of Erlangen, Germany).

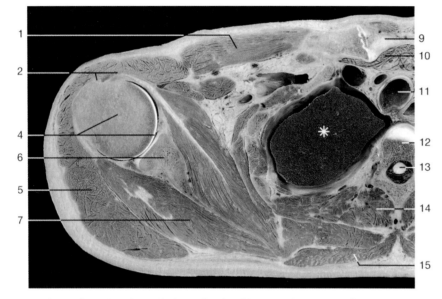

Horizontal section through the right shoulder joint (section 1; inferior aspect).
* = Upper lobe of lung.

1   Pectoralis major muscle
2   Greater tubercle and tendon of biceps muscle
3   Lesser tubercle
4   Head of humerus and articular cavity of shoulder joint
5   Deltoid muscle
6   Scapula
7   Infraspinatus muscle
8   Serratus anterior muscle
9   Sternum
10 Infrahyoid muscles
11 Trachea
12 Body of thoracic vertebra
13 Vertebral canal and spinal cord
14 Deep muscles of the back
15 Trapezius muscle
16 Brachialis muscle
17 Radial nerve and profunda brachii vessels

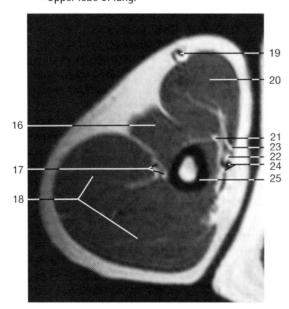

Axial section through the middle of the right arm (section 2; MRI scan; inferior aspect).

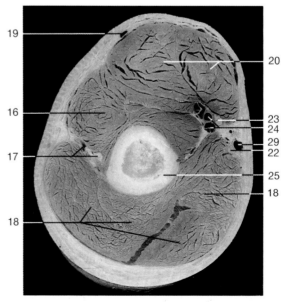

Axial section through the middle of the right arm (section 2; inferior aspect).

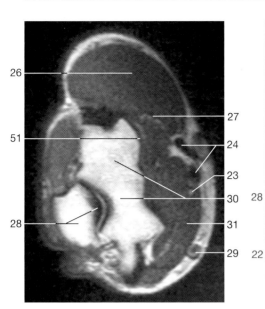

Axial section through the right elbow joint (section 3; MRI scan; inferior aspect).

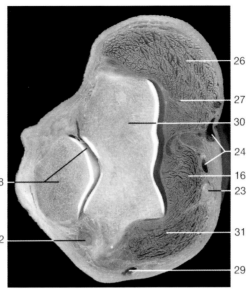

Axial section through the right elbow joint (section 3; inferior aspect).

18 Triceps brachii muscle
19 Cephalic vein
20 Biceps brachii muscle
21 Musculocutaneous nerve
22 Ulnar nerve
23 Medianus nerve
24 Brachial artery and vein
25 Shaft of humerus
26 Brachioradialis muscle
27 Radial nerve
28 Olecranon and articular cavity
   of elbow joint
29 Basilic vein
30 Humerus
31 Pronator teres muscle
32 Extensor muscles of forearm
33 Ramus profundus of
   radialis nerve
34 Anterior interosseus
   vessels and nerve
35 Interosseous membrane
36 Ulna
37 Radius
38 Radial artery and superficial
   branch of radial nerve
39 Flexor pollicis longus muscle
40 Flexor digitorum
   superficialis and profundus
   muscles
41 Ulnar nerve, ulnar artery, and
   vein
42 Flexor carpi ulnaris muscle
43 Radial artery
44 Metacarpal bones III and IV
45 Carpal canal with tendons of
   flexor digitorum muscles
46 Hypothenar muscle
47 Median nerve
48 Interosseous muscles
49 First metacarpal bone
50 Thenar muscles
51 Articular cavity of
   humeroradial joint

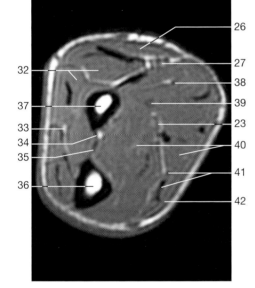

Axial section through the middle of the right forearm (section 4; MRI scan; inferior aspect).

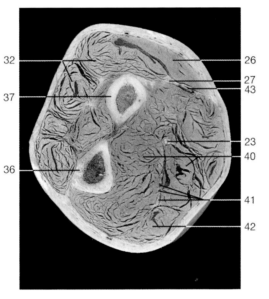

Axial section through the middle of the right forearm (section 4; inferior aspect).

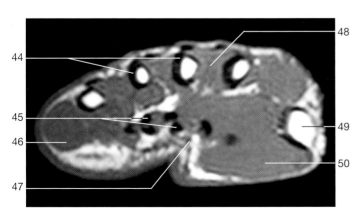

Axial section through the right hand at the level of the metacarpus (section 5; MRI scan; inferior aspect).

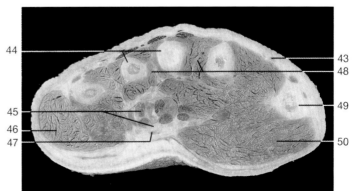

Axial section through the right hand at the level of the metacarpus (section 5; inferior aspect).

8 Lower Limb

The lower limb (extremity) is specialized for support of the upright posture, locomotion, and maintaining balance. In contrast to the upper limb, the lower limb is more restricted in its movements, and the joints are tighter and fixed by strong ligaments. The hip joint is a ball-and-socket type of synovial joint between the head of the femur and acetabulum. The knee joint is a hinge type of synovial joint that permits only limited rotation. The talocrural joint is a hinge joint between the talus, fibula, and tibia, only allowing movements of flexion and extension.

The long axis of the foot is at a right angle to that of the leg, thus forming an effective arch for the upright stance of the body.

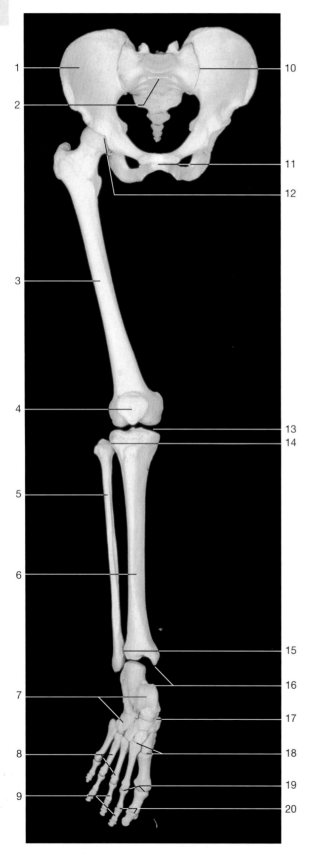

Skeleton of pelvic girdle and lower limb (anterior aspect). The ankle joint has been dislocated.

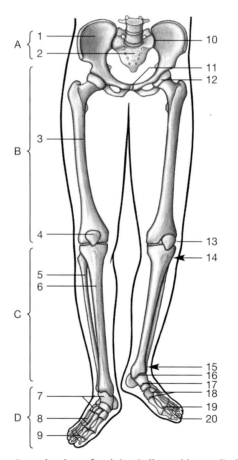

A = pelvic girdle
B = thigh
C = leg
D = foot

Organization of pelvic girdle and lower limb.

1	Right hip bone	11	Pubic symphysis
2	Sacrum	12	Hip joint
3	Femur	13	Knee joint
4	Patella	14	Proximal tibiofibular joint
5	Fibula	15	Distal tibiofibular joint
6	Tibia	16	Ankle joint
7	Tarsal bones	17	Talocalcaneonavicular joint
8	Metatarsal bones	18	Tarsometatarsal joints
9	Phalanges	19	Metatarsophalangeal joints
10	Sacro-iliac joint	20	Interphalangeal joints

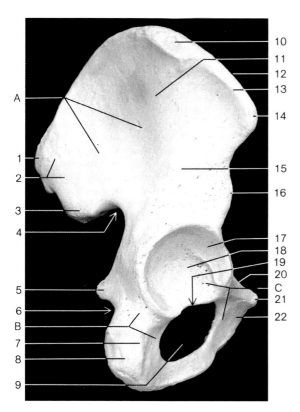

Right hip bone (lateral aspect).

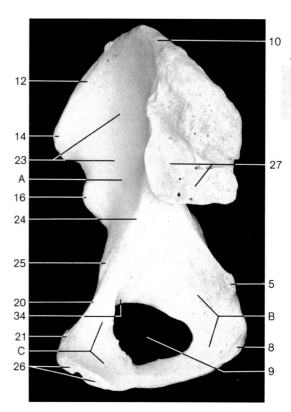

Right hip bone (medial aspect).

A = ilium
B = ischium
C = pubis

1   Posterior superior iliac spine
2   Posterior gluteal line
3   Posterior inferior iliac spine
4   Greater sciatic notch
5   Ischial spine
6   Lesser sciatic notch
7   Body of ischium
8   Ischial tuberosity
9   Obturator foramen
10 Iliac crest
11 Anterior gluteal line
12 Internal lip of iliac crest
13 External lip of iliac crest
14 Anterior superior iliac spine
15 Inferior gluteal line
16 Anterior inferior iliac spine
17 Lunate surface of acetabulum
18 Acetabular fossa
19 Acetabular notch
20 Pecten pubis
21 Pubic tubercle
22 Body of pubis
23 Iliac fossa
24 Arcuate line
25 Iliopubic eminence
26 Symphysial surface of pubis
27 Auricular surface
28 Pelvic surface of sacrum
29 Superior articular process of sacrum
30 Dorsal sacral foramina
31 Sacral tuberosity
32 Lateral sacral crest
33 Median sacral crest
34 Obturator groove
35 Coccyx

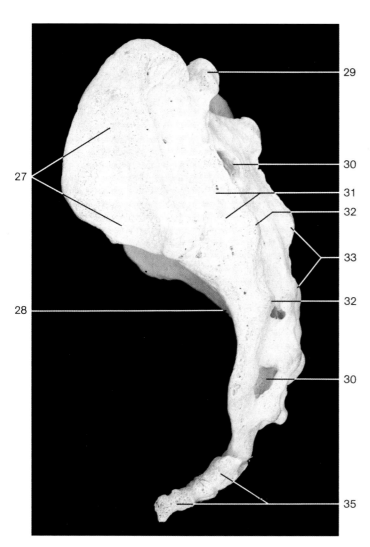

Sacrum and coccyx (lateral aspect).

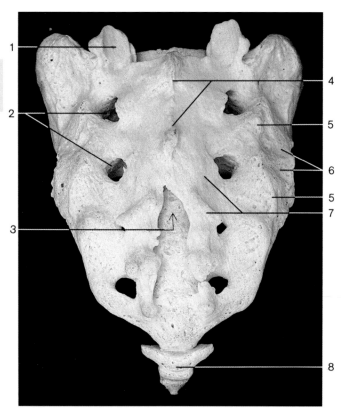

Sacrum (posterior aspect).

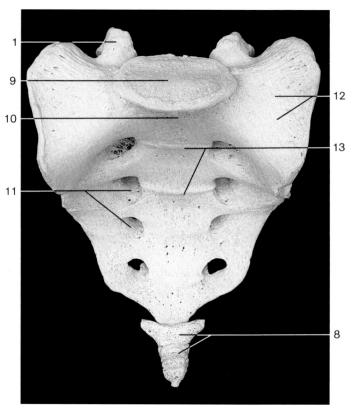

Sacrum (anterior aspect).

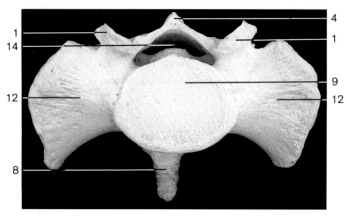

Sacrum (superior aspect).

1 Superior articular process of sacrum
2 Dorsal sacral foramina
3 Sacral hiatus
4 Median sacral crest
5 Lateral sacral crest
6 Sacral tuberosity
7 Intermediate sacral crest
8 Coccyx
9 Base of sacrum
10 Sacral promontory
11 Anterior sacral foramina
12 Lateral part of sacrum (ala)
13 Transverse line of sacrum
14 Sacral canal
15 Linea terminalis
16 True conjugate
17 Diagonal conjugate
18 Transverse diameter
19 Oblique diameter
20 Inferior pelvic aperture or outlet

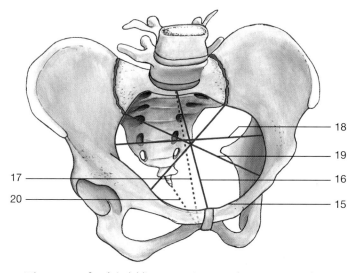

Diameters of pelvis (oblique superior aspect).
(Schematic drawing.)

The pelvic girdle is firmly connected to the vertebral column at the sacro-iliac joint. Therefore, the body can be kept upright more easily even if only one limb is used for support (as in walking). The mobility of the lower limb is more limited than that of the upper limb.

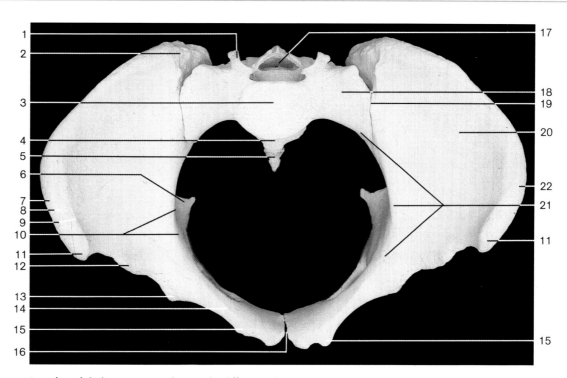

Female pelvis (superior aspect). Note the differences between the male and female pelvis, predominantly in the form and dimensions of the sacrum, the superior and inferior apertures, and the alae of the ilium.

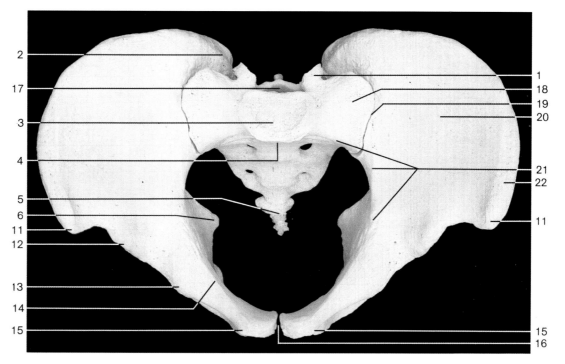

Male pelvis (superior aspect). Compare with the female pelvis (depicted above).

1	Superior articular process of sacrum	12	Anterior inferior iliac spine
2	Posterior superior iliac spine	13	Iliopubic eminence
3	Base of sacrum	14	Pecten pubis
4	Sacral promontory	15	Pubic tubercle
5	Coccyx	16	Pubic symphysis
6	Ischial spine	17	Sacral canal
7	External lip ⎫ of iliac	18	Ala of sacrum
8	Intermediate line ⎬ crest	19	Position of sacro-iliac joint
9	Internal lip ⎭	20	Iliac fossa
10	Arcuate line	21	Linea terminalis
11	Anterior superior iliac spine	22	Iliac crest

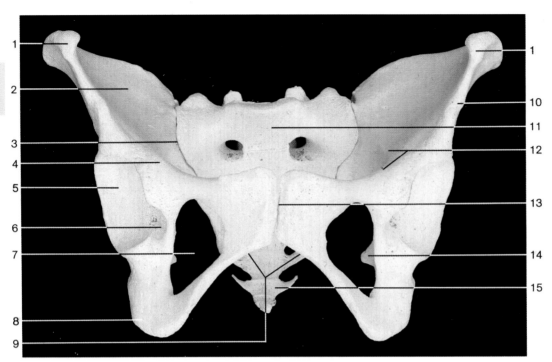

Female pelvis (anterior aspect). Note the differences between the form and dimensions of the male and female pelvis. The female pubic arch is wider than the male. The obturator foramen in the female pelvis is triangular, while that in the male pelvis is ovoid.

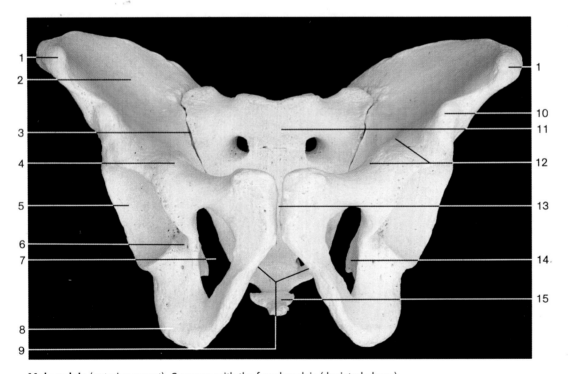

Male pelvis (anterior aspect). Compare with the female pelvis (depicted above).

1	Anterior superior iliac spine	9	Pubic arch
2	Iliac fossa	10	Anterior inferior iliac spine
3	Position of sacro-iliac joint	11	Sacrum
4	Iliopubic eminence	12	Linea terminalis (at margin of superior aperture)
5	Lunate surface of acetabulum	13	Pubic symphysis
6	Acetabular notch	14	Ischial spine
7	Obturator foramen	15	Coccyx
8	Ischial tuberosity		

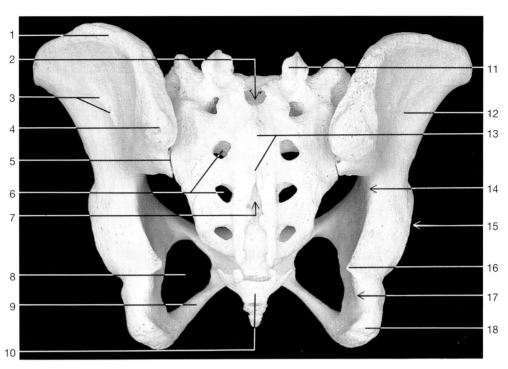

Female pelvis (posterior aspect). Note the differences between the female and male pelvis, especially with respect to the inferior aperture, the shape of the sacrum, the two sciatic notches, and the pubic arch.

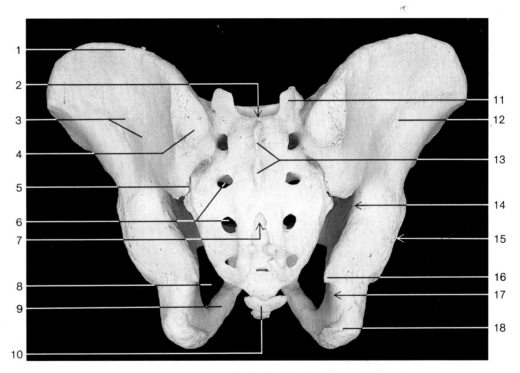

Male pelvis (posterior aspect). Compare with the female pelvis (depicted above).

1	Iliac crest	10	Coccyx
2	Sacral canal	11	Superior articular process of sacrum
3	Posterior gluteal line	12	Gluteal surface of ilium
4	Posterior superior iliac spine	13	Median sacral crest
5	Position of sacro-iliac joint	14	Greater sciatic notch
6	Dorsal sacral foramina	15	Position of acetabulum
7	Sacral hiatus	16	Ischial spine
8	Obturator foramen	17	Lesser sciatic notch
9	Ramus of ischium	18	Ischial tuberosity

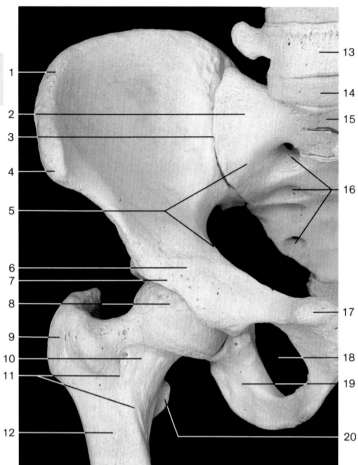

1 Iliac crest
2 Lateral part of sacrum (ala)
3 Position of sacro-iliac joint
4 Anterior superior iliac spine
5 Linea terminalis
6 Iliopubic eminence
7 Bony margin of acetabulum
8 Head of femur
9 Greater trochanter
10 Neck of femur
11 Intertrochanteric line
12 Shaft of femur
13 Fifth lumbar vertebra
14 Imitation intervertebral disc between fifth lumbar
   vertebra and sacrum
15 Sacral promontory
16 Anterior sacral foramina
17 Pubic tubercle
18 Obturator foramen
19 Ramus of ischium
20 Lesser trochanter
21 Dorsal sacral foramina
22 Greater sciatic notch
23 Ischial spine
24 Pubic symphysis
25 Pubis
26 Ischial tuberosity
27 Intertrochanteric crest
28 Symphysial surface

Bones of right hip joint (anterior aspect).

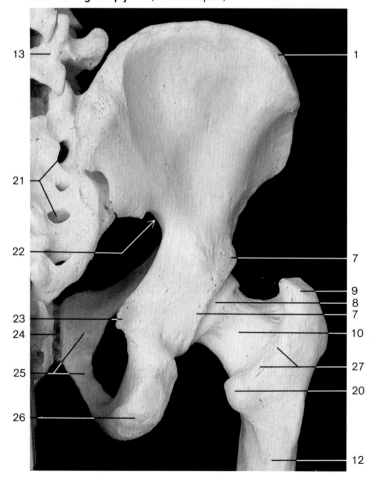

Bones of right hip joint (posterior aspect).

Diameters of the pelvis
A = true conjugate (11–11.5 cm) (conjugata vera)
B = diagonal conjugate (12.5–13 cm)
C = largest diameter of pelvis
D = inferior pelvic aperture
E = pelvic inclination (60°)

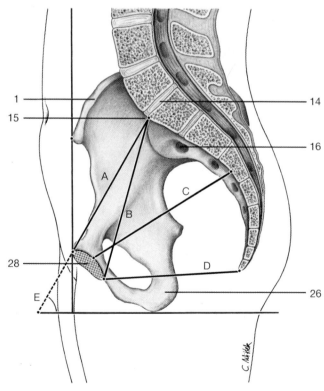

Inclination and diameters of the female pelvis,
right half (medial aspect).

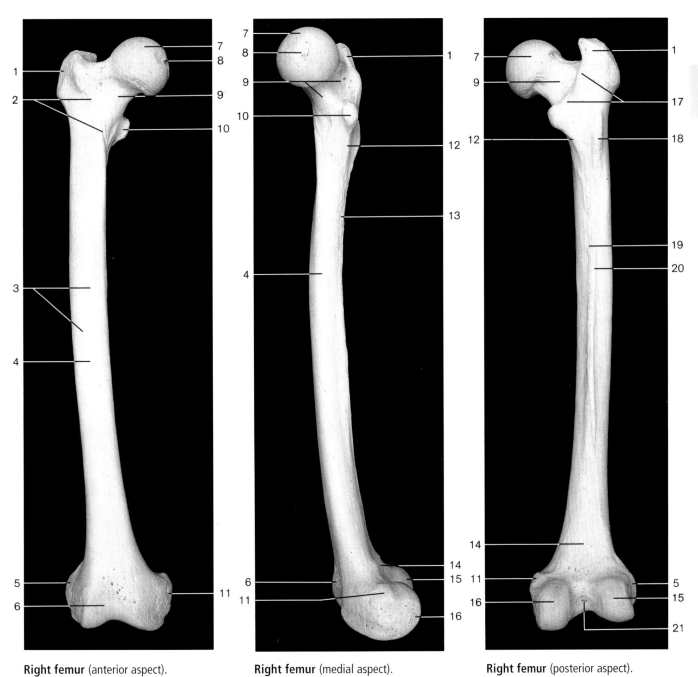

Right femur (anterior aspect).

Right femur (medial aspect).

Right femur (posterior aspect).

1	Greater trochanter	8	Fovea of head	15	Lateral condyle
2	Intertrochanteric line	9	Neck	16	Medial condyle
3	Nutrient foramina	10	Lesser trochanter	17	Intertrochanteric crest
4	Shaft of femur (diaphysis)	11	Medial epicondyle	18	Third trochanter
5	Lateral epicondyle	12	Pectineal line	19	Medial lip of linea aspera
6	Patellar surface	13	Linea aspera	20	Lateral lip of linea aspera
7	Head	14	Popliteal surface	21	Intercondylar fossa

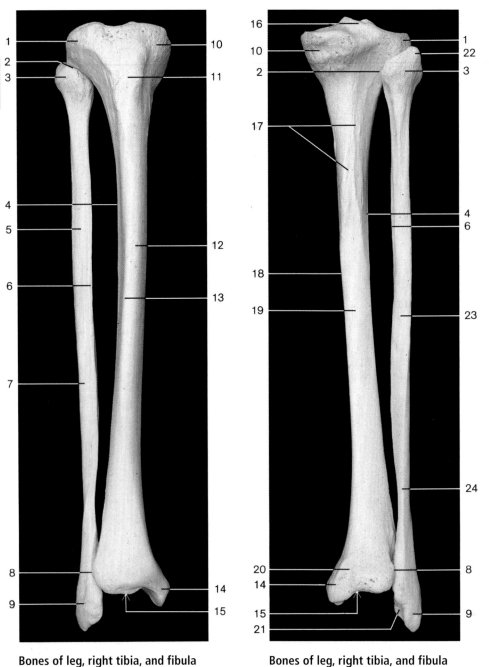

1 Lateral condyle of tibia
2 Position of tibiofibular joint
3 Head of fibula
4 Interosseous border of tibia
5 Shaft of fibula
6 Interosseous border of fibula
7 Lateral surface of fibula
8 Position of tibiofibular joint
9 Lateral malleolus
10 Medial condyle of tibia
11 Tuberosity of tibia
12 Shaft of tibia (diaphysis)
13 Anterior margin of tibia
14 Medial malleolus
15 Inferior articular surface
   of tibia
16 Intercondylar eminence
17 Soleal line
18 Medial border of tibia
19 Posterior surface of tibia
20 Malleolar sulcus of tibia
21 Malleolar articular surface
   of fibula
22 Apex of head of fibula
23 Posterior surface of fibula
24 Posterior border of fibula
25 Medial intercondylar tubercle
26 Posterior intercondylar area
27 Anterior intercondylar area
28 Lateral intercondylar tubercle

Bones of leg, right tibia, and fibula
(anterior aspect).

Bones of leg, right tibia, and fibula
(posterior aspect).

Upper end of right tibia with fibula
(from above), anterior margin of tibia above.
Superior articular surface of tibia.

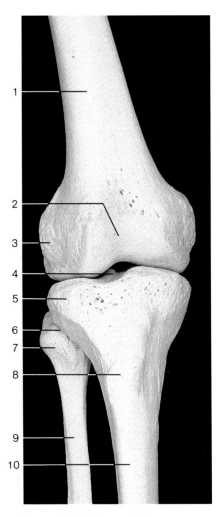

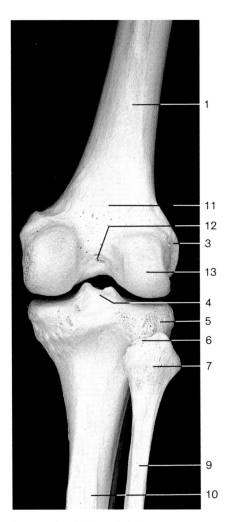

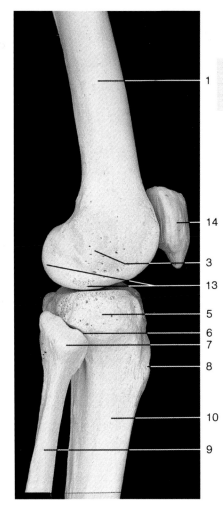

Bones of right knee joint
(anterior aspect).

Bones of right knee joint
(posterior aspect).

Bones of right knee joint
(lateral aspect).

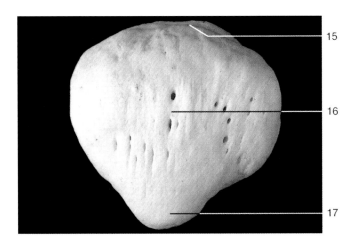

Right patella (anterior aspect).

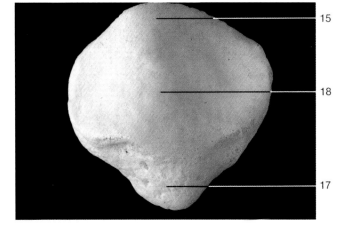

Right patella (posterior aspect).

1 Femur	10 Shaft of tibia
2 Patellar surface of femur	11 Popliteal surface of femur
3 Lateral epicondyle of femur	12 Intercondylar fossa of femur
4 Intercondylar eminence of tibia	13 Lateral condyle of femur
5 Lateral condyle of tibia	14 Patella
6 Position of tibiofibular joint	15 Base of patella
7 Head of fibula	16 Anterior surface of patella
8 Tuberosity of tibia	17 Apex of patella
9 Fibula	18 Articular surface of patella

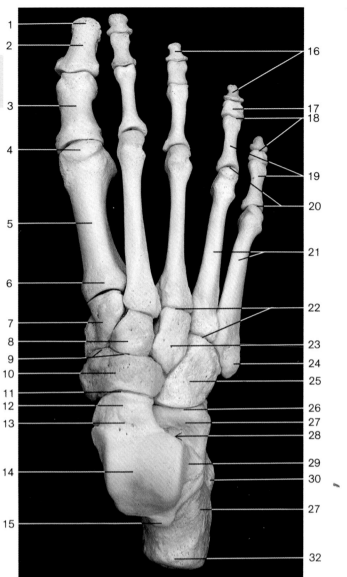

Bones of right foot (dorsal aspect).

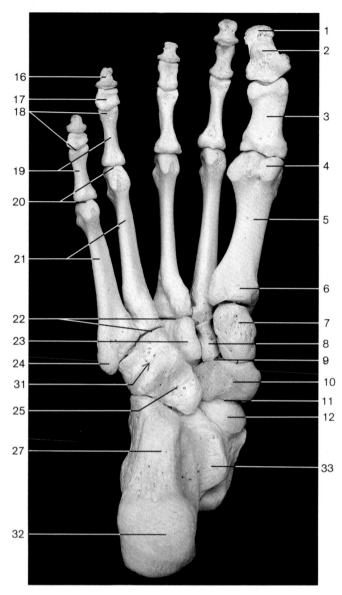

Bones of right foot (plantar aspect).

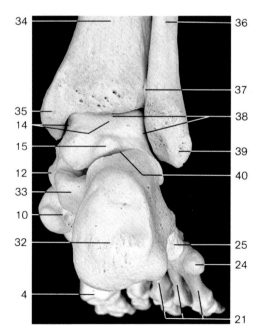

Bones of right foot together with tibia
and fibula (posterior aspect).

1 Tuberosity of distal phalanx of great toe
2 Distal phalanx of great toe
3 Proximal phalanx of great toe
4 Head of first metatarsal bone
5 First metatarsal bone
6 Base of first metatarsal bone
7 Medial cuneiform bone
8 Intermediate cuneiform bone
9 Position of cuneonavicular joint
10 Navicular bone

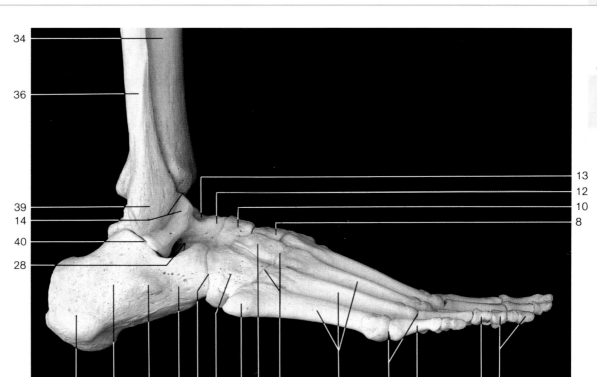

Bones of right foot, tibia, and fibula (lateral aspect).

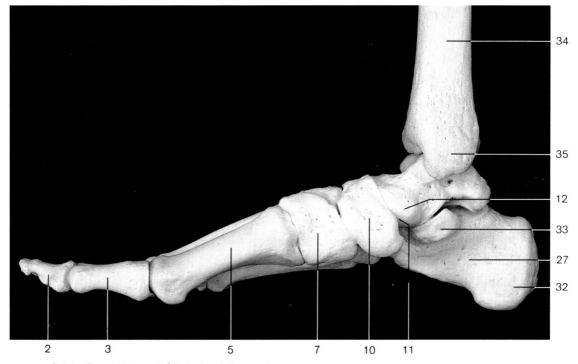

Bones of right foot, tibia, and fibula (medial aspect).

11	Position of talocalcaneonavicular joint	21	Metatarsal bones	31	Groove for tendon of peroneus longus
12	Head of talus	22	Position of tarsometatarsal joints	32	Calcaneal tuberosity
13	Neck of talus	23	Lateral cuneiform bone	33	Sustentaculum tali
14	Trochlea of talus	24	Tuberosity of fifth metatarsal bone	34	Tibia
15	Posterior talar process	25	Cuboid bone	35	Medial malleolus
16	Distal phalanges	26	Position of calcaneocuboid joint	36	Fibula
17	Middle phalanges	27	Calcaneus	37	Position of tibiofibular syndesmosis
18	Position of interphalangeal joints	28	Tarsal sinus	38	Position of ankle joint
19	Proximal phalanges	29	Lateral malleolar surface of talus	39	Lateral malleolus
20	Position of metatarsophalangeal joints	30	Peroneal trochlea of calcaneus	40	Position of subtalar joint

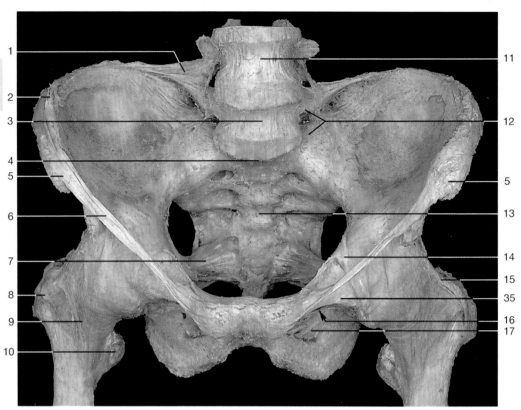

Ligaments of pelvis and hip joint (anterior aspect).

1	Iliolumbar ligament	13	Sacrum
2	Iliac crest	14	Iliopectineal arch
3	Fifth lumbar vertebra	15	Iliofemoral ligament (horizontal band)
4	Sacral promontory	16	Obturator canal
5	Anterior superior iliac spine	17	Obturator membrane
6	Inguinal ligament	18	Greater sciatic foramen
7	Sacrospinous ligament	19	Sacrospinous ligament
8	Greater trochanter	20	Sacrotuberous ligament
9	Iliofemoral ligament (vertical band)	21	Lesser sciatic foramen
10	Lesser trochanter	22	Ischial tuberosity
11	Fourth lumbar vertebra	23	Ischiofemoral ligament
12	Iliolumbar and ventral sacro-iliac ligaments	24	Intertrochanteric crest
		25	Femur

26 Articular capsule of hip joint
27 Dorsal sacro-iliac ligaments
28 Coccyx with superficial dorsal sacrococcygeal ligament
29 Head of femur
30 Articular cartilage of head of femur
31 Articular cavity of hip joint
32 Acetabular lip
33 Spongy bone
34 Ligament of head of femur
35 Pubofemoral ligament
36 Zona orbicularis

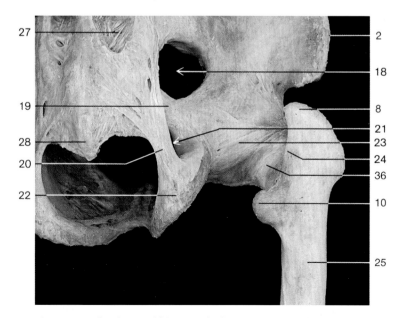

Ligaments of pelvis and hip joint (right posterior aspect).

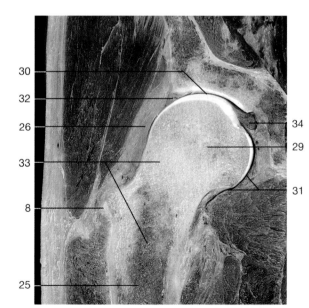

Coronal section of right hip joint (anterior aspect).

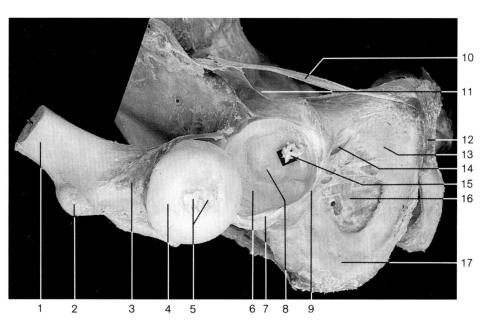

1   Femur
2   Lesser trochanter
3   Neck of femur
4   Head of femur
5   Fovea of head with cut edge of ligament of head
6   Lunate surface of acetabulum
7   Acetabular lip
8   Acetabular fossa
9   Transverse acetabular ligament
10 Inguinal ligament
11 Iliopectineal arch
12 Pubic symphysis
13 Pubic bone
14 Obturator canal
15 Ligament of head of femur
16 Obturator membrane
17 Ischium
18 Anterior longitudinal ligament (level of fifth lumbar vertebra)
19 Sacral promontory
20 Iliolumbar ligament
21 Iliac crest
22 Anterior superior iliac spine
23 Iliofemoral ligament (horizontal band)
24 Iliofemoral ligament (vertical band)
25 Greater trochanter
26 Pubofemoral ligament
27 Anterior inferior iliac spine
28 Ventral sacro-iliac ligaments
29 Sacrospinous ligament
30 Sacrotuberous ligament
31 Intertrochanteric line
32 Ischiofemoral ligament
33 Zona orbicularis

Right hip joint, opened (latero-anterior aspect). The ligament of the head of the femur has been divided, and the femur has been posteriorly reflected.

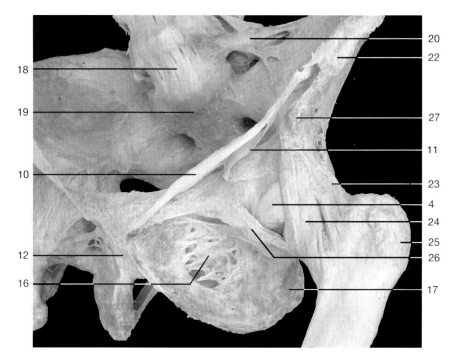

◁ **Ligaments of the pelvis and hip joint** (antero-lateral aspect).

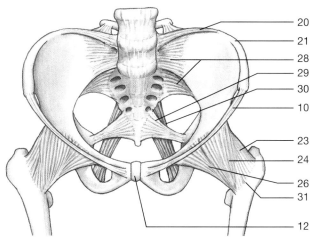

Ligaments of hip joint (anterior aspect, schematic drawing).

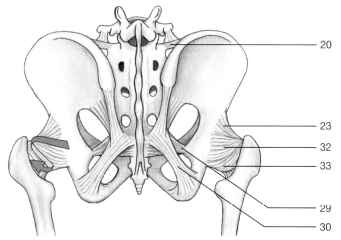

Ligaments of hip joint (posterior aspect, schematic drawing).

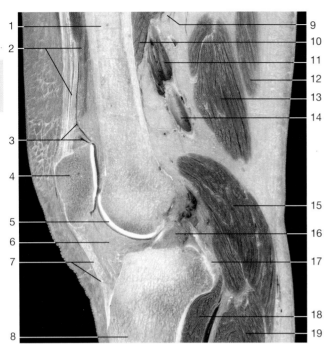

Sagittal section through the knee joint (lateral aspect). Anterior surface to the left.

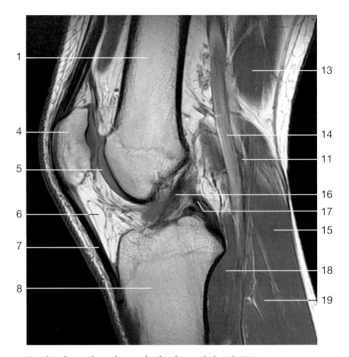

Sagittal section through the knee joint (MRI scan; from Heuck et al., MRT-Atlas, 2009).

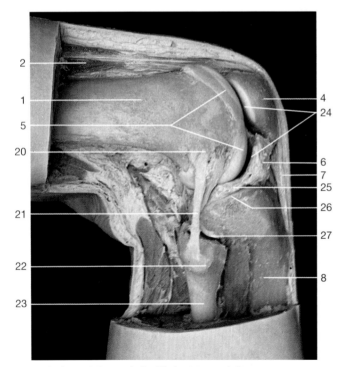

Right knee joint and tibiofibular joint with ligaments (lateral aspect). Note the position of the lateral meniscus.

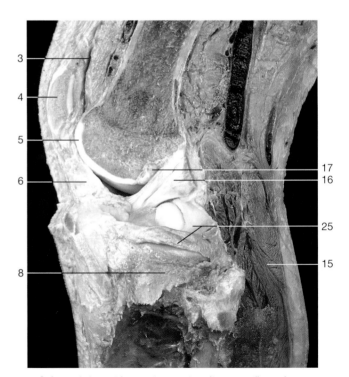

Left knee joint with anterior cruciate ligament (lateral aspect).

1 Femur	10 Adductor magnus muscle	19 Soleus muscle
2 Quadriceps femoris muscle	11 Popliteal vein	20 Lateral epicondyle of femur
3 Suprapatellar bursa and articular cavity	12 Semitendinosus muscle	21 Fibular collateral ligament
4 Patella	13 Semimembranosus muscle	22 Head of fibula
5 Articular cartilage of femur	14 Popliteal artery	23 Fibula
6 Infrapatellar fat pad	15 Gastrocnemius muscle	24 Articular cavity of knee joint
7 Patellar ligament	16 Anterior cruciate ligament	25 Lateral meniscus of knee joint
8 Tibia	17 Posterior cruciate ligament	26 Lateral condyle of tibia
9 Tibial nerve	18 Popliteus muscle	27 Tibiofibular joint

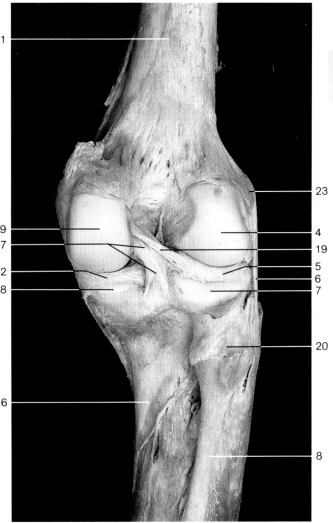

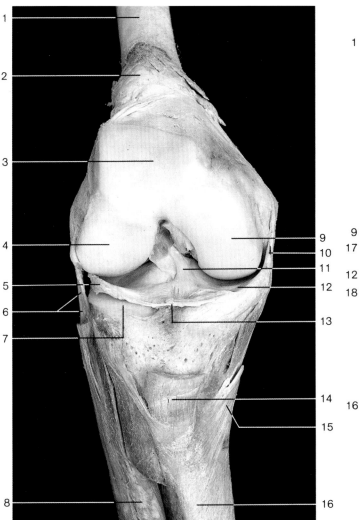

Right knee joint (opened) with ligaments (anterior aspect). The patella and articular capsule have been removed and the femur slightly flexed.

Right knee joint with ligaments (posterior aspect). The joint is extended and the articular capsule has been removed.

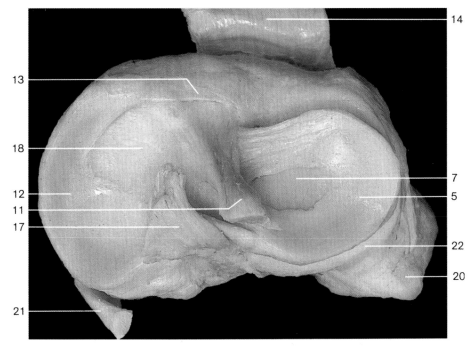

Articular surface of right tibia, menisci, and cruciate ligaments (superior aspect). Anterior margin of tibia above.

1   Femur
2   Articular capsule with suprapatellar bursa
3   Patellar surface
4   Lateral condyle of femur
5   Lateral meniscus of knee joint
6   Fibular collateral ligament
7   Lateral condyle of tibia (superior articular surface)
8   Fibula
9   Medial condyle of femur
10 Tibial collateral ligament
11 Anterior cruciate ligament
12 Medial meniscus of knee joint
13 Transverse ligament of knee
14 Patellar ligament
15 Common tendon of sartorius, semitendinosus, and gracilis muscles
16 Tibia
17 Posterior cruciate ligament
18 Medial condyle of tibia (superior articular surface)
19 Posterior meniscofemoral ligament
20 Head of fibula
21 Tendon of semimembranosus muscle
22 Posterior attachment of articular capsule of knee joint
23 Lateral epicondyle of femur

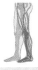

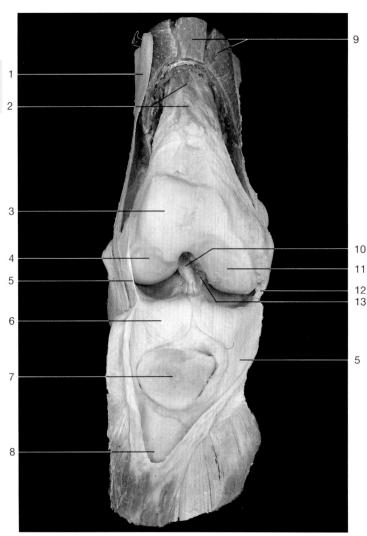

Right knee joint, opened (anterior aspect). Patellar ligament with patella reflected.

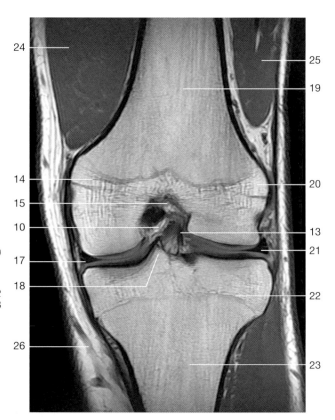

Coronal section through the knee joint (MRI scan; from Heuck et al., MRT-Atlas, 2009).

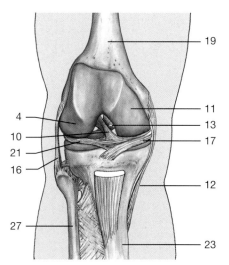

Ligaments of the right knee joint (anterior aspect).

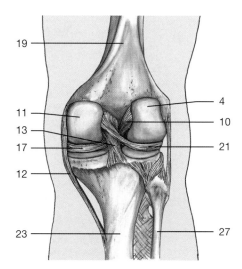

Ligaments of the right knee joint (posterior aspect).

1   Iliotibial tract
2   Articular muscle of knee
3   Patellar surface
4   Lateral condyle of femur
5   Articular capsule
6   Infrapatellar fat pad
7   Patella (articular surface)
8   Suprapatellar bursa
9   Quadriceps femoris muscle
10 Anterior cruciate ligament
11 Medial condyle of femur
12 Tibial collateral ligament
13 Posterior cruciate ligament
14 Medial epicondyle of femur
15 Intercondylar fossa of femur
16 Fibular collateral ligament
17 Medial meniscus of knee joint
18 Medial intercondylar tubercle
19 Femur
20 Lateral epicondyle of femur
21 Lateral meniscus of knee joint
22 Epiphysial line of tibia
23 Tibia
24 Vastus medialis muscle
25 Vastus lateralis muscle
26 Great saphenous vein
27 Fibula

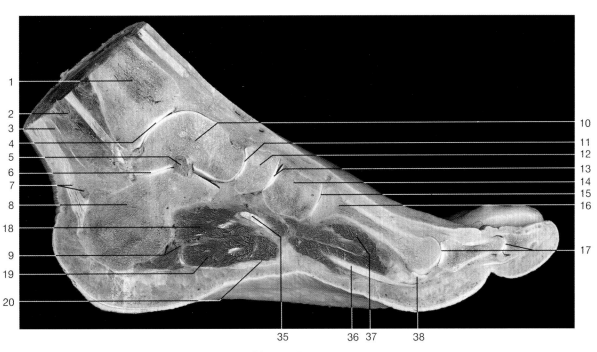

Sagittal section through the foot at the level of first phalanx.

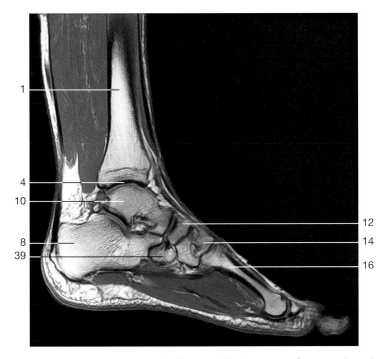

Sagittal section through the foot and leg (MRI scan; from Heuck et al., MRT-Atlas, 2009).

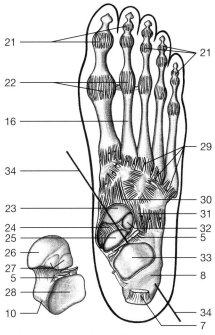

Talocalcaneonavicular joint. The talus has been rotated to show the articular surfaces of the joint.

1 Tibia
2 Deep flexor muscles
3 Superficial flexor muscles
4 Ankle joint
5 Interosseous talocalcaneal ligament
6 Subtalar joint
7 Calcaneal or Achilles tendon and bursa
8 Calcaneus
9 Vessels and nerves of foot
10 Talus
11 Talocalcaneonavicular joint
12 Navicular bone
13 Cuneonavicular joint
14 Intermediate cuneiform bone
15 Tarsometatarsal joints

16 Metatarsal bones
17 Metatarsophalangeal and interphalangeal joints
18 Quadratus plantae muscle with flexor tendons
19 Flexor digitorum brevis muscle
20 Plantar aponeurosis
21 Articular capsules of interphalangeal joints
22 Articular capsules of metatarsophalangeal joints
23 Articular surface of navicular bone
24 Plantar calcaneonavicular ligament
25 Middle talar articular surface of calcaneus
26 Navicular articular surface of talus

27 Anterior and middle calcaneal surfaces of talus
28 Posterior calcaneal surface of talus
29 Dorsal tarsometatarsal ligaments
30 Talonavicular ligament
31 Bifurcate ligament
32 Anterior talar articular surface of calcaneus
33 Posterior talar articular surface of calcaneus
34 Axis for inversion and eversion
35 Tendon of tibialis posterior muscle
36 Tendon of flexor hallucis longus muscle
37 Flexor hallucis brevis muscle
38 Sesamoid bone
39 Cuboid bone

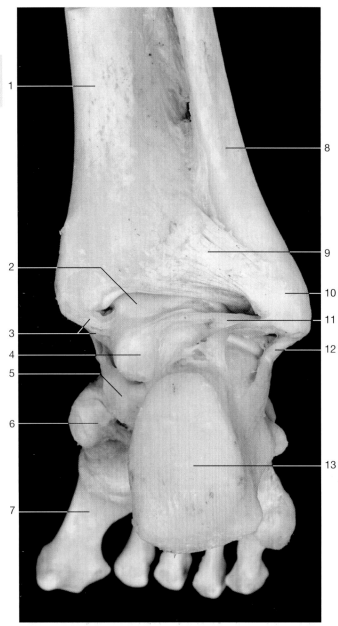

Ligaments of ankle joint, right foot (posterior aspect).

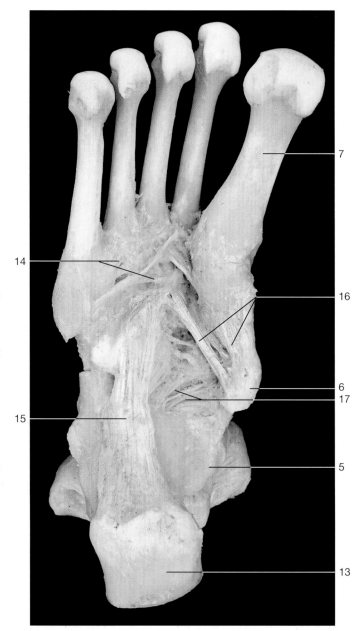

Deep ligaments of the foot, right foot (plantar aspect).
The toes have been removed.

1 Tibia	9 Posterior tibiofibular ligament
2 Trochlea of talus	10 Lateral malleolus
3 Deltoid ligament of ankle (posterior tibiotalar part)	11 Posterior talofibular ligament
4 Talus	12 Calcaneofibular ligament
5 Sustentaculum tali	13 Calcaneal tuberosity
6 Navicular bone	14 Plantar tarsometatarsal ligaments
7 First metatarsal bone	15 Long plantar ligament
8 Fibula	16 Plantar cuneonavicular ligaments
	17 Plantar calcaneonavicular ligament

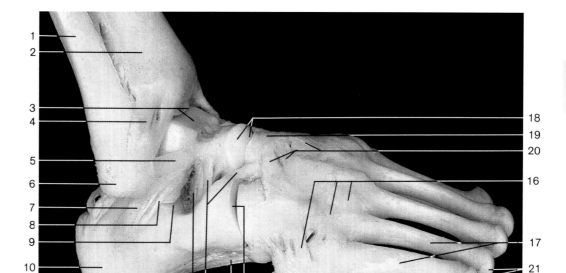

Ligaments of right foot (lateral aspect).

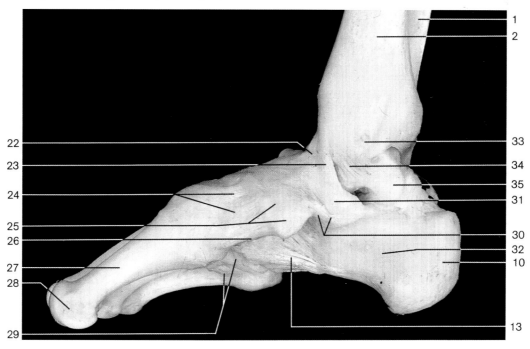

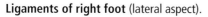

Ligaments of right foot (medial aspect).

1	Fibula	19	Navicular bone
2	Tibia	20	Dorsal cuneonavicular ligaments
3	Trochlea of talus and ankle joint	21	Heads of metatarsal bones
4	Anterior tibiofibular ligament	22	Medial or deltoid ligament of ankle (tibionavicular part)
5	Anterior talofibular ligament	23	Medial or deltoid ligament of ankle (tibiocalcaneal part)
6	Lateral malleolus	24	Dorsal cuneonavicular ligaments
7	Calcaneofibular ligament	25	Navicular bone
8	Lateral talocalcaneal ligament	26	Plantar cuneonavicular ligament
9	Subtalar joint	27	First metatarsal bone
10	Tuber calcanei	28	Head of first metatarsal bone
11	Interosseous talocalcaneal ligament	29	Plantar tarsometatarsal ligaments
12	Bifurcate ligament	30	Plantar calcaneonavicular ligament
13	Long plantar ligament	31	Sustentaculum tali
14	Calcaneocuboid joint	32	Calcaneus
15	Tuberosity of fifth metatarsal bone	33	Medial malleolus
16	Dorsal tarsometatarsal ligaments	34	Medial or deltoid ligament of ankle (posterior part)
17	Metatarsal bones	35	Talus
18	Head of talus and talocalcaneonavicular joint		

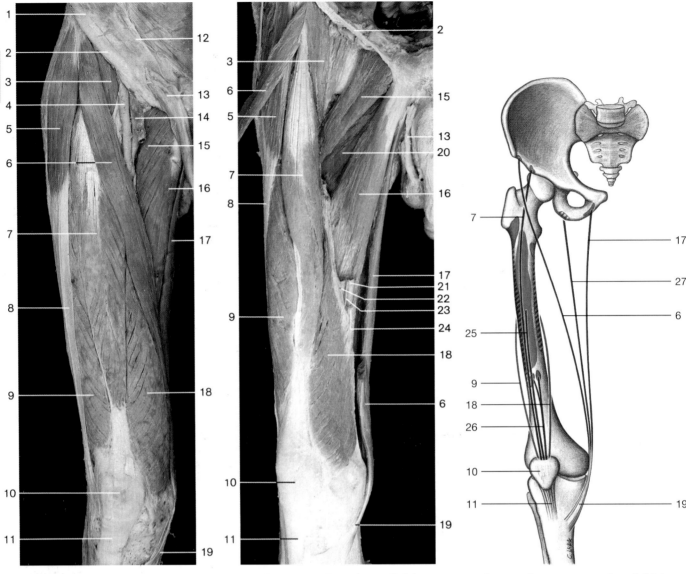

Extensor and adductor muscles of thigh, right thigh (anterior aspect).

Quadriceps muscle and superficial layer of adductor muscles, right thigh (anterior aspect). The sartorius muscle has been divided.

Course of extensor muscles of thigh and muscles inserting with common tendon on tibia (schematic drawing).

1	Anterior superior iliac spine
2	Inguinal ligament
3	Iliopsoas muscle
4	Femoral artery
5	Tensor fasciae latae muscle
6	Sartorius muscle
7	Rectus femoris muscle
8	Iliotibial tract
9	Vastus lateralis muscle
10	Patella
11	Patellar ligament

12	Aponeurosis of external abdominal oblique muscle
13	Spermatic cord
14	Femoral vein
15	Pectineus muscle
16	Adductor longus muscle
17	Gracilis muscle
18	Vastus medialis muscle
19	Common tendon of sartorius, gracilis, and semitendinosus muscles (pes anserinus)

20	Adductor brevis muscle
21	Femoral artery ⎫ entering the
22	Femoral vein ⎬ adductor canal
23	Saphenous nerve ⎭
24	Fascia of adductor canal
25	Vastus intermedius muscle
26	Articularis genus muscle
27	Semitendinosus muscle

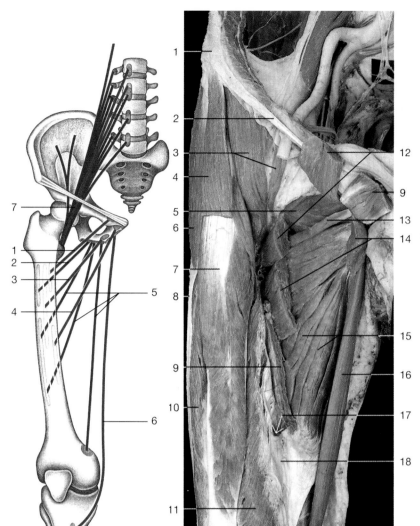

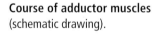

Course of adductor muscles (schematic drawing).

1 Pectineus muscle (blue)
2 Adductor minimus muscle (red)
3 Adductor brevis muscle (blue)
4 Adductor longus muscle (blue)
5 Adductor magnus muscle (red)
6 Gracilis muscle (blue)
7 Iliopsoas muscle (red/blue)

Adductor magnus muscle and deep layer of adductor muscles, right thigh (anterior aspect). Pectineus, adductor longus, and brevis muscles have been divided.

1 Anterior superior iliac spine
2 Inguinal ligament
3 Iliopsoas muscle
4 Sartorius muscle
5 Obturator externus muscle
6 Tensor fasciae latae muscle
7 Rectus femoris muscle
8 Iliotibial tract
9 Adductor longus muscle (divided)
10 Vastus lateralis muscle
11 Vastus medialis muscle
12 Pectineus muscle (divided)
13 Adductor minimus muscle
14 Adductor brevis muscle (cut)
15 Adductor magnus muscle
16 Gracilis muscle
17 Adductor hiatus
18 Vasto-adductor membrane
19 Diaphragm
20 Quadratus lumborum muscle
21 Iliacus muscle
22 Vastus intermedius muscle

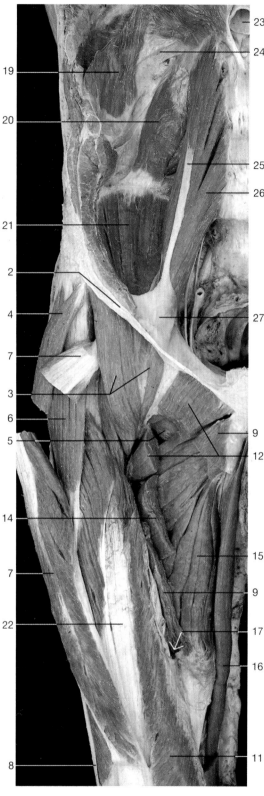

Iliopsoas muscle and deepest layer of adductor muscles, right thigh (anterior aspect). Pectineus, adductor longus and brevis, and rectus femoris muscles have been divided.

23 Aorta in aortic hiatus
24 Twelfth rib
25 Psoas minor muscle
26 Psoas major muscle
27 Iliopectineal arch

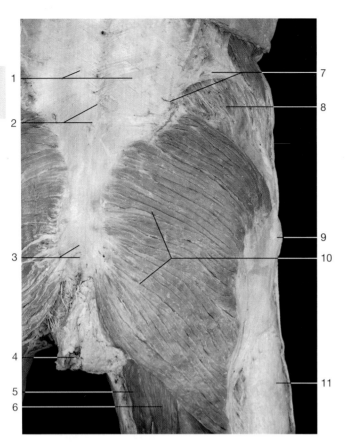

Gluteal muscles, superficial layer (posterior aspect).

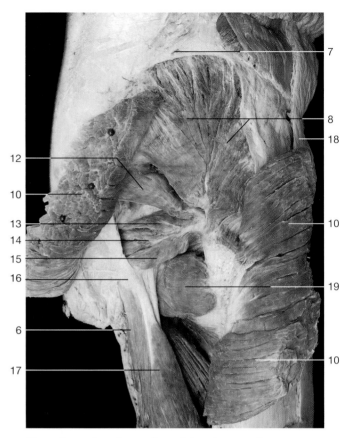

Gluteal muscles, deeper layer (posterior aspect).

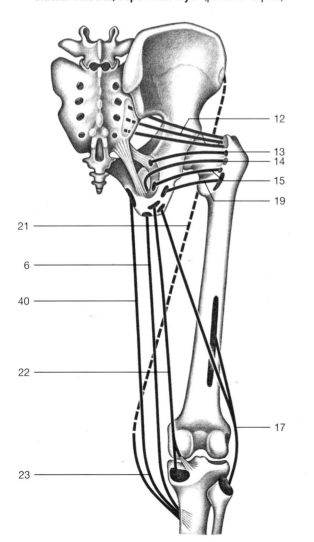

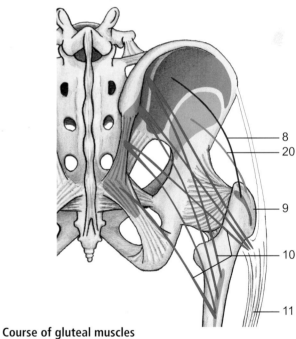

Course of gluteal muscles
(posterior aspect; schematic drawing).

◁

Course of gluteal muscles (deeper layer)
and of ischiocrural muscles (posterior aspect).
Sartorius muscle is indicated by a dotted line
(schematic drawing).

1 Thoracolumbar fascia
2 Spinous processes of lumbar vertebrae
3 Coccyx
4 Anus
5 Adductor magnus muscle
6 Semitendinosus muscle
7 Iliac crest
8 Gluteus medius muscle
9 Greater trochanter
10 Gluteus maximus muscle
11 Iliotibial tract
12 Piriformis muscle
13 Superior gemellus muscle
14 Obturator internus muscle
15 Inferior gemellus muscle
16 Ischial tuberosity
17 Biceps femoris muscle
18 Tensor fasciae latae muscle
19 Quadratus femoris muscle
20 Gluteus minimus muscle
21 Sartorius muscle
22 Semimembranosus muscle
23 Tendon of gracilis muscle
24 Tibial nerve
25 Medial head of gastrocnemius muscle
26 Common peroneal nerve
27 Tendon of biceps femoris muscle
28 Lateral head of gastrocnemius muscle
29 Rectus femoris muscle
30 Vastus medialis muscle
31 Vastus intermedius muscle
32 Vastus lateralis muscle
33 Sciatic nerve
34 Gluteus maximus muscle (insertion)
35 Great saphenous vein
36 Femoral artery
37 Femoral vein
38 Adductor longus muscle
39 Femur
40 Gracilis muscle
41 Septum between semitendinosus and semimembranosus muscles

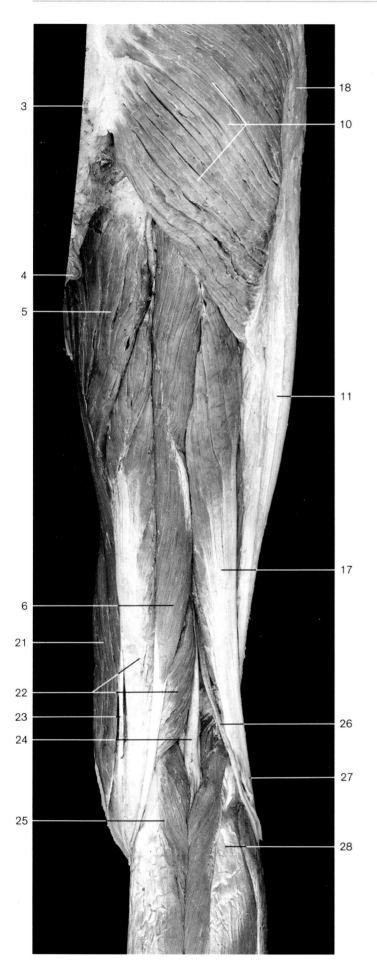

Flexors of the right thigh, superficial layer (posterior aspect).

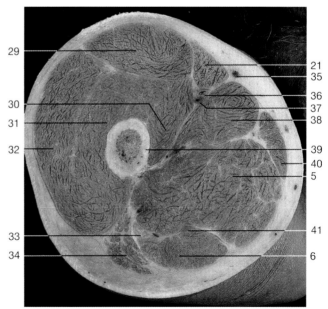

Cross section of right thigh (inferior aspect).
Anterior side on top.

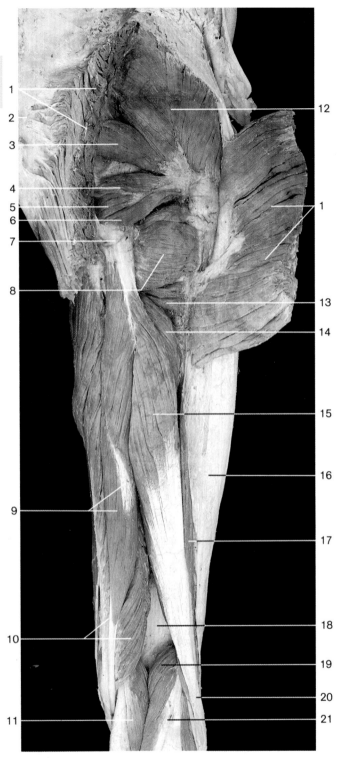

Dorsal muscles of right thigh (posterior aspect).
The gluteus maximus muscle has been cut and reflected.

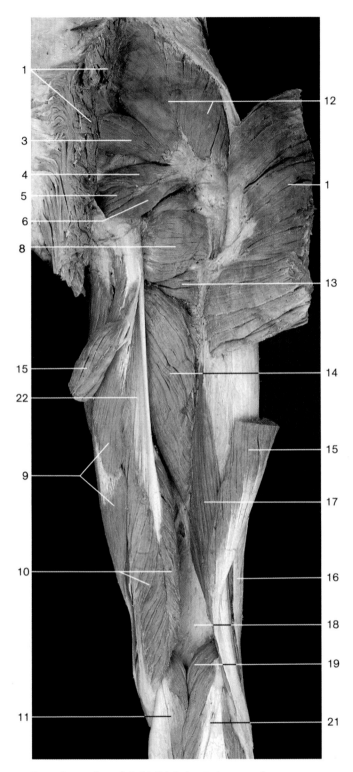

Dorsal muscles of right thigh (posterior aspect).
The gluteus maximus muscle and the long head of biceps
femoris muscle have been divided and displaced.

1 Gluteus maximus muscle (divided)	9 Semitendinosus muscle with intermediate tendon	17 Short head of biceps femoris muscle
2 Position of coccyx	10 Semimembranosus muscle	18 Popliteal surface of femur
3 Piriformis muscle	11 Medial head of gastrocnemius muscle	19 Plantaris muscle
4 Superior gemellus muscle	12 Gluteus medius muscle	20 Tendon of biceps femoris muscle
5 Obturator internus muscle	13 Adductor minimus muscle	21 Lateral head of gastrocnemius muscle
6 Inferior gemellus muscle	14 Adductor magnus muscle	22 Membranous part of
7 Ischial tuberosity	15 Long head of biceps femoris muscle	semimembranosus muscle
8 Quadratus femoris muscle	16 Iliotibial tract	

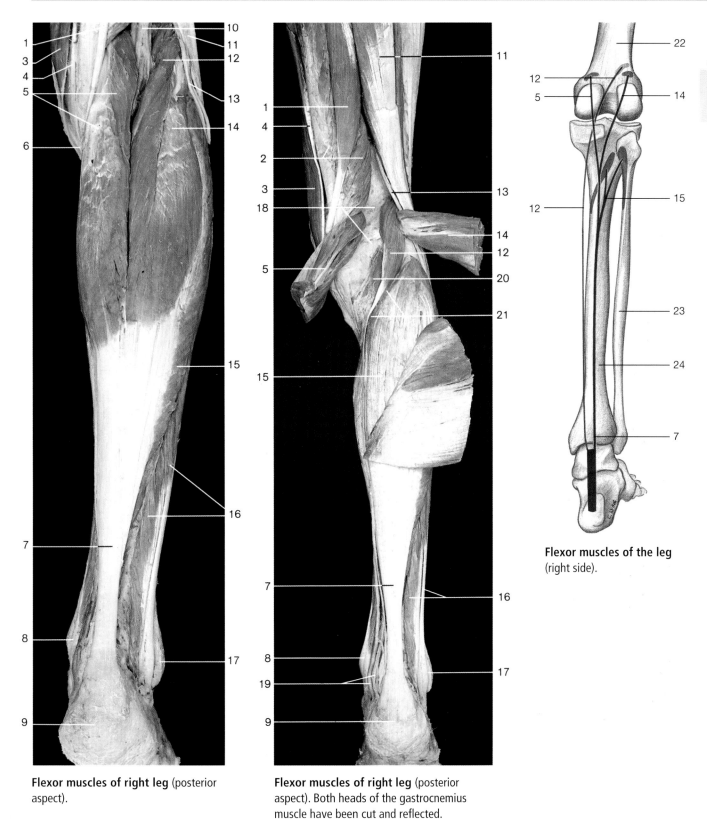

Flexor muscles of the leg (right side).

Flexor muscles of right leg (posterior aspect).

Flexor muscles of right leg (posterior aspect). Both heads of the gastrocnemius muscle have been cut and reflected.

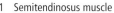

1 Semitendinosus muscle	9 Calcaneal tuberosity	18 Popliteal fossa
2 Semimembranosus muscle	10 Tibial nerve	19 Tibial nerve and posterior tibial
3 Sartorius muscle	11 Biceps femoris muscle	artery
4 Tendon of gracilis muscle	12 Plantaris muscle	20 Popliteus muscle
5 Medial head of gastrocnemius muscle	13 Common peroneal nerve	21 Tendinous arch of soleus muscle
6 Common tendon of gracilis,	14 Lateral head of gastrocnemius muscle	22 Femur
sartorius, and semitendinosus muscles	15 Soleus muscle	23 Fibula
7 Calcaneal or Achilles tendon	16 Peroneus longus and brevis muscles	24 Tibia
8 Medial malleolus	17 Lateral malleolus	

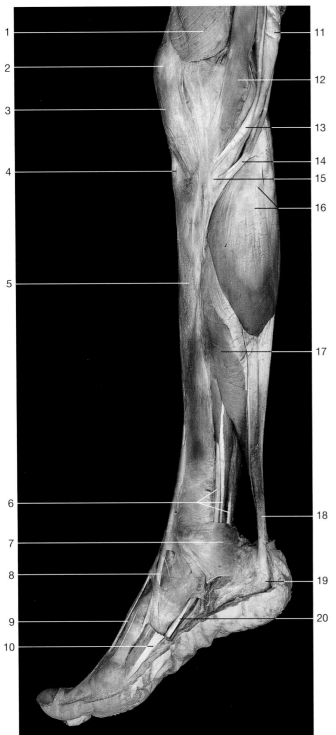

Muscles of right leg and foot (medial aspect).

Popliteal region with plantaris and soleus muscles, right side (dorsal aspect). Notice the insertion of the tendon of semimembranosus muscle.

1	Vastus medialis muscle	
2	Patella	
3	Patellar ligament	
4	Tibial tuberosity	
5	Tibia	
6	Tendons of deep flexor muscles (from anterior to posterior: 1. tibialis posterior; 2. flexor digitorum longus; 3. flexor hallucis longus muscles)	
7	Flexor retinaculum	
8	Tendon of tibialis anterior muscle	
9	Tendon of extensor hallucis longus muscle	
10	Abductor hallucis muscle	

11	Semimembranosus muscle
12	Sartorius muscle
13	Tendon of gracilis muscle
14	Tendon of semitendinosus muscle
15	Common tendon of gracilis, semitendinosus, and sartorius muscles
16	Medial head of gastrocnemius muscle
17	Soleus muscle
18	Calcaneal or Achilles tendon
19	Calcaneus muscle
20	Tendon of flexor hallucis longus muscle
21	Quadriceps femoris muscle (divided)
22	Tendon of adductor magnus muscle (divided)

23	Medial condyle of femur
24	Popliteal artery and vein, tibial nerve
25	Tibia
26	Femur
27	Lateral epicondyle of femur
28	Oblique popliteal ligament
29	Lateral (fibular) collateral ligament
30	Plantaris muscle
31	Tendon of biceps femoris muscle (divided)
32	Tendinous arch of soleus muscle

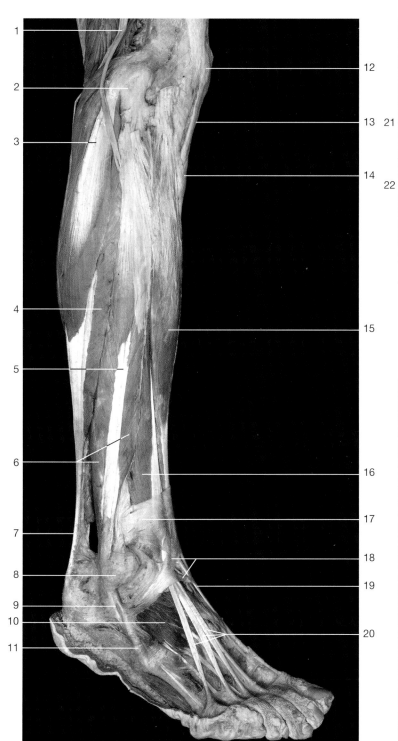

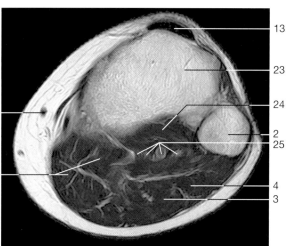

Axial section of the right leg distally of the knee joint (MRI scan; from Heuck et al., MRT-Atlas, 2009).

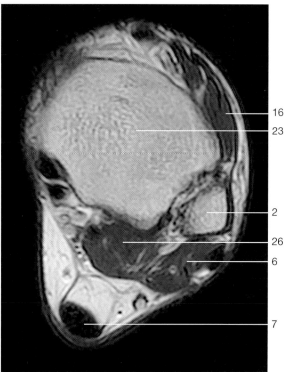

Muscles of right leg and foot (lateral aspect).

Axial section of the right leg cranially of the ankle joint (MRI scan; from Heuck et al., MRT-Atlas, 2009).

1	Common peroneal nerve	11	Tendon of peroneus brevis muscle	20	Tendons of extensor digitorum longus muscle
2	Head of fibula	12	Patella	21	Great saphenous vein
3	Lateral head of gastrocnemius muscle	13	Patellar ligament	22	Medial head of gastrocnemius muscle
4	Soleus muscle	14	Tuberosity of tibia	23	Tibia
5	Peroneus longus muscle	15	Tibialis anterior muscle	24	Popliteus muscle
6	Peroneus brevis muscle	16	Extensor digitorum longus muscle	25	Tibial nerve, popliteal artery, and veins
7	Calcaneal or Achilles tendon	17	Superior extensor retinaculum	26	Flexor hallucis longus muscle
8	Lateral malleolus muscle	18	Inferior extensor retinaculum		
9	Tendon of peroneus longus muscle	19	Tendon of extensor hallucis longus muscle		
10	Extensor digitorum brevis muscle				

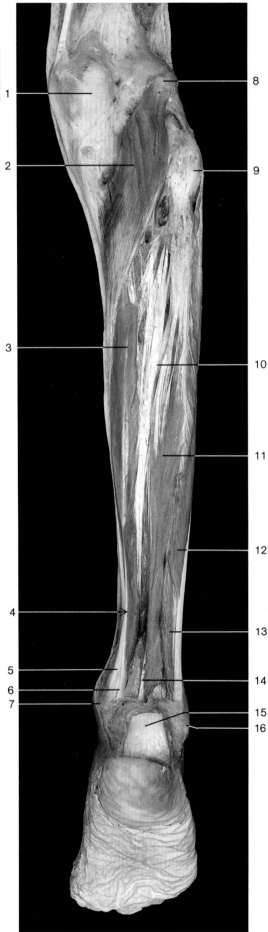

1 Medial condyle of femur
2 Popliteus muscle
3 Flexor digitorum longus muscle
4 Crossing of tendons in leg
5 Tendon of tibialis posterior muscle
6 Tendon of flexor digitorum longus muscle
7 Medial malleolus
8 Lateral condyle of femur
9 Head of fibula
10 Tibialis posterior muscle
11 Flexor hallucis longus muscle
12 Peroneus longus muscle
13 Peroneus brevis muscle
14 Tendon of flexor hallucis longus muscle
15 Calcaneal tendon (divided)
16 Lateral malleolus

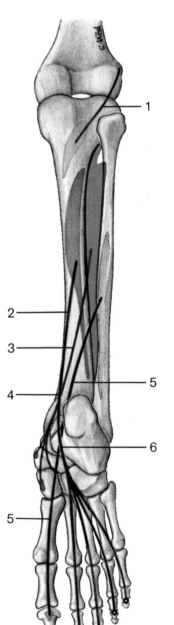

1 Popliteus muscle (blue)
2 Flexor digitorum longus muscle (blue)
3 Tibialis posterior muscle (red)
4 Crossing of tendons in leg
5 Flexor hallucis longus muscle (blue)
6 Crossing of tendons in sole

Deep flexor muscles of right leg and foot
(posterior aspect).

Course of deep flexor muscles of leg (schematic drawing).

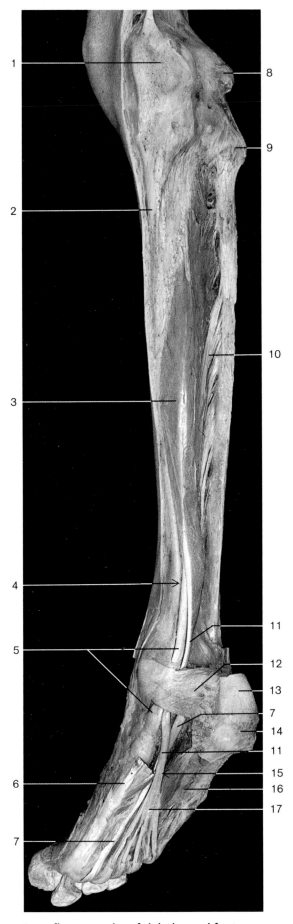

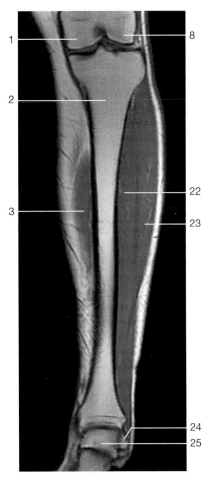

1 Medial condyle of femur
2 Tibia
3 Flexor digitorum longus muscle
4 Crossing of tendons in leg
5 Tendon of tibialis posterior muscle
6 Abductor hallucis muscle
7 Tendon of flexor hallucis longus muscle
8 Lateral condyle of femur
9 Head of fibula
10 Tibialis posterior muscle
11 Tendon of flexor digitorum longus muscle
12 Flexor retinaculum
13 Calcaneal tendon
14 Calcaneal tuberosity
15 Crossing of tendons in sole
16 Quadratus plantae muscle
17 Tendons of flexor digitorum longus muscle
18 Tendon of tibialis anterior muscle
19 Area of insertion of tibialis posterior muscle
20 Lumbrical muscles
21 Flexor hallucis longus muscle
22 Tibialis anterior muscle
23 Extensor hallucis longus muscle
24 Lateral malleolus of fibula
25 Trochlea of talus

Coronal section of the leg
(MRI scan; from Heuck et al., MRT-Atlas, 2009).

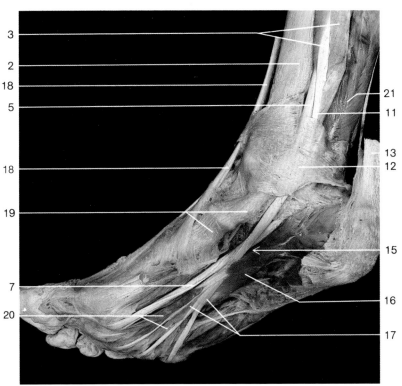

Deep flexor muscles of right leg and foot
(posterior oblique medial aspect). Flexor digitorum brevis and flexor hallucis longus muscles have been removed.

Sole of foot with tendons of long flexor muscles (oblique medial and inferior aspect).

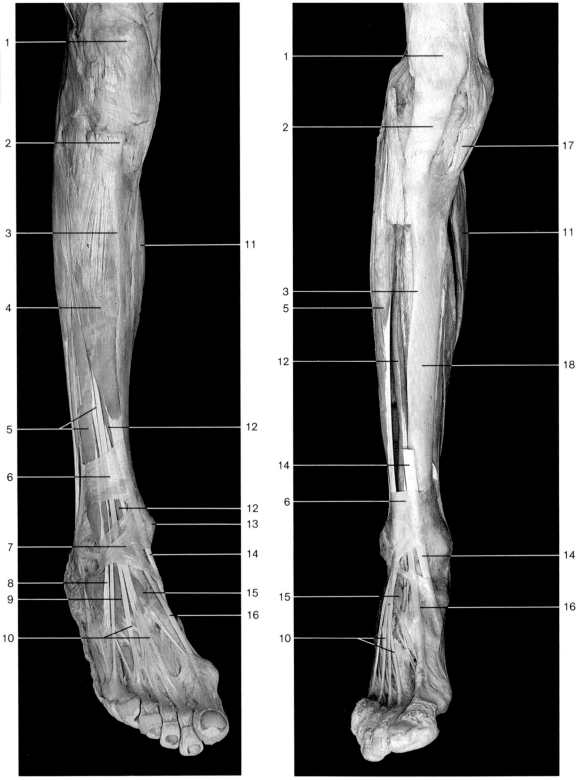

Extensor muscles of right leg and foot
(oblique antero-lateral aspect).

Extensor muscles of right leg and foot (anterior aspect). Part of the tibialis anterior muscle has been removed.

1 Patella	8 Tendon of peroneus tertius muscle	14 Tendon of tibialis anterior muscle
2 Patellar ligament	9 Extensor digitorum brevis muscle	15 Extensor hallucis brevis muscle
3 Anterior margin of tibia	10 Tendons of extensor digitorum	16 Tendon of extensor hallucis
4 Tibialis anterior muscle	longus muscle	longus muscle
5 Extensor digitorum longus muscle	11 Gastrocnemius muscle	17 Common tendon of gracilis,
6 Superior extensor retinaculum	12 Extensor hallucis longus muscle	semitendinosus, and sartorius muscles
7 Inferior extensor retinaculum	13 Medial malleolus	18 Tibia

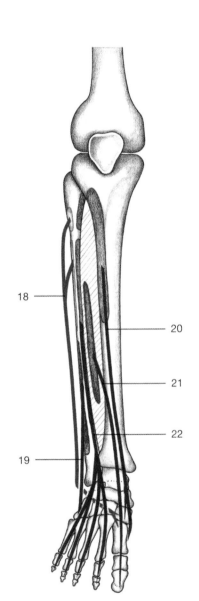

Extensor muscles of the leg (right side).

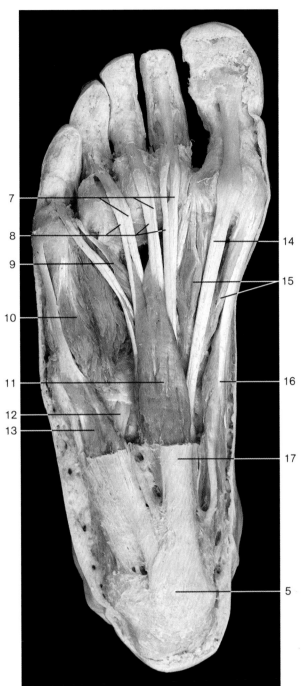

Muscles of sole of foot, first layer (from below). The plantar aponeurosis and the fasciae of the superficial muscles have been removed.

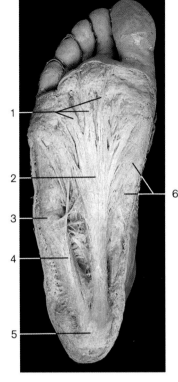

Sole of foot, plantar aponeurosis (from below).

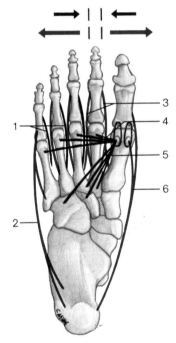

Course of abductor and adductor muscles of foot (schematic drawing). Red arrows = abduction. Black arrows = adduction.

1 Longitudinal bands of plantar aponeurosis
2 Plantar aponeurosis
3 Position of tuberosity of fifth metatarsal bone
4 Muscles of fifth toe with fascia
5 Calcaneal tuberosity
6 Muscles of great toe with fascia
7 Tendons of flexor digitorum longus muscle
8 Tendons of flexor digitorum brevis muscle
9 Lumbrical muscle
10 Flexor digiti minimi brevis muscle
11 Flexor digitorum brevis muscle

12 Tendon of peroneus longus muscle
13 Abductor digiti minimi muscle
14 Tendon of flexor hallucis longus muscle
15 Flexor hallucis brevis muscle
16 Abductor hallucis muscle
17 Plantar aponeurosis (cut)
18 Peroneus longus muscle
19 Peroneus brevis muscle
20 Tibialis anterior muscle
21 Extensor hallucis longus muscle
22 Extensor digitorum longus muscle

1 Plantar interossei muscles (black)
2 Abductor digiti minimi muscle (red)
3 Dorsal interosseous muscles (red)
4 Transverse head of adductor muscle (black)
5 Oblique head of adductor muscle (black)
6 Abductor hallucis muscle (red)

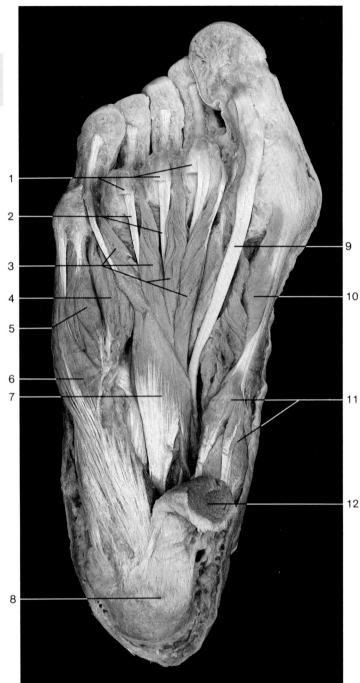

Muscles of sole of foot, second layer (from below). The flexor digitorum brevis muscle has been divided.

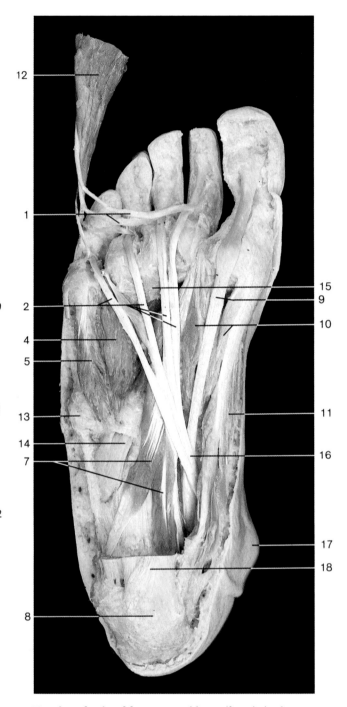

Muscles of sole of foot, second layer (from below). The tendons of the flexor muscles and the crossing of tendons are displayed. The flexor digitorum brevis muscle has been divided and reflected.

1 Tendons of flexor digitorum brevis muscle	6 Abductor digiti minimi muscle	13 Tuberosity of fifth metatarsal bone
2 Tendons of flexor digitorum longus muscle	7 Quadratus plantae muscle	14 Tendon of peroneus longus muscle
	8 Calcaneal tuberosity	15 Transverse head of adductor hallucis muscle
3 Lumbrical muscles	9 Tendon of flexor hallucis longus muscle	16 Crossing of tendons in sole of foot
4 Interossei muscles	10 Flexor hallucis brevis muscle	17 Medial malleolus
5 Flexor digiti minimi brevis muscle	11 Abductor hallucis muscle	18 Plantar aponeurosis (divided)
	12 Flexor digitorum brevis muscle (divided)	

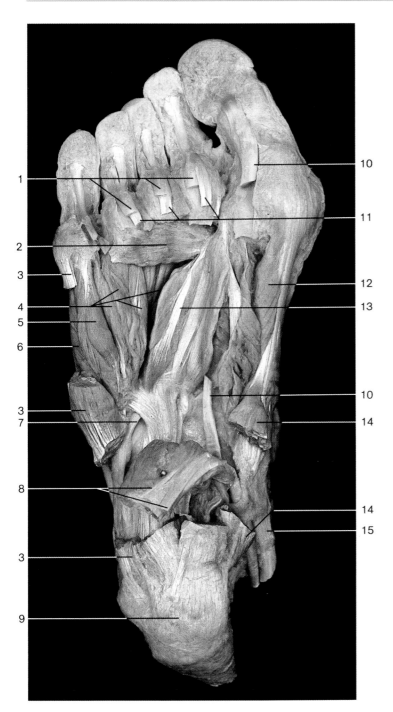

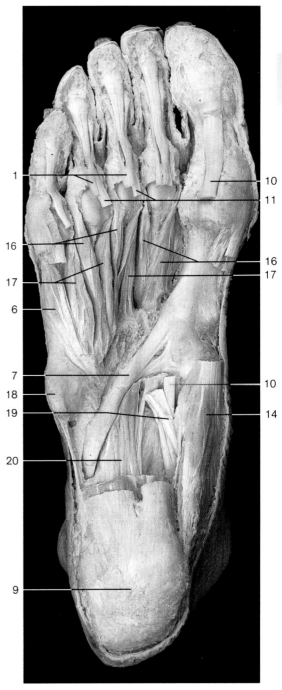

Muscles of sole of foot, third layer (from below). The flexor digitorum brevis muscle has been removed, and the quadratus plantae, abductor hallucis, and digiti minimi muscles have been divided.

Muscles of sole of foot, fourth layer (from below). The interosseous muscles and the canal for the tendon of peroneus longus muscle are shown.

1   Tendons of flexor digitorum brevis muscle
2   Transverse head of adductor hallucis muscle
3   Abductor digiti minimi muscle
4   Interossei muscles
5   Flexor digiti minimi brevis muscle
6   Opponens digiti minimi muscle
7   Tendon of peroneus longus muscle

8   Quadratus plantae muscle with tendon of flexor digitorum longus muscle
9   Calcaneal tuberosity
10 Tendons of flexor hallucis longus muscle (divided)
11 Tendon of flexor digitorum longus muscle
12 Flexor hallucis brevis muscle
13 Oblique head of adductor hallucis muscle
14 Abductor hallucis muscle (cut)

15 Tendon of tibialis posterior muscle
16 Dorsal interossei muscles
17 Plantar interossei muscles
18 Tuberosity of fifth metatarsal bone
19 Tendon of flexor digitorum longus muscle (crossing of plantar tendons)
20 Long plantar ligament

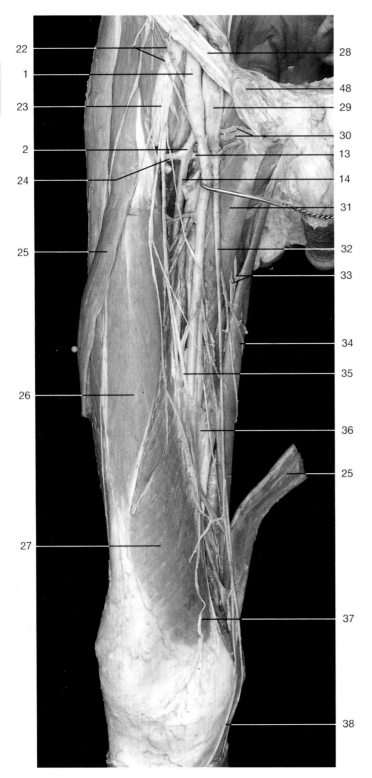

22	28
1	48
23	29
	30
2	13
24	14
	31
25	32
	33
	34
	35
26	36
	25
27	
	37
	38

Main arteries and nerves of right thigh (anterior aspect). Sartorius muscle has been divided and reflected. The femoral vein has been partly removed to show the deep femoral artery. Notice: the vessels enter the adductor canal to reach the popliteal fossa.

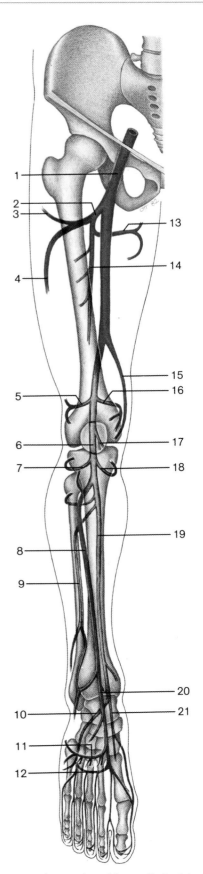

Main arteries of lower limb, right side (anterior aspect, schematic drawing).

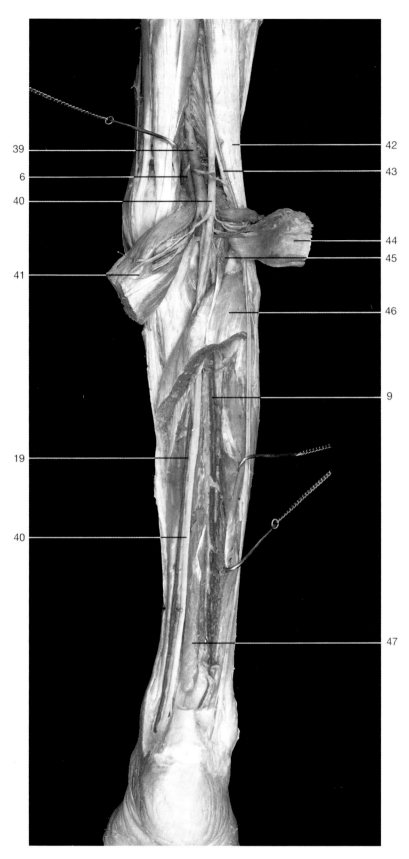

1 Femoral artery
2 Profunda femoris artery
3 Ascending branch of lateral circumflex femoral artery
4 Descending branch of lateral circumflex femoral artery
5 Lateral superior genicular artery
6 Popliteal artery
7 Lateral inferior genicular artery
8 Anterior tibial artery
9 Peroneal artery
10 Lateral plantar artery
11 Arcuate artery with dorsal metatarsal arteries
12 Plantar arch with plantar metatarsal arteries
13 Medial circumflex femoral artery
14 Profunda femoris artery with perforating arteries
15 Descending genicular artery
16 Medial superior genicular artery
17 Middle genicular artery
18 Medial inferior genicular artery
19 Posterior tibial artery
20 Dorsalis pedis artery
21 Medial plantar artery
22 Superficial and deep circumflex iliac arteries
23 Femoral nerve
24 Lateral circumflex femoral artery
25 Sartorius muscle (cut and reflected)
26 Rectus femoris muscle
27 Vastus medialis muscle
28 Inguinal ligament
29 Femoral vein (cut)
30 External pudendal artery and vein
31 Adductor longus muscle
32 Great saphenous vein
33 Obturator artery and nerve
34 Gracilis muscle
35 Saphenous nerve
36 Tendinous wall of adductor canal
37 Anterior cutaneous branch of femoral nerve
38 Infrapatellar branch of saphenous nerve
39 Popliteal vein
40 Tibial nerve
41 Medial head of gastrocnemius muscle
42 Biceps femoris muscle
43 Common peroneal nerve
44 Lateral head of gastrocnemius muscle
45 Plantaris muscle
46 Soleus muscle
47 Flexor hallucis longus muscle
48 Spermatic cord

Arteries of the right leg (posterior aspect).

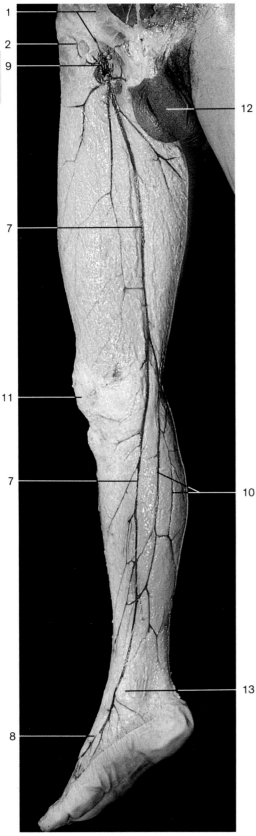

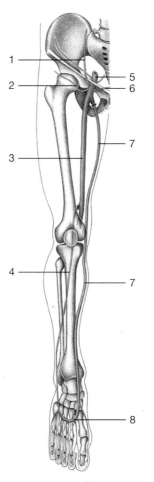

Main veins of lower limb, right side (anterior aspect, schematic drawing).

1   Superficial epigastric vein
2   Superficial circumflex iliac vein
3   Femoral vein
4   Small saphenous vein
5   External iliac vein
6   External pudendal vein
7   Great saphenous vein
8   Dorsal venous arch
9   Saphenous opening with femoral vein
10   Venous anastomoses of small saphenous vein with great saphenous vein
11   Patella
12   Penis
13   Medial malleolus
14   Popliteal fossa
15   Perforating veins
16   Lateral malleolus
17   Dorsal digital veins of foot
18   Dorsal venous arch of foot
19   Dorsal metatarsal veins
20   Anterior tibial artery and veins
21   Tibia
22   Posterior tibial artery and veins
23   Fibula
24   Peroneal artery and vein
25   Deep layer of crural fascia
26   Superficial layer of crural fascia
27   Perforating veins I–III (of Cockett)
28   Tibial nerve
29   Arcuate vein
30   Saphenous nerve
31   Medial dorsal cutaneous nerve (branch of superficial peroneal nerve)
32   Posterior tibial vein

Superficial veins of lower limb, right side (medio-anterior aspect). The veins have been injected with red solution.

Medial malleolar region. Dissection of ▷ tibial nerve, posterior tibial vessels, and great saphenous vein (veins injected with blue resin).

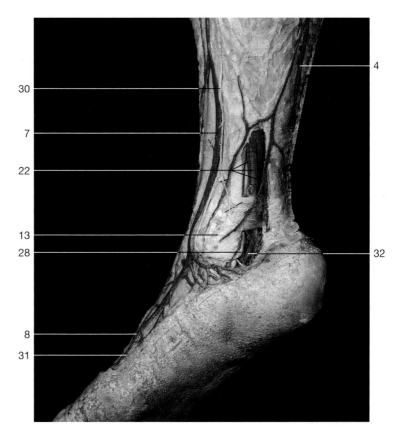

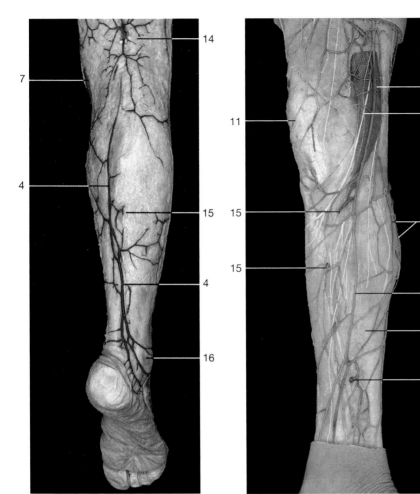

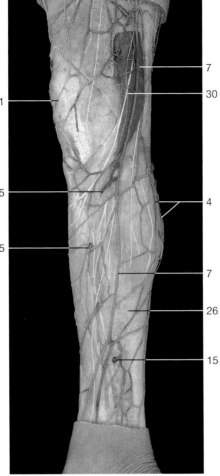

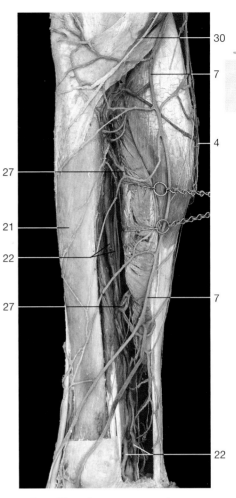

Superficial veins of leg (posterior aspect; veins injected with blue resin).

Superficial veins of leg. The perforating veins of Cockett have been dissected (left side, medial aspect).

Veins of leg. The anastomoses between superficial and deeper veins are dissected (left side, medial aspect).

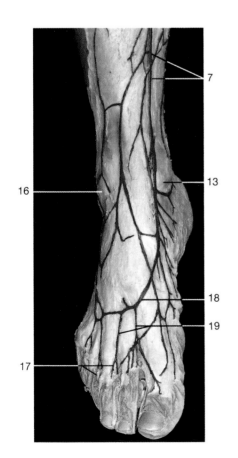

Anastomoses between superficial ▷ **and deep veins of the leg** (schematic drawing, after Aigner).
Arrows: directions of blood flow.

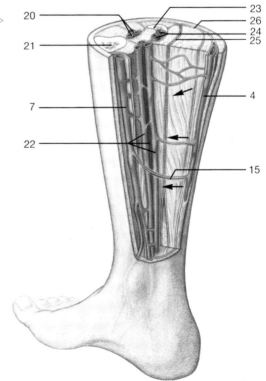

◁

Superficial veins on dorsum of foot (veins injected with blue resin).

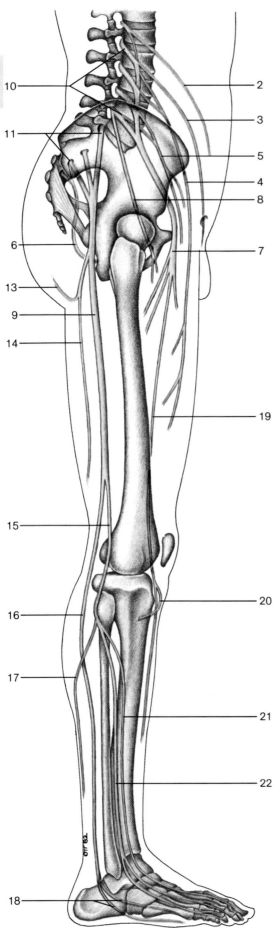

1   Subcostal nerve
2   Iliohypogastric nerve
3   Ilio-inguinal nerve
4   Lateral femoral cutaneous nerve
5   Genitofemoral nerve
6   Pudendal nerve
7   Femoral nerve
8   Obturator nerve
9   Sciatic nerve
10 Lumbar plexus (L$_1$–L$_4$)
11 Sacral plexus (L$_4$–S$_4$)   } lumbosacral plexus
12 "Pudendal" plexus (S$_2$–S$_4$)
13 Inferior cluneal nerves
14 Posterior femoral cutaneous nerve
15 Common peroneal nerve
16 Tibial nerve
17 Lateral sural cutaneous nerve
18 Medial and lateral plantar nerves
19 Saphenous nerve
20 Infrapatellar branch of saphenous nerve
21 Deep peroneal nerve
22 Superficial peroneal nerve
23 Anterior cutaneous branch of iliohypogastric nerve
24 Lateral cutaneous branch of iliohypogastric nerve
25 Femoral branch of genitofemoral nerve
26 Lateral cutaneous branches of intercostal nerve
27 Anterior cutaneous branches of intercostal nerve
28 Genital branch of genitofemoral nerve
29 Anterior scrotal nerve

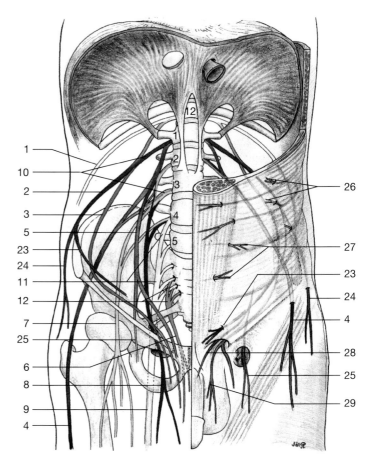

Nerves of lower limb, right side (lateral aspect).
(Schematic drawing.)

Main branches of lumbosacral plexus (ventral aspect).
(Schematic drawing.)

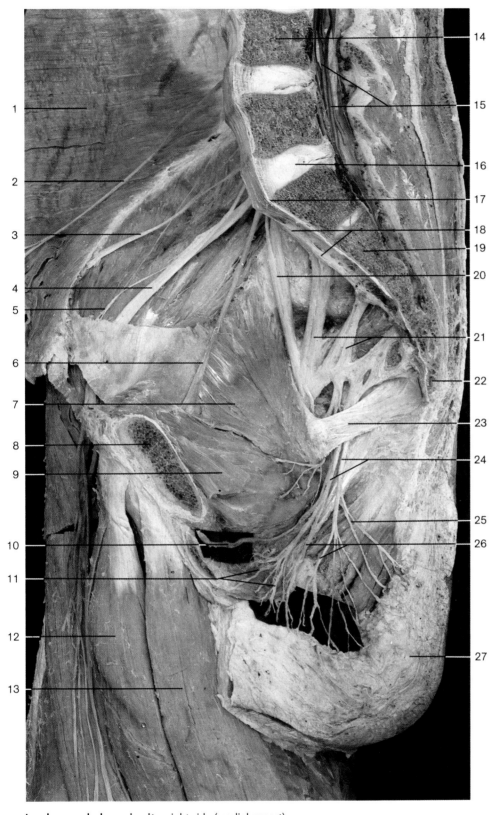

1   Transversus abdominis muscle
2   Iliohypogastric nerve
3   Ilio-inguinal nerve
4   Femoral nerve
5   Lateral femoral cutaneous nerve
6   Obturator nerve
7   Obturator internus muscle
8   Pubic bone (cut edge)
9   Levator ani muscle (remnant)
10 Dorsal nerve of penis
11 Posterior scrotal nerves
12 Adductor longus muscle
13 Gracilis muscle
14 Body of fourth lumbar vertebra
15 Cauda equina
16 Intervertebral disc
17 Sacral promontory
18 Sympathetic trunk
19 Sacrum
20 Lumbosacral trunk
21 Sacral plexus
22 Coccyx
23 Sacrospinous ligament
24 Pudendal nerve
25 Inferior rectal nerves
26 Perineal nerves
27 Subcutaneous fat tissue
    of gluteal region

Lumbosacral plexus in situ, right side (medial aspect).
Pelvic organs with peritoneum and part of the levator ani muscle have been removed.

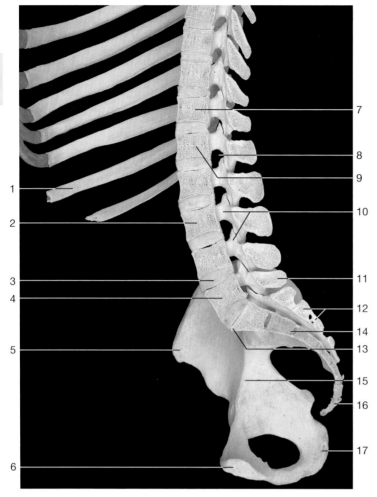

Lumbar part of vertebral column with pelvis
(sagittal section, medial aspect).

1   Eleventh rib
2   Body of third lumbar vertebra
3   Intervertebral disc
4   Body of fifth lumbar vertebra
5   Anterior superior iliac spine
6   Symphysial surface
7   Body of twelfth thoracic vertebra
8   Intervertebral foramen
9   Body of first lumbar vertebra
10 Vertebral canal
11 Spinous process of fifth lumbar vertebra
12 Sacrum (median sacral crest)
13 Promontory (promontorium)
14 Sacrum
15 Arcuate line
16 Coccyx
17 Ischial tuberosity
18 Sympathetic trunk with ganglia
19 Ureter
20 Iliohypogastric nerve (Th$_{12}$, L$_1$)
21 Ilio-inguinal nerve (L$_1$)
22 Femoral nerve (L$_2$–L$_4$)
23 Genitofemoral nerve (L$_1$, L$_2$)
24 Inferior hypogastric plexus
25 Ductus deferens
26 Urinary bladder
27 Medullary cone of spinal cord
28 Root filaments of spinal nerves
29 Subarachnoid space
     (filled with cerebrospinal fluid) (blue)
30 Terminal filament of spinal cord
31 Sacral plexus
32 Pelvic splanchnic nerves (nervi erigentes)
33 Rectum

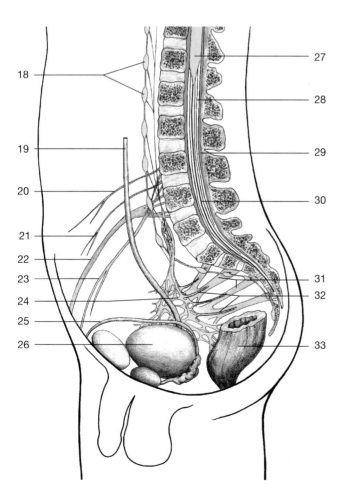

Vertebral canal with spinal cord and root filaments.
Note the high location of the medullary cone. Sacral plexus and inferior hypogastric plexus are schematically shown.

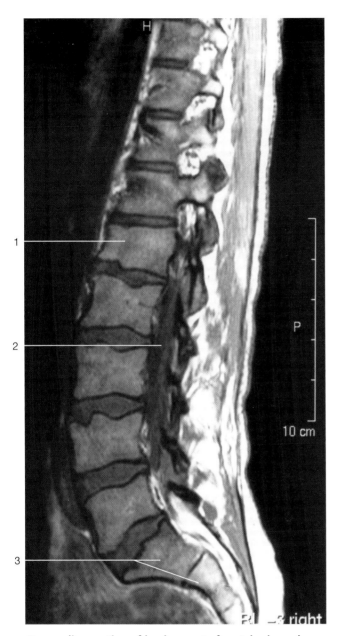

Paramedian section of lumbar part of vertebral canal
(MRI scan, dotted line in the schematic drawing below; courtesy of Prof. Bautz, Erlangen, Germany).

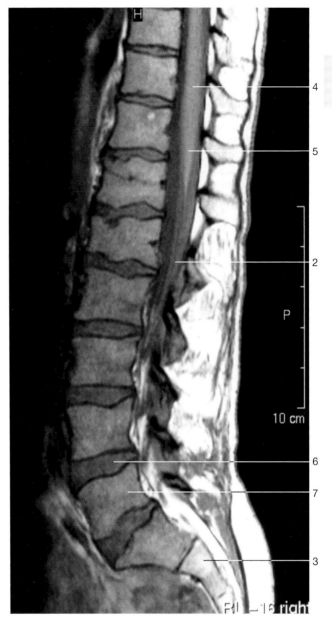

Median section of lumbar part of vertebral canal at the level of the medullary cone (MRI scan, continuous line in the schematic drawing below; courtesy of Prof. Bautz, Erlangen, Germany).

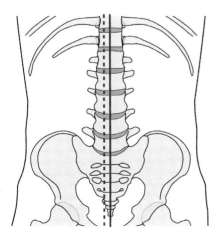

1   First lumbar vertebra
2   Root filaments of spinal nerves
3   Sacrum
4   Spinal cord
5   Medullary cone of spinal cord
6   Intervertebral disc between fourth and fifth lumbar vertebra
7   Fifth lumbar vertebra

Location of the sections shown above through the vertebral canal.

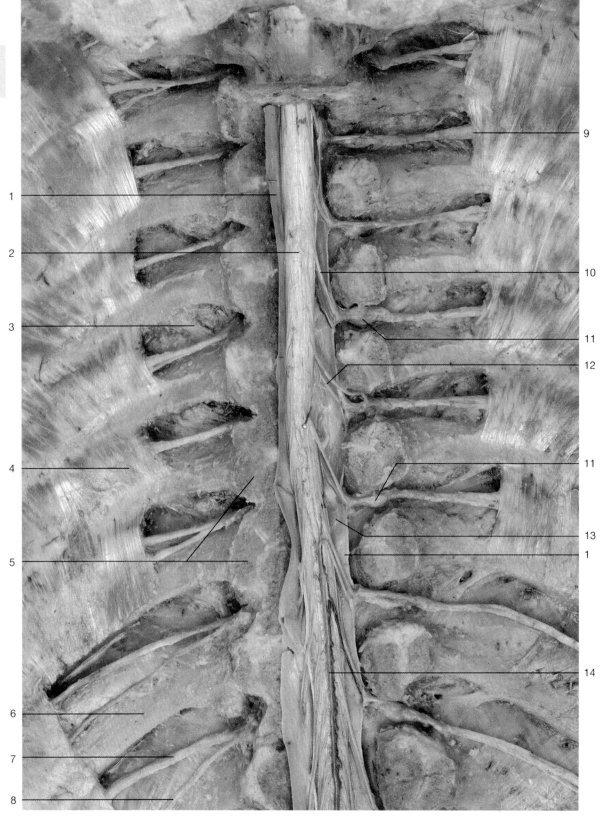

Spinal cord with intercostal nerves. Inferior thoracic region (anterior aspect). Anterior portion of thoracic vertebrae removed, dural sheath opened, and spinal cord slightly reflected to the right to display the dorsal and ventral roots.

1 Dura mater	6 Eleventh rib	10 Anterior root filaments
2 Spinal cord	7 Intercostal nerve	11 Spinal (dorsal root) ganglion
3 Costotransverse ligament	8 Collateral branch of intercostal nerve	12 Posterior root filaments
4 Innermost intercostal muscle	9 Intercostal nerve (entering the	13 Arachnoid mater and denticulate ligament
5 Vertebral arches (cut surfaces)	intermuscular interval)	14 Anterior spinal artery

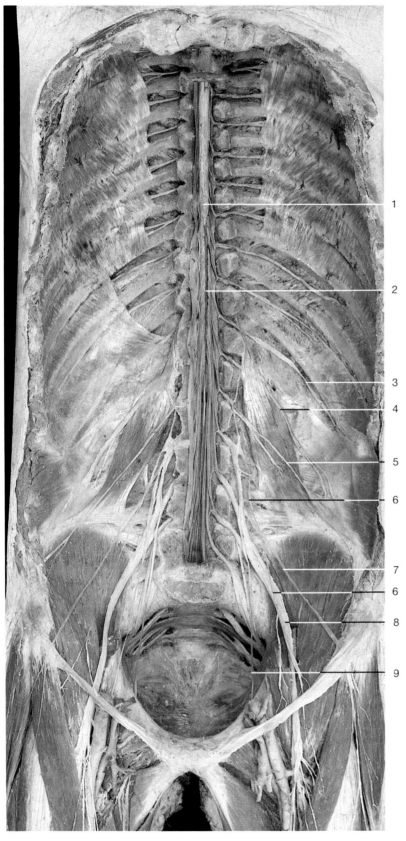

Spinal cord and lumbar plexus in situ (anterior aspect).

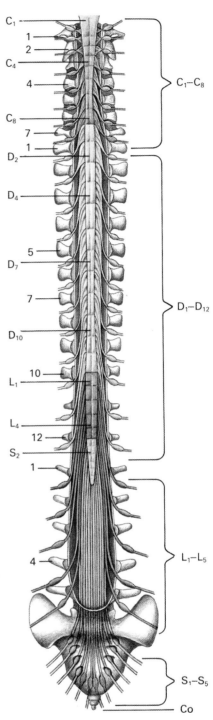

Organization of spinal cord segments in relation to the vertebral column (anterior aspect).
C = cervical; D = thoracic;
L = lumbar; S = sacral segments;
Co = coccygeal bone.
Numbers indicate the related vertebrae.

1	Conus medullaris	
2	Filum terminale	
3	Subcostal nerve	
4	Iliohypogastric nerve	
5	Ilio-inguinal nerve	
6	Genitofemoral nerve	
7	Lateral femoral cutaneous nerve	
8	Femoral nerve	
9	Obturator nerve	

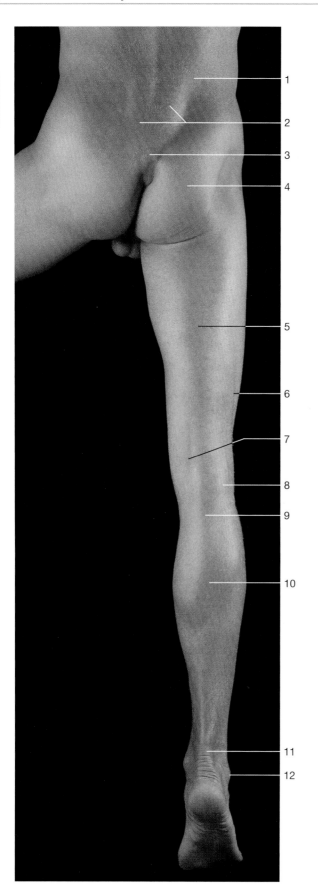

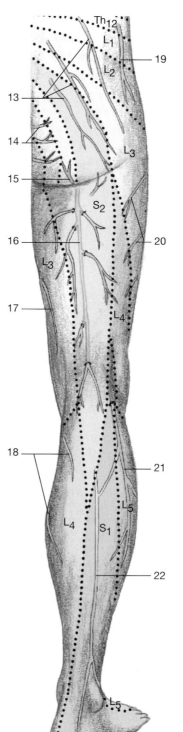

1 Iliac crest
2 Sacrum
3 Coccyx
4 Gluteus maximus muscle
5 Dorsal muscles of the leg
6 Iliotibial tract
7 Tendon of semimembranosus muscle
8 Tendon of biceps femoris muscle
9 Popliteal fossa
10 Triceps surae muscle
11 Calcaneal or Achilles tendon
12 Lateral malleolus
13 Superior cluneal nerves
14 Middle cluneal nerves
15 Inferior cluneal nerves
16 Posterior femoral cutaneous nerve
17 Obturator nerve
18 Saphenous nerve
19 Iliohypogastric nerve
20 Branch of lateral femoral cutaneous nerves
21 Common peroneal nerve
22 Sural nerve

Cutaneous nerves of the lower limb (posterior aspect).
Dotted lines = border of segments.

Surface anatomy of the right leg (posterior aspect).
Gluteal muscles contracted.

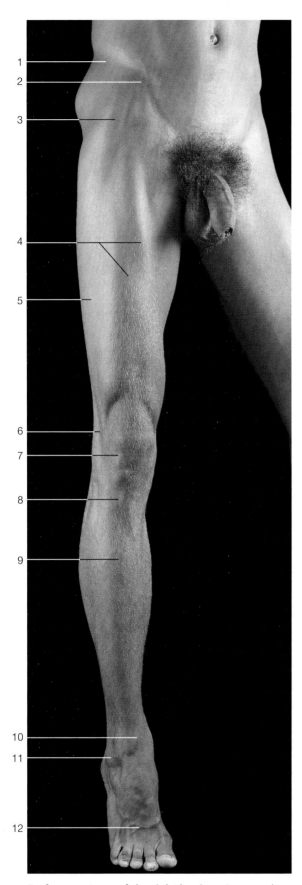

Surface anatomy of the right leg (anterior aspect).

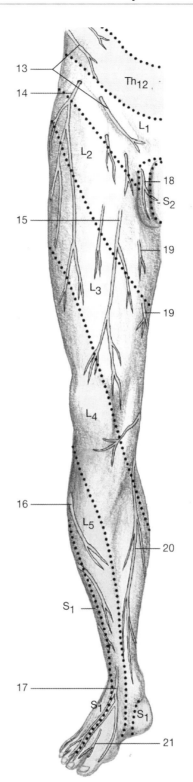

Cutaneous nerves of the lower limb (anterior aspect).
Dotted lines = border of segments.

1 Iliac crest
2 Anterior superior iliac spine
3 Tensor fasciae latae muscle
4 Quadriceps femoris muscle
5 Iliotibial tract
6 Tendon of biceps femoris muscle
7 Patella
8 Patellar ligament
9 Tibia
10 Tendon of tibialis anterior muscle
11 Lateral malleolus
12 Venous network of dorsum of foot
13 Iliohypogastric nerve
14 Lateral femoral cutaneous nerve
15 Femoral nerve
16 Common peroneal nerve
17 Superficial peroneal nerve
18 Ilio-inguinal nerve
19 Obturator nerve
20 Saphenous nerve
21 Deep peroneal nerve

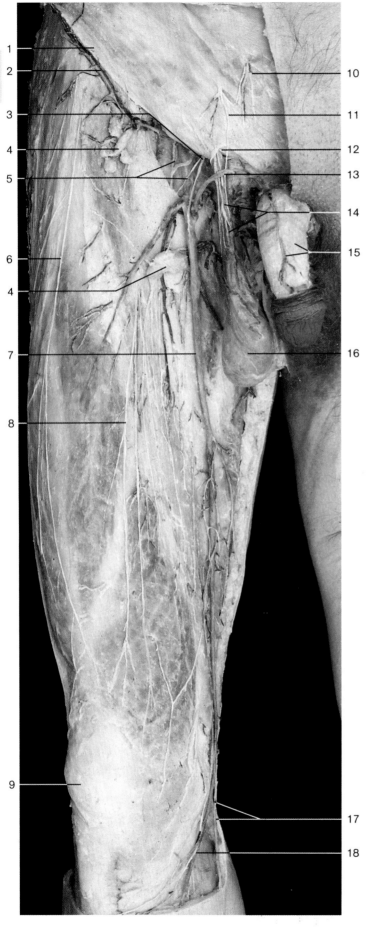

Cutaneous nerves and veins of thigh (anterior aspect).

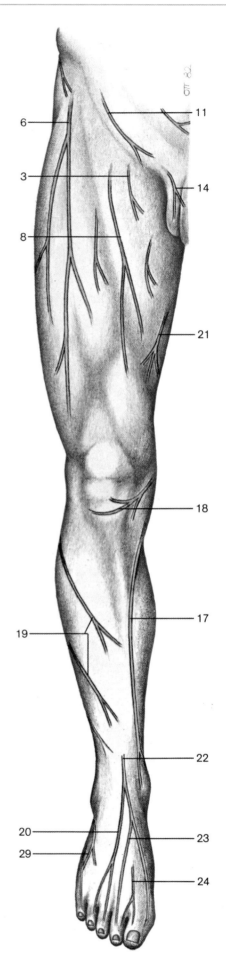

Cutaneous nerves of lower limb (anterior aspect).
(Schematic drawing.)

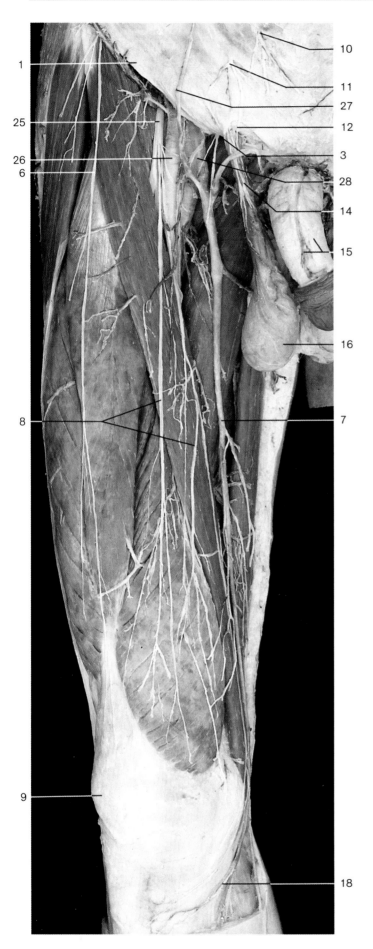

1 Inguinal ligament
2 Superficial circumflex iliac vein
3 Femoral branch of genitofemoral nerve
4 Superficial inguinal lymph nodes
5 Saphenous opening with femoral artery and vein
6 Lateral femoral cutaneous nerve
7 Great saphenous vein
8 Anterior cutaneous branches of femoral nerve
9 Patella
10 Terminal branches of subcostal nerve
11 Terminal branches of iliohypogastric nerve
12 Superficial inguinal ring
13 External pudendal vein
14 Spermatic cord with genital branch of genitofemoral nerve
15 Penis with superficial dorsal vein of penis
16 Testis and its coverings
17 Saphenous nerve
18 Infrapatellar branch of saphenous nerve
19 Lateral sural cutaneous nerves
20 Intermediate dorsal cutaneous branch of superficial peroneal nerve
21 Cutaneous branch of obturator nerve
22 Superficial peroneal nerve
23 Medial dorsal cutaneous branch of superficial peroneal nerve
24 Deep peroneal nerve
25 Femoral nerve
26 Femoral artery
27 Superficial epigastric vein
28 Femoral vein
29 Lateral dorsal cutaneous branch of sural nerve
30 Inguinal nodes (enlarged)
31 Lympathic vessels
32 Sartorius muscle

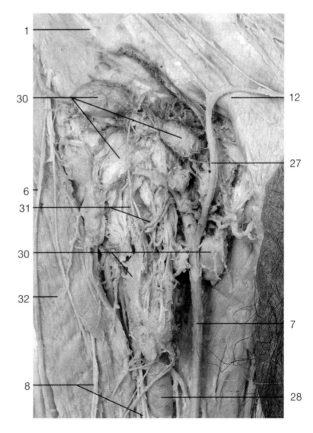

Cutaneous nerves and veins of thigh (anterior aspect). The fascia lata and fasciae of the thigh muscles have been removed.

Inguinal nodes with lymphatic vessels (anterior aspect).

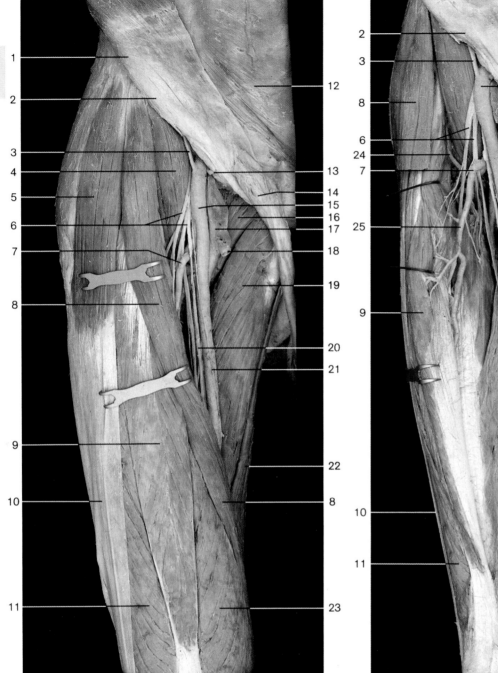

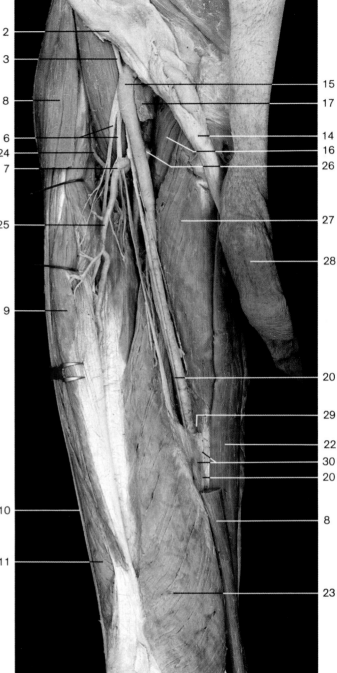

Anterior region of right thigh (anterior aspect). The fascia lata has been removed, and the sartorius muscle has been slightly reflected.

Anterior region of right thigh (anterior aspect). The fascia lata has been removed, and the sartorius muscle has been divided.

1   Anterior superior iliac spine
2   Inguinal ligament
3   Deep circumflex iliac artery
4   Iliopsoas muscle
5   Tensor fasciae latae muscle
6   Femoral nerve
7   Lateral circumflex femoral artery
8   Sartorius muscle
9   Rectus femoris muscle
10 Iliotibial tract
11 Vastus lateralis muscle
12 Anterior sheath of rectus abdominis muscle
13 Inferior epigastric artery
14 Spermatic cord
15 Femoral artery

16 Pectineus muscle
17 Femoral vein
18 Great saphenous vein (divided)
19 Adductor longus muscle
20 Saphenous nerve
21 Muscular branch of femoral nerve
22 Gracilis muscle
23 Vastus medialis muscle
24 Ascending branch of lateral circumflex femoral artery
25 Descending branch of lateral circumflex femoral artery
26 Medial circumflex femoral artery
27 Adductor longus muscle
28 Penis
29 Entrance to adductor canal
30 Vasto-adductor membrane of fascia beneath sartorius muscle

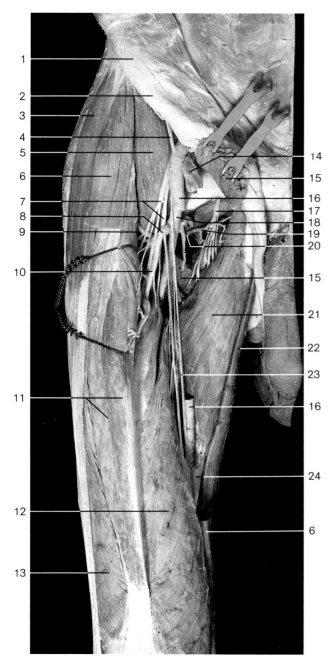

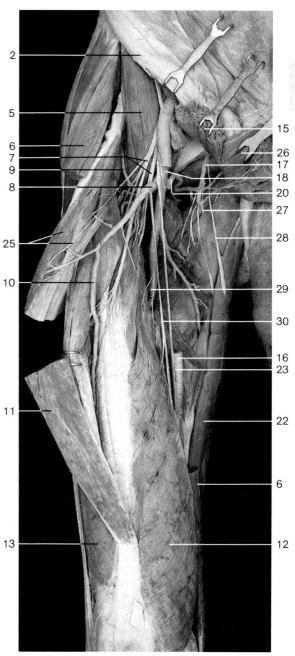

Anterior region of right thigh (anterior aspect).
The fascia lata has been removed. Sartorius muscle,
pectineus muscle, and femoral artery have been cut to
display the deep femoral artery with its branches.
The rectus femoris muscle has been slightly reflected.

1 Anterior superior iliac spine
2 Inguinal ligament
3 Tensor fasciae latae muscle
4 Deep circumflex iliac artery
5 Iliopsoas muscle
6 Sartorius muscle (cut)
7 Femoral nerve
8 Lateral circumflex femoral artery
9 Ascending branch of lateral circumflex femoral artery
10 Descending branch of lateral circumflex femoral artery
11 Rectus femoris muscle
12 Vastus medialis muscle
13 Vastus lateralis muscle
14 Femoral vein
15 Pectineus muscle (cut)
16 Femoral artery (cut)

Anterior region of right thigh (anterior aspect).
The sartorius, pectineus, adductor longus, and rectus
femoris muscles have been divided and reflected.
The greater part of the femoral artery has been
removed.

17 Obturator nerve
18 Profunda femoris artery
19 Ascending branch of medial circumflex femoral artery
20 Medial circumflex femoral artery
21 Adductor longus muscle
22 Gracilis muscle
23 Saphenous nerve
24 Distal part of vasto-adductor membrane
25 Rectus femoris muscle with muscular branch of
   femoral nerve
26 Adductor longus muscle (divided)
27 Posterior branch of obturator nerve
28 Anterior branch of obturator nerve
29 Point at which perforating artery branches off from
   profunda femoris artery
30 Muscular branch of femoral nerve to vastus medialis muscle

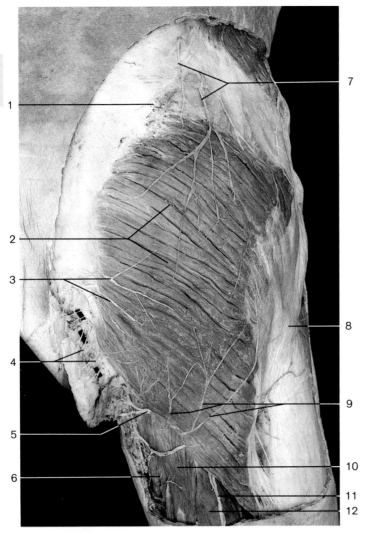

1 Iliac crest
2 Gluteus maximus muscle
3 Middle cluneal nerves
4 Anococcygeal nerves
5 Perineal branch of posterior femoral cutaneous nerve
6 Adductor magnus muscle
7 Superior cluneal nerves
8 Position of greater trochanter
9 Inferior cluneal nerves
10 Semitendinosus muscle
11 Posterior femoral cutaneous nerve
12 Long head of biceps femoris muscle

Gluteal region, right side (posterior aspect).

A	**Suprapiriform foramen** (of greater sciatic foramen) Superior gluteal artery, vein, and nerve
B	**Infrapiriform foramen** (of greater sciatic foramen) Sciatic nerve Inferior gluteal artery, vein, and nerve Posterior femoral cutaneous nerve Internal pudendal artery and vein Pudendal nerve
C	**Lesser sciatic foramen** Pudendal nerve Internal pudendal artery and vein

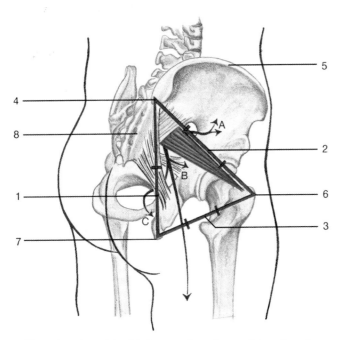

Gluteal region, right side (postero-lateral aspect). Location of sciatic foramina in relation to the bones (schematic drawing).

Red lines

1 Spine-tuber line:
   the infrapiriform foramen is situated in the middle of this line
2 Spine-trochanter line:
   the suprapiriform foramen is located in the upper third
3 Tuber-trochanter line:
   the ischiadic nerve can be found between the middle and posterior third

Other structures

4 Posterior superior iliac spine
5 Iliac crest
6 Greater trochanter
7 Ischial tuberosity
8 Sacrum

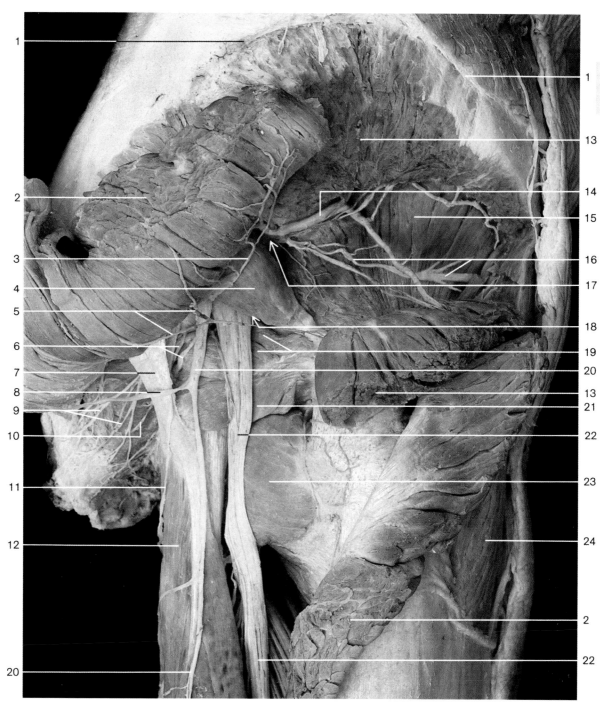

Gluteal region, right side (posterior aspect). The gluteus maximus and gluteus medius muscles have been divided and reflected. Notice the position of the foramina above and below the piriformis muscle and the lesser sciatic foramen.

1 Iliac crest
2 Gluteus maximus muscle (cut)
3 Inferior gluteal nerve
4 Piriformis muscle
5 Muscular branches of inferior gluteal artery
6 Pudendal nerve and internal pudendal artery within the lesser sciatic foramen (entrance to the pudendal canal)
7 Sacrotuberous ligament
8 Inferior cluneal nerve
9 Inferior rectal nerves
10 Inferior rectal arteries
11 Perforating cutaneous nerve
12 Long head of biceps femoris muscle

13 Gluteus medius muscle (cut)
14 Deep branch of superior gluteal artery
15 Gluteus minimus muscle
16 Superior gluteal nerve
17 Suprapiriform foramen ⎫ greater sciatic foramen
18 Infrapiriform foramen ⎭
19 Tendon of obturator internus and superior gemellus muscles
20 Posterior femoral cutaneous nerve
21 Inferior gemellus muscle
22 Sciatic nerve
23 Quadratus femoris muscle
24 Tensor fasciae latae muscle

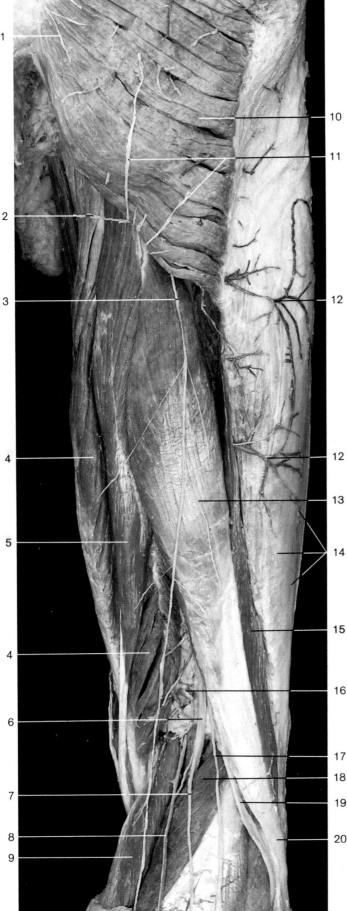

1 Middle cluneal nerves
2 Perineal branch of posterior femoral cutaneous nerve
3 Posterior femoral cutaneous nerve
4 Semimembranosus muscle
5 Semitendinosus muscle
6 Tibial nerve
7 Medial sural cutaneous nerve
8 Small saphenous vein
9 Medial head of gastrocnemius muscle
10 Gluteus maximus muscle
11 Inferior cluneal nerves
12 Cutaneous veins
13 Long head of biceps femoris muscle
14 Iliotibial tract
15 Short head of biceps femoris muscle
16 Popliteal fossa
17 Lateral sural cutaneous nerve
18 Lateral head of gastrocnemius muscle
19 Common peroneal nerve
20 Tendon of biceps femoris muscle
21 Inferior gluteal nerve
22 Sacrotuberous ligament
23 Inferior rectal branches of pudendal nerve
24 Anus
25 Gluteus medius muscle
26 Piriformis muscle
27 Sciatic nerve
28 Inferior gluteal artery
29 Gluteus maximus muscle (cut)
30 Quadratus femoris muscle
31 Sciatic nerve dividing into its two branches: the common peroneal nerve and the tibial nerve
32 Muscular branches of sciatic nerve to hamstring muscles
33 Popliteal artery
34 Popliteal vein
35 Small saphenous vein (cut)
36 Long head of biceps femoris muscle (cut)
37 Superficial peroneal nerve

Cutaneous nerves of thigh (posterior aspect).
The fascia lata and the fasciae of muscles have been removed.

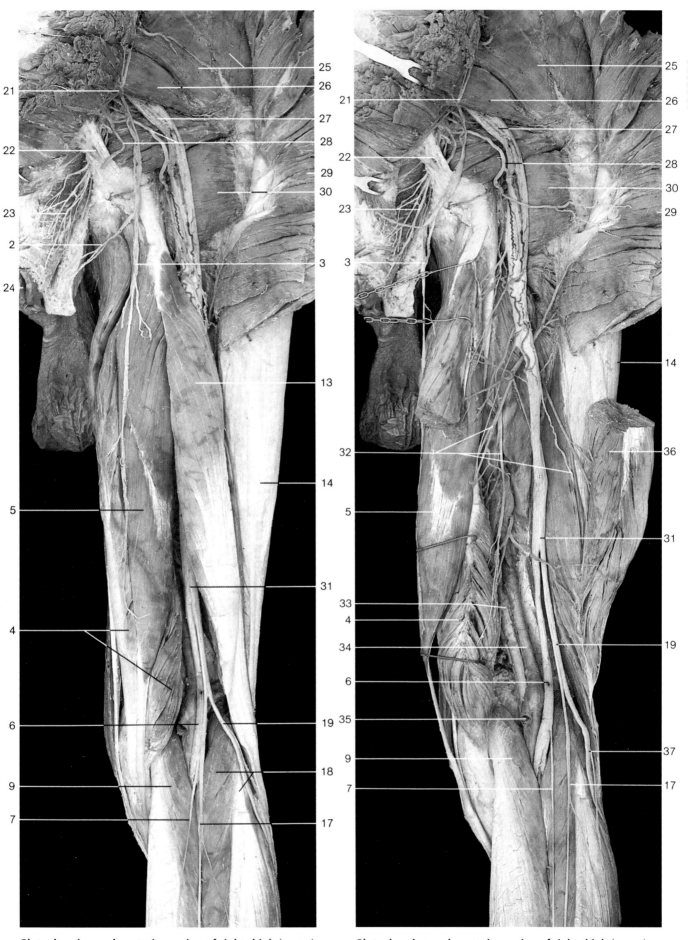

Gluteal region and posterior region of right thigh (posterior aspect). The gluteus maximus muscle has been divided and reflected.

Gluteal region and posterior region of right thigh (posterior aspect). The gluteus maximus muscle and the long head of the biceps femoris muscle have been divided and reflected.

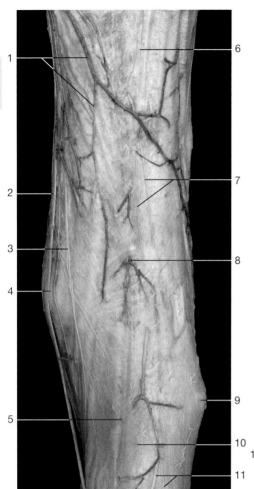

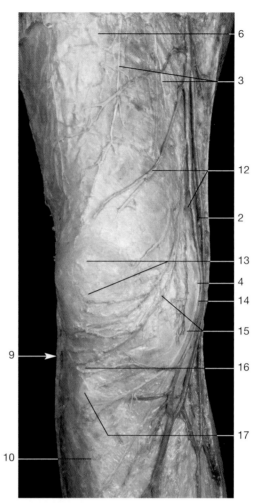

1   Cutaneous veins (tributaries of great saphenous vein)
2   Great saphenous vein
3   Cutaneous branch of femoral nerve
4   Position of medial condyle of femur
5   Position of small saphenous vein
6   Fascia lata
7   Terminal branches of posterior femoral cutaneous nerve
8   Cutaneous veins of popliteal fossa
9   Position of head of fibula
10   Superficial layer of fascia cruris
11   Lateral sural cutaneous nerve
12   Venous network around knee
13   Patella
14   Saphenous nerve
15   Infrapatellar branch of saphenous nerve
16   Patellar ligament
17   Position of tuberosity of tibia
18   Sartorius muscle
19   Semimembranosus muscle
20   Gastrocnemius muscle
21   Popliteal vein
22   Tibial nerve
23   Biceps femoris muscle
24   Popliteal artery
25   Lateral inferior genicular artery
26   Fibula

Posterior region of right knee, cutaneous nerves and veins (posterior aspect).

Anterior region of right knee, cutaneous nerves and veins (anterior aspect).

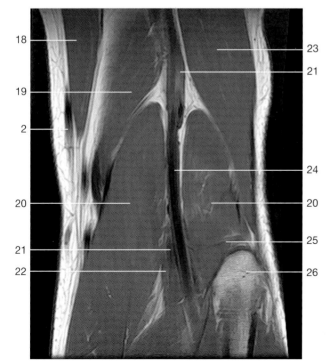

Coronal section of popliteal fossa (MRI scan; from Heuck et al., MRT-Atlas, 2009).

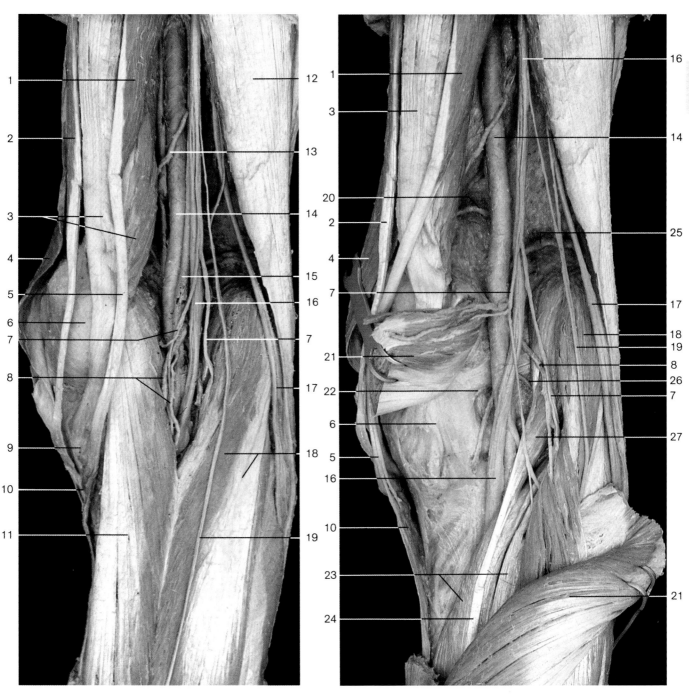

Right leg, popliteal fossa, middle layer (posterior aspect). The gastrocnemius muscle has been divided and reflected.

Right leg, popliteal fossa, deep layer (posterior aspect). The gastrocnemius and the soleus muscles have been divided and reflected.

1 Semitendinosus muscle
2 Gracilis muscle
3 Semimembranosus muscle
4 Sartorius muscle
5 Tendon of semitendinosus muscle
6 Position of medial condyle of femur
7 Muscular branches of tibial nerve
8 Sural arteries and veins
9 Tendon of semimembranosus muscle
10 Common tendon of gracilis, semitendinosus, and sartorius muscles
11 Medial head of gastrocnemius muscle
12 Biceps femoris muscle
13 Muscular branch of popliteal artery

14 Popliteal artery
15 Popliteal vein
16 Tibial nerve
17 Common peroneal nerve
18 Lateral head of gastrocnemius muscle
19 Medial sural cutaneous nerve
20 Medial superior genicular artery
21 Medial head of gastrocnemius muscle (cut and reflected)
22 Medial inferior genicular artery
23 Soleus muscle
24 Tendon of plantaris muscle
25 Lateral superior genicular artery
26 Lateral inferior genicular artery
27 Plantaris muscle

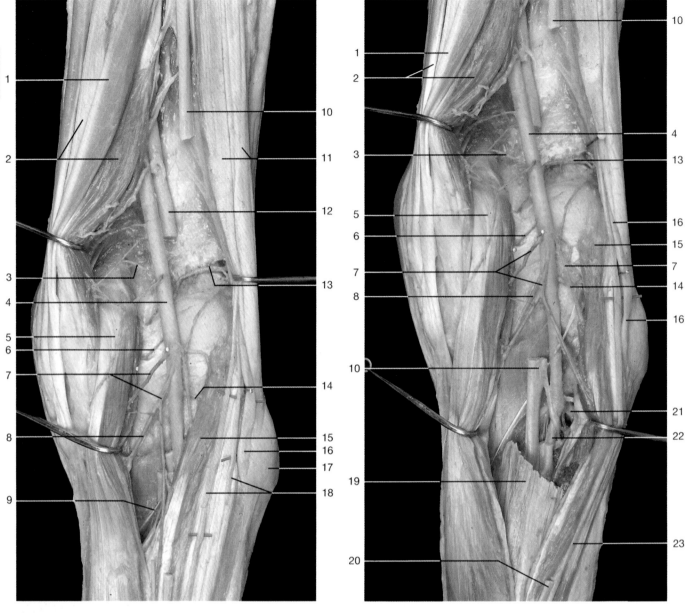

Right leg, popliteal fossa, deep layer (posterior aspect).
The muscles have been reflected to display the genicular arteries.

Right leg, popliteal fossa, deepest layer (posterior aspect).
Tibial nerve and popliteal vein have been partly removed
and a portion of the soleus muscle was cut away to display the
anterior tibial artery.

1	Semitendinosus muscle	12	Popliteal vein (cut)
2	Semimembranosus muscle	13	Lateral superior genicular artery
3	Medial superior genicular artery	14	Lateral inferior genicular artery
4	Popliteal artery	15	Lateral head of gastrocnemius muscle
5	Medial head of gastrocnemius muscle	16	Common peroneal nerve
6	Middle genicular artery	17	Head of fibula
7	Muscular branches	18	Lateral sural cutaneous nerves
8	Medial inferior genicular artery	19	Soleus muscle
9	Tendon of plantaris muscle	20	Medial sural cutaneous nerve
10	Tibial nerve (cut)	21	Anterior tibial artery
11	Biceps femoris muscle	22	Posterior tibial artery
		23	Lateral sural cutaneous nerve

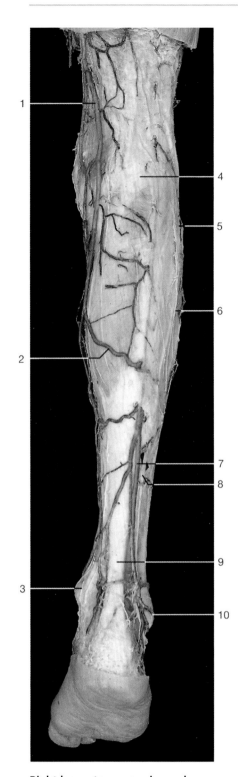

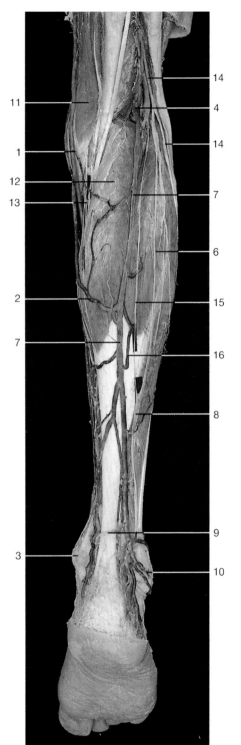

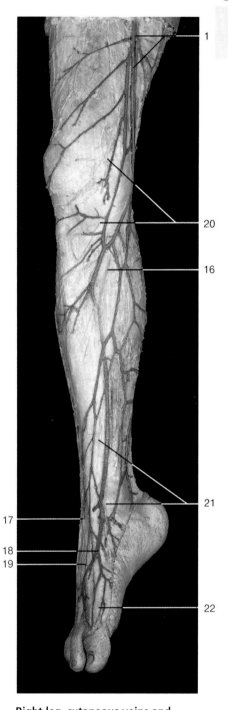

Right leg, cutaneous veins and nerves (posterior aspect).

Right leg, cutaneous veins and nerves (posterior aspect).
The superficial layer of the crural fascia has been removed.

Right leg, cutaneous veins and nerves (antero-medial aspect).

1 Great saphenous vein
2 Venous anastomosis between small and great saphenous veins
3 Medial malleolus
4 Popliteal fossa
5 Position of head of fibula
6 Lateral sural cutaneous nerve
7 Small saphenous vein

8 Sural nerve
9 Calcaneal tendon
10 Lateral malleolus
11 Semitendinosus muscle
12 Medial head of gastrocnemius muscle
13 Saphenous nerve
14 Common peroneal nerve
15 Medial sural cutaneous nerve

16 Perforating veins
17 Superficial peroneal nerve
18 Dorsal venous arch
19 Intermediate dorsal cutaneous nerve
20 Infrapatellar branches of saphenous nerve
21 Terminal branches of saphenous nerve
22 Medial dorsal cutaneous nerve

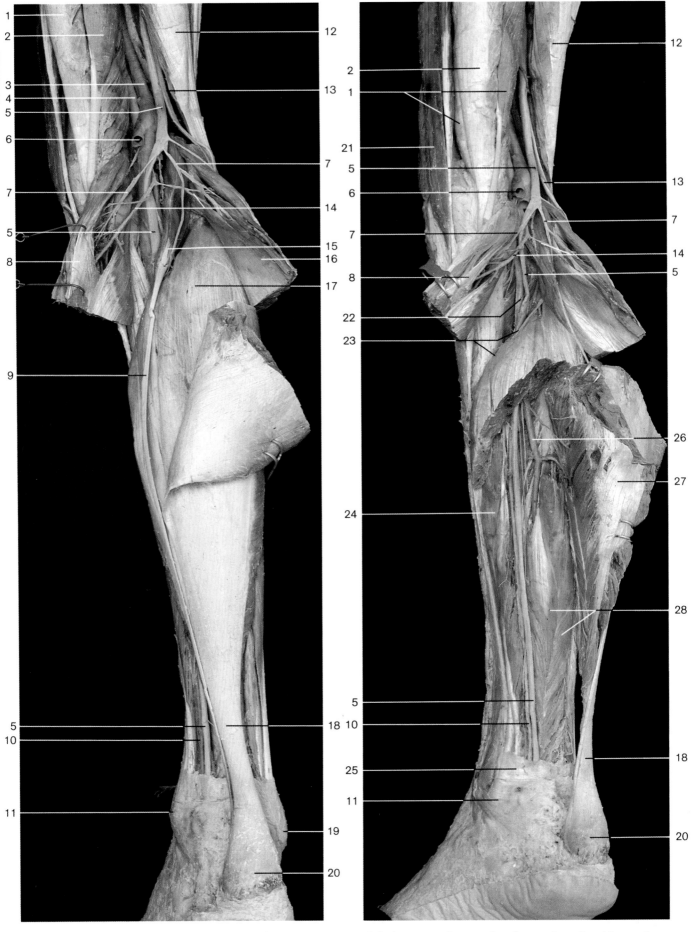

Right leg, posterior crural region, and popliteal fossa, middle layer (posterior aspect). The cutaneous veins and nerves have been removed.

Right leg, posterior crural region, and popliteal fossa, deep layer (posterior aspect). The medial head of gastrocnemius muscle has been divided and reflected.

1 Semimembranosus muscle
2 Semitendinosus muscle
3 Popliteal vein
4 Popliteal artery
5 Tibial nerve
6 Small saphenous vein (cut)
7 Muscular branch of tibial nerve
8 Medial head of gastrocnemius muscle
9 Tendon of plantaris muscle
10 Posterior tibial artery
11 Medial malleolus
12 Biceps femoris muscle
13 Common peroneal nerve
14 Sural arteries
15 Plantaris muscle
16 Lateral head of gastrocnemius muscle
17 Soleus muscle
18 Calcaneal tendon
19 Lateral malleolus
20 Calcaneal tuberosity
21 Sartorius muscle
22 Popliteal artery
23 Tendinous arch of soleus muscle
24 Flexor digitorum longus muscle
25 Flexor retinaculum
26 Peroneal artery
27 Soleus muscle
28 Flexor hallucis longus muscle
29 Anterior tibial artery
30 Muscular branches of tibial nerve
31 Tibialis posterior muscle
32 Communicating branch of peroneal artery
33 Tendon of tibialis anterior muscle
34 Tibia
35 Tendon of extensor hallucis longus muscle
36 Tendons of extensor digitorum longus muscle
37 Anterior tibialis artery
38 Fibula
39 Tendons of peroneus longus and brevis muscles

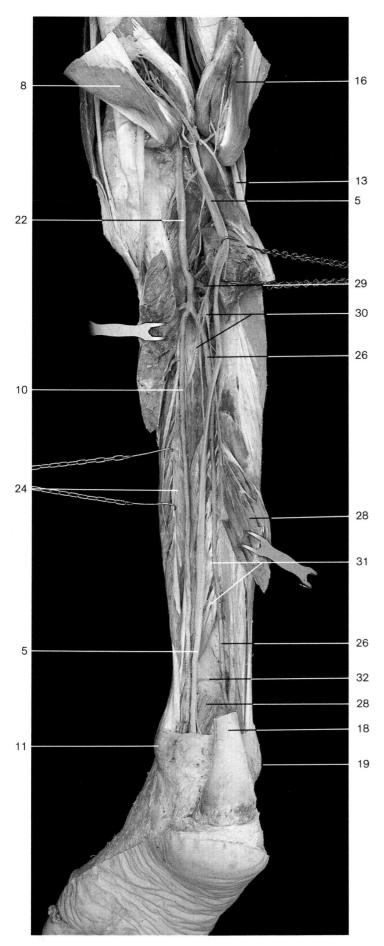

Right leg, posterior crural region, deepest layer (posterior aspect). Triceps surae (gastrocnemius and soleus) and flexor hallucis longus muscles have been cut and reflected.

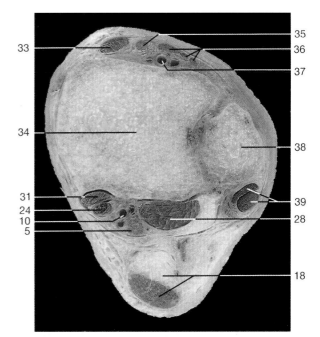

Cross section of the leg, superior to the malleoli (from below).

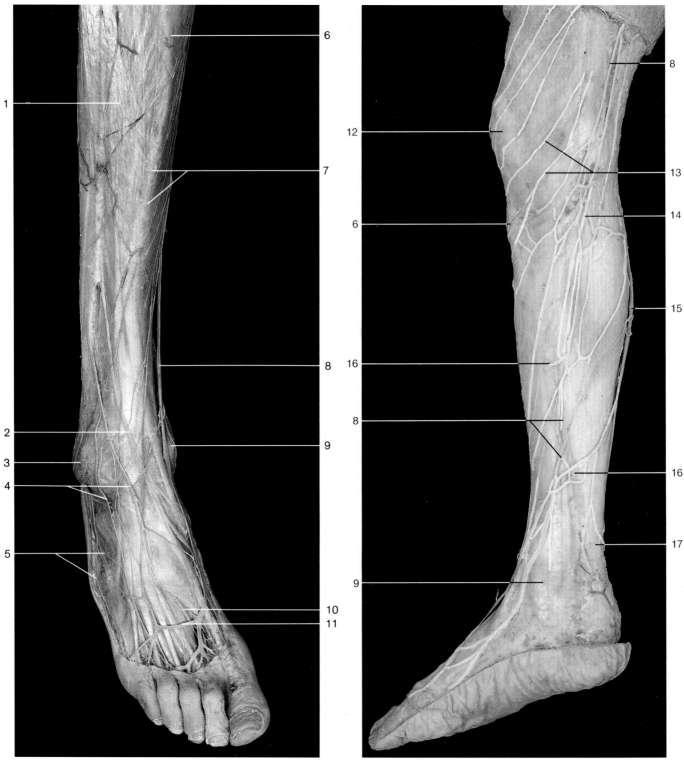

Right leg and foot, anterior crural region and dorsum of foot (anterior aspect). Cutaneous nerves and veins.

Right leg and foot (medial aspect). Cutaneous nerves and veins.

1 Superficial crural fascia
2 Medial cutaneous branch of superficial peroneal nerve
3 Lateral malleolus
4 Lateral cutaneous branch of superficial peroneal nerve
5 Cutaneous branch of sural nerve
6 Position of tuberosity of tibia
7 Anterior margin of tibia
8 Great saphenous vein
9 Medial malleolus

10 Deep peroneal nerve
11 Venous arch of dorsum of foot
12 Position of patella
13 Infrapatellar branches of saphenous nerve
14 Saphenous nerve
15 Small saphenous vein
16 Perforating vein
17 Calcaneal tendon

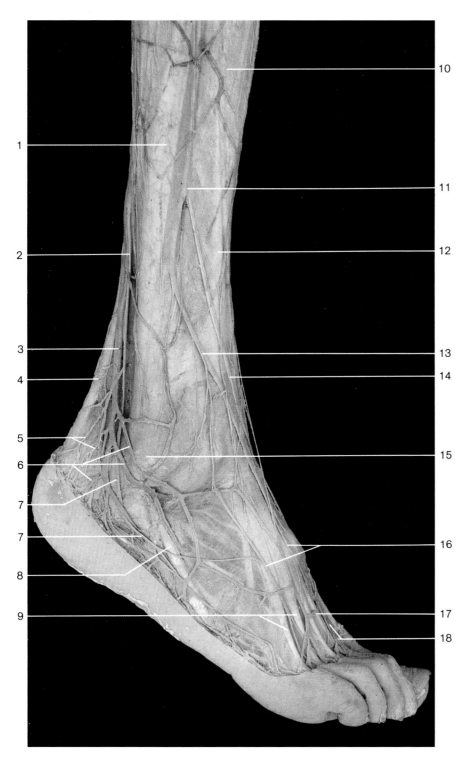

Right leg and foot (lateral aspect). Cutaneous nerves and veins.

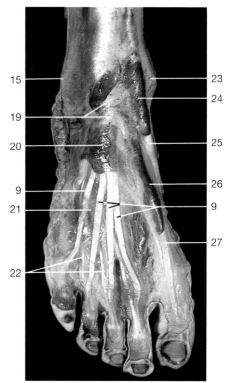

Right foot with synovial sheaths of extensor muscles (dorsal aspect). The synovial sheaths have been injected with blue solution.

1   Position of fibula
2   Sural nerve
3   Small saphenous vein
4   Calcaneal tendon
5   Lateral calcaneal branches of
     sural nerve
6   Venous network at lateral malleolus
7   Cutaneous branch of sural nerve
8   Tendon of peroneus brevis muscle
9   Tendons of extensor digitorum
     longus muscle
10   Fascia cruris

11   Superficial peroneal nerve
12   Position of tibia
13   Lateral cutaneous branch ⎤ of superficial
14   Medial cutaneous branch ⎦ peroneal nerve
15   Lateral malleolus
16   Dorsal digital nerves
17   Dorsal venous arch
18   Deep peroneal nerve
19   Inferior extensor retinaculum
20   Common synovial sheath of
     extensor digitorum longus muscle
21   Extensor digitorum brevis muscle

22   Tendons of extensor digitorum
     brevis muscle
23   Medial malleolus
24   Synovial sheath of tendon of
     tibialis anterior muscle
25   Tendon of tibialis anterior muscle
26   Synovial sheath of tendon of
     extensor hallucis longus muscle
27   Tendon of extensor hallucis longus
     muscle

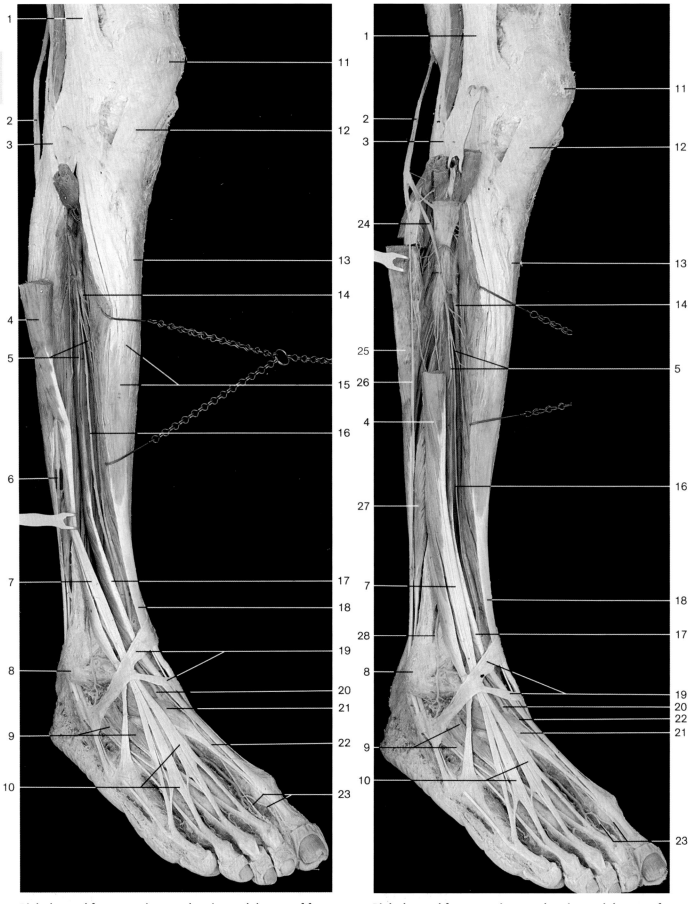

Right leg and foot, anterior crural region and dorsum of foot, middle layer (antero-lateral aspect). The extensor digitorum longus muscle has been divided and reflected laterally.

Right leg and foot, anterior crural region and dorsum of foot, deep layer (antero-lateral aspect). The extensor digitorum longus and peroneus longus muscles have been divided or removed. The common peroneal nerve has been elevated to show its course around the head of fibula.

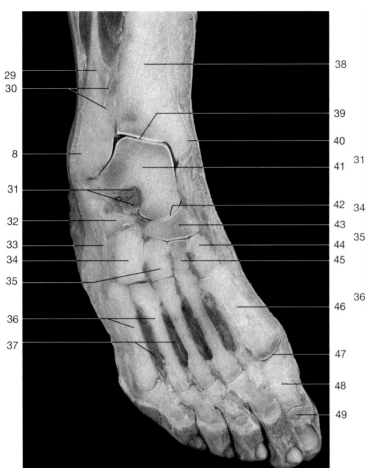

Coronal section through the foot and ankle joint (anterior aspect).

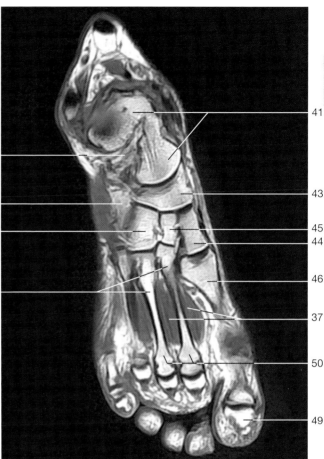

Coronal section through the foot and ankle joint (MRI scan; from Heuck et al., MRT-Atlas, 2009).

1 Iliotibial tract
2 Common peroneal nerve
3 Position of head of fibula
4 Extensor digitorum longus muscle
5 Muscular branches of deep peroneal nerve
6 Superficial peroneal nerve
7 Tendon of extensor digitorum longus muscle
8 Lateral malleolus
9 Extensor digitorum brevis muscle
10 Tendons of extensor digitorum longus muscle
11 Patella
12 Patellar ligament
13 Anterior margin of tibia
14 Anterior tibial artery
15 Tibialis anterior muscle
16 Deep peroneal nerve
17 Extensor hallucis longus muscle
18 Tendon of tibialis anterior muscle
19 Extensor retinaculum
20 Dorsalis pedis artery
21 Extensor hallucis brevis muscle
22 Deep peroneal nerve (on dorsum of foot)
23 Dorsal digital nerves (terminal branches of deep peroneal nerve)
24 Deep peroneal nerve
25 Peroneus longus muscle (cut)

26 Superficial peroneal nerve (with peroneal muscles laterally reflected)
27 Peroneus brevis muscle
28 Lateral anterior malleolar artery
29 Fibula
30 Distal tibiofibular joint (syndesmosis)
31 Talocalcaneal interosseous ligament
32 Calcaneus
33 Tendon of peroneus brevis muscle
34 Cuboid bone
35 Lateral cuneiform bone
36 Metatarsal bones
37 Dorsal interosseous muscles
38 Tibia
39 Ankle joint
40 Medial malleolus
41 Talus
42 Talocalcaneonavicular joint
43 Navicular bone
44 Medial cuneiform bone
45 Intermediate cuneiform bone
46 First metatarsal bone
47 Metatarsophalangeal joint of great toe
48 Proximal phalanx of great toe
49 Distal phalanx of great toe
50 Heads of metatarsal bones II–III

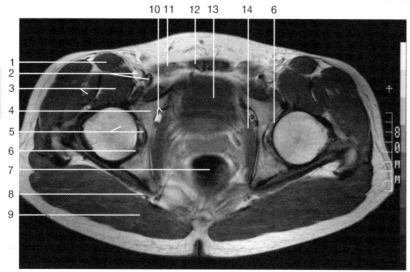

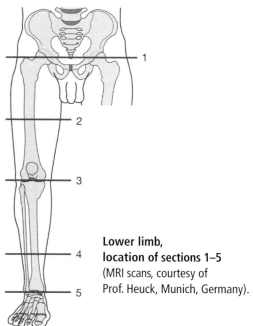

Axial section through the pelvis and the hip joints
(section 1; MRI scan; inferior aspect).

**Lower limb,
location of sections 1–5**
(MRI scans, courtesy of
Prof. Heuck, Munich, Germany).

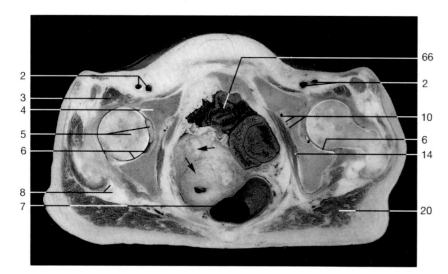

Axial section through the pelvis and the hip joints in the female
(section 1; inferior aspect). Arrows: uterus, myometrium with myoma.

1 Sartorius muscle
2 Femoral artery and vein
3 Iliopsoas muscle
4 Pubis (os pubis)
5 Femoral head with ligament of femoral head
6 Articular cavity
7 Rectum
8 Sciatic nerve and accompanying artery
9 Gluteus maximus muscle
10 Obturator vessels and obturator nerve
11 Rectus abdominis muscle
12 Pyramidalis muscle
13 Urinary bladder
14 Obturator internus muscle
15 Rectus femoris muscle
16 Vastus intermedius and vastus lateralis of quadriceps femoris muscle

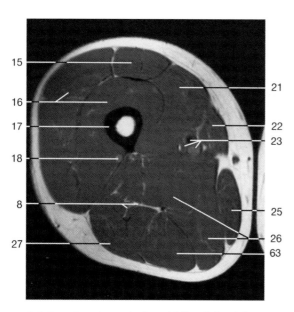

Axial section through the middle of the right thigh (section 2; MRI scan; inferior aspect).

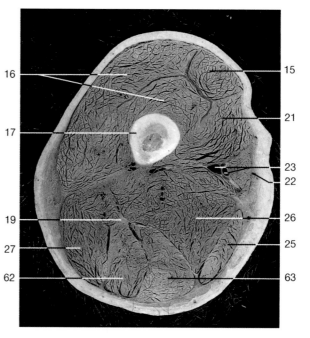

Axial section through the middle of the right thigh (section 2; inferior aspect).

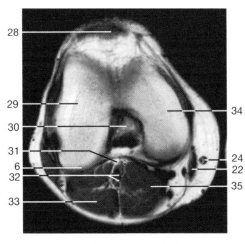

Axial section through the right knee joint (section 3; MRI scan; inferior aspect).

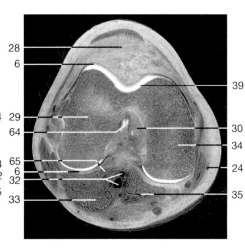

Axial section through the right knee joint (section 3; inferior aspect).

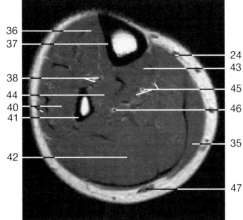

Axial section through the middle of the right leg (section 4; MRI scan; inferior aspect).

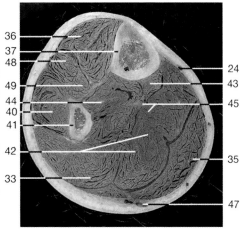

Axial section through the middle of the right leg (section 4; inferior aspect).

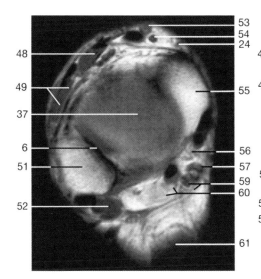

Axial section through the end of the right leg (section 5; MRI scan; inferior aspect).

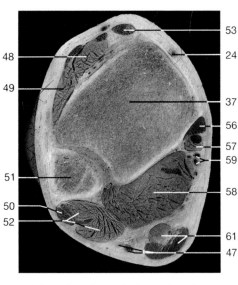

Axial section through the end of the right leg (section 5; inferior aspect).

17 Femur
18 Perforating artery
19 Sciatic nerve
20 Gluteus maximus muscle (insertion)
21 Vastus medialis muscle
22 Sartorius muscle
23 Femoral artery and vein
24 Great saphenous vein
25 Gracilis muscle
26 Adductor muscles
27 Biceps femoris muscle
28 Patellar ligament
29 Lateral condyle of femur
30 Posterior cruciate ligament
31 Tibial nerve
32 Popliteal artery and vein
33 Lateral head of gastrocnemius muscle
34 Medial condyle of femur
35 Medial head of gastrocnemius muscle
36 Tibialis anterior muscle
37 Tibia
38 Deep peroneal nerve, anterior tibial artery, and vein
39 Patellar surface
40 Peroneus longus and brevis muscles
41 Fibula
42 Soleus muscle
43 Flexor digitorum longus muscle
44 Tibialis posterior muscle
45 Posterior tibial artery and vein and tibial nerve
46 Peroneal artery
47 Small saphenous vein and sural nerve
48 Extensor hallucis longus muscle
49 Extensor digitorum longus muscle
50 Tendon of peroneus longus muscle
51 Lateral malleolus (fibula)
52 Peroneus brevis muscle
53 Tibialis anterior muscle (tendon)
54 Dorsalis pedis artery
55 Medial malleolus (tibia)
56 Tibialis posterior muscle (tendon)
57 Flexor digitorum longus muscle (tendon with synovial sheath)
58 Flexor hallucis longus muscle
59 Posterior tibial artery and vein
60 Lateral and medial plantar nerves
61 Calcaneal tendon
62 Semitendinosus muscle
63 Semimembranosus muscle
64 Anterior cruciate ligament
65 Plantaris muscle
66 Small intestine

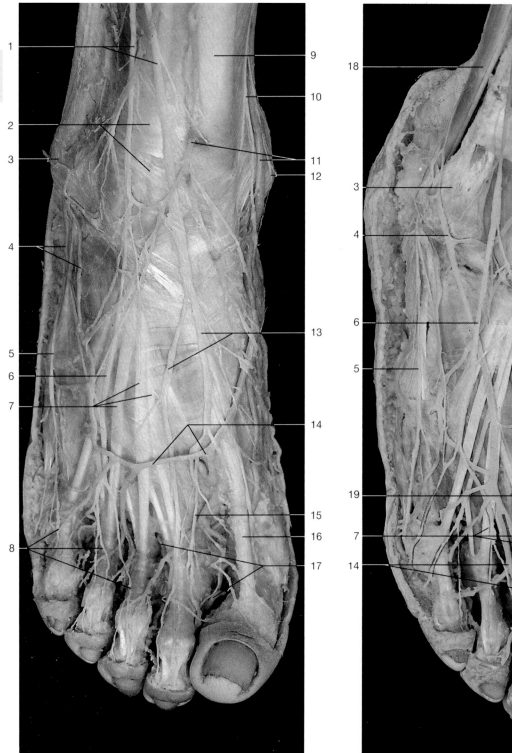

Dorsum of the right foot, superficial layer (anterior aspect).

Dorsum of the right foot, superficial layer (anterior aspect). The fascia of the dorsum has been removed.

1 Superficial peroneal nerve	9 Tendon of tibialis anterior muscle	17 Dorsal digital arteries
2 Superior extensor retinaculum	10 Saphenous nerve	18 Peroneal muscles
3 Lateral malleolus	11 Venous network of medial malleolus and	19 Deep plantar branch of dorsalis pedis
4 Venous network of lateral malleolus and	tributaries of great saphenous vein	artery anastomosing with plantar arch
tributaries of small saphenous vein	12 Medial malleolus	20 Extensor digitorum longus muscle
5 Lateral dorsal cutaneous nerve (branch of	13 Medial dorsal cutaneous nerves	21 Extensor hallucis longus muscle
sural nerve)	14 Dorsal venous arch	22 Inferior extensor retinaculum
6 Intermediate dorsal cutaneous nerve	15 Dorsal digital nerve (of deep peroneal	23 Extensor hallucis brevis muscle
7 Tendons of extensor digitorum longus muscle	nerve)	
8 Dorsal digital nerves	16 Tendon of extensor hallucis longus muscle	

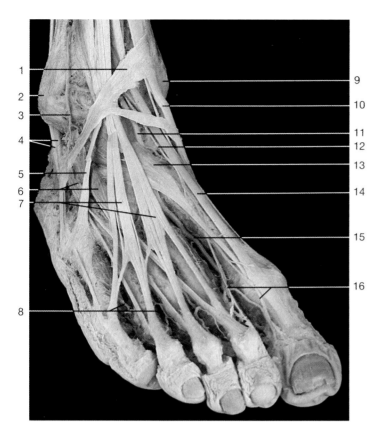

1   Extensor retinaculum
2   Lateral malleolus
3   Lateral anterior malleolar artery
4   Tendons of peroneal muscles
5   Tendon of peroneus tertius muscle
6   Extensor digitorum brevis muscle
7   Tendons of extensor digitorum longus muscle
8   Dorsal metatarsal arteries
9   Medial malleolus
10 Tendon of tibialis anterior muscle
11 Dorsalis pedis artery
12 Deep peroneal nerve (on dorsum of foot)
13 Extensor hallucis brevis muscle
14 Tendon of extensor hallucis longus muscle
15 Dorsalis pedis artery with deep plantar branch to
    the plantar arch
16 Dorsal digital nerves (terminal branches of deep
    peroneal nerve)
17 Lateral tarsal artery
18 Extensor digitorum brevis muscle (divided)
19 Arcuate artery
20 Dorsal interosseous muscles
21 Deep peroneal nerve
22 Medial cuneiform and first metatarsal bone
23 Tendon of peroneus longus muscle
24 Abductor hallucis and flexor hallucis brevis muscles
25 Medial plantar artery, vein, and nerve
26 Fourth and fifth metatarsal bone
27 Adductor hallucis muscle (oblique head)
28 Tendons of flexor digitorum longus muscle
29 Lateral plantar artery, vein, and nerve
30 Flexor digitorum brevis muscle
31 Plantar aponeurosis

Dorsum of the right foot, middle layer (antero-lateral aspect).
The cutaneous nerves have been removed.

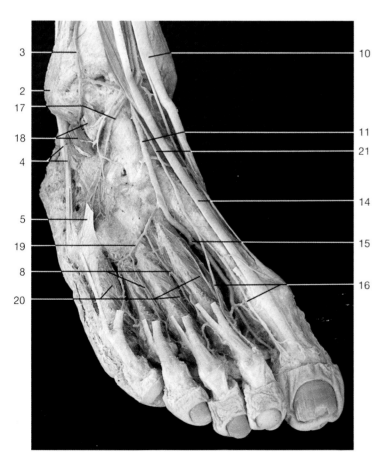

Dorsum of the right foot, deep layer (antero-lateral aspect).
The extensor digitorum and hallucis brevis muscles have
been removed.

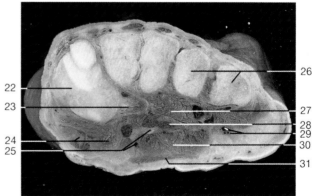

Cross section of the right foot at the level of the
metatarsal bones (posterior aspect).

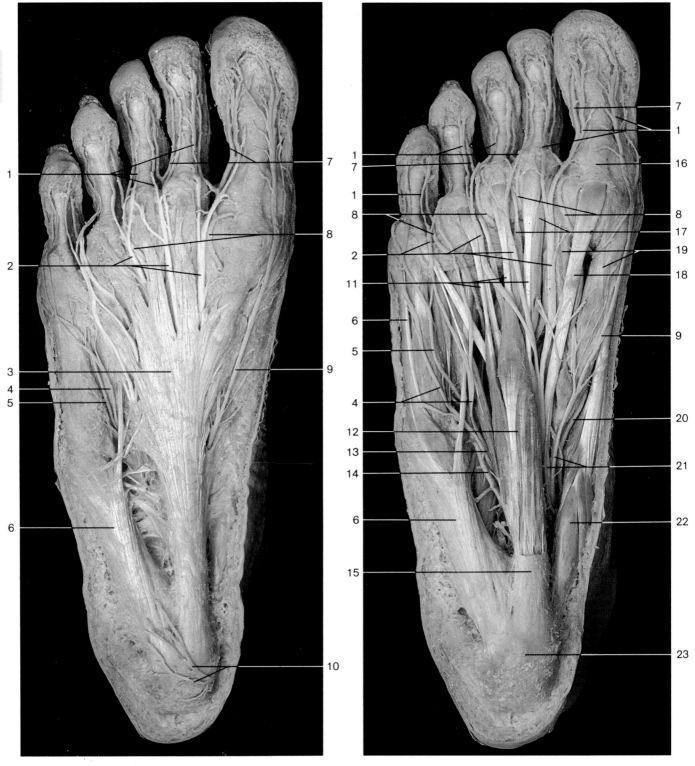

Sole of the right foot, superficial layer (from below).
Dissection of cutaneous nerves and vessels.

Sole of the right foot, middle layer (from below).
The plantar aponeurosis has been removed.

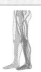

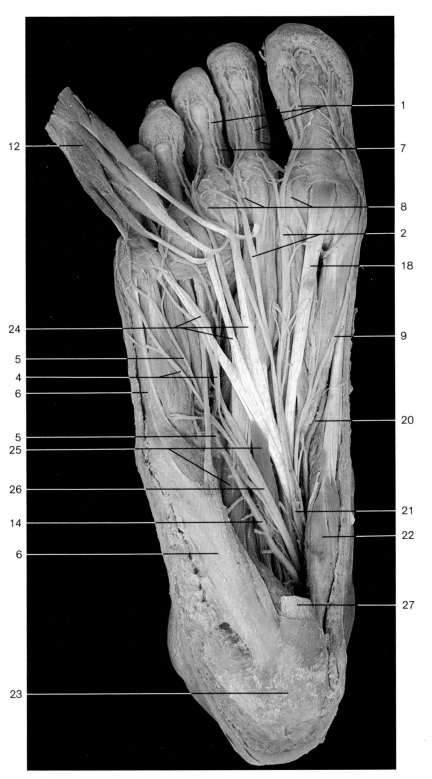

1 Proper plantar digital nerves
2 Common plantar digital nerves
3 Plantar aponeurosis
4 Superficial branch of lateral plantar nerve
5 Superficial branch of lateral plantar artery
6 Abductor digiti minimi
7 Proper plantar digital arteries
8 Common plantar digital arteries
9 Digital branch of medial plantar nerve to great toe
10 Medial calcaneal branches
11 Tendons of flexor digitorum brevis muscle
12 Flexor digitorum brevis muscle
13 Superficial branch of lateral plantar nerve
14 Lateral plantar artery
15 Plantar aponeurosis (remnant)
16 Digital synovial sheath
17 Lumbrical muscles
18 Tendon of flexor hallucis longus muscle
19 Flexor hallucis brevis muscle
20 Medial plantar artery
21 Medial plantar nerve
22 Abductor hallucis muscle
23 Calcaneal tuberosity
24 Tendons of flexor digitorum longus muscle
25 Quadratus plantae muscle
26 Lateral plantar nerve
27 Flexor digitorum brevis muscle (cut)
28 Synovial sheaths
29 Plantar arch

Sole of the right foot, middle layer (from below). Dissection of vessels and nerves. The flexor digitorum brevis muscle has been divided and anteriorly reflected.

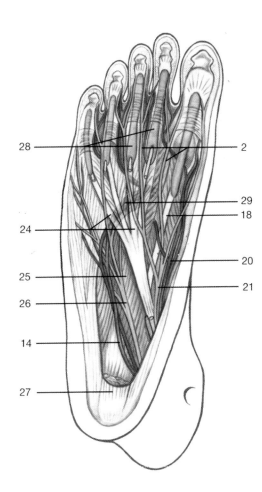

Sole of the right foot. Synovial sheaths of flexor tendons indicated in light blue (schematic drawing).

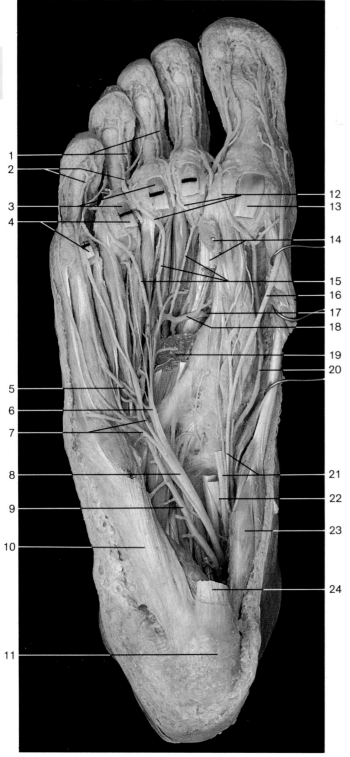

1   Proper plantar digital arteries
2   Proper plantar digital nerves
3   Tendons of flexor digitorum brevis muscle
4   Tendons of flexor digitorum longus muscle
5   Superficial branch of lateral plantar artery
6   Deep branch of lateral plantar nerve
7   Superficial branch of lateral plantar nerve
8   Lateral plantar nerve
9   Lateral plantar artery
10 Abductor digiti minimi muscle
11 Calcaneal tuberosity
12 Common plantar digital arteries
13 Tendon of flexor hallucis longus muscle
14 Insertion of both heads of adductor hallucis muscle
15 Plantar metatarsal arteries
16 Medial plantar nerve of great toe
17 Deep plantar branch of dorsalis pedis artery
    (perforating branch)
18 Plantar arch
19 Oblique head of adductor hallucis muscle (cut)
20 Medial plantar artery
21 Medial plantar nerve
22 Crossing of tendons in sole of foot (flexor hallucis
    longus and flexor digitorum longus muscles)
23 Abductor hallucis muscle
24 Origin of flexor digitorum brevis muscle

Sole of the right foot, deep layer (from below). Dissection
of vessels and nerves. The flexor digitorum brevis muscle, the
quadratus plantae muscle with the tendons of the flexor digitorum
longus muscle, and some branches of the medial plantar nerve
have been removed. The flexor hallucis brevis and adductor
hallucis muscles have been cut and portions removed to show the
somewhat atypical course of the medial plantar artery and deep
muscles of the foot.

Index

Page numbers in **bold** indicate main discussions.

A

Abdomen, parasagittal section 298
Abdominal organs 291 ff
– position 292, 306
– upper 301, 312 ff
– – arteries 314 f
– – blood supply 316
– vessels 302 ff
Abduction of fingers 395
Acetabulum 188, 345, 432
– bony margin 438
– lunate surface 433, **436**, 445
Achilles tendon 449, **457 ff**, 489, 491 ff
– surface anatomy 476
Acromion 15, 188 f, **369 ff**, 378, 382, 384 f
Adduction of fingers 395
Adductor hiatus 453
Adhesion, interthalamic 86, **107**
Adnexa of uterus 359 ff
Air cells
– ethmoidal 28, 36, **38**, 41 f, 44 f, **48**, 53, 135
– – openings 144
– mastoid 70, 125 ff
Ala s. also Wing
– of central lobule of vermis 102
– of ilium 435
– of sacrum **434 f**, 438
– of vomer 37, 45, **48 f**
Amnion 359
Ampulla 128 f
– bony 129
– of ductus deferens **336 ff**, 342, 344
– of rectum 342, 354
– of uterine tube 358, 361, 366
Amygdala (amygdaloid body) **107**, 110 f, **114 f**, 116
Anastomoses, portocaval 303
Aneurysm, infrarenal, of aorta 348
Angiogram(-graphy)
– fluorescent, of eye 134
– internal carotid artery 95 f
Angle
– costal 192
– inferior, of scapula **370 f**, 382 f
– infrasternal 7, 192, 248
– – surface anatomy 204
– lateral, of scapula 188, **370 f**
– of mandible 21, **52**
– of ribs 370
– sphenoidal, of parietal bone 29
– sternal 192 f
– superior, of scapula 371
– venous

– – left 17
– – right 17, 398
Ankle joint 432, **443**, **449 ff**, 495
Ansa
– cervicalis 71, **163**, 177, **181 f**, 266
– – muscular branches 181, 265
– – root
– – – inferior 184
– – – superior 69, 71, **82 f**, 152, 179
– lenticular 116
– subclavia of sympathetic trunk 169
– thyroid, of sympathetic trunk 169
Antihelix 124
Antitragus 124
Antrum
– mastoid 127
– pyloric 294, 324
– tympanic 126
Anulus
– fibrosus 198
– inguinalis s. Ring, inguinal
– tympanic, of newborn 33
Anus 350 ff, 354, 361 ff, 366
Aorta 16 f
– abdominal 16, 210, **245**, 256, 278, 292, 296, 300, 302, 329 ff, **348**, 359 f
– – subtraktion angiography 328
– ascending 243, 245, **252 ff**, 260, 266, 272, 284, 396
– – bypass vessel 263
– – of fetus 288
– – horizontal section 286
– descending 244, 252 f, 276
– – of fetus 288 f
– – horizontal section 286
– – main branches 281
– relation to bronchial tree 275
– thoracic 253, 274, **281**
Aperture
– lateral, of fourth ventricle 112
– of Luschka 112
– of Magendie 94, **112**
– median, of fourth ventricle 94, **112**
– nasal, anterior 22 f, 45
– pelvic, inferior 434, **438**
Apex
– of cochlea 125
– of head of fibula 440
– of heart **252**, 257 f, 262 f
– of lung 248 f, 271
– of patella 441
– of petrous part of temporal bone 27, 127
– of sacrum 191
– of urinary bladder 337, 339, 357
Aponeurosis 388 ff
– of abdominal wall 187
– bicipital **387 f**, 416, 423
– of external abdominal oblique muscle 217, 362

– of levator palpebrae superioris muscle 142
– palmar 388, 423
– – transverse fasciculi 388
– plantar 449, **463**, 499, 501
– – longitudinal bands 463
Apparatus
– auditory 22, **122 ff**, 129
– lacrimal 142
– masticatory 22
– vestibular **122 ff**, 129
– visual 132 ff
Appendix(-ces) 304
– of epididymis 343
– epiploicae 306
– fibrosa 299
– of testis 343
– vermiform 291, 304, **306 f**, 310, 318, 324
– – Head's area 205
– – orifice 310
– – variations in the position 307
Aqueduct
– cerebral 65, 73 ff, **86**, 90, 94, 99, **112**, 116, 121
– of cochlea 129
– of vestibule 27, **129**
Arachnoid mater 84 f, **89**, 92, 100, 118
– spinal 230, **232**, 474
Arbor vitae of cerebellum 94, 116
Arch
– anterior, of atlas 165, 200, 203
– aortic 95, 154, 169, 177, **245**, 253, 256 f, 273 f, 279, **284**
– – of fetus 288 f
– azygos 273 f, 276, 283
– of cervical vertebra 239 f
– costal 3 f, 188, **192 ff**, 196, 212 f, 243 f, 264 f, **370**
– – surface anatomy 204
– of cricoid cartilage 158
– dental 52
– iliopectineal 444 f, **453**
– palatoglossal 147
– palatopharyngeal 147
– palmar
– – deep 427, **429**
– – superficial 396, 423, **426 ff**
– plantar 467, 501 f
– posterior
– – of atlas **200**, 239
– – of axis 239
– pubic 436 f
– tendinous
– – of flexor digitorum superficialis muscle 418
– – of soleus muscle 457, 491
– venous
– – dorsal, of foot **468**, 489, 492 f, 498
– – jugular 170, **172**, 398, 406
– of vertebra 191, 231, 474

Page numbers in **bold** indicate main discussions.

Arch
- zygomatic 20, **33**, 52, **54**, 60 f, 79
- – coronal section 62
- – of newborn 33
Arcus costalis (s. also Arch, costal) 194
Area
- of acoustic centers 131
- bare, of liver 299, 318
- calcarina 138
- cortical
- – acoustic 101
- – premotor 101
- – reading comprehension 101
- – sensory speech 101
- – somatomotor 101
- – somatosensory 101
- – visuosensory 101
- – of Wernicke 101
- cribriform, of renal papilla 326
- intercondylar, anterior, of tibia 440
- muscle-free, of pharynx 167
- of primary acoustic centers 131
- vestibular, superior 123, 130
Areola **204**, 290
Arm (s. also Limb, upper) 368
- arteries 396 f
- axial section 430
- MRI scan 386
- muscles 382 ff, **386 f**
- nerves 399 f, **414 ff**
- – cutaneous 400
- sagittal section 386
- surface anatomy 401 f
- veins 398
Arteriole
- afferent, of glomerulus 329
- efferent, of glomerulus 329
Artery(-ies) **16**, 98, 241, 399 ff
- alveolar
- – inferior 63, 80, **81 ff**
- – superior posterior 63, 82
- angular 77, 79, 82, **168**
- appendicular 302, 304, 310
- arcuate
- – of foot 467, 499
- – of kidney 329
- auricular
- – deep 63
- – posterior 80
- axillary **168**, 170, **186**, 207, 252, 387, **396**, 411 f, 414 f
- basilar 31, 74, 86, 89, **93 ff, 98**, 116, 121
- brachial 387, **396**, 403, 410, 412, 414 ff, 418, 423
- – profunda **396**, 404
- buccal 63, **80**
- of bulb of penis 341, 351
- capsular, lower, of kidney 328
- carotid 154

- – common 83, 95, 97, 152, **157**, **163**, 165, **168 ff**, 252 f, 255, 266, **281**, 396, 414
- – – of fetus 288
- – external 63, 67, 69, 79, **97**, 152, 163, **164**, **168 ff, 396**
- – internal 31, 62, 67, 69, **73 f**, 87, 92 ff, 97 f, 122, 124, **168 ff, 396**
- – – Angiogram 95 f
- – – loop 96
- cerebellar
- – inferior
- – – anterior **93 f**, 96, 98
- – – posterior **93 f**, 96, 98, 116
- – superior **93 f**, 96
- cerebral 92 ff
- – anterior 86, **92 ff**, 97 f, 111
- – – area of blood supply 96
- – circle of Willis 93, 98
- – middle 92 ff, 98
- – – area of blood supply 96
- – – parietal branch 94
- – – temporal branch 94
- – MRI angiograph 95
- – posterior **92 ff**, 97 f
- – – area of blood supply 96
- cervical
- – ascending **168**, 170, 185, 396, 414
- – deep **168**, 237
- – superficial **168**, 170, 236
- – transverse **168**, 170, 264, 396, 414
- – – deep branch 235
- – – superficial branch 235
- ciliary
- – anterior **93**, 133 f
- – posterior 93
- – – long 133 f
- – – short 133 f
- colic
- – left 304, 308
- – – anastomosis with middle colic artery 308
- – middle **302 ff**, 308 f, 316 f, 328
- – right 302 ff, 309
- collateral
- – medial 408
- – middle 396, 409
- – radial 396, 408 f
- – ulnar
- – – inferior 396, 415
- – – superior 396, 416, 423
- communicating
- – anterior 93, 98
- – posterior 92 ff, 98
- coraco-acromial 411
- coronary 262 f
- – left 253, 258, **261 f**, 284, 286 f
- – – circumflex branch 254, **262 f**
- – – diagonal branch 262
- – – interventricular branch 253

- – – – anterior 254 f, 263
- – – septal branch 254
- – – right 243, **253 ff**, 257 f, 263, 270, 287
- – – – posterior interventricular branch 262
- cortical, radiating 329
- cystic 299, 316, 317
- deep
- – of clitoris 362, 365
- – of penis 339, 341, **346**, 347
- digital
- – dorsal, of foot 498
- – palmar 396, **428**
- – – common 396, 423, **427 f**
- – – proper 425, **427 f**
- – – – of thumb 427
- – – of thumb 428
- – plantar
- – – common 501 f
- – – proper 501 f
- dorsal
- – of clitoris 365
- – of penis 341 f, 346 f, 352
- dorsalis pedis 467, 499
- – deep plantar branch 498 f, 502
- of ductus deferens 343
- epigastric 265
- – inferior 208, 212, 214, 216, 219, 293, 480
- – – pubic branch **218**, 220
- – superficial 208, 216
- – superior 206, 208, **214**, 216, 264 ff
- ethmoidal 94
- – anterior 31, 134, 141, **146**
- – – nasal branch 146
- – posterior 134
- facial 63, 77, **79**, 81, 97, 152, **168**, 170, 398
- – transverse 63, **77**, 80, **168**, 170
- femoral 214, 216 f, 293, 340, 360, 367, 452, **466 f**, 480, 496
- – circumflex
- – – lateral 467, **480 f**
- – – – ascending branch 480 f
- – – – descending branch 467, 480 f
- – – medial 467, **480 f**
- – – – ascending branch 481
- – entering the adductor canal 452
- gastric
- – left 315 ff
- – – esophageal branches 315
- – right 304, **315 ff**
- – short 315 f
- gastroduodenal 296, **315 ff**
- gastro-epiploic 315 f
- gastro-omental 315 f
- genicular
- – descending 467
- – inferior
- – – lateral 467, 487 f
- – – medial 467, 487
- – middle 467

Page numbers in **bold** indicate main discussions.

– – superior
– – – lateral 467, 487 f
– – – medial 467, 487
– gluteal
– – inferior 346 f, **360**, 484
– – superior 347, **360**
– – – deep branch 483
– helicine 341
– hepatic
– – common 296, 315 f
– – of fetus 289
– – proper 279, 296, 299 f, **304**, 316 f
– – – left branch 315
– – – right branch 315
– humeral, circumflex
– – anterior 170, 396
– – posterior 383, 396, 404 f, **408 f**
– ileal 303 ff, **309**
– ileocolic 302 ff, **309 f**
– iliac
– – circumflex
– – – deep 208, 216, 338, **467**, 480
– – – superficial 208, 216, **467**
– – common **281**, 308, 330 f, 346 f, 358 f
– – external 293, 330, 332, 338, **346 f**
– – internal 332, **346 f**, 360, 366
– – – main branches 347
– iliolumbar 347
– infra-orbital 63, 142
– intercostal 206, **210 f**
– – anterior 207
– – highest 208, **281**
– – medial branches 290
– – posterior 214, 276, **279 ff**
– – – dorsal branches 408
– – superior 168
– interlobar, of kidney 329
– interlobular, of kidney 328 f
– interosseous
– – anterior 396, 418, 423
– – – posterior branch 421
– – posterior 396, 421, **424**
– interventricular, anterior 257, 262, 270
– – bypass vessel 263
– iridial 134
– jejunal 302 ff, **308 f**
– labial
– – inferior 168
– – superior 168
– of labyrinth 31, **93**, 98
– lacrimal **93**, 141
– laryngeal, superior 152, 166, 169
– lingual 146, **152**, **168**
– – deep 153
– lumbar 335
– macular, superior 134
– malleolar, anterior, lateral 495, 499
– mandibular, inferior 63
– masseteric 63, **79**

– maxillary **62 f**, 79 f, **81 ff**, 97, **168**
– – branches 63
– – – deep temporal 63
– – – pterygoid 63
– meningeal
– – anterior 31
– – base of skull 31
– – middle 31, 63, 82 f, 85, 87 f, 126, 141
– – – parietal branch 88
– – posterior 31
– meningolacrimal 141
– mesenteric 308 f
– – inferior **281**, 304 f, **308**, 329
– – superior **281**, 283, 292, 296, 300, **302 ff**, **309**, 316 f, 328 f
– metacarpal, dorsal 424
– metatarsal
– – dorsal 467, 499
– – plantar 467, 502
– musculophrenic 206, 208, 216
– nasal
– – dorsal 168
– – inferior, of retina 134
– – superior, of retina 134
– obturator **346 f**, 360, 366, 467
– occipital 63, **81 f**, **85**, **168**, 223, 235, 237 f, **240 ff**
– – occipital branch 170
– ophthalmic **73**, **93 f**, 98, 132, **134**, 141, 146
– ovarian 328, 360
– – ovarian branch 360
– – tubal branch 360
– palatine
– – descending 63, **146**
– – greater 146
– – lesser 146
– pallidostriate 92
– pancreaticoduodenal
– – inferior 316 f
– – superior 315
– – – anterior 316
– – – posterior 316
– perforating 467
– pericardiacophrenic 272, 281
– perineal 346, 352
– – superficial 351
– peroneal 467 f, 491
– pharyngeal, ascending 146, 165
– phrenic, inferior 315, 328
– plantar 499
– – lateral **467**, 499, 501 f
– – – superficial branch 501
– – medial **467**, 499, 501 f
– popliteal 446, **467**, 484, **486 ff**, 491
– princeps pollicis 396, **427**
– profunda
– – brachii 409, 415
– – – anastomosis with posterior humeral
        circumflex artery 408 f

– – femoris 467, 481
– of pterygoid canal 63
– pudendal
– – external **220**, 467
– – internal 341, **346 f**, 351 f, 360, 362, 364, 483
– pulmonary 16, 252 f, 260, 273, **274 ff**, 281
– – branches 246
– – of fetus 288 f
– radial 388, **396**, **414 ff**, 419, 421, 423 f, 428
– – dorsal carpal branch 424
– – superficial palmar branch 396
– rectal
– – inferior 346 f, **351 f**, 483
– – middle 347
– – superior 304, 308
– recurrent
– – radial 396, **416 ff**
– – ulnar 418
– renal **281**, **326 f**, 331, 335
– – anterior branch 328
– – left 292
– – posterior branch 328
– – superior 329
– retinal 134
– – central **93**, 133 f
– of round ligament 360
– sacral
– – lateral 347
– – median 333
– – middle 360
– scapular
– – circumflex 378, 404 f, **408 ff**, 412
– – descending **168**, 396, 404
– – dorsal 168
– scrotal, posterior 351
– segmental, inferior, anterior, of kidney 328
– septal 146
– sphenopalatine 63
– sigmoid 304, 308, 346
– spinal
– – anterior 31, 93, 98, 232, 474
– – posterior 31, 93, 98, 232
– spiral, of renal pelvis 329
– splenic 279, 296, 300, **309**, 315 f, 328 f
– – posterior pancreatic branch 316
– subclavian 95, 97, 170, **177**, 184, 206, 208, 252, 271, 273 ff, **281**, 396, 414
– – of fetus 288
– subcortical, of kidney 329
– submental 152, **168**
– subscapular 396, 412, 415
– supra-orbital 134, **168**
– – medial branch 82
– suprarenal
– – inferior 328 f
– – middle 328
– – superior 328
     suprascapular 168, 170, 378, **396**, 404 f, 414

Page numbers in **bold** indicate main discussions.

Artery(-ies)
– suprascapular
– – anastomosis with circumflex scapular artery 404
– supratrochlear 93, 134, **168**
– sural 487, 491
– tarsal, lateral 499
– temporal
– – deep 80, **82**
– – – anterior 81
– – inferior, of retina 134
– – middle 168
– – superficial 63, **77**, **81 ff**, 85, **168**, 170, 183
– – – anterior articular branch 80
– – – frontal branch 79 f, **168**
– – – parietal branch 79 f, **168**
– – superior, of retina 134
– testicular 218, 328, 341, **343**, 346
– thalamic 92
– thoracic
– – internal **168**, 177, 206, **208**, **214**, 216, **264 ff**, 272, 396, 398
– – lateral 168, 170, 196, **207 f**, **214**, 396, 410, 412
– – superior 396, 412
– – thoraco-acromial 168, 170, **184 f**, 207, 264, 396, 407
– – acromial branch 407
– – pectoral branch 407
– thoracodorsal 396, 404, **407**, 410, 412, 415
– thyroid
– – inferior **168 f**, 177, 185, 396
– – superior 152, **168 ff**, 177, 185, 396
– tibial 468
– – anterior 467 f, 491, 495
– – posterior 457, **467 f**, 488, 491
– tympanic
– – anterior 126
– ulnar 388, **396**, 415 ff, 419, 423, 425, 428
– umbilical 289, **346 f**
– – obliterated 293
– – remnant 219
– uterine 360, 366
– – ovarian branch 360
– vaginal 360
– vertebral 31, 62, 69, 71, 89, **93 ff**, 96 ff, 165, **168 f**, 174, 177, 200, **237**, 240, 414
– – muscular branch 237
– vesical
– – inferior 347
– – superior 346 f
– zygomatico-orbital 85
Articulation s. Joint
Atlas 53, 159, 165, **188 ff**, **192 ff**, **200 ff**, 240, 369 f
– articulation with dens of axis 200
Atrium
– left, of heart **245**, **252 ff**, 256 ff, 273, 281, 285
– – midsagittal section 322

– – orifices of pulmonary veins 285
– nasal 144
– right, of heart 244 f, **252 f**, 255 ff, 259, 261 ff, 270 f, 273, 283 f
– – of fetus 288
Auditory apparatus **122 ff**, 129
Auditory pathway 131
Auricle 122 ff
– of left atrium **252**, 258, 260 ff
– – of fetus 288
– of right atrium **244**, **252**, 255 f, 258, **260 ff**, 269, 271, 283
– – of fetus 288
Axilla, lymphatics 290
Axis 159, **188 ff**, 192 ff, **200 ff**, 369 f

B

Back
– innervation 229
– muscles 221 ff
– – deep 292
– – deepest layer 224
– nerves **226 ff**, 229
Ball-and-socket joint 10, 432
Band, longitudinal
– inferior, of cruciform ligament 200 f
– superior, of cruciform ligament 200 f
Base
– of cochlea 123, 125, **129**
– of coracoid process 371
– of mandible 22 f
– of metacarpal bone 376 f
– of metatarsal bone 442
– of patella 441
– of proximal phalanx 376 f
– of sacrum **191**, 434 f
– of skull 20, **30 ff**, 84, 97, 203
– – angulation 19, 37, 143
– – bones 23
– – canals 34
– – cranial nerves **31**, **75**, 98
– – fissures 34
– – foramina 34
– – inferior aspect 32 f
– – internal aspect **30 f**, 34
– – of newborn **33**, 35
– of stapes 128
– of urinary bladder 367
Bicuspid
– first 50
– second 50
Bifurcation
– of atrioventricular bundle 261
– of trachea 18, **246**, **274 ff**, 281
Bile duct(s) 296 f
– common 292, **296 f**, 299 f, 317

– extrahepatic 296 f, **301**, **316**
Bladder, urinary s. Urinary bladder
Blindness 139
Body
– amygdaloid **107**, 110 f, **114 ff**
– of axis 200
– carotid 164 f
– cavernous s. Corpus cavernosum
– of cervical vertebra 53, 177, **194 f**
– – MRI scan 201, 203
– ciliary 133
– of clitoris 361 f, 365
– of corpus callosum 99, **107**
– of epididymis 343
– of fifth lumbar vertebra 189
– of first lumbar vertebra 189, 211
– of fornix 106 f, 113
– of gallbladder 297
– geniculate 107
– – lateral 131, 137
– – medial 115, 131, 137
– of hyoid bone **150**, 158
– of incus 128
– of ischium 433
– of lumbar vertebra **190 f**, 194, **198 f**
– mamillary 65 f, 86, 94, 99, 103, **107**, 137
– of mandible 22 f, **52**
– of maxilla 21 f
– – nasal surface 42
– of metacarpal bone 376
– of pancreas 296 f, **316**
– perineal 350 f, 362
– pineal 86, 99, 107, 115, 120
– of pubis 433
– restiform 116
– retrosternal 398
– of rib 192, **197**
– of sphenoidal bone 26
– of sternum 188 f, 192 f, **264**, **369 f**
– of stomach 294, 316
– of thoracic vertebra 192
– trapezoid 131
– of twelfth thoracic vertebra 189
– of uterus 357
– of vertebra 53, 177, **191 f**, **194 f**, 199
– vitreous 133, **148**
Bone(s) 42, 155
– capitate **376 f**, 380
– – coronal section 425
– carpal 7, **368**, **375 ff**, 427
– cranial 20 ff
– – of newborn 35
– cuboid 443, 449, 495
– cuneiform
– – intermediate **442**, 449, 495
– – lateral 443
– – medial 495
– ethmoidal 20 ff, 23, 34, **37 f**, **40 ff**, 44 f, 47
– – of newborn 35

Page numbers in **bold** indicate main discussions.

– – orbital part 21
– facial 20, **28**
– – lateral aspect 52
– frontal 7, 19 ff, 23, **28 f**, 34, 36 f, 42, **44 f**, 47, 52
– – of newborn 35
– – squamous part 28, **44 f**
– – temporal surface 44
– hamate **376 f**, 380
– – coronal section 425
– hyoid 20, 22, 55, **60 f**, 67, 69, 86, **150 f**, 154 f, **158 ff**, 161, **166**, 169, 175
– incisive **33**, 45
– lacrimal 20 ff, 23, 28, 37, 47, 52, 132
– lunate **376 f**, 380
– – coronal section 425
– metacarpal 7, **368**, 375 ff, 427
– – axial section 431
– – coronal section 425
– – first **375 ff**, 380, 425
– – of newborn 9
– – of thumb 375 f
– metatarsal 7, 432, **442 f**, 449 ff, 495
– – first 450
– – of newborn 9
– nasal 20 ff, 23, 37, **47 f**, 52, **144**
– of nasal cavity 48
– navicular **442**, 449 ff, 495
– – articular surface 449
– occipital 7, 20 f, **24 ff**, **27 ff**, 33 f, 37, **38 ff**, 42, 46 f, 194
– – basilar part 25, 33
– – lateral part 33, 39
– – of newborn 33, **35**
– – squamous part 20 f, 25, 28, 33, 39 ff, 44
– – – lower part 27
– – – upper part 27
– palatine 20, **33**, 37, **39 ff**, 42, **44 f**, 48, 49
– parietal 7, 20 ff, 23, **29**, 34, 37
– – of newborn 33
– pisiforme **377**, 381, 389 f, 394
– pubic 346, 355
– scaphoid **376 f**, 380
– – coronal section 425
– sesamoid 449
– of skull 20 ff
– sphenoidal 20 ff, 23, **24 ff**, 28, 33 f, 37, **38 ff**, **41 f**, 44 f
– – of newborn 35
– tarsal 7, 432
– temporal 20 ff, 23, **27 ff**, 33 f, 37, 46 f, 52, **125**
– – of newborn 35, 125
– – petromastoid part 125
– – petrous part 20, 33 f, 37, 122, 127, 130
– – squamous part 20 f, **27 f**, 125
– – – of newborn 35
– – tympanic part 20 f, 27
– trapezium 376 f
– – coronal section 425

– trapezoid **376 f**, 380
– – coronal section 425
– triquetral **376 f**, 380
– – coronal section 425
– zygomatic 7, 19 ff, 23, 28, 33, 37, 45, 47, 52, 54
– – orbital surface 45
Border
– anterior, of spleen 300
– inferior, of lung 249
– interosseous
– – of fibula 440
– – of tibia 440
– lateral, of scapula 370 f
– medial
– – of scapula 371, 382
– – of tibia 440
– posterior, of fibula 440
– superior, of scapula 371
Brachium of inferior colliculus 115, 131
Brain 3, **99 ff**
– areas of blood supply 96
– arterial blood supply 92
– coronal section 92, **116 f**
– cross section 116 f
– dissections 104 ff
– divisions 91
– horizontal section 118 ff
– inferior aspect 65, **99**
– median section 90 f
– ventricular cavities 112
Brain stem **67**, **69 ff**, 84, **91**, **114 f**, 139
– auditory pathway 131
– median section 90 f
Breast, lymphatics 290
Breast tissue 290
Bronchial tree 246 f, 275
– mediastinal dissection 247
Bronchus(-i) **246**, 249
– primary
– – left 276, 278 f, 281
– – – of fetus 288
– – right 280
– secondary 278
– segmental 246
Bulb 147
– of aorta 244, 252, 259, 261
– olfactory 31, **65 f**, **75**, 89, 99, 103, **107**, **146 f**
– of penis **336 f**, 339, **342**, 345
– of vestibule 355, **360 ff**, 364
Bulla, ethmoidal 37, 53, 145
Bundle
– atrioventricular 261
– of His 261
Bursa
– of Achill tendon 449
– omental 292, **311 ff**
– – horizontal section 324
– – isthmus 318

– – midsagittal section 322
– – splenic recess 318
– – superior recess 318
– suprapatellar 446 ff
Bypass vessel 263

C

Calcaneus 7, **443**, 449, 451, 495
– articular surface
– – talar
– – – anterior 449
– – – middle 449
– – – posterior 449
– of newborn 9
Calcar avis 104, 106, **110**
Calvaria **29**, 53, 87 ff, 97, 149
Calyx, renal 326 f
– major 326
– minor 326 f
Canal
– adductor 452
– – entrance 480
– – tendinous wall 467
– anal 3, **336 f**
– – coronal section 345
– – midsagittal section 322
– carotid 27, 31, **33**, 46, 98, 125, 127, **164**
– central 86, 91, 116
– cervical 357
– condylar 25, 27, **33**, 39
– facial 31, 125 f, 129 f
– gastric 294
– for greater petrosal nerve, hiatus 27
– hypoglossal 25, **30 f**, 33, 36, 39, 46, 201
– incisive **33**, 42, 145, 147
– infra-orbital 46
– inguinal 217 f
– – in the female **220**, 323
– – in the male 217 ff
– mandibular 165
– – entrance **52**, 83
– musculotubal 129
– nasolacrimal **46 f**, 132
– obturator 444 f
– optic 23, 25 f, **30 f**, 34, 38, 44, 46 f, 132, **138**
– osseus semicircular
– – anterior **123 ff**, 129 f
– – lateral **123 ff**, 127, **129 f**
– – posterior 124 f, **129 f**
– palatine
– – greater 40, 46
– – lesser 46
– pterygoid 25, **33**, 45 f, 146, 164
– pudendal, entrance 483
– pyloric 294
– sacral 434 f, **437**

Page numbers in **bold** indicate main discussions.

Canal
– of Schlemm 133
– spiral, of cochlea 125
– vertebral 88, 188, **230 ff**, 472
– – sagittal section 232
Canaliculus
– chordae tympani 125
– cochlear 27
– lacrimal, inferior 142
– mastoid 27, 125
Canalis
– carpi 14, **389**, 394 f, 427, 429
– musculotubarius 27
Canine 50 f
– permanent 51
Capitulum of humerus 373, 375, 379, 391
Capsula adiposa perirenalis 296, 300, 324
Capsule
– articular 12
– – of atlanto-occipital joint 200
– – of elbow joint 379, **391**
– – of hip joint 444
– – of interphalangeal joint
– – – of fingers 381
– – – of toes 449
– – of knee joint 12, 447 f
– – of metacarpophalangeal joint 381
– – – of thumb 381
– – of metatarsophalangeal joint 449
– – of shoulder joint 378
– – of temporomandibular joint 53 f
– – of wrist joint 380
– external **116**, 120
– fibrous, of kidney 326
– – vessels 329
– internal 92, **105**, 109 f, **111**, 113, 115 f
– – anterior limb 120
– – posterior limb 120
Cardia 296, 300
Carotid sheath 174
Carotid sinus nerve 164 f
Carpal tunnel 14, **389**, 394 f, 427, 429
Cartilage(s)
– alar
– – greater 49
– – lesser 49
– articular
– – of condylar process of mandible 54
– – of knee joint 12
– – of shoulder joint 15
– arytenoid 158 f
– corniculate 158
– costal 7, 189, 192
– cricoid 155, 157, **158 f**
– of larynx 158
– nasal 49
– – lateral 49
– septal 49
– thyroid 151, 154 f, **158 f**, 255

– tracheal 158 f
Cauda equina **230**, 232, 471
– horizontal section 320, 324
Cavity(-ies) 345
– abdominal 1, **291 ff**
– – coronal section 1
– – CT scan 321
– – frontal section 309
– – horizontal section 320 f, 324
– – midsagittal section 313
– – MRI scan 309, 320
– – parasagittal section 325
– – posterior 332 f
– – veins of posterior wall 279
– articular 12
– – elbow joint 431
– – hip joint 496
– – humeroradial joint 431
– – knee joint 446
– – shoulder joint 10, **15,** 378
– cranial 84 ff
– – coronal section 62
– glenoid 188 f, **369 ff**, 378
– nasal 7, 22, 31, 84, **88**, 90, **143 ff**
– – arteries 146 f
– – bones 48
– – coronal section 62
– – horizontal section 148
– – lateral wall 145 ff
– – – nerves 147
– – median section 145
– – nerves 146 f
– oral **50**, 84, 143, **150 ff**, 163
– – coronal section 50, 62
– – floor 150 f
– – median section **88**, 145
– – transverse section 82
– pelvic
– – in the female 366 f
– – horizontal section 4
– – in the male
– – – coronal section 345
– – – MRI scan 342, 345
– – – nerves 349
– – – parasagittal section 346
– – – sagittal section 342
– – – vessels 346 f
– – MRI scan 4 f
– of septum pellucidum 104, 120
– thoracic
– – coronal section 1
– – parasagittal section 325
– – posterior 332 f
– – veins of posterior wall 279
– tympanic 69, 120, **122 ff, 128 ff**
– – medial wall 126 f
– – roof 123
– uterine 367
– ventricular, of brain 112

Cecum 291 f, 304, 307, 318
– horizontal section 320
Center, acoustic 131
Cerebellum 66, 74 f, 84, 86, 90, 94, **102 f**
– median section 90 f
Cerebrum 18, **99 ff**, 233
– in neonate 233
Cervix of uterus 354, **356 f**, 359
– vaginal portion 322, 356 f, 360
Chamber, anterior, of eyeball 134
Chiasma, optic 65 f, **73 f**, 86, 90 f, 99, 103, **138 f**
– lesion 139
Choana 45, 146, 163, **164**
– of newborn 33
Chondrocranium 22
Chord, oblique 379
Chorda(-ae)
– tendineae 253, 256, 258
– tympani 62, 68 ff, 77, **124 ff**, 128, 146
– – extracranial part 126
– – intracranial part 126
Chorion 359
Circle
– arterial, of Willis 93, 98
– greater, of iris 134
– lesser, of iris 134
Circulation
– collateral, of shoulder 404
– lymphatic 16
– portal 16
– pulmonary 16
– systemic 16
Circulatory system 16
– fetal 288 f
– shunts 288
Circumference, articular
– of radius 374 f
– of ulna 374 f
Cistern
– cerebellomedullar 85 f, 89, **112**, **145**, 230, 240 f
– chiasmatic 85
– interpeduncular 85
– of lateral cerebral fossa 89
– of pons 201
Cisterna chyli 17, 332
Claustrum 92, 116, 120
Clava 115
Clavicle 3, 7, 168, 174, 177, 187 ff, **206 ff, 264**, 284, **368 ff**
– articular facet
– – for acromion 369
– – for sternum 369
– end
– – acromial **369 f**, 378
– – sternal 369 f
– surface anatomy **204**, 401 f
Clitoris 354, **360 ff**
Clivus 25, 27, **30**, 38

Page numbers in **bold** indicate main discussions.

– Dura mater 89
Coccyx 3, 7, 189, **191**, **193**, 195, 350, **433 ff**, 437, 472
– surface anatomy 476
Cochlea **122 ff**, 127, 129
Cockett veins 468 f
Colliculus(-i)
– facial 115
– inferior of midbrain 67, 103, 111, **114 ff**, 131
– of midbrain 67, 86, 90 f, 99, 107
– seminal **338 f**, 344 f
– superior of midbrain 114 ff
Colon 3
– ascending 302, 304, 307
– descending 210, 304, 310
– Head's area 205
– sigmoid 292, 304, 306 f, 310, 322
– transverse 244, 291 f, 302, 306 ff
– – midsagittal section 322
Column
– of fornix 103, 105, 107, **114 ff**, 119 f
– lateral, of erector spinae muscle 212
– medial, of intrinsic muscles of back 212, **225**
– renal 326
– vertebral s. Vertebral column
Commissure
– anterior 86, 90 f, 94, **99**, **107**, 110, 116, 137
– of fornix 104
– habenular 107
– labial, posterior 361
Concha
– of auricle 122, **124**
– nasal
– – inferior 20, 22 f, 36 f, 42, 44, 46, **48**, 53, **86**, 90, 142, **143 ff**, 147 f
– – – inferior border 48
– – middle 22 f, 33, 36 f, **38**, 40, 44 f, **48**, **86**, **143 ff**
– – superior 36 f, **48**, **86**, 145
Condyle
– lateral
– – of femur 9, 439, **441**, 447
– – of tibia **440**, 446 f
– medial
– – of femur 9, **439**, 447
– – of tibia 440
– occipital 21, 25, 27, **33**, 36, 46, 62, 202
Cone, medullary, of spinal cord 472 f
Confluence of sinuses 75, **85**, **87 f**, 241
Conjugate
– diagonal 434, **438**
– true 434, **438**
Conjunctiva
– of eyeball 133
– palpebral, of lower lid 142
Connection, intertendinous 392
Conus
– arteriosus 256, 258
– – horizontal section 286

– elasticus 158
– medullaris 230, 232 f, **475**
– – midsagittal section 322
– – in neonate 233
Cord
– spermatic 204, 211 ff, 217, **219**, **337**, 340, **343**, 346, 479 f
– spinal s. Spinal cord
– umbilical 233, 359
– urachus 219
Cornea **132 f**, 135 f
Cornu s. also Horn
– greater, of hyoid bone 61, 67, 149, **150**, 158, 167
– inferior, of thyroid cartilage 159
– lesser, of hyoid bone **150**, 158
– sacral 191
– superior, of thyroid cartilage 158 f
Corona
– of glans penis 342
– radiata 109 f
Corpus
– callosum 62, 85 f, 233
– – coronal section 116
– – fiber system 104
– – median section 90 f, 233
– – in neonate 233
– cavernosum
– – of clitoris 356, 360
– – of penis **336 ff**, 339 f, **341 f**, 347
– spongiosum of penis 336 f, **339 ff**
– sterni 194
Cortex
– cerebral 85, 92, **118 ff**
– insular 113
– of kidney 326
– limbic 99
– striate 121
– of suprarenal gland 326
– of temporal lobe 116
– visual 121, **138**
Costae fluctuantes 194
Cowper's gland 336 f, 339, 342, **344**
Crest
– conchal 40, 42, 44
– frontal 28, **30**
– of greater tubercle of humerus 373
– iliac 3, 189, 330, **433**, 435, 482 f
– – surface anatomy 476 f
– infratemporal 52
– – of sphenoid 21, 25 f, 38
– intertrochanteric 438 f
– lacrimal
– – anterior 41
– – posterior 22
– of lesser tubercle of humerus 373
– nasal 40, 42, 44 f
– of nasal septum 146

– occipital
– – external 25
– – internal 27, **30**, 39, 42
– sacral
– – intermediate 191, 434
– – lateral 191, 433 f
– – median **191**, 195, 433 f, **437**, 472
– sphenoidal 25
– supraventricular 271
– transverse 123
– urethral 338
Crista
– galli **30**, 34, 37, **38**, 40 f, 49, 53, 86
– spiralis ossea 127
– terminalis of right atrium 258, 283
Crossing of tendons
– in leg 460 f
– in sole of foot 460 f, **464 f**, 502
Crus
– anterior, of stapes 128
– cerebri 73
– of clitoris 356, **361 f**, 364
– commune 129
– of fornix **105**, 106
– lateral, of superficial inguinal ring 217, 362
– long, of incus 126, 128
– medial, of superficial inguinal ring 362
– penis 337, 339, **342**, 345, 352
– posterior, of stapes 128
– right of lumbar part of diaphragm 282 f, 335
– short, of incus 126, 128
Culmen of vermis 102
Cuneus 137
Cupula 125, **129**
Curvature
– cervical 193
– greater, of stomach 294 f, **311 f**, 316
– lesser, of stomach 294 f, **311 f**
– – longitudinal muscle layer 295
– lumbar 193
– thoracic 193
Cusp 261
– anterior, of tricuspid valve 258
– semilunar
– – anterior, of pulmonary valve 259
– – left
– – – of aortic valve 259
– – – of pulmonary valve 259
– – posterior, of aortic valve 259
– – right
– – – of aortic valve 259
– – – of pulmonary valve 259
– septal, of tricuspid valve 259, 261
Cuspid (canine) 50 f
– permanent 51

Page numbers in **bold** indicate main discussions.

D

Declive of vermis 102
Decussation
– of pyramidal tracts 109, **114**
– of superior cerebellar peduncle 103
Demifacet
– inferior, for head of rib 191, **197**
– superior, for head of rib 191, **197**
Dens of axis 53, 86, 89 f, 165, **191**, 195, **200 f,** 203
– articulation with atlas 200
Dentition 50
Desmocranium 22
Diameter
– largest, of pelvis 438
– oblique 434
– transverse 434
Diaphragm 3, 16, 206, 244, 255, **264 ff,** 269 ff, 273, 276, 279 f, **281 ff,** 284 f, **292 f,** 307, 320
– central tendon **278,** 283, 298, 329
– changes of position during respiration 282
– costal part 278, 282 f
– lumbar part **282,** 315, 327
– – right crus 282 f
– midsagittal section 322
– oral 150
– pelvic
– – in the female 362 f
– – in the male 350 ff
– sternal part 278, 283
– superior aspect 283
– urogenital
– – fascia inferior 350
– – in the female 362 ff
– – in the male 337, 347, 350 ff, **353**
Diaphragma sellae 75
Diaphysis s. Shaft
Diastole 260
Diencephalon 91
Digestive system, organization 291
Digitations, hippocampal 107, **110**
Diploe 30, 53, 85, 87
Direction of the body 4 f
Disc
– articular
– – fibrocartilagenous 12
– – of sternoclavicular joint 177
– – of temporomandibular joint 54, 56 f, 79
– – of wrist joint 380, **425**
– intervertebral 7, 89, 193, **197 ff,** 472 f
– – inner core 198 f
– – midsagittal section 322
– – MRI scan 195, 201, 203, 232
– – outer portion 198
– optic 133 f
Dorsum
– of foot 492 ff, **498 f**
– sellae 25 f, **30,** 34, **36,** 38, 41, 46, 75

– – of newborn 35
Douglas' pouch **354,** 357 ff, 366 f
Duct **128 ff, 219**
– cystic **296 f,** 299 f, 317
– ejaculatory 336 ff, **344**
– endolymphatic 128 f
– epidymal 343
– hepatic 296 f
– – common 297, 299, 317
– lymphatic, right 332
– nasofrontal 145
– nasolacrimal 135, **142,** 145
– – opening 145
– pancreatic **296 f, 300 f,** 317
– – accessory 297, **301,** 317
– parotid 54, 58, 61, **77,** 82, 151, **153,** 168
– perilymphatic 129
– semicircular
– – anterior **122,** 127 f
– – lateral **122,** 127 f
– – posterior **122,** 127 f
– submandibular 152 f
– thoracic 17, 170, **172 f,** 184 f, 276, 279, **332**
Ductus 338
– arteriosus Botalli 263, **288 f**
– – remnant 253, 256
– deferens 218 f, 330, **336 ff, 341 ff,** 344
– venosus 288 f
Duodenum 291 f, 296, 300, 302, 316
– descending part 297, **311 f**
– Head's area 205
– horizontal part 309, 317
– superior part 312
Dura mater **84 ff,** 87, **88 f,** 97, 118, 133, 200
– spinal 69, 71, **198,** 230 f, **232,** 474

E

Ear
– inner 31, 122 ff, 128 ff
– middle **122 ff,** 128
– outer 122 ff
Elbow joint 10, **368, 374 f, 379**
– axial section 431
– axis
– – of extension 391
– – of flexion 391
– – of rotation 391
– bones 374 f
– coronal section 10, 379
– ligaments 10, **379**
– MRI scan 10, 379
– of newborn 9
Eminence
– arcuate 27, **122**
– carpal
– – radial 394

– collateral 107
– frontal 35
– iliopubic 433, **435,** 438
– intercondylar 440 f
– parietal 29, **35**
Epicardium 273
Epicondyle
– lateral
– – of femur 439, **441,** 446
– – of humerus **373,** 379, 391 f
– medial
– – of femur 439
– – of humerus **373,** 379, 387 f, 415
Epididymis 218, 330, **336 f,** 339, 341, **343**
– longitudinal section 343
Epiglottis 86, 89 f, 146, 155, **158,** 161, 163
Epiphysis 114
Epithelium
– conjunctival 133
– corneal 133
– pigmented, retinal 133
Equator of lens 133
Esophagus 86, 154 f, 157, 244 f, **273 ff,** 279, 291
– abdominal part 278, **282**
– Head's area 205
– horizontal section 286
– relation to bronchial tree **275**
– thoracic part 278, 281
Eustachian valve (Valve of inferior vena cava) 288
Exostosis 380
Extremity s. also Limb
– caudal, of caudate nucleus 110 f, 114
Eye 84, **133 ff**
Eyeball 68 f, **72 ff, 133,** 142
– anterior segment 133 f
Eyelid 142
– upper 142

F

Facet, articular
– for acromion 369, 371
– inferior, of vertebra 191
– for sternum 369
– superior
– – of atlas 191, 200
– – of vertebra **191,** 197
Falx
– cerebelli 86
– cerebri 67, **74 f, 86 f,** 97, 120, 241
– inguinalis 218
Fascia
– of adductor canal 452
– antebrachial 388, 423
– – distal part 428
– cervical 178 ff

Page numbers in **bold** indicate main discussions.

– – lamina
– – – pretracheal 174, 179 f
– – – prevertebral 174
– – – superficial 174, 178
– cremasteric 341
– crural 493
– – superficial 468, 486, **492**
– deep, of penis 339
– of external abdominal oblique muscle 213
– of Gerota 324 f
– inferior, of urogenital diaphragm 350
– lata **218**, 486
– pectoral 290
– pharyngobasilar 164, 167
– renal
– – anterior layer 324 f
– – posterior layer 324 f
– spermatic
– – external 218, 340
– – internal 218, 340, **343**
– temporal **58 ff**, 79
– thoracolumbar 212, 214, 223, **455**
– transversalis 210, 212 f
Fasciculus(-i)
– longitudinal
– – dorsal 107
– – medial 116
– mamillotegmental 107
– mamillothalamic 107 f
– of Schütz 107
– transverse, of palmar aponeurosis 389
– of Vicq d'Azyr 107 f
Fastigium 102
Fat
– capsular, perirenal 300
– epicardial 252
Fat pad
– buccal 168
– infrapatellar 446, 448
Fatty tissue
– orbital 132
– subcutaneous 210
Femur 7, 12, 432, **438 f**, 441, 446 ff
– coronal section 8 f
– MRI scan 8
– of newborn 9
– ossification 9
– proximal end 8
– X-ray 8
Fenestra 126
– cochleae **125 f**, 128
– vestibuli **125**, 129
Fiber(s)
– arcuate, cerebral 109, 116
– corticospinal 116
– intercrural 217 f, **220**, 362
– pontine, transverse 109, 116
– radiating, of corpus callosum 104

– zonular 133
Fibula 7, 12, 432, **440 ff**, 446 f, 493
– of newborn 9
– upper end 440
Filum(-a)
– radicularia posteriora 98, 239, **241**
– terminale 230 ff, **475**
Fimbria(-ae)
– hippocampal 106 f
– of uterine tube 354, **356 ff**
Finger 368
– joints 381
– ligaments 381
Fissure 23
– cerebral, longitudinal 66, **99 f, 104**
– horizontal
– – of cerebellum 101
– – of right lung **244**, **246**, 248 f, 267 f
– oblique
– – of left lung **246**, 248 f
– – of right lung **244**, **246**, 248 f, 267
– orbital
– – inferior 22 f, 33, 41, **47**, 132
– – superior 22 f, 25, **30 f**, 34, 38, 40 f, **47**
– petrotympanic 27, 125
Flexure
– colic
– – left 284 f, **302**, **304**, 312, 316
– – right 311 f
– duodenojejunal 296, 302 ff, 306, **309 f**, 317 f
Flocculus of cerebellum 66, **102**, 114
Floor of the oral cavity 150 f
Fluid, cerebrospinal 84 f
– flow 85, **112**
Fluorescent angiography of eye 134
Fold(s)
– ary-epiglottic **150**, 160 f, 163
– axillary
– – anterior 385
– – posterior 385
– duodenal
– – inferior 310
– – superior 310
– gastropancreatic 312
– ileocecal 310
– interureteric 338, **355**
– iridial 134
– of mucous membrane
– – of gallbladder 297
– – of stomach 294
– – of urinary bladder 355
– recto-uterine 366 f
– salpingopalatine 145
– salpingopharyngeal 144 f
– umbilical
– – content 293
– – lateral **219**, 337
– – medial **219**, 337 f
– – median **219**, 293, 338, 354

– vestibular 161
– vocal 86, 89, **155**, **161**
Fontanelle
– anterior 35
– antero-lateral 33, **35**
– mastoid 33, **35**
– posterior 35
– postero-lateral 33, **35**
– sphenoidal 33, **35**
Foot 442 f
– axis
– – for eversion 449
– – for inversion 449
– – long 432
– coronal section 495
– cross section 499
– ligaments 450 f
– MRI scan 449, 495
– of newborn, X-ray 9
– sagittal section 449
– skeleton 442 f
Foramen(-ina)
– alveolaria 41, 46
– cecum 28, **30**, 149
– epiploic **311 ff**, 315, 317 f
– – midsagittal section 322
– ethmoidal 132
– – anterior 28, 46 f
– – posterior 46 f
– infra-orbital 22 f, 41 f, 44 f, **47**, 68, **142**
– infrapiriform 482 f
– interventricular, of Monro 86, **94**, 99, **105**, **112 f**
– intervertebral 193, **197 ff**, **472**
– jugular **30 f**, **33 f**, 201
– lacerum 26, **30**, 127, 164
– magnum 25, **27**, **30 f**, **33 f**, 39, 62, 89, 201 f
– mandibular 36, **52 f**
– mastoid 27
– mental 20 ff, 23, 51, **52**, 68 f
– nasal, of nasal bone 47
– nutrient 439
– obturator 188 f, **433**, **436**
– ovale 25 f, **30 f**, **33 f**, 38, 125, 164, 288 f
– palatine
– – greater 33, 37, 45, 164
– – lesser 33, 45, 164
– parietal 29
– rotundum 25 f, **30 f**, 34, 38, 45, 46, 72
– sacral
– – anterior **434**, 438
– – dorsal **191**, 195, **433 f**, 437
– sciatic
– – greater 444, **482 f**
– – lesser 444, **482 f**
– singulare 123
– sphenopalatine 46
– spinosum 25 f, **30 f**, 34, 38
– stylomastoid 27, 31, **33**, 70, 77, 127, 164

Page numbers in **bold** indicate main discussions.

Foramen(-ina)
– supra-orbital 42, **44 f**
– suprapiriform 482 f
– transversarium 157, **191**
– – of atlas 200
– – of axis 200
– vertebral 191
– zygomaticofacial 28
Forceps
– major of corpus callosum 104
– minor of corpus callosum 104
Forearm 368
– anterior region 423
– arteries 397, 421
– axial section 419, 431
– blood vessels 419, 421
– bones 374 f
– muscles 388 ff, 419
– – extensor 392 f
– – flexor 389 ff
– nerves 419 ff
– – cutaneous 420
– position to manual skills 368
– posterior region 420 f
Forebrain 91
Foreskin 336
Formation, reticular 116
Fornix 90, **99**, **114**
– anterior, of vagina 354, **357**
– conjunctival 148
– – inferior 132
– – superior 132
– posterior, of vagina 354
Fossa
– acetabular 433, 445
– axillary 385
– canine 41, 45, 52
– cerebellar 25, 27
– cerebral 25, 27
– condylar 25
– coronoid **373**, 379
– cranial
– – anterior 30 f
– – middle 30 f
– – posterior **30 f**, 39
– hypophysial 25 f, **30**, 34, 36 ff, 49, 75, 88
– – of newborn 35
– iliac 433, **435**
– incisive 45
– infraspinous 371
– infratemporal 31, 52
– inguinal, lateral 293
– intercondylar 439, **441**, 448
– interpeduncular 66, 99, **103**
– ischiorectal 345
– jugular 27, 127, 155
– for lacrimal gland 28
– mandibular 27, 28, **33**, **50**, **54**, 126, 164
– navicular, of urethra 336

– ovalis 258, 283
– popliteal **457**, 468, 484, **487**, 489
– – coronal section 486
– – surface anatomy 476
– pterygopalatine 31, 37, **46**, **72 f**
– radial, of humerus **373**, 379
– retromandibular 168
– rhomboid 67, 69, 71, 115 f, 163
– scaphoid 124
– sublingual 52
– submandibular 52
– supraspinous 371
– supravesical 293
– temporal 20, 52
– triangular 124
– trochlear 28
Fovea
– centralis 134
– of head of femur 439, **445**
– submandibular 36
Frenulum
– of clitoris 362
– of ileocecal valve 310
– veli 115
Fundus
– of bladder 339
– of eye 134
– of gallbladder 297 ff, 311, 316
– of stomach **294 f**, 312
– of uterus 356 ff

G

Galea aponeurotica **55 ff**, 60, 63, 79, 85, 234 ff
Galen's vein 145
Gallbladder **296 f**, 299 f, 302, 311 f, 317 f
– Head's area 205
Ganglion(-ia) 164
– autonomic 334
– celiac 302, 323, **327**, 331, **335**
– cervical
– – middle **162**, 185
– – superior, of sympathetic trunk 71, 146, 162 ff, 165, 168, 183 f
– ciliary 68 f, 72 f, 136, 141
– geniculate **70**, 77, 123 f, 127, 146
– impar 335
– intramural 18
– otic 69
– prevertebral 18
– pterygopalatine 68 f, **146**
– spinal 69, **98**, 229 f, 240
– – dorsal root 474
– – dural sheath 71
– – meningeal covering 231
– spirale 131
– stellate 185

– submandibular 81, 151
– sympathetic 279 f, 327, 335
– trigeminal 31, **68 f**, 72 ff, 140, 146
Genital organs
– female 354 ff
– – external 361 ff
– – – cavernous tissue 362
– – internal **358 ff**, 366 f
– – arteries 360
– – lymph vessels 360
– – position 354
– male 336 ff
– – arteriography 341
– – external 340 ff
– – internal 343 f
– – nerves 349
– – vessels 340, **346 f**, 351
– position 323
Genu s. also Knee
– of corpus callosum 99, 104 f, **107**, 118, 120
– of facial nerve 70
– of internal capsule 120
– of optic radiation 137
Gerota's fascia 324 f
Gingiva of upper jaw 61
Glabella 21 f
Gland(s)
– accessory, of male genital organs 344
– bulbo-urethral 336 f, 339, 342, **344**
– of Cowper 336 f, 339, 342, **344**
– lacrimal 69, 72, 140, 142
– mammary 208, **290**
– palatine **50**, 165
– parathyroid 167
– parotid 58, **77 f**, **152 f**, 178
– pituitary (Hypophysis) 86 ff, 121, **148**
– salivary 153
– sublingual 50, 149, **152 f**
– submandibular 62, 69, **77**, **152 ff**, 177
– suprarenal 300, 311, 324, **326 f**, 331
– – arteries 328
– thyroid 154, 161 f, 167, 169, 176, **266 ff**, 275 ff
– – pyramidal lobe 184
– vestibular, greater 360, **361 f**, 366
Glans
– of clitoris 356, **361 f**
– penis 336, **339**, 341
Globus pallidus 116, 120
Glomerulus 329
Glottis 161
Granulations, arachnoid, of Pacchioni **85**, 100, 112
Gray matter 116, **118 f**
Groove
– of aortic arch 249
– for auditory tube 33
– of azygos arch 249
– chiasmatic 25
– deltopectoral 170, **290**, 387, 398, **406**

Page numbers in **bold** indicate main discussions.

– of esophagus 249
– for greater petrosal nerve 30
– infra-orbital 39 ff, 42, 44 f, 47
– lacrimal 41 f, 52
– for middle meningeal artery 27, 29, 34, **36**, 49
– mylohyoid 36, 53
– nasolacrimal 39
– obturator 433
– for occipital artery 33
– for radial nerve 373
– for sigmoid sinus 27, **30**, 34, 36, **53**
– of subclavian artery 249
– for superior petrosal sinus 27, **30**
– for superior sagittal sinus 25, 27 f, 42
– for tendon of peroneus longus muscle 443
– of thoracic aorta 249
– for transverse sinus 25, 27, **30**, 42
– for ulnar nerve 373
Gubernaculum testis 343
Gyrus(-i)
– angular 101
– cingulate **99**, 103
– dentate 106
– frontal
– – inferior 101
– – middle 100 f
– – superior 101
– of Heschl 131
– long, of insula 109
– occipitotemporal
– – lateral 99
– – medial 66, 99
– orbital 66, 99
– parahippocampal 66, **99**, 106
– postcentral 99 f
– precentral 99 ff
– rectus 99
– short, of insula 109
– straight 66
– of striate cortex 137
– supracallosal 107
– supramarginal 101
– temporal
– – inferior 101
– – middle 101, 131
– – superior 101, 131
– – transverse 131

H

Hamulus
– of hamate bone 377, 394
– pterygoid **25 f**, 37, 144, 164
Hand
– anterior region 423, 426
– arteries 396 f, **426 ff**
– arteriogram 427

– axial section 425, 431
– coronal section 380, 425
– innervation 423 f
– ligaments 380 f
– longitudinal section 426
– MRI scan 380, 425 f
– muscles 388 ff
– – extensor 392 f
– – flexor 389 ff
– nerves 399 f, 423 f, **426 ff**
– – cutaneous 400
– of newborn, X-ray 9
– posterior region 420 f, 424 f
– surface anatomy 401 f
– synovial sheaths of flexor tendons 14
– transverse section 395
– veins 398
Handle of malleus 126, 128
Haustra 307
Head 7, **145 ff**, 458
– arteries 168 ff
– of caudate nucleus **104 ff**, 110, 113, 115 f, 120
– coronal section 149
– CT scan 121
– deep, of flexor pollicis brevis muscle 394
– of epididymis 339, **343**
– of femur 367, 432, **438 f**, 445, 496
– – coronal section 345, 355, 367
– – frontal section 293
– – horizontal section 367
– – ossification center 9
– – trajectorial lines 8
– of fibula 440, 446
– horizontal section 1, **118 ff**, 138, 148
– humeral, of pronator teres muscle 418
– of humerus 15, **372 f**, 378, 430
– lateral
– – of gastrocnemius muscle 455 ff, 484, **487 f**, 491
– – of triceps brachii muscle 382, 401, 408 f
– long
– – of biceps brachii muscle 207, **384 f**, 407, 412
– – of biceps femoris muscle 456, 482 ff
– – of triceps brachii muscle **382 f**, 387, 403 ff, 408 f
– lymph vessels 172 f
– of malleus 126, **128**
– of mandible 50, **52**, 62, 79
– medial
– – of gastrocnemius muscle 455 ff, 458, **487 f**, 491
– – of triceps brachii muscle 382, 387, 401
– median sagittal section 143
– median section 90 f, 145, 233
– – in neonate 233
– of metacarpal bone 376 f
– of metatarsal bone 442, 451, 495

– midsagittal section 85
– MRI scan 90, **118 f**, 149
– muscles 19
– oblique
– – of adductor hallucis muscle 463, 499, 502
– – of adductor pollicis longus muscle 394, 429
– of optic nerve 138, **148**
– of pancreas 297, 312, **316 f**, 320
– of proximal phalanx 376 f
– of radius **374**, 379
– of rib 191, **197**
– sagittal section 84
– short
– – of biceps brachii muscle 384 f, **407**, 411 f
– – of biceps femoris muscle 456, 484
– of stapes 128
– superficial, of flexor pollicis brevis muscle 388, 394
– of talus 443, 451
– transverse
– – of adductor hallucis muscle 463 f
– – of adductor pollicis longus muscle 394, 429
– of ulna **374**, 380
– ulnar, of pronator teres muscle 418
– veins **170 f**, 398
– vessels 262 f
Head's areas 205
Heart **16**, **252 ff**, **268 ff**, 306
– blood flow 256
– – fetal circulatory system 288
– conducting system 261
– electron beam tomographic image 254
– of fetus 288
– function 260
– Head's area 205
– left 16
– left lateral aspect 281
– movements 260
– MRI scan 256
– position 3, 243, **252**
– right 16
– right lateral aspect 280
– valves 255 ff
Helix **122**, 124
Hemianopsia
– binasal 139
– bitemporal 139
– homonymous 139
Hemisphere
– cerebellar 89, **102 f**, 116
– cerebral
– – auditory areas 130
– – frontal pole 89
– – lateral aspect 100
– – median aspect 99
– – occipital pole 88 f
– – temporal pole 89
Hernia
– femoral 218

Page numbers in **bold** indicate main discussions.

Hernia
– inguinal 217 ff
Hiatus
– adductor 453
– aortic **282**, 453
– esophageal **282**, 298
– maxillary 36 f, 42, 46, **48**, **144**
– sacral 434, **437**
– semilunar 53, 145
Hilum of spleen 300
Hindbrain 91
Hindgut 291
Hinge joint 10, **11**, 432
Hip bone 188 f, 432
Hip joint 432
– axial section 496
– bones 438
– coronal section 444
– ligaments 444
– MRI scan 5, 8
– X-ray 8
Hippocampus 138
Hook of hamate bone 377, 394
Horn s. also Cornu
– anterior, of lateral ventricle **104 f**, 110, **112**, 118 ff
– inferior, of lateral ventricle **105 f**, **112**, 116
– – entrance 119
– posterior, of lateral ventricle **104 ff**, 110, **112 f**, 120
Humerus 7, 10, 15, **368**, **372 ff**, 378, 430
– antero-lateral surface 373
– antero-medial surface 373
– of newborn 9
– posterior surface 373
Hymen 354, 356, **361**
Hyoid s. Bone, hyoid
Hypophysis 86 ff, 121, **148**
Hypothalamus 90 f, **108**, 116
Hypothenar muscles **390 f**, 395, **423**
– axial section 431
Hypotympanon 127

I

Ileum 302, 304, 306
– terminal 307
Ilium 7, **433**
– gluteal surface 437
– horizontal section 320
Impression(s)
– cardiac, of lung 249
– for costoclavicular ligament 369
– digitate **30**, 34
– trigeminal 27, 34
Incisor
– central 37, 45, **50**

– lateral 50
– permanent 51
Incisura
– angularis 294 f
– tentorii 75
Incisure
– of pancreas 297
– of tympanic ring 125
Inclination, pelvic 438
Incus 20, **122 f**, 126, **128 f**
Indusium griseum 104
Infundibulum
– of hypophysis 65, 74 f, 93 f, 99, **114**, 116, 148
– of right ventricle 256
– of uterine tube 354, **356 f**, 361, 366
Insula **94**, 116, 119 f
Intersections, tendinous, of rectus abdominis muscle **211**, 213, 293
Intestine, small s. Small intestine
Iris 133 f
– pupillary margin 134
Ischium 7, **433**
Isthmus
– of lesser sac 318
– oropharyngeal 246
– of uterine tube 354

J

Jejunum 292, 302 ff, 306
Joint
– acromioclavicular **368 ff**, 372, 378
– of ankle 432, **443**, **449 ff**, 495
– atlanto-axial 200 f
– – lateral 200 ff
– – median 53, 145, 165, **200**, 202
– atlanto-occipital 53, 194, **200 ff**
– biaxial 11
– calcaneocuboid 443, 451
– carpometacarpal **368**, 375
– – coronal section 425
– – of thumb 11, **368**, 375, 377
– costotransverse 191 f, **197**, **199**, 372
– – effect of intercostal muscles 196
– – of first rib 194
– costovertebral 191, 195, **197**, **199**
– – effect of intercostal muscles 196
– crico-arytenoid 158
– cricothyroid 158
– cuneonavicular 442, 449
– of fingers 10
– hip (s. Hip joint) 5
– humeroradial **374 f**, 420, 431
– humero-ulnar 10, **374 f**
– interphalangeal
– – of fingers **368**, 375, 381, **425**
– – of toes 432, **443**, **449**

– knee s. Knee joint
– metacarpophalangeal 10 f, **368**, 375, 381, 394, **425**
– – of thumb 425
– metatarsophalangeal 432, **443**, **449**
– – of great toe 495
– midcarpal **368**, 375
– monaxial 11
– multiaxial 11
– radio-ulnar 10
– – distal 375, 381, **425**
– – proximal **374 f**, 379
– sacro-iliac 432, **434 f**, **437**
– of shoulder 378
– sternoclavicular 177, **368 f**, 406
– subtalar **443**, **449**, 451
– synovial 12
– talocalcaneonavicular 432, 443, **449**, 451, 495
– talocrural 432
– tarsometatarsal **443**, **449**
– temporomandibular 19, **53 ff**, 63, 120
– – effect of masticatory muscles 55
– – ligaments 52 f
– tibiofibular
– – distal **432**, 440, 495
– – proximal 432, **440 f**, 446
– zygapophysial 195
Joint capsule s. Capsule, articular
Joint cavity s. Cavity, articular
Juga
– alveolaria 41, 45
– cerebralia 28
Junction
– costochondral 196
– ileocecal 310

K

Kerckring's fold 297
Kidney 296, 300, **326 ff**
– arteries 328 f
– arteriography 328
– coronal section 326
– Head's area 205
– horizontal section 320, 324
– left 17, 292, **330 ff**
– position 3, 323 ff
– right 292, 311, **330 ff**
– segments 326
– ultrasound image 327
– upper pole 328
– vascular system 329
– veins 329
Killian's triangle 167
Knee (s. also Genu) 486 f
Knee joint 432, 446 ff
– articular capsule 12

Page numbers in **bold** indicate main discussions.

– axial section 497
– bones 441
– coronal section 12
– ligaments 447 f
– MRI scan 4, 446
– of newborn 9
– sagittal section 4, 446

L

Labium 355
– majus 354, **361**
– minus 354 ff, **361 ff**, 364
Labrum, glenoid 378
Labyrinth 128 ff
– bony 130
– membranous 130
Lacrimal apparatus 142
Laimer's triangle (area prone to developing
    diverticula) 167
Lamina
– affixa 104 f, 115
– of axis 200
– cribrosa **30 f**, 34, **38**, 49
– of cricoid cartilage 158
– pretracheal, of cervical fascia 174, 179 f
– prevertebral, of cervical fascia 174
– superficial, of cervical fascia 174, 178
– terminalis 91, **108**
– of thyroid cartilage 159
– of vertebra 191
Laryngopharynx **150**, 155
Larynx 143, 154, **158 ff**, 165, 233, 255
– cartilages 158 f
– coronal section 161
– entrance 246
– horizontal section 161
– MRI scan 203
– muscles 160
– – internal, action 160
– nerves 162
– position 159
– sagittal section 161
Layer, subcutaneous 204
Leg s. also Limb, lower
– axial section 459, **497**
– bones 440 f
– coronal section 461
– cross section 491
– long axis 432
– surface anatomy
– – anterior aspect 477
– – posterior aspect 476
Lemniscus
– lateral 131
– medial 103, 116
Lens 121, **132 f**

– anterior pole 133 f
– posterior pole 133
Ligament(s) 484
– acetabular, transverse 445
– alar 200 f
– annular, of proximal radio-ulnar joint 379
– anococcygeal 350, 353, 364 f
– anterior, of malleus 126
– arcuate, medial 282 f
– bifurcate 449 f
– broad, of uterus 356, 367
– calcaneofibular 450 f
– calcaneonavicular, plantar 449 ff
– carpal, radiating 380 f
– carpometacarpal
– – dorsal 380
– – palmar 380
– collateral
– – carpal, ulnar 380
– – of elbow joint 379
– – fibular 446 ff
– – of interphalangeal joint 381
– – of knee joint 12, 446 ff
– – radial 379 f
– – tibial 447 f
– – ulnar 379
– coraco-acromial 378
– coronary, of liver 299
– costoclavicular, impression of clavicle 369
– costotransverse 474
– – lateral 199
– – superior 197 ff
– crico-arytenoid, posterior 158
– cricothyroid 158
– cruciate 12
– – anterior 446 ff, 497
– – posterior 446 ff
– cruciform 200
– cuneonavicular
– – dorsal 451
– – plantar 450 f
– deltoid 450 f
– – posterior part 450 f
– – tibiocalcaneal part 451
– – tibionavicular part 451
– denticulate 231, 240
– of elbow joint 10, **379**
– falciform, of liver 244, 268, 278, 293, **298 f**,
    306 f, 311 f, 318, 320
– – free margin 293
– of foot 450 f
– fundiform, of penis 212
– gastrocolic 298, 306 f, **311 f**, 315
– gastrosplenic 300, 311
– of hand 380 f
– of the head of femur 345, 351, 367, **444**, 496
– hepatoduodenal **311 f**, 318
– – content 291
– of hip joint 444

– iliofemoral 444 f
– iliolumbar 444 f
– of inferior vena cava 299
– inguinal 3, 187, 209, 211, 213 f, **216 ff, 220,**
    444 f, 452 f, 479 f
– – surface anatomy 204
– intercarpal
– – deep 380
– – dorsal 380
– interfoveolar 218, 293
– interspinous 198 f
– intertransverse **197 ff**, 225, 240
– intra-articular 197, 199
– ischiofemoral 444 f
– of knee joint 446 ff
– of larynx 158
– lateral, of temporomandibular joint 53 f
– lienorenal 311
– longitudinal
– – anterior 197 ff
– – posterior **198 f**, 201
– medial, of ankle s. Ligament, deltoid
– meniscofemoral, posterior 447
– metacarpal
– – dorsal 380
– – palmar 380
– – transverse
– – – deep 381
– – – superficial 423
– of ovary 356 ff
– palmar
– – of interphalangeal joint 381
– – of metacarpophalangeal joint 381
– palpebral
– – lateral 142
– – medial 142
– patellar **446 f,** 452, 458 f, 462, 486, 495
– – surface anatomy 477
– of pelvis 444
– pisohamate 380 f
– pisometacarpal 380 f
– plantar, long 450 f, **465**
– pubofemoral 444 f
– puboprostatic 344
– pulmonary 249
– radiate 197, 199
– radiocarpal
– – dorsal 380
– – palmar 380 f
– round 220
– – fatty tissue 363
– – of liver **292 f**, 298, 303 f, 306, 317
– – of uterus 220, 354, **356 ff**, 359 f, **362,**
    366
– sacro-iliac
– – dorsal 444
– – ventral 445
– sacrospinous 346, 444 f, 471
– sacrotuberous 346, 353, 444 f, **483 f**

Page numbers in **bold** indicate main discussions.

Ligament(s)
- scapular, transverse, superior 404
- of shoulder 378
- sphenomandibular **53**, 153
- stylomandibular 53 f
- superior, of malleus 122
- supraspinous **198 f**, 224
- suspensory
- - of clitoris 362
- - of ovary 356 ff, 360 f, 366
- - of penis 211, 218, **342**
- talocalcaneal
- - interosseous 449, 451, 495
- - lateral 451
- talofibular
- - anterior 451
- - posterior 450
- talonavicular 449
- tarsometatarsal
- - dorsal 449, 451
- - plantar 450 f
- thyro-epiglottic 158
- thyrohyoid 161
- - lateral 158
- tibiofibular
- - anterior 451
- - posterior 450
- transverse
- - of atlas 200 f
- - of knee 447
- trapezoid 378
- triangular 299
- ulnocarpal, palmar 380 f
- umbilical 330
- - lateral 366
- - medial 330, 347, 366
- - median 336, 357, **361**
- vocal 158, **161**
- of wrist of hand 380 f
Ligamentum
- arteriosum 162, **252 f**, 256
- flavum 198
- nuchae **235**, 403
- teres
- - hepatis **292 f**, 298, 303 f, 306, 317
- - uteri 220, **356 ff**, 359 f, **362**, 366
- - - fatty tissue 363
Limb(s) 477
- anterior, of internal capsule 120
- lower (s. also Leg; s. also Thigh) 7, 432 ff
- - arteries 466 f
- - nerves 466 f
- - - cutaneous 476 ff
- - of newborn, X-ray 9
- - organization 432
- - skeleton 432
- - surface anatomy 476 f
- - - anterior aspect 477
- - - posterior aspect 476

- - veins 468 f, 478 f
- - - superficial 468 f
- - - - anastomoses with deep veins 469
- ossification 9
- posterior, of internal capsule 120
- upper (s. also Arm; s. also Forearm) 7, 368 ff
- - arteries 396 f
- - bones 368
- - joints 368
- - muscle(s) 14
- - - extensor 14
- - - flexor 14
- - nerves 399 ff
- - - cutaneous 400
- - of newborn, X-ray 9
- - organization 368
- - regional anatomy 408
- - skeleton 10, 368
- - surface anatomy 401 f
- - veins 398
- - - superficial 398
Limbic system 107
Limen
- insulae 109
- nasi 53
Line(s)
- arcuate 212, **216**, 293
- - of ilium **433**, 435, 472
- axillary 217
- - anterior 2
- - posterior 3
- epiphysial
- - of humerus 378
- - of tibia 448
- of Gennari 137
- gluteal
- - anterior 433
- - inferior 433
- - posterior 437
- intertrochanteric **438 f**, 445
- median 217
- midclavicular **2**, 217
- mylohyoid 36, **52**, 53
- nuchal
- - inferior 25, **27**, 29, **33**
- - superior 25, 27, **33**
- oblique, of mandible 52
- of orientation
- - dorsal 3
- - ventral 2
- parasternal **2**, 217
- paravertebral 3
- pectinal 439
- regional, ventral 2
- scapular 3
- semilunar 216
- soleal 440
- sternal, lateral 217
- temporal

- - inferior 20, 44
- - superior 20, 29
- trajectorial, of femoral head 8
- transverse, of sacrum 434
- trapezoid 369
- umbilical-pelvic 2
Linea
- alba 187, 204, 209, 211, **212 f**, 265
- aspera 439
- terminalis, of pelvis 356, **434 ff**, 438
Lingula
- cerebellar 102
- of lung 249, 268, 270
- of mandible 36, **52**
- sphenoidal 25 f, 38
Lip
- external, of iliac crest 433, 435
- intermediate, of iliac crest 435
- internal, of iliac crest 433, 435
- lateral, of linea aspera 439
- lower 53
- medial, of linea aspera 439
Liver 243 f, 278 f, 291 f, 296, **298 ff**
- bare area 299, 318
- coronal section 284
- of fetus 289
- Head's area 205
- midsagittal section 322
- position 3
- sagittal section 245
- segmentation 299
Lobe 149
- caudate, of liver 299, 304, **311 f**, 317
- - midsagittal section 322
- frontal 65, 68, 72, 84 f, 89, 97, **99 f**
- - coronal section 149
- - horizontal section 148
- - median section 90 f
- insular 92
- left, of liver 278, 292, **298 f**, 304, 306, 317
- lower
- - of left lung **244**, **246**, 248 f, **267 ff**, 284
- - of right lung **244**, **246**, 248 f, **267 ff**
- - - of fetus 288
- middle, of right lung **244**, **246**, 248, **249 ff**, **267 ff**, 273, 306
- occipital 65 ff, 74, 84, **99 f**, 101, 113
- - median section 90 f
- parietal 90, **99 f**, 101
- postcentral 99 f
- precentral 99 f
- pyramidal, of thyroid gland 184
- quadrate, of liver 299, 306
- right, of liver **298 f**, 315
- temporal 65 f, **99 f**, 107, 148
- - area of acoustic centers 131
- upper
- - of left lung **244**, **246**, 248, **249 ff**, **267 ff**, 273, 284 f, 306

Page numbers in **bold** indicate main discussions.

– – of right lung 244, **246**, 248, **249 ff**, **267 ff**, 272, 284 f
– – – of fetus 288
Lobe bronchus
– inferior
– – left 246
– – right 246
– lower
– – of left lung 251
– – of right lung 251
– middle, of right lung 246, **251**
– upper
– – of left lung 246, **251**
– – of right lung 246, **251**
Lobule
– of auricle **122**, 124
– biventral, of cerebellum 102
– central, of vermis 102
– semilunar, inferior, of cerebellum 102
Lobus insularis **94**, 116, 119 f
Lung 3, 177
– cardiac impression 249
– groove
– – of aortic arch 249
– – of azygos arch 249
– – of esophagus 249
– – of subclavian artery 249
– – of thoracic aorta 249
– horizontal section 286 f
– impressions of rib 249
– left 243, **249 ff**, **267 ff**, 274
– – bronchopulmonary segments **251**
– position 243
– right **249 ff**, **267 ff**, 274
– – bronchopulmonary segments **251**
– surface projection of the thorax wall 248
Lymph node(s) 17
– axillary 17, 290
– – deep 411
– – superficial 410
– bronchopulmonary 275
– cervical 172 f
– – deep 173, **180**
– – superficial 172, 175, **182**
– – superior 173
– iliac
– – common 332 f
– – external 332 f, 360
– – internal 360
– infraclavicular 172 f
– inguinal 17, 360
– – superficial 210, 212, **218**, **220**, 479
– jugulodigastric 172 f
– jugulo-omohyoid 172 f, 332
– lumbar 332, **360**
– mediastinal 332
– – superior 172
– mesenteric 309
– occipital 173

– parasternal 265
– parotid 173
– – superficial 172
– retro-auricular 172 f
– sacral 332, **360**
– submandibular 172 f, 179
– submental 172 f
– supraclavicular 172
– tracheal 275
– tracheobronchial, superior 275
Lymph trunk, lumbar 335
Lymph vessels 290
– iliac 335
– inguinal **218**, 479
– of internal female genital organs 360
– of neck 172
– of trunk 17
Lymphatic system 17

M

Macula
– lutea 134
– of saccule 129
– of utricle 129
Main bronchus
– left 244, **246**
– right 244, **246**
Malleolus
– lateral 440, **443**, 451, 457
– – surface anatomy 476 f
– medial 440, **443**, 451, 457
Malleus 20, 71, **122 f**, **128 f**
Mandible 7, 19 ff, **22**, 33, 37, 49, **50 ff**, 53 ff, 63, 159, 194
– coronal section 62
Manubrium of sternum 3, 159, 177, 188 f, **192 ff**, **369**
Margin 39, **265 f**
– anterior, of tibia 440, 462, 492, 495
– bony, of acetabulum 438
– costal s. Arch, costal
– frontal, of parietal bone 29
– infra-orbital, of maxilla 39 f
– lambdoid, of occipital bone 39
– lateral, of scapula 370 f
– mastoid, of occipital bone 39
– medial, of scapula 234 ff, 382, 403
– nasal, of frontal bone 28
– occipital
– – of parietal bone 29
– – of temporal bone 27
– parietal
– – of frontal bone 28
– – of temporal bone 27
– pupillary, of iris 134
– sagittal, of parietal bone 29

– sphenoidal, of temporal bone 27
– squamous, of parietal bone 29
– superior, of spleen 300
– supra-orbital 21 ff, 28, 45
Marshall's vein 262
Mass, intermediate 90, **99**
Masticatory apparatus 22
Maxilla 7, 19 ff, **22 f**, 28, 33, 36 f, **39 ff**, 42 ff, 45, 47, 52, 54, 132
– orbital surface 39 ff
Meatus
– acoustic
– – external 19 ff, 27 f, **54**, 55 f, 68 f, 72, 120, **122**, 126
– – – of newborn 33
– – internal 27, **30 f**, 34, 36, 46, 53, 164, 201
– – – bony base 124
– nasal
– – inferior 36, 42, 48, 53, **144**
– – middle 42, 53, **144**
– – superior 144
Mediastinum 274 ff
– anterior portion **245**, 266
– content 245
– middle portion **245**, 266
– posterior **245**, **278 f**, 281
– – inferior segment 279
– superior **245**, **281**
– testis 343
Medulla
– of kidney 326
– oblongata 31, 67, 86, 101, **114 f**, **240 f**
– – median section 90 f
– – MRI scan 203
– of suprarenal gland 326
Membrana tectoria 201
Membrane
– intercostal, external 196, **207**
– interosseous, of forearm 379 ff, **390 f**
– mucous, of uterus 357
– mucous, of urinary bladder 338 f, 355
– obturator 444 f
– thyrohyoid **158**, 160
– tympanic 69, 120, **122 f**, **126 ff**
– vasto-adductor 453, **480**
Meniscus 12
– lateral, of knee joint 446 ff
– medial, of knee joint 447 f
Mesencephalon s. Midbrain
Mesentery 306 f, 310
– midsagittal section 322
– root 306
Meso-appendix 307, **310**, 318
– root 318
Mesocolon, transverse 304, 306, **309 f**
– midsagittal section 322
– root 312, **318**
Mesosalpinx 356 ff
Mesosigmoid 310

Page numbers in **bold** indicate main discussions.

Mesosigmoid
– root 318
Mesovarium 356 f
Metacarpals s. Bones, metacarpal
Metacarpus, axial section 431
Metatarsals s. Bones, metatarsal
Metencephalon 91
Midbrain 65, 73 f, **91**
– cross section 117
– inferior portion 91
– median section 90 f
Moderator band 258
Modiolus 127
Molar 50 f
– permanent 51
Monro foramen 86, **94**, 99, **105**, **112 f**
Mons pubis 204, **364**, 367
MRI angiograph, cerebral arteries 95
Mucosa of wall of stomach 294
Muscle(s) **13 f**, 62, 161, **196**, 225, 395, 463, 498
– abductor 375
– – digiti minimi
– – – of foot 463 f, 501 f
– – – of hand 388, 390, **394 f**, 425, **427 f**
– – of foot 463 ff
– – hallucis 463 f, 499, 501 f
– – pollicis
– – – brevis 388, 394 f, **427 ff**
– – – longus 392 f, **424**
– – – – tendon 427
– adductor 344, 350
– – brevis 365, **453**
– – – of thigh 452 f
– – of foot 463
– – great 364
– – hallucis
– – – oblique head 463, 499, 502
– – – transverse head 463 f
– – longus, of thigh 365, **452 f**, 455, 480
– – magnus 351, 446, **453**, 455 f, 482
– – minimus **453**, 456
– – pollicis 390, 395, 402, **425**
– – – longus 394
– – – oblique head 429
– – – transverse head 429
– – of thigh 452 f
– anal sphincter
– – external 336 f, 345
– – internal 336, 345
– anconeus 392, 392 f, 419
– of arm 382 ff, **386 f**
– articular, of knee 448, 452
– ary-epiglottic 160
– arytenoid 155
– – transverse 160 f
– auricular, superior 85, 168
– of back 204, **221 ff**
– – deepest layer 224
– biceps 416

– – brachii 14, **384 ff**, 387, 393, **416 ff**, 431
– – – fascia 416
– – – long head 207, 384 f, 407, 412
– – – – tendon 378, **387**, 415 f, 419
– – – short head 384 f, **407**, 411 f
– – – – tendon 387
– – – surface anatomy 402
– – femoris **455 ff**, 491
– – – long head **456**, 482 ff
– – – short head 456, 484
– – – tendon 455 f, 484
– bicipital 13
– bipennate 13
– brachialis 14, **384 ff**, 387, 389, 393, 415
– brachioradialis 14, **387**, 390, 392 f, 416
– broad 13
– buccinator 50, 54, **55 ff**, 58, 60 f, 63, 68, 82 f, **151**, 167
– bulbospongiosus 350 ff, 361
– calcaneal 458
– ciliary 133
– coccygeus 351
– constrictor
– – inferior, of pharynx 60 f, 161, **164 f**, **167**, 182
– – – cricopharyngeal part 166
– – – thyropharyngeal part 166
– – middle, of pharynx 61, 67, **151**, **164 f**, **167**
– – superior, of pharynx 60 f, **151**, 164, 166, **167**
– coracobrachialis **384 ff**, 387, 411
– corrugator supercilii 58
– cremaster 218, 340, 341, **343**
– crico-arytenoid
– – lateral 160 f
– – posterior 160
– cricothyroideus 160, **166 f**, 266
– dartos 218, **343**
– deep, of back 214
– deltoid 14 f, 204, **209 ff**, 290, 378, **385**, **403 ff**, 408 f, 430
– – acromial part 384, 387
– – clavicular part 384 f, 387
– – posterior fibers 382
– – scapular part 387
– depressor
– – anguli oris 58, 60, **77 f**, 167
– – labii inferioris 58, 167
– – supercilii 58
– digastric **13**, 63
– – anterior belly **55**, 60 ff, 68, **77 f**, 150, 152, **156**, **166**, 168, 175, 181
– – posterior belly 54, **55**, 60, 67 f, 80, **81 f**, 151, **156**, 163, 165, **166 f**, 168, 175, 181
– dorsal
– – of leg, surface anatomy 476
– – of shoulder 382 f
– erector spinae
– – lateral tract 210

– – medial tract 210
– extensor 14
– – carpi
– – – radialis
– – – – brevis 389, **392 f**, 419
– – – – longus 387, **392 f**, 419
– – – ulnaris 392 f, 419
– – – – tendon 424
– – digiti minimi of hand 392 ff
– – digitorum
– – – brevis of leg 459, 462, 493, 499
– – – of hand 392 ff, 419, **424**
– – – longus of leg 459, **462 f**, 498
– – – – tendon 498
– – of foot 462
– – of forearm 392 f
– – – surface anatomy 401
– – hallucis
– – – brevis 462, 498 f
– – – longus **462 f**, 495, 498
– – – – tendon 458 f, **498**
– – of hand 392 f
– – indicis 393
– – – tendon 392
– – of leg 462 f
– – pollicis
– – – brevis 392 f, **424**
– – – – tendon 388
– – – longus 393
– – – – tendon 424
– – of thigh 452
– – of thumb 393 f
– extra-ocular 135 f
– – action 135
– – innervation 72
– facial 19, **58 f**
– of fifth toe 463
– flexor(s) 14
– – of arm 385
– – carpi
– – – radialis **388 f**, 416 f, 419, **423**
– – – – tendon 380, **427 f**
– – – ulnaris **388 f**, 416, 419, **423**
– – – – tendon 380, **427 f**
– – deep, of leg 460 ff
– – digiti minimi brevis
– – – of foot 463 f
– – – of hand 389 f, 394, **428**
– – digitorum
– – – brevis of foot 449, **463 f**, 501
– – – – origin 502
– – – of hand 389, 427
– – – – longus of foot 460 f, 464, 491, 499
– – – profundus of hand 389, 418 f, 423, 425, 427
– – – superficialis of hand **388 f**, 391, 416, 418 f, **423**, 425, **427 f**
– – – – tendon 389
– – of forearm 389 ff

Page numbers in **bold** indicate main discussions.

– – hallucis
– – – brevis 449, **464**, 499, 501
– – – longus 459 ff, 491
– – – – tendon 449, **460 f**, 463, 501 f
– – of hand 389 ff
– – of leg 457
– – pollicis
– – – brevis 427
– – – – deep head 429
– – – – superficial head 388, **427 ff**
– – – longus **388 f**, 418, 423
– – of thigh 455 f
– of foot 457 ff, **463 ff**
– of forearm 388 ff, 419
– fusiform 13
– gastrocnemius 446, **455 f**, 462
– – lateral head 455 ff, 484, **487 f**, 491
– – medial head 455 ff, 458, **487 f**, 491
– gemellus
– – inferior 455 f, 483
– – superior 455 f
– genioglossus 50, 86, **149 ff**, 155, 166
– geniohyoid 62, 86, **150 ff**, 155
– gluteus 454 f
– – maximus 225, 350 ff, 362, **455 f, 482 ff**
– – – surface anatomy 476
– – medius 320, **455 f**, 483 f
– – minimus **455**, 483
– gracilis 350, 365, **452 f**, 455, 480, 487
– – tendon 447, 452, **455**, 457
– of great toe 463
– hamstring 484
– of hand 388 ff
– – deep layer 395
– of head 19
– hyoglossus 61 f, **150 ff**, 160, 166 f
– iliacus 330, 453
– – horizontal section 320
– iliococcygeus 351
– iliocostalis 210 f, **221 ff**, 320, 324
– – cervicis 222
– – insertion 222
– – lumborum 222
– – origin 222
– – tendons 225
– – thoracis 222, 236
– iliopsoas 293, 338, 367, **452 f**, 480, 496
– of index finger 394
– infrahyoid 60 f, **151**, 174, **175**, 182
– infraspinatus 223, 240, **242**, **382 f**, 403 f, 408 f, 430
– intercostal
– – effect
– – – on costotransverse joint 196
– – – on costovertebral joint 196
– – external **196**, 207, 222, 403, 412
– – innermost **206**, 474
– – internal **196**, **206 f**, 210 f, 264

– – – of larynx, action 160
– interosseus(-i)
– – dorsal
– – – of foot 463, 495, 499
– – – of hand 380, 393 ff, **424**
– – of foot 464
– – of hand 425, 427
– – – actions 394 f
– – palmar 394 f, **429**
– – plantar 463
– interspinal, lumbar 224
– intertransversarius(-i) 221, **225**
– – cervical, posterior 225
– – lumborum 224 f
– intrinsic, of back, medial column 212, **225**
– ischiocavernous 345, 349, **350 ff**, 364
– ischiocrural 454
– latissimus dorsi 196, 207, 211, 223, 228, 234, 324, **382 f**, 385, **403**, 408 f
– of leg 457 ff
– levator(es) 351
– – anguli oris 58, 167
– – ani 337, 344 f, **350 f**, 355, 362, 364
– – costarum **223 f**, 225, 241
– – labii superioris 58, 167
– – – alaeque nasi 58, 167
– – palpebrae superioris **73**, 132, 135 f, 140
– – scapulae 181, 184, 222 ff, **235 ff**, 240, **382 f**, 403 ff
– – veli palatini 62, **122 f**, 147, 167
– long, of back 221 f
– longissimus 210 f, **221 ff**, 320
– – capitis **222**, 225
– – cervicis 222, 236
– – insertion 222
– – origin 222
– – thoracis 222, 236
– longitudinal
– – inferior, of tongue 50, **149** 166
– – superior, of tongue 50, 62, **86**, **149**
– longus
– – capitis 60 f, 157, 165
– – colli 157, 174, **185**
– lumbrical
– – of foot 461, **463 f**, 501
– – of hand 389, 394 f, **429**
– masseter 19, 54, **55 ff**, 58, 62, **77 ff**, 168
– masticatory 19, **55 ff**
– – effect on the temporomandibular joint 55
– mentalis 58, 167
– multicaudal 13
– multifidus 211, 223 ff, 324
– multiventral 13
– mylohyoid 55, 60 ff, **77 f**, 86, **150 ff**, 152, 155, **156**, **166**, 175
– nasalis 77, 167
– – alar part 58
– – transverse part 58

– of neck 203
– oblique
– – abdominal
– – – external 187, 196, 204, **208 ff**, 212 f, 264, 300
– – – internal 187, 204, 210 ff
– – inferior **72**, 132, **135 f**
– – superior **72 f**, 132, **135 f**, 140
– obliquus capitis
– – inferior 222 f, 225, **237 f**
– – superior 223, **237**
– obturator
– – externus 344 f, 453
– – internus 344 f, **350**, 351, 353, 355, 367, 455 f
– occipitofrontalis
– – frontal belly **56 ff**, 60, 79, 85, 168
– – occipital belly 58, 70, **77**, 85, 234 ff, **237 ff**
– ocular, external 133
– omohyoid 60 f, **77 f**, 81, 151, **156 f**, 174 f, 264, 266
– – intermediate tendon 179
– opponens
– – digiti minimi 394, **428**
– – – of foot 465
– – – of hand 389
– – pollicis 390, 394
– orbicularis
– – oculi **58 ff**, 61, 70, 77, 79, 85, **142**, 167
– – – orbital part 58, 60, 168
– – – palpebral part 58, **142**
– – oris 58, 77, 167
– palatopharyngeus 163
– palmaris
– – brevis 388, **423**
– – longus 388, 416, 419, 423
– – – tendon 388, 423, **428**
– papillary 253, 261
– – anterior 256, 258 f, 271
– – – of right ventricle of fetus 288
– – posterior 258, 271
– – septal 258
– pectineus 344, 367, **452 f**, 480
– pectoral 384 f
– pectoralis
– – major 14, 187, 207 f, **209 ff**, 264 f, 290, **384 f**, 387, 410, 412
– – – abdominal part 384
– – – clavicular head 185, 384
– – – insertion 411
– – – sternocostal part 384
– – – surface anatomy **204**, 402
– – minor 168, 204, 207, **264 ff**, **384 f**
– – – insertion 411
– perineus transverse
– – deep 345, 350, **351 ff**, 362, 364
– – superficial 350, 364
– peroneal 498

Page numbers in **bold** indicate main discussions.

Muscle(s)
– peroneus
– – brevis **457**, 460, 495
– – longus **457**, 460, 495
– – – tendon 462
– piriform 455 f, **483**
– plantaris 456 ff, **487**, 491
– popliteus 446, 457, **460**
– procerus 58
– pronator
– – quadratus **390 f**, 395
– – teres 387, **389**, **391**, 416, 419
– – – humeral head 418
– – – ulnar head 418
– psoas
– – major 210 f, 282 f, 292, 325, **330 f**, 333, 335, 355, **359**, **453**
– – minor 453
– pterygoid
– – lateral 53 f, **55**, **57**, 62, 80
– – – connection with articular disc of temporomandibular joint 57
– – medial 54, **55**, 57, 62, 68, 80, 83, **146**, 165 ff
– – – connection with articular disc of temporomandibular joint 57
– pubococcygeus 351
– puborectalis 351
– pyloric sphincter 295
– pyramidalis 211 f, 367
– quadratus
– – femoris **455 f**, 483 f
– – lumborum 210 f, 282, 330, 453
– – – horizontal section 320
– – plantae 449, **464**, 501
– quadriceps femoris 446, **448**, 452, 458
– – surface anatomy 477
– quadricipital 13
– rectus
– – abdominis 206, 208, 210, 212 f, **216**, **264 ff**, 292 f, 320, 324, 385
– – – surface anatomy **204**
– – capitis posterior
– – – major 222 f, 225, **237**
– – – minor 222 f, 225, **237 f**
– – femoris **452 f**, 455, **480 f**
– – inferior 72, 132, **135 f**
– – lateral 69, **71 ff**, 74, 121, 132, **135 f**, 138, 148
– – medial 74, 132, **135 f**, 148
– – superior **72 f**, 132, **135 f**, 140
– rhomboid
– – major 222 f, 225, 234 f, 238, **382 f**, 387, 403 ff, 408
– – minor 235, 238, **382 f**
– ring-like 13
– risorius 58
– rotator 225
– – lumbar 224

– sartorius 218, 344, 367, **452 ff**, 455, 457, 479 f, 487, 496
– – tendon 447, 452
– scalenus 60
– – anterior 162, 168, 170, **181**, **184 f**, 269, 271
– – medius 162, 180, **184 f**
– – posterior 162, **181**, **184 f**
– semimembranosus 446, **455 ff**, 484, 487
– – membranous part 456
– – tendon 447
– semispinalis
– – capitis 165, **222**, 225, **228**, 235, 238
– – cervicis **222 ff**, 225, 238
– – thoracis 225, 228
– semitendinosus **13**, 446, 452, **455 ff**, 482, 484, 487
– – tendon 447, 452, 487
– – – intermediate 456
– serrated 13
– serratus
– – anterior 196, 204, **207 ff**, 264, 290, 300, **384 f**, 410
– – posterior
– – – inferior 222, 403
– – – superior 228, **235**, 238, 404 f
– of shoulder 382 ff
– of sole of foot 463 ff
– soleus 446, **457 f**, 487, 491
– – tendinous arch 457, 491
– sphincter s. also Sphincter; s. also Sphincter muscle
– – urethrae 349
– spinalis **221**, 223 f
– – thoracis 222, 225
– spinotransversal **221**
– splenius
– – capitis 70, 77, 179 f, 228, 234 ff, 383, **403 ff**
– – cervicis 228, 235 f, **403**, 405
– stapedius 127
– sternocleidomastoid 58, 60 f, 63, 68, **77 ff**, 81 f, 85, 152, 154, **156 f**, 174, 178, 206, 209, 234 ff, 264, 384 f, 403, 405 ff
– – clavicular head 175
– – sternal head 175
– – surface anatomy 401
– sternohyoid 60 f, **78**, 97, **151**, **156 f**, 174 f, 209, 264
– sternothyroid 151, **156**, 174 f, **206**, 265
– styloglossus 60, 71, **151**, **166**, 167
– stylohyoid **55**, 60, 68, 71, **78**, **150 ff**, **166 f**, 175
– stylopharyngeus 61, 67, **167**
– subclavius **156**, 207, 384 f
– subscapularis 196, **384**, **386 f**
– supinator 389, **391**, 393
– suprahyoid 60 f, **151**, **175**
– supraspinatus 15, **382 f**
– – tendon 378

– temporalis 19, 54, **55 ff**, 62 f, 79
– – insertion 56
– – tendon 60 f, 80, 82
– temporoparietalis 58, **77**
– tensor
– – fasciae latae 452 f, **455**, 480, 483
– – – surface anatomy 477
– – tympani **122 f**, 127
– – veli palatini **60 ff**, 147, 167
– teres
– – major **223**, 225, 234, **242**, 378, **382 f**, 387, 403 ff, 408 f
– – minor **382 f**, 403 ff, 408 f
– of thigh 452 ff
– thyro-arytenoid 160
– thyro-epiglottic 160
– thyrohyoideus 60 f, **151 f**, **156 f**, 160, **166 f**
– tibialis
– – anterior 459, **461 ff**, 495
– – – tendon 458, 461, 491, **498**
– – posterior 460 f, 491
– – – tendon 460
– transverse
– – of tongue 50, 62, **149**
– – of trachea 160
– transversospinal 221, 225
– transversus
– – abdominis 206, 210 ff, **214**, 293
– – thoracis 206, 264
– trapezius 15, 77, 157, 225, 378, **382 f**, 408
– – ascending fibers 234, **382**, 403
– – descending fibers 234, **382**, 403
– – surface anatomy 402
– – transverse fibers 234, **382**, 403
– triceps
– – brachii 14, 387, 389
– – – lateral head 382, 401, 408 f
– – – long head **382 f**, 387, 403, 408 f
– – – – tendon 378 f
– – – medial head 382, 387, 401
– – – surface anatomy 401
– – – tendon 387
– – surae, surface anatomy 476
– tricipital 13
– unipennate 13
– vastus
– – intermedius **452 f**, 455
– – lateralis 344, 448, **452 f**, 455, 480 f
– – medialis 448, **452 f**, 455, 458, 480 f
– vertical, of tongue 62, **86**, **149**
– vocalis 160 f
– zygomaticus
– – major 58, **77 ff**, 168
– – minor 58
Muscle fibers, oblique, of stomach 295
Muscular coat
– of gallbladder 297
– of stomach 295
Myelencephalon 91

Page numbers in **bold** indicate main discussions.

Myocardium 256 ff, 259 f, 284
Myometrium 359, 367

N

Nasopharynx 62, **150**, 155
Neck **154 ff**, 403
– anatomical, of humerus 372 f
– anterior region **174 ff**, 406
– arteries 168 ff
– of bladder 338
– coronal section 195, 201
– cross section 157, 174, 176
– of femur 9, **438 f**
– of gallbladder 297
– horizontal section 203
– lateral region 178 ff
– lymph nodes 172 f
– lymph vessels 172 f
– of malleus 128
– MRI scan 157, 176, 195, 201
– muscles 203
– nerves 183, 414
– of radius 374
– posterior region **234 ff**, 403
– of scapula 371
– surgical, of humerus 372 f
– of talus 443
– veins **170 f**, 398
– vessels 183
Nerve(s) 147, **180**, 400, 415, 423, 477
– abducent 31, 64, 66, 69, **72 f**, 75, 93, 97 f,
    111, 114, 136, 140
– accessory 31, 63 f, 66 f, 69, 71, **81**, 98, 111,
    114 f, 163 ff, 225, 235 f, 242, 403 ff, 407
– – intracranial portion 67
– alveolar
– – inferior 62, 68 f, 71, 80, **81 ff**, 150
– – superior
– – – middle 69
– – – posterior 68 f, 72, **80**
– anococcygeal 351, 482
– of arm 414 ff
– auricular
– – great 63, **77 ff**, 80 f, 174, 178 f, 229, 234,
    236, 403 f
– – posterior 70, **77**
– auriculotemporal 63, 68 f, 72, **77**, **79 ff**, 82 f,
    85, 168
– – communicating branches to facial nerve 80
– axillary 383, **399**, 404, 408 f, **413 f**
– – cutaneous branch of arm 226, 409
– of back 226 ff
– buccal 63, 68 f, 72, **79 f**, 81 f
– cardiac, cervical
– – inferior 278 f
– – middle 162

– – superior 278
– carotid sinus 165
– cervical, transverse 63, **78 f**, 174, 178, 186,
    242
– chorda tympani 62
– ciliary
– – long 141
– – short 68, **72 f**, 140
– cluneal
– – inferior **226**, 229, 351 f, **470**, 476, 482 ff
– – middle **226**, 229, 476, 482, 484
– – superior 223, **226 f**, 229, 476, 482
– cranial 18, **64 ff**, 98, **114 f**
– – base of skull 31
– – nuclei 114
– cutaneous 416
– – brachial, medial 186
– – dorsal
– – – intermediate, of foot 489, 498
– – – lateral, of foot 498
– – – medial, of foot 468, 489, 498
– – femoral
– – – lateral **214**, 218, **470 f**, 475 ff, 479
– – – posterior 226, 351 f, **470**, 476, 482, 484
– – – – perineal branch 482, 484
– – lateral
– – – of forearm 399 f, 415 ff, **420**, 424
– – – lower, of arm 399 f, 409
– – – upper, of arm 226, **400**, 403, **408 f**
– – medial
– – – of arm 399, 409 f
– – – of forearm 399 f, **408 ff**, 413, 415 ff
– – perforating 483
– – posterior
– – – of arm **399 f**, 403
– – – of forearm 399 f, 409, **420**, 424
– – of region of knee 486
– – sural
– – – lateral **470**, 479, 484, 486, 488 f
– – – medial 484, 487 ff
– digital
– – dorsal
– – – of foot 493, 498 f
– – – of hand 399 f
– – palmar 427
– – – common 399, 423, **427**
– – – proper 423, **428**
– – – supplied regions 424
– – – of thumb 400
– – plantar
– – – common 501
– – – proper 501 f
– dorsal
– – of clitoris 364
– – of penis 217, **341**, 352, 471
– erigentes 349, **472**
– ethmoidal, anterior 31, 141, **146**
– – external nasal branch 68
– – internal nasal branches 147

– facial 31, 64, 66 f, 69, **70**, **77 ff**, 81, 98, 111,
    114 f, 146, 165, 168
– – buccal branches **70**, **77**, 178
– – cervical branch **70**, **77 ff**, 174, 177 f, 186
– – communicating branches to
    auriculotemporal nerve 80
– – marginal mandibular branch **70**, **77**, 79,
    152, 178
– – temporal branch 70, 77
– – zygomatic branch 70, 77
– femoral 214, 293, 340, 367, 444 f, 467, **470 ff**,
    475, 477, **479 ff**
– – cutaneous branch 486
– – – anterior 467, 479
– – muscular branch 480 f
– of forearm 419 ff
– frontal 69, 73
– – lateral branch 140
– genitofemoral 216, **330**, 333, 359, **470**, 472,
    475
– – femoral branch 216, **340**, **470**, 479
– – genital branch 216 f, **340**, **470**, 479
– glossopharyngeal 31, 64, 66 f, 69, 71, 98, 111,
    114 f, 151, 162 f, 165
– – carotid sinus branch 71
– – lingual branch 71
– gluteal
– – inferior 483 f
– – superior 483
– hypogastric 349
– hypoglossal 31, 33, 63 f, 66, 69, **78**, 81, 97 f,
    114 f, 151 f, 162, 164 ff, 183
– – intracranial portion 67
– – lingual branch 71, 183
– – omohyoid branch 183
– – thyroid branch 183
– iliocostalis 230
– iliohypogastric 212 f, 216, 329 f, 444 f, **470 ff**,
    475 ff
– – cutaneous branch
– – – anterior 470
– – – lateral 470
– ilio-inguinal 212, 214, 216 ff, 331, 333, **340**,
    359, 362, **470 ff**, **475**
– infra-orbital 68 f, 72, 79, 82, 136, 142
– – terminal branches 68
– infratrochlear 69
– intercostal 206 f, 214, 216, 279, **474**
– – collateral branch 474
– – cutaneous branches
– – – anterior 207, **209**, 211, **214**, 229, 385,
    400, 411, **470**
– – – lateral **196**, 207, **209**, **214**, 229, 385,
    408 ff, 412, **470**
– – mammarian branches, medial 290
– – perforating branches, anterior **208**
– intercostobrachial 186, 196, 207, **290**, 410,
    412, 414 f
– – terminal branches 400

Page numbers in **bold** indicate main discussions.

Nerve(s)
– interosseous
– – anterior, of forearm 399
– – posterior, of forearm 421, 424
– labial, posterior 364 f
– lacrimal 68 f, **72 f,** 140 f
– laryngeal
– – inferior 160, 163
– – recurrent 177, 185
– – – inferior laryngeal branch 162
– – – left **162,** 255, 266, 269 ff, 272 ff, 276, 279, **335**
– – – right **162,** 276, **335**
– – superior **162,** 165 f
– – – external branch 162
– – – internal branch 151, 163, 173
– lingual 62 f, 68 f, 71, 81, 146, **151 f**
– mandibular 31, 53, 68 f, 72, **83**
– – inferior 63
– – meningeal branch 31
– masseteric 63, 72, **79 f**
– maxillary 31, 68 f, 72, 136, **147**
– medial 417
– median 168, **186,** 207, 387 f, 391, 396, 399, **413 ff,** 419, 423, 425
– – axillary region 410, 412
– – cubital region 416 ff
– – palmar branch 399 f, 423, **427**
– – – digital 400
– – – – common 423, **428**
– – roots 399, **411,** 415
– meningeal, recurrent 31
– mental 68 f, **79**
– musculocutaneous 399, 410, **413 f**
– mylohyoid 68 f, **77 f,** 80, 152
– nasociliary 72 f, 141
– nasopalatine 146 f
– obturator 333, **346 f,** 366, 467, **470 f,** 475 ff, 481
– occipital 85
– – greater 63, 70, **77, 81,** 85, 223, 226, 229 f, **234 ff,** 238 ff, 403 f
– – lesser **77,** 81, 178, **179,** 226, 229, 234 ff, 237 f, 403 ff
– – third 226, 234 ff, 237, 404 f
– – – cutaneous branch 403
– oculomotor 31, 64 ff, 68 f, **72 ff,** 97 f, **114 ff,** 136 f, 140, **148**
– – inferior branch 69, **71 f,** 136
– – superior branch 141
– olfactory 31, 64, **147**
– ophthalmic 31, 68 f, **72 ff,** 136
– optic 31, 62, 64 ff, 68 f, **72 f,** 75, 84, 98, 114 f, 121, **132 ff, 135 ff, 138,** 146, 148
– – destruction 139
– – dural sheat **133,** 138, 148
– – extracranial part 135, 140
– – intracranial part 135, 140
– of the orbit 72 f

– palatine 146
– – greater 146 f
– – lesser 146
– parapharyngeal 164 ff
– parasympathetic 334
– pectoral
– – lateral 207, 407, **412,** 415
– – medial 177, 207, **214,** 407, 415
– perineal 471
– peroneal
– – common 455, 457, **467, 470,** 476 f, 484, 489, 491, 495
– – deep 470, 477, **479,** 492 f, 495, 499
– – superficial 470, 477, **479,** 484, 489, 493, 495, 498
– – – dorsal cutaneous branch
– – – – intermediate 479
– – – – lateral 492 f
– – – – medial 479, 492 f
– petrosal
– – deep 147
– – greater 31, 77, 123, 127, **147**
– – lesser 31, 127
– phrenic 170, 177, 185 f, 266 f, **269 ff,** 274 ff, **280 f,** 396, 413
– – accessory 185
– plantar
– – lateral 470, 499, 501 f
– – – superficial branch 501 f
– – medial 470, 499, 501 f
– – – of great toe 502
– of pterygoid canal 146
– pterygopalatine 68, 72
– pudendal 346, **351 f,** 364, **470,** 471, 483
– – inferior rectal branches 484
– – perineal branch 352
– radial 399, 404, 408, **413 ff**
– – axillary region 410
– – cubital region 416
– – deep branch 391, **399,** 414, 417 ff, 420 f
– – dorsal digital branch 400, **420,** 424
– – main branches 399
– – posterior interosseous branch 421
– – superficial branch 399 f, **414 f,** 418 ff, 424, 427
– – superficial palmar branch 427
– rectal, inferior 351 f, 364 f, **471,** 483
– recurrent 160
– saphenous 467 f, **470,** 476 f, 479 f, 486, 492, 498
– – entering the adductor canal 452
– – infrapatellar branch 467, **470,** 479, 486, 492
– scapular, dorsal 235, 237, 404
– sciatic 344, 351, 367, 444 f, 455, **470, 483 f,** 496
– – branches 484
– scrotal
– – anterior 470
– – posterior 351 f, **471**

– spinal 18, **98, 226 ff,** 229, 234
– – cervical 66, 154, 183
– – – dorsal root 157
– – – ventral rami 18
– – – ventral root 157
– – cutaneous branch 224
– – – lateral 226
– – – medial 226, 234
– – dorsal branches 403
– – dorsal root 71, 214, 230, **240**
– – lateral branches of dorsal rami 223, 226, 228 ff
– – lumbar, ventral rami 18
– – medial branches of dorsal rami 223, 226, 228 f
– – meningeal covering 231
– – ramus
– – – dorsal 214, 231, 240
– – – – cutaneous branch 400
– – – – lateral branches 408
– – – – medial branches 408
– – – ventral 18, 230
– – root filaments 472 f
– – – anterior 474
– – – posterior 474
– – sacral 231
– – – ventral rami 18
– – thoracic 229
– – – dorsal root 231
– – ventral root 214
– splanchnic
– – greater 279 f, 327, **335**
– – lesser 327, **335**
– – lumbar 335
– – pelvic 349, **472**
– – sacral 335
– subcostal 329, **470, 475**
– suboccipital 229, 238, **241**
– supraclavicular 63, **77,** 81, 207, 209, 242, 274
– – anterior 81, 180
– – intermediate 270, 400
– – lateral **174,** 178, **383**
– – medial 174 f, 178, **214,** 400
– – middle **174 ff,** 178 ff, 406
– – posterior **179 ff,** 400, 403, 408
– supra-orbital 63, 68, 72, **77,** 81, **136**
– – lateral branch 69, **73,** 85, 141
– – medial branch 69, **73,** 79, 85, 141
– suprascapular 170, 186, 378, 404, **414**
– supratrochlear **73,** 82
– sural 476, **479,** 489, 493
– – cutaneous branch 492
– – lateral calcaneal branches 493
– sympathetic 334
– temporal, deep 72, **82**
– thoracic, long 186, 196, **207, 214,** 407, 412 f
– thoraco-abdominal 212, **214,** 216
– thoracodorsal 186, 196, 207, **407,** 412, 415
– tibial 446 f, **455,** 457, 467 f, **470,** 484, 491

Page numbers in **bold** indicate main discussions.

- trigeminal 31, 64, 66, **68 f,** 71 ff, 98, **114 ff,** 146
- – main branches 69
- – motor root 146
- trochlear 31, 64 ff, 67 ff, 71, **72 ff,** 98, 114 f, 136
- – intracranial part 140
- – intra-orbital part 140
- ulnar **186,** 207, 396, 399, 403, **413 ff,** 419, 420, 423 f, 427
- – axillary region 410 f
- – cubital region 416 ff
- – deep branch 399, **427**
- – dorsal branch 399 f, 421, 427
- – palmar branch 423
- – palmar cutaneous branch 400
- – palmar digital branch 400
- – – common 423, **428**
- – – proper 423 f
- – superficial branch 399, 423, **427**
- vagus 18, 31, 64, 66 f, 69, 71, 98, 111, **114 f,** 146, 154, 162 f, 165, 169, 244, 255, 264, 266, 274 f, 278, **280, 335**
- – cardiac branch 165, 185
- – – cervical
- – – – inferior 274, 276, **280**
- – – – superior 274, 276
- – esophageal branches 278
- vestibulocochlear 31, 64, 66 f, 69, 98, 111, 114 f, **122 f,** 131
- – cochlear part 123
- zygomatic 68 f, **72**
Nervous system 18
- autonomic **18, 334 f**
- cranial part 18
Network
- capillary, of finger 427
- venous
- – of dorsum
- – – of foot 477
- – – of hand 398, 420
- – around knee 486
- – of lateral malleolus 498
- – of medial malleolus 498
Nipple **204,** 290, 410 f
Node
- atrioventricular 261
- sinu-atrial 260 f
Nodule of vermis 102
Nostril 49
Notch
- acetabular 433, **436**
- angular, of stomach 294 f
- cardiac, of left lung 248, **268**
- cardial, of stomach 294 f
- clavicular 192
- ethmoidal, of frontal bone 28
- frontal 42, 45
- interarytenoid 161

- intercondylar 9
- intertragic 124
- jugular 192
- mandibular **52,** 54, 79
- mastoid 27, 29, **33**
- parietal, of temporal bone 27
- pterygoid 25
- radial, of ulna 374
- scapular 371 f
- sciatic
- – greater 433, **437,** 438
- – lesser 433, **437**
- sphenopalatine 39 f, 42
- supra-orbital 22, 28
- tentorial 73 ff
- thyroid, superior 159
- trochlear, of ulna 374
- vertebral
- – inferior 191, 197
- – superior 191
Nucleus(-i)
- abducent 114
- ambiguus 114
- of Burdach 116
- caudate 62, 92, 104 ff, **111, 114,** 118 f
- cochlear
- – dorsal 131
- – ventral 131
- of cranial nerve 114
- cuneate 116
- dentate 103, 116
- dorsomedial, of hypothalamus 108
- emboliform 116
- facial 70, **114**
- of Goll 116
- gracilis 116
- hypoglossal **114,** 116
- hypothalamic 108
- lentiform **109, 111, 114 f,** 119
- motor
- – of oculomotor nerve 114
- – of trigeminal nerve 114
- oculomotor 116
- olivary, inferior 116
- paraventricular 108
- posterior, of hypothalamus 108
- pre-optic 108
- pulposus **198 f,** 232
- red 99, **103,** 107, 116
- salivatory 114
- sensory, of trigeminal nerve 114
- solitarius 116
- spinal, of accessory nerve 114
- subcortical, of brain 105, **109 ff**
- supra-optic 108
- trochlear 114
- ventromedial, of hypothalmus 108
- vestibular **114,** 116
- visceral

- – of glossopharyngeal nerve 114
- – of vagus nerve 114

O

Obex 131
Occlusion, centric 50
Olecranon **374,** 379, 387, 392
- fossa 373
- surface anatomy 401
Olfactory system 107
Olive, inferior 66, 103, **111,** 114 f, 131
Omentum
- greater 292, 298, **302,** 306, 312, 318
- – midsagittal section 322
- lesser 311 f
- – midsagittal section 322
Opening
- abdominal, of uterine tube 357
- pharyngeal, of auditory tube 86, 246
- saphenous 210, 217 f, 358, **468,** 479
Operculum
- frontal 109
- frontoparietal 109
- temporal 109
Ora serrata 133
Orbit 7, 31, **46 f, 132,** 140 f
- bones 132
- horizontal section 148
- nerves 72 f
Organs
- abdominal s. Abdominal organs
- genital s. Genital organs
- inner, position 2
- mediastinal 274 ff
- of neck 154
- of posterior mediastinum 278 f
- respiratory 247
- retroperitoneal 323 ff
- – vessels 305
- thoracic 243 ff
- – position 243 ff
- – regional anatomy 264 ff
- urinary, position 323 f
Orifice
- internal, of uterus 359
- ureteric 336 f, 355
- urethral
- – external 336, 355, 361 f
- – internal 336, **338 f,** 345, **355**
- – vaginal 356, 360, **361 f,** 364
Oropharynx **150,** 155, 246
Ossicles, auditory 20, 22, **122,** 125, **128**
- movements 128
Ossification, bones of limb 9
Ossification center 9
Outlet, pelvic 434

Page numbers in **bold** indicate main discussions.

Ovary 354, **356 ff**, 359 ff, 366 f
– position 323

P

Palate
– hard **50**, 53, 143 f, **146 ff, 150**, 164
– soft 53, 62, **88 f**, 143 f, 150, 163, 165
Palm of hand 368
Pancreas 279, 292, 294, **296 f**, 300, 302, 304,
 316 f
– Head's area 205
– horizontal section 324
Papilla(-ae)
– circumvallate 149
– duodenal
– – greater **296 f**, 300, 317, 320
– – lesser **296 f**, 300, 317
– filiform 149
– foliate 149
– fungiform 149
– renal 326 f
– sublingual 153
Patella 7, 432, **441**, 446, 452, 486, 492
– articular surface 448
– surface anatomy 477
Pecten pubis 433, **435**
Pedicle 191, 197
– of axis 200
Peduncle
– cerebellar
– – inferior **102 f**, 115
– – middle **102 f**, 111, **114 f**, 131
– – superior **102 f**, 111, 115
– cerebral 65, 71, **103**, 108, 114 ff, 131
Pelvic girdle 434
– organization 432
– skeleton 432
Pelvis 7, 188 f, 194 f
– aperture, inferior 437
– axial section 496
– female **359**, 435 ff
– – diameters 434, 438
– – inclination 438
– ligaments 444
– male **344 ff**, 435 ff
– renal **326 f**, 336
– – horizontal section 324
– skeleton 435 ff
Penis 336 ff
Perforated substance, anterior 66
Pericardium 170, 244 f, 255, 257, 265, **266 ff**,
 269 f, **272 f**, 280 f
– diaphragmatic part 272
– reflection 255, **273**
Pericranium 85
Periorbita **72**, 132

Periosteum
– of skull 85
– of vertebral canal 232
Peritoneum 210, 213
– of posterior abdominal wall 310
– reflections from organs 318
Pes
– anserinus 452
– hippocampi 105 f
Phalanx(-ges) 368
– distal
– – of fingers 375 ff, **425**, 427
– – of great toe 442, 495
– – of thumb 376 f
– – of toe 443
– of foot 7, 432
– of hand 7
– middle
– – of fingers 375 ff, **425**, 427
– – of toe 443
– of newborn 9
– proximal
– – of fingers 375 ff, **425**, 427
– – of great toe 442, 495
– – of thumb 376 f, **425**
– – of toe 443
Pharynx 67, 86, 143, 154, 161, **164 ff**
– muscles 166 f
– oral part 90, 165
Pia mater 84 f, **89, 92**, 100, 118
– spinal 98, 231, **232**
Pivot joint 10, **11**
Placenta 289, 359
Plane
– axial 4
– of the body 4 f
– coronal 5
– frontal 5
– horizontal 4
– median 5
– midsaggital 5
– nuchal 27, **33**
– sagittal 4
– transpyloric 217
– transtubercular 217
– transverse 4
Plate
– cribriform, of ethmoidal bone **30 f**, 34, **38**, 49
– horizontal, of palatine bone **39 ff**, 42, 44 f, 49,
 144
– orbital
– – of ethmoidal bone 38, 40 ff, 44 f, 46 f, 132
– – of frontal bone 28
– perpendicular **38 ff**, 41 f, 44, 47, 49
– pterygoid
– – lateral 21, 25 f, **33**, 36 ff, 41, 44 ff, 60 f, 125,
 164
– – medial 25 f, **33**, 36 f, 41, 45, 144, **146**,
 164

– tarsal
– – inferior 132
– – superior 132, 148
– tympanic 21
Platysma muscle 50, **55 ff, 58 f**, 62, **77**, 149,
 174, 290, 385
Pleura
– costal 264 ff
– surface projection of the thorax wall 248
Plexus
– alveolar, superior 72
– aorticorenal 335
– autonomic 323
– brachial 18, 77, 97, 154, 168, 170, 177, **186**,
 206, 264, 269, 281, 335, 396, **399, 412 ff**
– – lateral cord 170, **399, 413**, 415
– – medial cord **399, 413**, 415
– – middle trunk 396
– – posterior cord **399, 413**, 415
– – roots 404, **413**
– carotid, internal 146
– celiac 279, **327**
– cervical 18, 97, 154, 177, **186, 413**
– – cutaneous branches 174, **178**, 186, 207,
 226, 234
– choroid 71, **112 f**
– – of fourth ventricle 115
– – of lateral ventricle **104 f**, 113, 115
– – of third ventricle 86, 105
– dental
– – inferior 68
– – superior 68
– esophageal 275 ff, 278 ff, 335
– gastric 335
– – anterior 279
– hepatic 279
– hypogastric
– – inferior **347**, 359, 472
– – superior 308, 331, **335**
– lumbar 470
– lumbosacral 18, **470 f**
– nervous, of autonomic system 18
– pelvic 349
– pharyngeal 165
– prostatic 345
– pudendal 470
– sacral 349, **470 ff**
– solar 18
– splenic 279
– venous
– – extradural 232
– – pampiniform 218, 340, **343**, 347 f
– – prostatic 347, 349, 351
– – thyroid, inferior 184
– – uterine 367
– – vesicoprostatic 341, 346
– – vesico-uterine 355
Plica circularis of duodenum 297
Points, palpable, ventral 2

Page numbers in **bold** indicate main discussions.

Polarity 1
Pons 66, 68, 86, 103, **114**
– cross section 121
– median section 90 f, 233
– MRI scan 203
– in neonate 233
Porta hepatis 299
Pouch 358
– of Douglas **354**, 357 f f, 366 f
– recto-uterine 322, **354**, 357 ff, 366 f
– rectovesical 337 f
– vesico-uterine 322, **354**, 356, 358 f, 366
Premaxilla 33
Premolar
– first 50
– second 50
Prepuce
– of clitoris 361 f, 364 f
– of penis 336, 341
Process(es)
– alveolar
– – of mandible 22, **52**, 90
– – of maxilla 22, 37, 39 ff, 42, 44 ff, **52**, 90
– articular
– – of cervical vertebra 157
– – inferior
– – – of axis 200
– – – of vertebra 191, 197
– – superior
– – – of sacrum 433 ff, **437**
– – – of vertebra 191, 197
– – of vertebra 191
– ciliary 133
– clinoid
– – anterior 25 f, **30**, 34, 36, **38**, 75
– – posterior 25 f, **30**, 34, **38**
– cochleariform 126 f
– condylar, of mandible 20 f, 36, **50**, **52**, 54, 56
– coracoid 188 f, **369 ff,** 372, 378, 411
– coronoid
– – of mandible 20 f, **52**, 54, 56, 79
– – of ulna **374**, 379
– costal 191, 195, **198**
– ethmoidal, of inferior nasal concha 48
– frontal
– – of maxilla 22, 28, 37, **39 ff**, 42, 45, 47, 132, **144**
– – of zygomatic bone 45, 52
– intrajugular 39
– jugular 25, 39
– lacrimal, of inferior nasal concha 48
– lateral, of malleus 128
– lenticular 126, 128
– mamillary, of vertebra 191
– mastoid 20 f, 27 ff, **33**, 53, 56, 122
– maxillary
– – of inferior nasal concha 42, **48**
– – of palatine bone 40
– muscular

– – of arytenoid cartilage 158
– – of vertebra 191
– odontoid, of axis 86
– orbital, of palatine bone 39 f, 42, 44, 132
– palatine, of maxilla 33, 41 ff, **48**, **144**
– perpendicular 49, **144**
– pterygoid 21, 36, 127
– – of newborn 33
– pyramidal 39 f, 42, 45
– sphenoidal, of palatine bone 39 f, 42
– spinous 3, 191 f, 194, **197**
– – of axis 53, **200**, 202, 222 f, 225, **237**
– – of cervical vertebra 157, 177, **191**, 193 f, **201**
– – of lumbar vertebra **191**, 193 f
– – of seventh cervical vertebra 222 f, 235 f
– – of thoracic vertebra **191**, 193
– styloid
– – of radius 374, **376 f**, 380 f
– – of temporal bone 27 f, 33, 53, **54**, 60 ff, 71, 126, **151**, 164, 166
– – of ulna 374, **376 f**, 381
– talar, posterior 443
– transverse
– – of atlas 200 ff
– – of axis 200
– – of cervical vertebrae 177
– – of thoracic vertebrae 225
– – of vertebra 191, 197
– uncinate
– – of ethmoidal bone 37, 46
– – of pancreas 297
– vaginal 219
– – remnant 218
– vocal, of arytenoid cartilage 158
– xiphoid 189, 192, 196, 206, 264, 306, **369**
– zygomatic
– – of frontal bone 28, **44 f**
– – of maxilla 22, 39 ff, 42, 44 f
– – of temporal bone 21, 27 f, 125
Prominence
– saccular 128
– utricular 128
Promontory
– sacral 188 f, 310, 330, **337**, **346 f**, 354 f, **434 f**, 438, 471
– – midsagittal section 322
– of tympanic cavity 125 ff
Pronation 368 f, **391**
Prosencephalon 91
Prostate 336 ff, 341, **344**
– coronal section 345
Protuberance
– mental 23, **52**
– occipital
– – external 21, 25, 27, 29, **33**, 223
– – internal 25, 27, **30**, 39, 42
Pubis 7, **433**, 438, 496
– symphysial surface 433, 438

Pulvinar of thalamus 110, 115, 137
Punctum nervosum 63, **77**, 242
Purkinje fibers 261
Putamen 92, 105, **110**, 116, 120
Pylorus **295 f**, 298, 311, 318
Pyramid 66, 127
– of vermis 102

R

Radiation 120
– acoustic 131
– of Gratiolet **109**, 119 f, **137 f**
– optic **109**, 119 f, **137 f**
Radius 7, 10, **368**, **374**, 376 f, 379 ff, 425, 427
– anterior surface 374 f
– articular surface 374
– axial section 419, 431
– of newborn 9
– posterior surface 374 f
Ramus
– communicans, of sympathetic trunk 279 f
– of ischium 437 f
– of mandible 22 f, **52**, 54, 150
– pubic, inferior 342
Raphe
– fibrous, of pharynx 167
– mylohyoid 156
– pterygomandibular 61, **166 f**
Recess
– costodiaphragmatic 248, **265**, 282
– duodenal
– – inferior 318
– – superior 310, 318
– elliptical 129
– epitympanic 125, 128
– hypotympanic 125, 128
– ileocecal 318
– inferior, of tympanic cavity 127
– infundibular 112
– intersigmoid 318
– lateral, of fourth ventricle **112**, 116
– optic **112**, 116
– paracolic 318
– peritoneal 318
– pharyngeal 144, 147
– pineal 112
– piriform 161, 163
– retrocecal 318
– of Rosenmüller 145
– spheno-ethmoidal 145
– spherical 129
– splenic, of lesser sac 318
– superior, of lesser sac 318
– suprapineal 112
Rectum 291, 310, 366 f

Page numbers in **bold** indicate main discussions.

Region(s)
– anal 352
– anterior, of neck **174 ff**, 406
– axillary 407 f, **409 ff**
– cervical 155
– – anterior 155, **174 ff**
– – lateral 155, **178 ff**
– – posterior 155
– crural 489 ff
– – anterior 492, 494
– – posterior 489 ff
– cubital 416 ff
– epigastric 217
– facial, deep 82
– femoral
– – in the male 219
– gluteal 482 ff
– hypochondriac 217
– hypogastric 217
– iliac 217
– infraclavicular 407
– inguinal
– – in the female 220
– – in the male 219
– of knee 486 f
– lateral
– – of head 76 ff
– – of neck 178 ff
– lumbar 217
– malleolar, medial 468
– nuchal 234 ff
– parapharyngeal 31, 83, **151**
– pharyngeal 81
– popliteal 458
– posterior, of neck **234 ff**, 403
– retromandibular 81 f
– retroperitoneal
– – horizontal section 325
– – lymph nodes 332
– – lymph vessels 332
– – nerves 333
– – vessels 333
– retropharyngeal 83
– scapular 409
– sublingual 151
– submandibular 183
– superficial, of the face 76
– of trunk 217
– umbilical 217
– urogenital
– – in the female 363
– – in the male 352
Respiration, changes of the position of diaphragm 282
Respiratory system 246 ff
Retina 133 f
Retinaculum
– extensor
– – of hand **392 ff**, 420 f, **424**

– – tunnels 392
– – inferior, of foot **459**, 493, 495, 498 f
– – superior, of foot **459**, 462, 498
– flexor
– – of foot **458 f**, 461, 491
– – of hand 14, **388**, 390 f, 395, 423, **427 f**
Rhombencephalon 91
– cross section 117
Rib(s) 7, **190**, **369**
– false 369
– first 159, 185, 188 f, **192 ff**, 206, 372
– floating 194, **369 f**
– true 194, **369**
– twelfth 188 f, 193, 453
Ridge, supracondylar
– lateral 373
– medial 373
Rima glottidis 161
Ring
– ciliary 133
– inguinal
– – crus, lateral 217
– – deep 212, **218**, 293, 337, **347**
– – superficial 211, 217 f, **220**, **340**, **362**, 479
– tendinous, common 135, 141
– tympanic 125
– umbilical 209, 213
Riolan's anastomosis 304
Roof of orbit 72
Root(s)
– aortic 254
– of brachial plexus 404, **413**
– dorsal, of cervical spinal nerve 157
– inferior, of ansa cervicalis 184
– of median nerve 399, 411, 415
– of mesentery 306, **318**
– of meso-appendix 318
– of mesosigmoid 318
– motor, of trigeminal nerve 146
– of penis 293, 342
– superior, of ansa cervicalis 69, 71, **82 f**, 152, 179
– of tongue 149 f, 161
– of transverse mesocolon 312, **318**
– ventral, of cervical spinal nerve 157
Root filaments, posterior 98
Rostrum, sphenoidal 25 f

S

Sac
– endolymphatic 129
– lacrimal 142
– lesser 292, **311 ff**
– – horizontal section 324
– – isthmus 318
– – midsagittal section 322

– – splenic recess 318
– – superior recess 318
– pericardial 273
– – upper margin 269
Sacrum 3, 7, 188 f, **190 f**, 193, 195, **432 ff**, 472, 482
– lateral part 191
– pelvic surface 433
– shape 437
– surface anatomy 476
Saddle joint **11**, 377
Scapula 7, 15, 188, 223, **368 ff**, 378
– anterior surface 371
– costal suface 371
– of newborn 9
– posterior surface 370, 372
Scarring of ovary 357
Sclera 132 ff
Segmentation 1
Segment(s)
– bronchopulmonary 246, **250 f**
– of kidney 326
– of liver 299
– of spinal cord 475
Sella turcica 25 f, **30**, 34, 36, 38, 46, 49, 53
– of newborn 35
Semicanal of auditory tube 130
Septum(-a)
– intermuscular
– – lateral, of arm **387**, 392
– – medial, of arm **387 f**, 416 ff, 423
– interventricular 256, 258 f, 261
– lingual 62, 149
– nasal 22, **49**, 53, **144**, 146
– – posterior border 48
– pectiniforme 342
– pellucidum 86, **94**, 103 ff, 116, 118 ff
– of penis 339
– of testis 343
Shaft
– of femur 9, **438 f**
– of fibula 440
– of radius 374
– of rib 191 f
– of tibia 440
Sheath(s) (s. also Synovial sheath) 394, 427
– fibrous
– – digital, of tendons of flexor digitorum muscle 389
– – of flexor tendons of hand 391, 394, **427 f**
– of rectus abdominis muscle 204
– – anterior layer **187**, 196, **208 ff**, 212, 214, **264 f**, 480
– – posterior layer 206, **212 ff**, 293
– of round ligament 220
– synovial s. Synovial sheath
Shoulder 403 ff
– collateral circulation 404
– joints 378

Page numbers in **bold** indicate main discussions.

– ligaments 378
– muscles 382 ff
– region
– – anterior 406 ff
– – posterior 403 ff
Shoulder girdle 7, **368**
– organization 368
– skeleton 369 ff
Shoulder joint 10, **15**, **368**, **378**, 382 ff
– coronal section 11, 378
– frontal section 15
– horizontal section 430
– MRI scan 11, 15, 378, 430
– of newborn 9
– X-ray 15
Shunt in fetal circulatory system 288
Sinus(es) 258
– aortic 261
– carotid 63, **396**
– cavernous 31, 62, **87**, 97, 124
– coronary 257 f, 261, 273, 284
– ethmoidal 121, **148**
– frontal 37, **46**, **48**, 53, 73, 84, 86, 88 f, **143 ff**
– – opening 144
– intercavernous 87
– lactiferous 290
– of larynx 86
– maxillary 37, 46, 132, **144**
– – innervation of mucous membrane 72
– oblique, of pericardium 272 f
– paranasal 144 f
– – openings 144 f
– pericardial, transverse 269, 272 f
– petrosal, superior 87
– of pulmonary trunk 252
– renal 326
– sagittal
– – inferior **85**, **87**, 112
– – superior 75, **85 ff**, 112, 241
– sigmoid 87
– sphenoidal 36 f, **48 f**, 53, 62, **86**, 88 f, 121, 144, **148**
– – opening 25
– straight 67, 75, **85 ff**, 112, 121
– tarsal 443
– transverse 67, 121, 241
– venous, dural 86 f
Skeleton 6 ff
– appendicular 7
– of arm 10
– axial 7
– of a child 7
– cranial, of newborn 35
– facial 23
– – of newborn 35
– of a female adult 6
– of foot 442 f
– of hand 11
– of leg 440

– of pelvis 435 ff
– of thorax 192 ff
– of trunk **188 f**, 221
– visceral 22
– of wrist 11
Skin
– of scalp **89**, 236
– of scrotum 218
Skull 1
– anterior aspect 22
– base s. Base of skull
– bones 20 ff
– lateral aspect 20 f
– median section 36 f
– of newborn 33, **35**
– paramedian section 46
– periosteum 85
Small intestine 3, 210, 291 f
– of fetus 289
– Head's area 205
Snuffbox, anatomical 394, 428
Solar plexus 323
Sole of foot 461, **500 ff**
Space
– epidural, spinal 232
– extradural, spinal 232
– infratentorial 88
– intercostal
– – nerve s. Nerve, intercostal
– – vessels s. Artery, intercostal; s. Vein, intercostal
– intervaginal, of optic nerve 112
– quadrangular, of axillary region 408 f
– subarachnoid **85**, 97, 133, 241
– – spinal **232**, 472
– subdural 118
– – spinal 232
– triangular, of axillary region 408 f
Sphincter
– lower, of esophagus 278
– middle, of esophagus 278
– of Oddi 297
– upper, of esophagus 278
Sphincter muscle s. also Muscle, sphincter
– anal
– – external 342, 349, **350 ff**, 354, 361
– – internal 361
– pyloric 294 f
– urethral 338
– – external 336
– – internal 336
Spinal cord **18**, 62, 84, 86, 89, 177, 214, **230 ff**, 240 f, **473 ff**
– lumbar portion 230
– median section 91
– meningeal coverings 232
– MRI scan 203
– relation to vertebral column 475
– segments 475

– terminal filament 472
– terminal part 230 ff
– thoracic portion 231
Spine 435
– frontal 42
– iliac
– – inferior
– – – anterior 433, 435 f
– – – posterior 188, **433**
– – superior
– – – anterior 3, 189, **216**, **433**, **435 f**, 438, 452 f, 480
– – – – surface anatomy **204**, 477
– – – posterior 188, **433**, 435, **437**, 482
– ischial 188, **433**, 435 f, 438
– mental 36, **52**
– nasal 28
– – anterior 20, 36, 39, 45, 46 f
– – of frontal bone 47
– of scapula 3, 188, 234, **370 ff**, 382 f, 408 f
– of sphenoid 25, 126
– trochlear 22
Spine-trochanter line 482
Spine-tuber line 482
Spleen 279, 291, 296, **300**, 303 f, 311, 316 f, 329
– border, anterior 300
– horizontal section 324
– margin, superior 300
Splenium of corpus callosum 65, 99, **104 ff**, 119 f
Squama
– of occipital bone 20 f
– of temporal bone 20 f
Stapes 20, **122 f**, 127, **128 f**
Sternum 7, 187, 194, 206, **264**, **368 f**
Stomach 244, 279, 284, 291 f, **294 f**, 303, 306, **311**
– cardial part 294 f, 329
– circular muscle layer 295
– of fetus 289
– Head's area 205
– horizontal section 320
– longitudinal muscle layer 295
– midsagittal section 322
– muscular coat 295
– position 3, 294
– pyloric part 295, 316
– sagittal section 245
Stria
– acoustic, dorsal 131
– longitudinal
– – lateral 104 ff, **107**, 113
– – medial 104 ff
– medullaris of thalamus 99, 107, 115
– olfactory
– – lateral 103, **107**, 137
– – medial 103, **107**, 137
– terminalis 103 ff, **107**, 115, 118
Substance, perforated
– anterior 66, 99, 103, 137

Page numbers in **bold** indicate main discussions.

Substance, perforated
– posterior 103, 137
Substantia nigra 65, 99, **103**, 116
Sulcus
– calcarine **99**, 103, 137
– – communication with parieto-occipital sulcus 99
– carotid **30**, 38
– central 89 f, 94, 100 f
– – of insula 72
– chiasmatic 25, **30**
– cingulate 99
– circular, of insula 109
– coronary 252, 257 f, 260 ff
– of corpus callosum 99
– frontal, superior 100
– infra-orbital 132
– intertubercular 373, 378
– interventricular 268
– – anterior **252**, 255, 257, 260, 262
– – posterior **252**, 257, 262
– lateral 89, 100
– – ascending ramus, anterior 100 f
– – horizontal ramus, anterior 100 f
– – posterior ramus 101
– lunate 100
– malleolar, of tibia 440
– median, of tongue 149
– mylohyoid 52
– occipital, transverse 92
– olfactory 66
– orbital, of frontal lobe 66
– parieto-occipital 99
– postcentral 100 f
– precentral **99 f**, 101
– temporal, inferior 66
– terminalis
– – cordis 256, 260 f
– – of tongue 149
Supination 368 f, **391**
Surface
– articular
– – calcaneal
– – – anterior, of talus 449
– – – middle, of talus 449
– – – posterior, of talus 449
– – inferior, of tibia 440
– – malleolar, of fibula 440
– – navicular, of talus 449
– – of navicular bone 449
– – of patella 441, 448
– – proximal, of tibia 447
– – superior
– – – of axis 200
– – – of tibia 440
– – talar
– – – anterior, of calcaneus 449
– – – middle, of calcaneus 449
– – – posterior, of calcaneus 449

– auricular, of sacrum 191, 433
– bare
– – of ascending colon 318
– – of descending colon 318
– costal 369
– diaphragmatic
– – of liver 298
– – of lung 249
– gluteal, of ilium 437
– lunate, of acetabulum 433, **436**, 445
– malleolar, lateral, of talus 443
– patellar, of femur 439, **441**, 447
– pelvic, of sacrum 433
– popliteal, of femur 439, **441**
– symphysial, of pubis 433, 438
Surface anatomy 204 f, 401 f, 476 f
Sustentaculum tali **443**, 450 f
Suture
– coronal 20 ff, **29**, **35**
– ethmoidolacrimal 20
– frontal 22 f, **35**
– frontomaxillary 23
– frontonasal 22
– frontosphenoid 21
– intermaxillary 22
– internasal 22 f
– lacrimomaxillary 20
– lambdoid 20 f, **29**, **35**
– nasomaxillary 20 ff, 23
– of newborn 35
– occipitomastoid 20 f, **29**
– palatine
– – median 33, 45
– – transverse 45
– palatomaxillary 33
– parietomastoid 20
– sagittal 29, 35
– sphenofrontal 20, 23
– sphenosquamosal 21
– sphenozygomatic 23
– squamomastoid 125
– squamous 20 f
– zygomaticomaxillary 22 f
Symmetry, bilateral 1
Symphysis, pubic 7, 188 f, 293, 354, 356, 432, **435 f**
– midsagittal section 322
Synchondrosis, spheno-occipital 27, **38**
Syndesmosis, tibiofibular 443, 495
Synovial fluid 12
Synovial sheath
– common
– – of extensor digitorum longus muscle 493
– – of flexor tendons of hand 390 f
– digital
– – of flexor tendons of hand 390 f
– – of foot 501
– of extensor tendons of hand 392
– of flexor tendons

– – of foot 501
– – of hand 390
– of hand 14
– of tendon
– – of extensor hallucis longus muscle 493
– – of flexor pollicis longus muscle 390 f
– – of tibialis anterior muscle 493
Systole 260

T

Taenia
– coli 306
– free, of colon 307 f, 310, 318
Tail
– of caudate nucleus 115
– of epididymis 343 f
– of pancreas 297, 300, 316
Talus **443**, 449 ff
– articular surface
– – calcaneal
– – – anterior 449
– – – middle 449
– – – posterior 449
– – navicular 449
– of newborn 9
Tectum 94, **108**, **114**
Telencephalon 91
Tendon 393, 415, 499
– of abductor pollicis longus muscle 388, **390**, 392, 394, 401, **427**
– annular, common 135, 141
– of biceps femoris muscle 455 f, 484
– – surface anatomy 476 f
– calcaneal 449, **457 ff**, 489, 491 ff
– – surface anatomy 476
– central
– – of diaphragm **278**, 283, 298, 329
– – of perineum **353**, 361
– of deep flexor muscles 458
– of extensor carpi radialis brevis muscle 392 ff
– of extensor carpi radialis longus muscle 392 ff
– of extensor carpi ulnaris muscle 392, **424**
– of extensor digiti minimi muscle 392
– of extensor digitorum brevis muscle of foot 493
– of extensor digitorum longus muscle of foot 459, 462, 491, 498 f
– of extensor digitorum muscle of hand 392 ff, 401, **424**
– of extensor hallucis longus muscle **458 f**, 491, 493, **498 f**
– of extensor indicis muscle 392, 394, 401
– of extensor muscles of hand 381
– of extensor pollicis brevis muscle 388, 392, 394, **427**
– of extensor pollicis longus muscle 392, 394, **424**

Page numbers in **bold** indicate main discussions.

– of flexor carpi radialis muscle 380 f, **389 f,** 394 f, **427 f**
– – surface anatomy 402
– of flexor carpi ulnaris muscle 380 f, 388, **390 f,** 394 f, **427 f**
– of flexor digitorum brevis muscle of leg 463 ff, 501 f
– of flexor digitorum longus muscle of leg 460, 463 ff, 501 f
– of flexor digitorum profundus muscle of hand **389 f,** 394 f, 425, 427
– of flexor digitorum superficialis muscle of hand **389 f,** 394 f, 425, **427 f**
– of flexor hallucis longus muscle 449, **460 f,** 463, 465, 501 f
– of flexor pollicis longus muscle 388, **390,** 394 f
– of gracilis muscle 447, 452, **455,** 457
– of iliocostalis muscle 225
– intermediate
– – of digastric muscle 150
– – of omohyoid muscle 179
– – of semitendinosus muscle 456
– of long head
– – of biceps brachii muscle 378, **387,** 415 f, 419
– – of triceps brachii muscle 378 f, 392
– of lumbrical muscle of hand 394
– of palmaris longus muscle 388, 402, 423, **428**
– of peroneus brevis muscle 491
– of peroneus longus muscle 462, **464,** 491
– of peroneus tertius muscle 462, 499
– of plantaris muscle 488
– of sartorius muscle 452
– of semimembranosus muscle 447
– – surface anatomy 476
– of semitendinosus muscle 447, 452, 487
– sheath s. Sheath, fibrous; s. Synovial sheath
– of short head of biceps brachii muscle 387
– of stapedius muscle 126, 128
– of superior oblique muscle 135 f, 140
– of supraspinatus muscle 378
– of temporalis muscle 60 f, 80, 82
– of tensor veli palatini muscle 126
– of tibialis anterior muscle 458, 461, 493, 495, **498 f**
– of tibialis posterior muscle 460 f
– of triceps brachii muscle 409
Tenon's space 132
Tentorium cerebelli 67, 75, **87 ff,** 97, 121
Testis 3, 218, 330, **336 f,** 339, 341, **343,** 351, 479
– Head's area 205
– longitudinal section 343
Thalamus 90 f, 99, 103 ff, 107, 113, 116, 120
Thenar muscles **390 f,** 395, **423**
– axial section 431
Thigh
– anterior region 478 ff
– arteries 480 f
– axial section 496

– muscles 480 f, 484 f
– nerves, cutaneous 478 f, 484
– posterior region 484 f
– veins 478 f
Thoracic cage, changes of position during respiration 282
Thorax 1, 7, 188 f, **369 ff**
– coronal section 253, **284 f**
– horizontal section 286 f
– MRI scan 253, **284 ff**
– paramedian section 283
– sagittal section 245, 263
– skeleton 192 ff
Thymus 155, 233, **265 ff,** 292
– remaining parts 245
Tibia 7, 12, 432, **440 ff,** 446
– of newborn 9
– upper end 440
Tissue
– adipose
– – encasing round ligament 363
– – perirenal 300, 324
– cavernous, of female external genital organs 362
Tongue 83, 84, 143
– innervation 31
Tonsil
– cerebellar 66, **102**
– lingual **149,** 161
– palatine 83, 143, **147, 149,** 153, 165
– pharyngeal 144
Tooth (teeth)
– deciduous 51
– lower 22, **50 ff**
– molar 42, **50 f**
– – permanent 51
– – third 37
– premolar 37, **50 f**
– upper 22, 41 f, 44 f, **50 ff**
Trabecula(-ae)
– carneae 259
– septomarginal 258
Trachea 154, 243, 255, **274 ff,** 285
Tract(s) 477
– cerebellorubral 103
– iliotibial 448, **452 f,** 455, **480,** 495
– – surface anatomy 476 f
– olfactory **65 f,** 69, **74 f,** 98 f, 103, **107, 114 f,** 146
– – lateral root 99
– – medial root 99
– olivocochlear 131
– optic 66, 71, 107, **137 f**
– pyramidal 109, 116
– – course 111
– – lateral 103
– of Rasmussen 131
– spiral, foraminous 123
Tractus solitarius 116

Tragus **122,** 124
Triad, portal 299
Triangle(s)
– carotid 155, 173, 178 f
– deltopectoral 384, **407**
– – surface anatomy 402
– lumbar 223
– lumbocostal 335
– of neck 155
– sternocostal 283
– submandibular 155
– suboccipital 237 f
– supraclavicular 155
Trigone
– of bladder 336, 338 f, **355**
– habenular 115
– hypoglossal 115
– olfactory 66, 115, 137
Trochanter
– greater 9, **438 f,** 482
– lesser 438 f
– third 439
Trochlea
– of humerus 373, 375, 379
– peroneal, of calcaneus 443
– of superior oblique muscle **72,** 135 f, **141**
– of talus 443, 450 f
Trunk 7, **187 ff**
– brachiocephalic 162, **168 f,** 252 f, 256 f, 263, 267 f, 274 f, **396, 414**
– bronchomediastinal 332
– celiac 279, 283, 300, 302, 316, **327 ff,** 330 f, 333, **335**
– – branches **311, 314 f**
– costocervical 168
– cross section 204
– horizontal section 210 f
– jugular 172 f
– lumbar 332
– lumbosacral 471
– lymph vessels 17
– median section 4, 233
– – in neonate 233
– midsagittal section 322, 354
– neuro-vascular segments 187
– parasagittal section 325
– pulmonary **245, 252 ff,** 260 ff, 266, 269, 271
– – of fetus 288
– – relation to bronchial tree 275
– reference lines 217
– regions 217
– sagittal section 5
– skeleto-motoric segments 187
– skeleton 221
– subclavian 184, 332
– sympathetic 18, 67, 146, 162, 164 f, 168, 185, 266, **279 ff,** 327, 333, **334 f,** 471 f
– – cervical part 174
– – Ramus communicans 280 f

Page numbers in **bold** indicate main discussions.

Trunk
– thyrocervical 162, **168 ff**, **177**, 271, 396, 404
– vagal 335
– – anterior 327
– – posterior 327
Tube
– auditory 120, **122 ff**, 126 f, 143
– – bony part 27
– – opening 145, **147**
– – pharyngeal opening 86, 144, 246
– uterine **354 ff**, 359 f, 366 f
– – position 323
Tuber
– calcanei 451
– cinereum 99
– frontal 35
– parietal 29, **35**
– of vermis 102
Tuber-trochanter line 482
Tubercle
– anterior
– – of atlas 191
– – of transverse process 191
– articular 21, 27 f, **50**, 54
– conoid 369
– corniculate 160
– cuneiform 160
– dorsal, of atlas 223
– genial 36, **52**
– greater, of humerus 372 f, 430
– infraglenoid 370 ff
– intercondylar
– – lateral, of tibia 440
– – medial, of tibia 448
– – posterior, of tibia 440
– jugular 25, 27, 39
– lesser, of humerus 373, 430
– olfactory 99
– pharyngeal 25, 27, **33**, 164
– posterior
– – of atlas 191, 200
– – of transverse process 191
– pubic 433, **435**
– of rib 191 f, **197**
– supraglenoid 370 f
– thyroid
– – inferior 159
– – superior 159
Tuberculum sellae 38
Tuberosity
– calcaneal 443, **450**, 457, 463, 491
– deltoid 373
– of distal phalanx 376 f
– – of great toe 442
– of fifth metatarsal bone 443
– ischial 188, 344, **433**, **436 f**, 455 f, 472, 482
– masseteric 52
– maxillary 39 ff, 46
– radial 374 f, 379

– sacral 433
– tibial **440 f**, 458 f
– ulnar 374
Tubules, seminiferous, convoluted 343
Tunica
– albuginea
– – of corpora cavernosa 339
– – of corpus spongiosum 339
– – of testis 341
– vaginalis
– – parietal layer 341, **343**
– – testis 218, **343**
– – visceral layer 341, **343**

U

Ulna 7, 10, **368**, **374**, 376 f, 379 ff, 425
– anterior surface 375
– axial section 419, 431
– of newborn 9
– posterior surface 374
Umbilicus 3, 187, **209**
Uncus
– hippocampi 99
– of parahippocampal gyrus 106
Urachus 289, 339, 354, 361
Ureter 3, 210, 296, 300, **326 ff**, **330 ff**, **336 ff**, 359
– abdominal part **326 f**, 330, 336
– Head's area 205
– pelvic part 330, 336
– position 323
Urethra
– female 354 f
– male 336 ff
– membranous part 336 ff, 342, 344
– prostatic part 336 ff, 344 f
– spongy 337 ff
Urinary bladder
– base 367
– of the female 354 f, 357 ff, 361
– of the fetus 289
– frontal section 293
– Head's area 205
– horizontal section 324
– of the male 336 ff
– midsagittal section 322
– mucous membrane 338 f
– position 323
Urinary organs, position 323 f
Urinary system 330 f
Urogenital system
– female 354 ff
– male 336 ff
Uterus **354 ff**, 358, **359 f**, 366 f
– position 323
Utricle, prostatic 338

Uvula 62, **86 f**, 144, 147, 163, 165
– of bladder 338
– of vermis 102

V

Vagina 322 f, 355, **356**, **358**, 360
Vallecula of epiglottis 149
Valve(s)
– aortic 253, **255 f**, 258 f, 261, 284
– atrioventricular
– – left **255 f**, 258 f
– – right **255 f**, 258 ff, 287
– bicuspid **255 f**, 258 f
– of heart 255 ff
– – position 255, **260**
– ileocecal 310
– – horizontal section 320
– of inferior vena cava 288
– mitral **255 f**, 258 f
– pulmonary **255 f**, 259 f, 271, 286, 325
– tricuspid **255 f**, 258 ff, 287
Vasa recta of renal medulla 329
Vein(s) 16, 468
– alveolar
– – inferior 83
– anastomotic
– – inferior 92
– – superior 89
– angular 170
– arcuate 329, 468
– axillary 170, **186**, 196, **214**, 252, 264, 398, 411
– azygos 244, 246, 276, **279 f**, 332
– basilic 398, 402, 410, 419
– brachial 398, 415
– – surface anatomy 402
– brachiocephalic 155, 170, **177**, 244, 252, 255, 265, 267, 271, 274, **396**, 398
– – of fetus 288 f
– cardiac
– – great 258, 262
– middle 262
– – minimal 262
– – small 262, 270
– cephalic **170 f**, 207, 209, 211, 265, 290, 398, **406**, 416
– – accessory 401 f
– – on forearm 398, 401 f, 419
– – surface anatomy 402
– cerebral 92
– – great 90, 145
– – inferior 89, **92**
– – internal 86
– – middle, superficial 92
– – superior 89, **92**
– of Cockett 468 f

Page numbers in **bold** indicate main discussions.

– coronary 262 f
– cubital, median 398, **402,** 416, 419
– – surface anatomy 402
– cutaneous
– – of leg 489
– – of popliteal fossa 486
– – of region of knee 486
– – of thigh 484
– digital
– – of foot 468
– – of hand 398
– dorsal
– – deep, of penis 217 f, **339 ff,** 342, 346
– – of penis 479
– – superficial, of penis 346
– epigastric
– – inferior 212, 219
– – superficial 210 f, 217, 468
– – superior 206, 208
– ethmoidal, anterior 31
– facial 77, **79,** 152, 170, 398
– femoral **214,** 293, 340, 367, 452, **467 f,** 480, 496
– – entering the adductor canal 452
– gastric, left 303
– gastro-omental 303
– hemiazygos 279
– – accessory 279, 287
– hepatic 283, 299, 303
– ileal 303
– ileocolic 303
– iliac
– – circumflex, superficial 210 f, 217, 468, **479**
– – common 359
– – external 293, **346,** 468
– – internal 279
– intercostal 206, **210 f**
– – anterior 207
– – posterior 276, 279 ff
– – – dorsal branches 408
– – superior 281
– interlobar, of kidney 329
– interlobular, of kidney 329
– jejunal 303
– jugular 154
– – anterior 170, 398
– – external **77,** 80, 170, **264 f,** 398
– – internal 80, 124, 127, 152, **157,** 165, **170 f,** 177, 179, 244, 252, **264 f,** 274 f, 398
– – – of fetus 289
– labial
– – inferior 170
– – superior 170
– of labyrinth 31
– lacrimal 140
– lumbar 335
– – ascending 279
– median, of forearm 402
– meningeal, middle 8 / f

– mesenteric
– – inferior 300, 303, 308
– – superior 296, 300, **302 ff, 309,** 316
– metacarpal, dorsal 398
– metatarsal, dorsal 468
– nasal, superior, of retina 134
– oblique, of left atrium of heart 262
– obturator 366
– occipital **85,** 170, 398
– ophthalmic, superior 31
– para-umbilical 303
– perforating 468, 492
– pericardiacophrenic 272, 281
– peroneal 468
– plantar
– – lateral 499
– – medial 499
– popliteal 446, **467,** 484, 486 ff
– portal 16, 296, 299, **303 f,** 315, 317
– – of fetus 289
– posterior, of left ventricle 262
– of posterior abdominal wall 279
– of posterior thoracic wall 279
– pudendal, external 467 f, 479
– – superficial 210, 217
– pulmonary 16, 252 f, 271
– – branches 246
– – of fetus 288 f
– – left 249, 262, 272 ff, 276, **281**
– – right 244, 249, 262, **272 ff,** 276, 283
– radial 419
– rectal
– – inferior 352
– – superior 303
– renal **326 f,** 331
– – left 292, 327
– – right 329 f
– retinal 134
– – central 133
– retromandibular 77, 152
– sacral, median 279
– saphenous
– – great 210 ff, **214,** 217 f, 340, 344, **467 f,** 479, 480, 486, 489, 492
– – small 468, 484, **489,** 492 f
– – – anastomoses with great saphenous vein 468, 489
– scapular, circumflex 378, **408 f**
– scrotal, posterior 351
– sigmoid 303
– spermatic 331
– splenic 294, 303, 317
– subclavian **170 f,** 184, 207, 244, 255
– – right 264 ff, 270
– subcortical of kidney 329
– submental 152, 170
– superficial
– – on dorsum of foot 469
– – of forearm 420

– – of leg 469
– – of lower limb 468 f
– supra-orbital 170
– suprascapular 378
– sural 487
– temporal
– – inferior, of retina 134
– – superficial **77,** 79, 85, **168,** 170, 183, **398**
– – superior, of retina 134
– testicular 341, 349
– thoracic
– – internal **208, 264 ff,** 398
– – lateral 196, 208, **290,** 398
– thoraco-epigastric 207, 410 f
– thymic 270
– thyroid
– – inferior 170, 181, 269, 272
– – superior 170
– tibial
– – anterior 468
– – posterior 468
– ulnar 425
– umbilical 289
– vorticose 133, 140
Velum medullary superior 102, 115
Vena
– cava
– – inferior 210, 252, 272, **283, 285,** 303 f, 311, 320, 327, 329, 330 f, 359
– – – of fetus 288 f
– – – opening 258, 288
– – superior 169 f, 177, 244, **252 f,** 255, 260 ff, 270 f, 280, **282,** 284 f, 396
– – – of fetus 288 f
– vorticosa 133, 140
Ventricle 269
– fourth 71, 86, 91 f, 94, 102, **112,** 116
– of larynx 161
– lateral 71, **104 f,** 116
– – central part **112,** 118
– left 16, 244 f, **252 f,** 255, 258, 262 f, **268 ff,** 271, 273, 285, 325
– – of fetus 288
– right 16, 243 ff, **252 ff,** 255, 262 f, **268 ff,** 273, 325
– – of fetus 288 f
– – horizontal section 287
– – midsagittal section 322
– third 86, 90 f, 99, 105, 107, **112,** 115 f, 119 f
– – inferior wall 73
Ventricular system 112
Vermis of cerebellum 66, 74 f, 94, **102 ff, 105,** 107, 116, 240
Vertebra 190
– cervical 7, 53, 159, **190,** 192 f, 369 f
– – joints 195
– – seventh 188 f, 193, **370**
– lumbar 7, 188, **190,** 199
– – fifth 438

Page numbers in **bold** indicate main discussions.

Vertebra
– lumbar
– – first 189, 211, **369 f**
– – joints 195
– prominens 188, 193, 222 f, 235, **370**
– thoracic 7, **190**, **197**
– – first 192, **369 f**
– – joints 195
– – twelfth 192, **369 f**
Vertebral column 84, 188 f, **193 ff**, **369**
– cervical 53, 193
– joints connecting to the head 200 f
– ligaments 197 f
– lumbar part 472 f
– – median section 473
– – MRI scan 473
– – paramedian section 473
– – sagittal section 472
– midsagittal section 322
– relation to spinal cord 475
– thoracic 193
Vertex of skull 84
Vesicle, seminal 336 ff, 341 f, **344 ff**
Vessels s. also Artery; s. also Vein
– of arm 415 ff
– gastro-omental 311 f
– lymphatic s. Lymph vessels
– retinal 134
Vestibular apparatus **122 ff**, 129
Vestibule
– of larynx 149
– of lesser sac 324
– nasal 53, **144 f**
– oral 50, 53, 83, **150**

– of vagina 355, **361**
Vidian canal 25, **33**, 45 f, 146, 164
Vinculum(-a)
– breve 394
– of flexor tendon 394
Visual apparatus 132 ff
Visual pathway 137 f
– injuries 139
Visual system, 3-D reconstruction 139
Vomer 20, 22 f, 33, 45, **47 ff**
Vortex, muscular, of right ventricle 257

W

Wall
– abdominal
– – anterior 187, 293
– – – arteries 208
– – – muscles 205
– – – – superficial 209
– – – segments **205**, 214
– – – surface anatomy 204 f
– – horizontal section 214
– – nerves 214 ff
– – posterior 316 ff
– – – veins 279
– – transverse section 213
– – vessels 214 ff
– thoracic 206 ff
– – anterior 187, 206 ff
– – – arteries 208

– – – muscles 205
– – – – superficial 209
– – – segments **205**, 214
– – – surface anatomy 204 f
– – position of spinal nerves 229
– – posterior
– – – MRI scan 229
– – – veins 279
White matter 118
Window, round 125 f, 128
Wing s. also Ala
– greater, of sphenoidal bone 20, 22 f, **25 f**, 34, **38**, 40 f, 47, 132
– – cerebral surface **25**, 52
– – maxillary surface 38
– – of newborn 35
– – orbital surface 25, **38**, 40 ff, 45
– – temporal surface 25, 42, 44
– lesser, of sphenoidal bone 22, 23, **25 f**, **30**, 34, **38**, 40 ff, 44, 132
Wrist 368
– coronal section 380
– ligaments 380 f
– MRI scan 380
– skeleton 376 f
Wrist joint **368**, 375
– coronal section 425

Z

Zona orbicularis 444 f